The Oxford Handbook of Auditory Science

Hearing

VOLUME 3

Edited by

Christopher J. Plack

Human Communication and Deafness Division
The University of Manchester

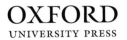

OXFORD
UNIVERSITY PRESS

OXFORD

UNIVERSITY PRESS

Great Clarendon Street, Oxford OX2 6DP

Oxford University Press is a department of the University of Oxford.
It furthers the University's objective of excellence in research, scholarship,
and education by publishing worldwide in

Oxford New York

Auckland Cape Town Dar es Salaam Hong Kong Karachi
Kuala Lumpur Madrid Melbourne Mexico City Nairobi
New Delhi Shanghai Taipei Toronto

With offices in

Argentina Austria Brazil Chile Czech Republic France Greece Guatemala
Hungary Italy Japan Poland Portugal Singapore South
Korea Switzerland Thailand Turkey Ukraine Vietnam

Oxford is a registered trade mark of Oxford University Press
in the UK and in certain other countries

Published in the United States
by Oxford University Press Inc., New York

British Library Cataloguing in Publication Data
Data available

Library of Congress Cataloging in Publication Data
Data available

Typeset in Minion by Glyph International, Bangalore, India
Printed in China
on acid-free paper through Asia Pacific Offset

ISBN 978–0–19–923355–7

10 9 8 7 6 5 4 3 2 1

Series Preface

Auditory science has been, over the last three decades, one of the fastest growing areas of biomedical research. Worldwide there are now perhaps 10,000 researchers whose primary job is auditory research, and ten times that number working in allied, mainly clinical hearing professions. This rapid growth is attributable to and, in turn, fuelled by several major developments in our understanding. While this Handbook focuses on fundamental research and underlying mechanisms, it does so from the perspective of understanding the impact of auditory science on our quality of life. That impact has been realized through the explosive growth of digital technology and microelectronics, and has been delivered by devices as diverse as MP3 compression for music listening (based on models of perceptual coding) to the latest instruments for the management of hearing loss, including digital hearing aids and multichannel cochlear implants. The discovery of otoacoustic emissions (OAEs) – sounds produced by the cochlea - has enabled a step change both in our understanding of ear function and in the development of a clinical tool for deafness screening in newborn infants.

Fundamental research on the inner *ear* has shown that an elaborate system of sound-induced active processes, acting through the outer hair cells, serves to improve sensitivity, sharpen frequency tuning, dynamically modulate the mechanical response of the ear to sound, and create sound energy that passes back out of the ear. Each of these processes is also influenced by descending neural input to the hair cells. Most recently, the molecular machinery underlying these incredible phenomena has been explored and described in detail. The development, maintenance and repair of the ear are also subjects of contemporary interest at the molecular level, as is the genetics of hearing disorders due to cochlear malfunctions. The *auditory brain* is responsible for sound (including speech) identification and localization. Through functional neuroimaging in humans, and the application of novel methods in animals, such as multichannel recordings of single unit activity, multiple cortical and subcortical areas necessarily involved in hearing and listening have now been identified and characterized. They occupy the superior (dorsal) temporal cortex, and extend into non-classical cortical regions, including the more rostral and ventral temporal lobe, the limbic system, and elsewhere in the frontal and parietal lobes. Understanding of subcortical processing has expanded through the use of molecular and cellular techniques *in vitro* and recordings in awake and behaving humans and animals *in vivo*. Increasingly, the widespread, descending pathways are being shown to have profound functional significance, and to influence the coding of both simple and complex sounds. Recent studies of *hearing* (auditory perception) have shown how our perceptions relate to the underlying physiological mechanisms. For example, behavioural measures of peripheral auditory function have lead to the development of sophisticated models of cochlear processing in humans. These models are having a widespread influence in our understanding of both normal and pathologic hearing. At the same time, there has been an increasing focus on auditory 'ecology', on complex sound perception in real (or virtual) environments. Traditional distinctions between spectral, temporal and binaural processing have evolved into more functional concerns, including auditory scene analysis and auditory object perception.

Here, then, are the three major domains of auditory science – the ear, the brain and hearing – and I am proud to present a corresponding three volume Handbook. However, as the volume editors and I started sifting through all the areas we wished to cover, a number of recent developments in our science became apparent that made us question the way in which we had decided to partition the field. Spurred on by ever-increasing knowledge, the availability of enabling technology, and cultural shifts in attitudes towards 'relevance' and 'interdisciplinary' research, the three domains have begun to merge into one. Several instances of this are hinted at above: a transition from more segmented to more holistic approaches to audition, a shift in focus from more simple to more complex and, hence, more realistic sounds, a drilling down across traditional disciplinary boundaries from the phenomenological to the mechanistic and generic. Dynamic properties of hearing are becoming more prominent across all three domains, and beyond, as lifespan development, adaptation and learning receive increasing recognition. Reciprocal influences of hearing on and from cognition (attention, memory and emotion), action and vision add to a picture of a powerful, working, integrated sense that is arguably the most important we possess for what makes us distinctly human - our social interaction with our world. Organizationally, researchers at all levels (peripheral, central and perceptual) now work increasingly together, with many major and several new interdisciplinary centres of auditory science dotted across the globe.

Our ambitious aim has been to deliver a working Handbook that would fill an unmet need for a single reference work spanning all of auditory science. We wanted it to offer a basic background for all those interested in the subject, from the curious undergraduate to the professional researcher and clinician, whilst also capturing the excitement, and some of the detail, of the most recent developments in this rapidly evolving discipline. Consequently, we set out with the conflicting aims of producing a comprehensive, even definitive work, but of completing it within the minimum time possible. We optimistically targeted this at one year, recognising that the finished product would have a finite lifespan. In fact, the preparation of the chapters, from commissioning to collection of the final versions of the final chapters, has taken about two years. Although disappointing to us, Martin Baum, our very helpful and ever-patient senior commissioning editor at Oxford University Press, has tried to console us, suggesting that even this effort has been something of a world record.

I knew at the outset of this project that its success would be completely dependent on the recruitment of the right volume editors. I feel incredibly lucky and humbled to have retained the services of four colleagues whose insight, experience, determination, interpersonal skills and sheer hard work have managed to get this Handbook together more quickly than some of my own previous book chapters have taken to be read by the book's editors, and more professionally than I had dreamed possible. Many, many thanks to all four – my dedication is to you.

David R Moore
MRC Institute of Hearing Research
Nottingham
April 2009

Contents

List of Contributors

Michael A. Akeroyd
MRC Institute of Hearing Research
(Scottish Section)
Glasgow Royal Infirmary
Glasgow

Sygal Amitay
MRC Institute of Hearing Research
Nottingham University
University Park
Nottingham

John F. Culling
School of Psychology
Cardiff University
Cardiff

Chris Darwin
Department of Psychology
University of Sussex
Falmer
Brighton

William J. Davies
Acoustics, Audio and Video
Newton Building
University of Salford
Salford
Greater Manchester

Alain de Cheveigné
Equipe Audition
Centre National de la Recherche
Scientifique, University Paris Descartes, and
Ecole Normale Supérieure
Paris
France

Hamid Djalilian
Otology, Neurotology and Skull Base Surgery
University of California Irvine Medical Center
Orange
USA

W. Jay Dowling
School of Behavioral and Brain Sciences
University of Texas at Dallas
Richardson, TX
USA

Benjamin J. Dyson
Department of Psychology
Jorgenson Hall 1033
Ryerson University
Toronto, ON
Canada

Michael Epstein
Department of Speech-Language
Pathology and Audiology (106A FR)
Institute for Hearing, Speech,
& Language
Northeastern University
Boston
USA

Lorna F. Halliday
Division of Psychology and
Language Sciences
University College London
London

Jeremy Marozeau
The Bionic Ear Institute
East Melbourne
Australia

Karen Mattock
Department of Psychology
Lancaster University
Lancaster

David R. Moore
MRC Institute of Hearing Research
Nottingham University
University Park
Nottingham

Andrew J. Niemiec
Department of Psychological Sciences
Kenyon College
Gambier
USA

Andrew J. Oxenham
Department of Psychology
Elliott Hall, N218
University of Minnesota
Minneapolis
USA

Christopher J. Plack
Human Communication and
Deafness Division
Ellen Wilkinson Building
The University of Manchester
Manchester

Valerio Santangelo
Neuroimaging Laboratory
Santa Lucia Foundation
Rome
Italy

William P. Shofner
Auditory Physiology Lab (C162)
Department of Speech and
Hearing Sciences
Indiana University
Bloomington
USA

Salvador Soto-Faraco
Parc Científic de Barcelona
Universitat de Barcelona
Spain; and
Institució Catalana de Recerca i Estudis
Avançats
Spain

Charles Spence
Department of Experimental Psychology
University of Oxford
South Parks Road
Oxford

Jesko L. Verhey
Carl von Ossietzky Universität Oldenburg
Fak. V, Institut für Physik
Oldenburg
Germany

Magdalena Wojtczak
Department of Psychology
University of Minnesota
Minneapolis
USA

Fan-Gang Zeng
Hearing and Speech Research Laboratory
University of California
Irvine
USA

Chapter 1

Overview

Christopher J. Plack

1.1 Introduction

The final volume in the series considers the perception of sound; that is, how humans and other animals experience the auditory world. Without a study of perception there would be little meaningful auditory science, since physiological mechanisms need to be understood in terms of the perceptual functions that they perform. For example, we want to understand the physiological mechanisms of frequency selectivity to explain the remarkable ability of listeners to separate and identify sounds.

Auditory psychophysics, or psychoacoustics, is the study of the relations between the physical characteristics of sounds and the evoked sensations. However, as well as providing mathematical formulae (and qualitative and quantitative models) that describe these relations without assuming any particular biological implementation, psychoacoustic research is increasingly directed to an understanding of perceptual phenomena in terms of the underlying physiology. Psychoacoustic research and physiological research are therefore strongly co-dependent, and throughout this volume you will read examples of psychoacoustic results being interpreted in terms of, and indeed informing, our understanding of the underlying biomechanical and neural mechanisms.

Traditionally, perceptions have been measured using psychoacoustic techniques in which participants are required to make behavioural responses (often by pressing a button on a response box) to indicate their experience of a sound. These techniques allow researchers to estimate basic subjective quantities such as the magnitude of a sensation, or to measure the limits of discrimination performance, for example the smallest frequency difference that is perceptible. However, the boundaries between psychoacoustics and physiology are becoming blurred by the use of human brain imaging techniques in combination with behavioural measures. These techniques include electroencephalography (EEG) and magnetoencephalography (MEG), which measure the electrical activity of neurons in the brain and have good temporal resolution (of the order of milliseconds) but poor spatial resolution; and functional magnetic resonance imaging (fMRI), that accurately localizes activity in the brain by measuring the increased blood oxygen levels in active regions, but has poor temporal resolution (of the order of seconds). By using brain imaging in combination with behavioural measures it is possible to link neural activity to sensation for individual listeners. In addition, brain imaging provides a connection between psychoacoustics and animal neurophysiology, bridging the gap between our understanding of human perception and our understanding of the responses of individual neurons. Being educated as a hardcore psychophysicist, I was surprised (pleasantly) by how many authors in this volume included brain imaging research in their discussions.

When considering human hearing it is important not to lose sight of the end goal of perception, which is to provide meaningful information about the world around us. To do this, the auditory system has to encode and analyse the different physical characteristics of sounds, separate the acoustic information from different sources, and identify and extract meaning from the sounds produced by a particular source, be it an inanimate object or the human voice. These topics of encoding, separation, and meaning provide a broad framework for the chapters in this volume.

1.2 **Chapter summary**

The overall flow of Chapters 2–11 in this volume is from our perception of the primary physical characteristics of sounds such as frequency and intensity, and basic measures of auditory sensation such as loudness and pitch, to the perception of complex sounds such as speech and music, and high-level, more cognitive, functions such as attention. In tandem, the discussions vary from processes that can be understood in terms of basic auditory physiology, to those that are dependent on vastly complex neural interactions in the cerebral hemispheres. The final chapters describe related topics including cross-modal interactions, auditory development, hearing and language disorders, and environmental sound.

Masking is a fundamental auditory phenomenon, and Chapter 2 (Oxenham and Wojtczak) considers the processes that determine whether one sound will obscure or mask another sound, with particular regard to the remarkable frequency selective mechanisms of the cochlea. Despite being one of the first areas of psychoacoustic investigation, there is currently considerable excitement in the field, as new behavioural techniques have allowed accurate measures of the complex non-linear response properties of the basilar membrane.

Chapter 3 (Epstein and Marozeau) is concerned with the auditory representation of sound intensity, and its perceptual correlate of loudness. The authors discuss intensity discrimination and the dynamic range of hearing, techniques for measuring loudness, and the complex relation of loudness to the physical characteristics of sounds. Important new developments in loudness modelling are described.

Pitch is the main perceptual dimension of western music, and has important roles in speech perception and in sound segregation. In Chapter 4, de Cheveigné describes how the sensation depends on the spectral, temporal, and binaural properties of sounds, and provides an overview of models of pitch perception. The author shows how our perceptions may relate to the physiological properties of auditory neurons, particularly their ability to 'phase lock' to periodic sounds, and describes recent hypotheses regarding neural pitch processing in the auditory brain.

The auditory system shows remarkable temporal resolution, having the ability to detect changes in sounds lasting just a few milliseconds (much faster than the visual system!). This acuity is necessary since information in sounds is often conveyed as a rapid sequence (e.g. speech). In Chapter 5 (Verhey) the main characteristics of auditory temporal resolution are described, as well as the specific mechanisms that process fluctuations in temporal envelope. The author also explains how the auditory system *combines* information over time in order to improve performance.

Frequency, intensity, periodicity, and temporal envelope can be regarded as fundamental physical characteristics of sounds. To these we might add spatial location as a fundamental characteristic of a sound *source*. Chapter 6 (Culling and Akeroyd) concerns spatial hearing; how we localize sound sources using binaural and monaural cues, and how we use echoes and reverberation to tell us about the nature of the listening space.

This volume, along with most perceptual research, focuses on human hearing. However, *H. sapiens* is not the only species to make use of acoustic information, and many insights have been provided from behavioural measurements on other animals. These advances are described in Chapter 7 (Shofner and Niemiec). As explained by the authors, this research provides a conceptual bridge between human psychophysics and animal neurophysiology, and allows us to understand human hearing in an evolutionary context.

Chapter 8 (Dyson) addresses the huge topic of auditory organization: How the auditory system separates out the sounds from different sources, and groups together the sounds from the same source into a coherent auditory stream. This vital stage in hearing, a prerequisite of sound identification, can be regarded as one of the most complex processing tasks accomplished by the auditory brain. The author shows how behavioural results are being combined with advances in neuroimaging to shed new light on the brain mechanisms involved.

Oral communication is perhaps the most important use of hearing for humans, allowing us to convey our thoughts and emotions with comparative ease. Chapter 9 (Darwin) considers many aspects of speech perception, including speech production, the representation of speech in the auditory system, grouping mechanisms, and speech recognition. It is shown how the auditory system copes remarkably well with severe distortions of the speech signal and the huge variability in speech across different contexts.

Music is arguably second only to speech as a means of acoustic communication (some might say higher than second!), and is an extremely rich and diverse product of human creativity. In Chapter 10, Dowling describes the dimensions of the music experience, how we organize the components of music, and how tension and relaxation are generated. The chapter emphasizes the importance of expectation and familiarity to our understanding and appreciation of a musical work.

Auditory attention is discussed in Chapter 11 (Spence and Santangelo). Through a series of ingenious experiments, the authors describe the limitations on our ability to analyse multiple streams of auditory information, how we direct our auditory attention, and how neuroimaging results have identified the brain regions involved in these complex processes.

Chapter 12 (Spence and Soto-Faraco) takes us beyond the purely acoustic world, and describes how auditory information combines and interacts with that from vision. What we hear is determined by much more than the sounds entering our ears, and the authors show how real-world perception needs to be understood as a multisensory experience.

In Chapter 13 (Mattock, Amitay, and Moore), the changing nature of auditory abilities is addressed. The authors describe how the developing auditory system learns how to make sense of the complex waveforms arriving at the ears, from the fetal stage, to infancy, and through childhood. The chapter also considers auditory learning; how the auditory brain changes and adapts to experience throughout life.

Hearing impairment is a very common disability, and improving the diagnosis and treatment of hearing disorders is the most important application for auditory research. In Chapter 14, Zeng and Djalilian describe the wide range of hearing disorders, and their underlying physiological and 'system level' bases. The authors also summarize the different treatments for hearing loss, including exciting recent developments.

Chapter 15 (Halliday and Moore) concerns the effects of hearing disorders, some of which may be quite subtle, on language and cognitive development. The links between auditory function and the development of higher-level abilities are still poorly understood, and present a considerable challenge to researchers. The authors present a balanced view of the evidence, and argue for an approach based on 'risk factors' rather than simplistic causal links.

In the final chapter (Chapter 16), Davies describes the mathematics and acoustics of sound production and propagation in the contemporary environment, including the different types of sound source, and the effects of human structures, including room acoustics. He also discusses the perception of environmental sound, and the recently reinvigorated concept of the 'soundscape'.

I am deeply indebted to the chapter authors for contributing their time and expertise to this volume. Together they have produced a wide-ranging, current, and stimulating account of auditory perception that should be an invaluable resource for students, educators, and researchers in the field.

Chapter 2

Frequency selectivity and masking

Andrew J. Oxenham and Magdalena Wojtczak

2.1 Introduction

Making sense of our acoustic environment is no trivial task. Sound—tiny and rapid variations in air pressure—is produced by sources of mechanical vibrations, such as a person's vocal apparatus or the body of a violin. When many sources are present at the same time, the single acoustic waveform that reaches a listener's eardrum can be a hodgepodge mixture that may not resemble any of the original source waveforms. In fact, the superposition of the different waveforms creates a new waveform that cannot be decomposed into the original source waveforms without prior knowledge of at least some of their properties. Furthermore, the acoustics of the environment, be it a room, hall, forest, or cave, will alter the waveform in many ways to make the task of separating and identifying the original sources even more complicated.

Fortunately for us, the auditory system seems ideally tailored to the task, and some of the important steps in segregating different sounds are achieved as early in the system as the inner ear, or cochlea. Sounds entering the cochlea are separated according to frequency content in a way that can be compared to a prism breaking up white light into its constituent wavelengths. The process of separating sound by frequency, and the extent to which the process is successful, is known as *frequency selectivity, frequency analysis*, or *frequency resolution*. These terms are often used interchangeably. In some cases, sounds can no longer be segregated from one another, and one sound (e.g. a running shower) may make it impossible to hear another (e.g. the phone ringing). This phenomenon is known as *masking*. Masking can often be considered a failure of frequency selectivity, in the sense that the frequencies comprising the masked sound (or target) cannot be resolved or separated from those of the masker. In fact, masking has been widely used in psychoacoustic research to probe the limits of frequency selectivity. This chapter reviews a number of phenomena related to frequency selectivity and masking, and explores the ways in which they can be related to what we know about the mechanics of the inner ear, primarily from physiological studies in other mammals. For earlier reviews of these and related areas, the reader is referred to the chapters of Scharf (1970), Patterson and Moore (1986), and Moore (1995).

2.2 Physiological underpinnings

2.2.1 Tonotopic organization and frequency selectivity in the cochlea and beyond

In 1961 the Nobel Prize in Physiology or Medicine was awarded to Georg von Békésy 'for his discoveries of the physical mechanism of stimulation within the cochlea'. Earlier scientists, most prominently Hermann von Helmholtz, had postulated that the cochlea acted as a frequency analyser, but von Békésy was the first to actually observe how this was achieved. He carefully drilled through the temporal bones of human cadavers to expose the cochlea, in particular the cochlear partition including the basilar membrane (BM). Using a light microscope, he found that each tone he presented resulted in a pattern of vibration along the BM known as a 'travelling wave'. The peak of the travelling wave reached a maximum at different places along the BM, depending on the tone's frequency. Here was a mechanical mechanism by which sound could be analysed in terms of its frequency content: low-frequency sounds produced maximum responses near the apical end of the cochlea, whereas high-frequency sounds produced maxima near the basal end (von Békésy, 1960). One remaining puzzle was that the frequency tuning exhibited in von Békésy's cochlear measurements was much poorer than that found in the responses of individual auditory nerve fibres (e.g. Kiang et al., 1965; Rose et al., 1968). There followed an extended period in the 1970s during which most researchers postulated and sought a 'second filter' that was thought to operate between the BM and the auditory nerve. The first indications that BM tuning itself may be much sharper than originally thought came with the measurements of BM motion in live squirrel monkeys, performed by Rhode (1971). The key differences between Rhode's experiments and those of von Békésy were (1) the animal was alive during the measurements and (2) the measurements using the Mössbauer technique were much more sensitive that those using a light microscope, meaning that less extreme sound levels were needed to elicit a measurable response. Rhode showed first that BM tuning was sharper than had previously been thought, and second that the responses were non-linear; in other words, a given change in input sound level did not always result in the same change in BM vibration level.

Rhode's results were met at first with a great deal of scepticism, and it took more than a decade before the concept of a sharply tuned non-linear cochlea became fully established. One criticism was that the Mössbauer technique itself is highly non-linear, and so there was some concern that the observed non-linearities were an artefact of the measurement technique, rather than a property of BM mechanics. However, Rhode's initial observations have stood the test of time. In fact, as measurement techniques and technologies have become more refined, the trend has been to find ever more sharply tuned and non-linear responses (e.g. Sellick et al., 1982; Ruggero, 1992; Rhode, 2007). Nevertheless, the responses measured in the auditory nerve still exhibit subtle differences from BM motion, such that neither the velocity nor the displacement of the BM can fully explain the responses in the auditory nerve. This is illustrated in Fig. 2.1, which compares iso-response curves, or tuning curves, in the auditory nerve with those obtained from the BM. Such curves are derived by presenting a single pure tone at a given frequency and adjusting its level until it produces a certain response (velocity or amplitude on the BM or firing rate in the auditory nerve), and then doing the same for a range of different frequencies while monitoring the same place on the BM or firing rate of the same auditory nerve fibre. It can be seen from Fig. 2.1 that neither BM velocity nor BM amplitude quite matches the tuning curve derived from the auditory nerve, which falls in between the two. It seems that some interactions between elements on the organ of Corti and the tectorial membrane may provide some form of 'second filter' after all (Ruggero et al., 2000).

Tonotopic organization is maintained beyond the cochlea, through brainstem structures, all the way to the primary auditory cortex. However, at all these stages convergence occurs, and different scales of frequency selectivity can be observed, with some units being as sharply tuned as those in the auditory nerve, and others being extremely broadly tuned, with bandwidths of several octaves. Responses in higher auditory centres tend also to be more complex and effects of wide-band neural inhibition are often observed, as are more complex time-dependencies than those found in the auditory nerve. These different scales of frequency selectivity, along with more complex responses, are presumably important in coding certain sound features, as well as maintaining perceptual constancy of sound objects at different distances and in different reverberant conditions. These different pathways and different scales imply parallel processing. In contrast, all

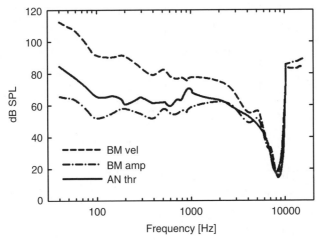

Fig. 2.1 Tuning measured on the BM. The dashed line shows levels of different frequency tones needed for a constant BM velocity, and the dashed–dotted line shows the levels needed for a constant amplitude of BM vibration at one selected place of the chinchilla cochlea. Tuning of the auditory nerve responses is shown by the solid line. Data replotted from Ruggero *et al.* (2000).

sounds must pass through the cochlea before being processed in higher stages—there is no alternative parallel route. This fact may explain in part why researchers in auditory perception have concentrated on identifying perceptual correlates and consequences of cochlear processing: it seems important to understand how sound is represented at this critical (and unavoidable) level because it will affect all subsequent processing.

2.2.2 The active cochlea: Gain, compression, and suppression

One of the most important insights to come from work on BM motion is that the sharp tuning and non-linear aspects of the response are physiologically vulnerable; cochlear damage or death leads to a loss of sharp tuning and non-linearity, resulting in observations resembling those originally made by von Békésy. More recent work has implicated the outer hair cells as being responsible for the so-called 'active mechanism', although the way in which they provide non-linear gain and tuning is still under some debate, with some groups pointing to the action of the cilia (the tiny hair bundles on top of the hair cells) (e.g. Martin *et al.*, 2000), and others pointing to movement (expansion and contraction) of the outer hair cells themselves (e.g. Dallos *et al.*, 2006). Regardless of how the non-linear amplification is achieved, it is undoubtedly critical to the normal functioning of the ear; in fact, a loss of this amplification may underlie many of the difficulties experienced by people with cochlear hearing loss, as discussed in Chapter 14 (Zeng and Djalilian, this volume).

Figure 2.2 shows some important aspects of BM response from two different perspectives. The left panel shows how the velocity of vibration, measured at one point along the BM, changes as a function of sound input level for a few selected tone frequencies. By definition, the BM response at low sound levels is greatest to a tone at the characteristic frequency (CF) of the place of measurement. This is seen in the left panel by the fact that the response to low-level tones is greatest for the tone at 10 kHz, which is at the CF of that place. As the level of the tone increases, so does the response of the BM. However, the rate at which the response increases depends on the tone frequency. For frequencies well below the CF of the measurement place (e.g. 5 kHz), response growth is roughly linear, with a 10-dB increase in response for every 10-dB increase in sound level.

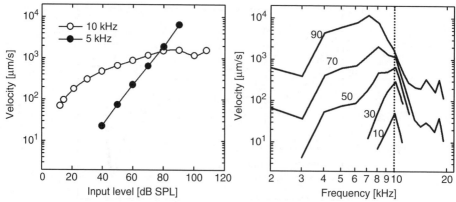

Fig. 2.2 BM responses measured in the chinchilla cochlea. The left panel shows growth of rms velocity (plotted on a logarithmic scale) with increasing level of the stimulating tone measured at a place with CF = 10 kHz. The open symbols show responses to stimulation by the CF (10-kHz) tone and the filled symbols show responses to a 5-kHz tone (a frequency an octave below CF). The right panel shows responses measured at the 10-kHz place to different frequency tones presented at the same level (iso-level responses), for a number of levels from 10 to 90 dB SPL. Data replotted from Ruggero *et al.* (1997).

For frequencies at or near CF, the response growth is compressive over a wide range of levels, meaning that a given increase in sound level leads to a smaller increase in BM response.

The right panel of Fig. 2.2 shows a different perspective of the same types of measurement. Now, the response of the BM at the same fixed measurement point is plotted as a function of the frequency of the tone for a range of different sound levels in 10-dB steps. The frequency selectivity of the BM is more apparent in this type of plot, as is the dependence of frequency selectivity on level. The principle behind these iso-level curves is similar to that of the iso-response tuning curves of Fig. 2.1; the difference is that the tuning curves are derived by keeping the response (or output) constant, while the iso-level curves are derived by keeping the sound level (or input) constant. Both, however, provide a measure of frequency selectivity. At low sound input levels, the BM is sharply tuned, with a much greater response to tones at or near CF ('on-frequency' tones) than to tones far away from CF ('off-frequency' tones); at high sound input levels, the BM is more broadly tuned, and the difference in response to on- and off-frequency tones is not as pronounced.

One of the most obvious functions for the non-linear, compressive response of the BM is to take a wide sound dynamic range of around 120 dB (or a ratio of $1:10^6$ in sound pressure) and squeeze it into a smaller range that is more amenable to neural coding. A loss of this gain and compression results in a smaller dynamic range, and an inability to hear quiet sounds; see Zeng and Djalilian (Chapter 14, this volume) and Oxenham and Bacon (2003).

The level-dependent gain observed for frequencies near the CF, but not below, has other implications than simply a change in tuning with level and a non-linear input–output function. One of the most prominent, and most widely researched, is a phenomenon known as 'two-tone inhibition' or 'two-tone suppression'. First observed in the response of auditory nerve fibres (Sachs and Kiang, 1968), the neural response to one tone can be reduced by the addition of a second tone. The term 'suppression' is now preferred over 'inhibition' because the mechanisms appear to be mechanical rather than neural. In the context of the two-path cochlear model, suppression occurs when the high level of the second tone reduces the gain of the active mechanism (and hence the response to the first tone), but the frequency of the second tone is far enough away from CF to be attenuated strongly relative to the first tone (Meddis *et al.*, 2001; Zhang *et al.*, 2001). Two-tone suppression is observed on the BM as well as in the auditory nerve, but differences in characteristics between the two forms of suppression again leave open the possibility that auditory nerve suppression reflects more complex interactions than simply BM motion (Geisler and Nuttall, 1997; Cai and Geisler, 1996).

All the physiological phenomena we have mentioned so far have correlates in perception, and the remainder of the chapter is devoted to studying them. Although it is encouraging to find agreement, and in some cases very close agreement, between physiological and perceptual data, it should always be remembered that these measurements are being taken at very different levels within the system. This caveat is particularly important when relating cochlear mechanics to perception, because in most cases the comparisons that can be made are from different species, with most cochlear-related measures coming from non-human (and in most cases non-primate) mammals, and most perceptual data coming solely from humans. As we shall see, the few studies that have made within-species comparisons of perceptual and physiological data provide encouragement that certain aspects of perception, in particular masking and frequency selectivity, can be related to cochlear physiology; however, no matter where and what the neural bases of masking and frequency selectivity are, they remain an important part of understanding human auditory perception in its own right.

2.3 Psychophysical masking

2.3.1 Experimental designs and theoretical frameworks

Masking is the process whereby one sound renders one or more other sounds inaudible. In the rest of this chapter we will typically use 'masker' and 'signal' to refer to the sound producing the masking and the sound being masked, respectively. To determine whether a sound is masked or not requires a behavioural test. The simplest behavioural test might be to play a signal in the presence of a masker and ask subjects whether they heard the signal. Although this may be satisfactory in some situations, it does not provide a very rigorous test of masking, because it does not separate 'sensitivity' from 'bias'. For instance, two subjects may be equally sensitive to the presence of a particular signal, but one subject may be much more willing to claim to have heard the signal than another more cautious subject in situations where some uncertainty exists. A common approach in psychophysical studies of masking is to play two or more (*N*) presentations of the masker, only one of which also contains the signal. In this so-called two-interval, two-alternative (or *N*-interval, *N*-alternative) forced-choice procedure, the subject must choose which interval contained the signal, and subjects are not required to say whether or not they actually heard the signal. This removes much of the potential scope for bias in the procedure and leads to a more objective measure of signal detection. The theory underlying signal detection has itself been the subject of much study (Green and Swets, 1966; Macmillan and Creelman, 2004).

In masking experiments, one is often interested in how high in level the signal needs to be in order for subjects to hear it. Typically, a 'threshold' signal level is estimated, which can be defined as the level at which a subject can just hear (or just not hear) a signal. This threshold can be defined and determined in many different ways, most of which are to some extent arbitrary. In a two-interval, two-alternative forced-choice procedure, subjects would get 50% correct, even if they could not hear the signal at all. Therefore, threshold must be defined as a level at which subjects get more than 50% but less than 100% correct. There are a family of automated adaptive tracking procedures that allow an experimenter to track a certain level of performance, be it

75% (Zwislocki and Relkin, 2001), 71%, 79%, or a number of other possibilities (Levitt, 1971). The function relating performance to signal level (or other variable) is known as the 'psychometric function'. Depending on the task, and the scientific question being posed, it may be necessary to determine the entire psychometric function, from chance to perfect performance. In other tasks it may be sufficient to just determine one point on the psychometric function, and compare the conditions needed to obtain that particular level of performance. Probably because the latter option—tracking a single level of performance—is less time-consuming, it is by far the most widespread method used in psychophysics today, in masking as well as many other types of perceptual studies. Various different forms of masking are reviewed below.

2.3.2 Categories of masking: Simultaneous masking, forward and backward masking, and the pulsation threshold

Masking is probably the most widely used of all phenomena in auditory perception research. It has been studied for its own sake, and as a tool to tell us about other aspects of auditory processing. Masking is typically divided into different categories, from an operational perspective (i.e. how the stimuli are generated and presented) but also from a functional perspective (i.e. how we think the masking occurs within the auditory system). The most commonly studied form of masking is simultaneous masking. This is understandable because it is certainly the most ubiquitous form of masking in our everyday environment, as anyone who has tried to hold a conversation in a noisy restaurant or bar can attest. Simultaneous masking covers all situations in which the masker is present for the entire duration of the signal. The masker may begin earlier than the signal or end later, but the important point is that the signal is never present when the masker is absent.

The other main category of masking is non-simultaneous masking, which can be further divided into forward masking and backward masking. Forward masking is when the signal occurs after the offset of the masker. Compared to the reductions in sensitivity to visual stimuli after a bright light, the auditory system recovers very rapidly after all but the most intense stimulation. In most cases, forward masking is no longer found when the gap between the end of the masker and the signal is longer than about 200 ms. Backward masking occurs when the signal precedes the masker in time, and is a much more fragile and variable effect than forward masking; typically, delays between the onset of the signal and the onset of masker that are longer than 10 ms elicit no backward masking, and there are some indications that backward masking, even at shorter delays, might diminish substantially with sufficient practice on the part of the subjects (e.g. Oxenham and Moore, 1994, 1995).

The final phenomenon, which has been referred to as the continuity illusion, auditory induction, or the pulsation threshold (Houtgast, 1972; Warren et al., 1972), is not really masking at all but shares many of the properties of non-simultaneous masking, particularly with respect to defining frequency selectivity, as is discussed in Section 2.4. The basic finding is that a quiet sound that alternates with a louder sound is sometimes heard as continuous (i.e. continuing through the louder sound) if the frequency content of the louder sound could mask the quieter sound, were they to be presented simultaneously.

2.3.3 Mechanisms of simultaneous masking

In psychoacoustics, simultaneous masking has been traditionally thought of as an 'excitatory' effect. According to this view, the masker produces enough BM and neural activity to render the additional activity due to the target undetectable. Conversely, a signal is heard when it produces a detectable overall increase in the neural response to the masker alone. The assumption that masking is excitatory, and that a signal is detected by virtue of an overall increase in neural activity underlies many models of masking and frequency selectivity, ranging from the earliest (e.g. Fletcher, 1940) to the more recent (Glasberg and Moore, 2000). The most important part of the assumption is that the level at threshold for a pure-tone signal tells us something about the activity produced by the masker at the place along the BM that responds best to the signal frequency. In its strongest (and most common) form, the assumption goes further to state that the level of the signal at threshold is proportional to the excitation produced by the masker at that place (Fletcher, 1940; Zwicker, 1970; Patterson, 1974; Glasberg and Moore, 1990). Although it has always been recognized that these are simplifying assumptions, they have turned out to be quite powerful, particularly in terms of enabling researchers to relate the masked thresholds that are measured in psychophysical experiments to the underlying patterns of neural activity. It remains, however, important to remember the nature of the assumptions and not to confuse them for fact. This is particularly important because there are other mechanisms that may underlie simultaneous masking in certain situations. For instance, along with excitation, suppression has been observed in responses along the BM and in the auditory nerve, as well as in psychophysical studies (e.g. Houtgast, 1974; Shannon, 1976).

Suppression is another possible mechanism for simultaneous masking: a masker could reduce the response to the signal to the extent that it is no longer distinguishable from the spontaneous neural activity in the absence of sound stimulation. As discussed above (Section 2.2.2), evidence for suppression has been found in BM and auditory nerve studies. However, very few physiological studies have examined masking (i.e. the inability to distinguish the presence from the absence of a signal), as opposed to simply a reduction in response. One exception is the study by Delgutte (1990), in which he measured the effect of a pure-tone masker on the auditory nerve response to a pure-tone signal, with the specific intention of distinguishing excitatory masking from suppressive masking. In his 'simultaneous masking' condition, he measured the responses of individual auditory nerve fibres to the masker alone and to the masker-plus-signal. Masked threshold for each fibre was estimated by determining the signal level necessary for the masker-plus-signal to produce a distinguishable change in the number of neural spikes generated by the masker alone. The operational definition of threshold was that the spike count in the masker-plus-signal interval exceeded the spike count in the masker-alone interval 75% of the time.

Delgutte's (1990) 'non-simultaneous masking' paradigm resembled pulsation thresholds more closely than forward or backward masking. In this case, the spike count in response to the masker alone was compared with that in response to the signal alone. Suppressive masking is assumed *not* to play a role here, because the masker is never present at the same time as the signal, and so cannot be expected to suppress the signal. Again, threshold was defined as the level at which the signal alone produced a higher spike count than the masker alone 75% of the time. Delgutte was able to compare thresholds in his simultaneous and non-simultaneous conditions in order to estimate the extent to which excitation or suppression were dominant in producing masking in the auditory nerve. The predictions were as follows: if suppressive masking is normally dominant in simultaneous masking, thresholds in the simultaneous masking conditions should be much higher than in the non-simultaneous conditions, where suppression should be absent; on the other hand, if excitatory masking is normally dominant, thresholds in the simultaneous and non-simultaneous conditions should be very similar. Delgutte found that at low masker levels (45 dB SPL) and at all masker levels for signals close to the masker frequency, excitatory masking seemed to dominate; at higher masker levels, for signals higher (> 0.5 octaves) than the masker, suppressive masking played an important role. However, even when suppressive masking was strong, it was rare for excitatory masking to be completely absent (as evidenced by no response to the masker alone).

Suppression effects have also been studied psychophysically to elucidate the possible mechanisms of simultaneous masking. Moore and Vickers (1997) and Oxenham and Plack (1998) addressed the question of whether suppression was the dominant form of masking for maskers well below the signal frequency, as was found in the auditory nerve by Delgutte (1990). The general approach of both studies was to compare the effectiveness of a low-frequency masker in simultaneous masking with its effectiveness in non-simultaneous masking (where suppression is thought to be absent). In line with the earlier physiological data (Delgutte, 1990), both psychoacoustic studies found strong evidence for a major component of suppressive masking for high-level maskers that were well below the signal in the frequency. However, in neither case did suppressive masking occur in the absence of any excitatory masking. Thus, in these cases masking always incorporates a component of excitatory masking and may also involve suppressive masking, depending on the level and frequency relationships between the masker and signal.

Both excitatory and suppressive accounts of masking generally assume that signal detection is achieved by an increase in neural response when the signal is present. However, it has been clear from the early days of psychoacoustic research that the detection of a signal is not always achieved in this way. In fact, even in the earliest quantitative studies of masking (e.g. Wegel and Lane, 1924) it was already noted that the temporal 'beating' effects that occur when two tones of similar frequency are presented simultaneously could make signal detection easier than might be predicted by the increase in overall response produced by the signal. 'Beating' is the term describing audible fluctuations in the temporal envelope of a sound when two pure tones are added. For instance, if two tones separated in frequency by 10 Hz (say tones of 1000 Hz and 1010 Hz) are combined, the resulting waveform will exhibit amplitude fluctuations that repeat at the difference frequency of 10 Hz. A related phenomenon of signal detection, which also cannot be explained simply by energy considerations, is that a tone is more readily masked by a band of noise in a narrow frequency range (a narrowband noise) than the converse, where a noise is masked by a tone (e.g. Hellman, 1972). Again it appears that amplitude fluctuations play a role: the presence of noise fluctuations are easily detected in a background of steady pure tone with no fluctuations, even when the change in the overall energy is small. In contrast, for the more commonly studied case of a pure-tone signal embedded in a noise masker, the overall increase in energy produced by the signal may be the most perceptually salient change. Similar asymmetries have been observed when comparing harmonic with inharmonic or noise stimuli (Treurniet and Boucher, 2001; Micheyl *et al.*, 2006).

Traditionally, masking experiments have treated these 'non-energy' cues as artefacts, and have sought to avoid them. The most common way to avoid potential temporal beating cues is to use a masker that has inherent fluctuations (such as a band of noise) so that the additional fluctuations produced by adding a signal are no longer audible (Egan and Hake, 1950). However, even in the 'simple' case of detecting a tone in noise, it is not always a change in energy that reveals the presence of the signal (e.g. Richards, 1992; Richards and Nekrich, 1993; Kohlrausch *et al.*, 1997). Alternative cues include a change in the envelope characteristics and a change in the temporal fine-structure characteristics, with temporal envelope becoming less modulated and the temporal fine structure becoming more periodic as the signal-to-noise ratio increases. It seems that all these cues can be used by subjects, and that substantial individual differences may exist in terms of how these different cues are weighted (Richards, 2002). Thus, while it may be a convenient simplification to assume that signals are detected by an overall increase in response, it should always be remembered that alternative cues may be available and, in some cases, may be more salient.

2.3.4 Mechanisms of non-simultaneous masking

As mentioned above, non-simultaneous masking has been used as a tool to probe the mechanisms of simultaneous masking and suppression, but what are the neural substrates of non-simultaneous masking itself? Forward masking has been studied much more thoroughly than backward masking, and there are at least three ways in which it might occur. The first explanation relies on the filtering properties of the BM. The impulse response of any filter (including cochlear filters) is finite, meaning that the filters will continue to respond for some period after the stimulus has ended (filter 'ringing'). If the filter ringing in response to a forward masker overlaps with the filter response to the subsequent signal, the result may essentially be simultaneous masking (Duifhuis, 1973). Peripheral filter ringing may account for some forward masking observed at very short delays between the end of the masker and the beginning of the signal, particularly for low signal frequencies. However, the ringing in the peripheral filters is generally thought to last only a few cycles of the filter's CF, whereas forward masking can extend out to 200 ms. Indeed, no evidence for interactions of consecutive stimuli through peripheral ringing has been found for frequencies of 1 kHz and above (Vogten, 1978; Gorga *et al.*, 1980; Carlyon, 1988). Thus, other mechanisms are necessary to account for forward masking.

The two other potential mechanisms underlying forward masking that have received the most attention can be termed 'neural adaptation' and 'neural persistence'. Neural adaptation relates to the fact that the neural response to a tone (i.e. the number of spikes generated) is reduced if the tone is preceded by another stimulus. This general neural phenomenon has been observed in the auditory nerve, which has been proposed as the potential site of psychophysical forward masking (Smith, 1977, 1979). Most studies of neural adaptation have measured only the reduction in response due to the masker, rather than the degree to which a signal is rendered less detectable by the presence of the masker. This is an important distinction: a reduction in response to the signal may be matched by an equivalent reduction in spontaneous neural activity. In this case, the forward masker may not produce any masking at all—just a decrease in the 'baseline' neural activity. A systematic study of neural masking, comparing the response to the masker-plus-signal to the response to the masker alone, concluded that forward masking in individual auditory nerve fibres of chinchillas was a relatively small effect, which could not account well for the forward masking observed psychophysically in humans (Relkin and Turner, 1988). The study concluded that 'forward masking must result from suboptimal processing of spike counts from auditory neurons at a location central to the auditory nerve.' Thus, it seems that adaptation in the auditory nerve cannot alone account for forward masking, although it is very possible that further adaptation and/or non-optimal processing of auditory nerve information at higher processing stages can explain psychophysical forward masking.

Neural persistence as an explanation for forward masking is probably less favoured among researchers in general but, with few exceptions (e.g. Dau *et al.*, 1996a,b), has formed the basis of most of the quantitative models of forward (and backward) masking. The idea that forward masking reflects a continuation of neural response to the masker, rather than reduction in response to the signal, goes back further than the early studies of auditory nerve responses, as is evidenced by the title of one such study, 'The rate of decay of auditory sensation' (Plomp, 1964b). Although there is no evidence of neural persistence in the auditory nerve, studies of auditory cortical responses have often found a persistence in neural activity after the end of a stimulus, consistent with longer integration times of higher level neurons. In some cases this may be continued sustained activity, whereas in other cases, it may involve a distinct response to the offset of a stimulus (e.g. Recanzone, 2000). The most common way to model the persistence is by assuming the presence of a sliding temporal integrator or 'temporal window', the output of which is a running weighted average of the rectified input (e.g. Moore *et al.*, 1988). The effect of the window is to smear the representation of the masker, so that it overlaps with the response to the signal. A simple linear temporal window is unable to account for the many non-linear effects of forward masking, such as its dependence on the level and duration of the masker, without assuming that the window changes shape as the input stimulus changes (Plack and Moore, 1990). However, a combination of a physiologically realistic 'front-end', incorporating BM-like compression, and a linear time-invariant temporal window can account for a number of the properties of forward masking, such as its level and duration dependence (Plack and Oxenham, 1998) and the effects of combining two non-overlapping forward maskers (Plack and O'Hanlon, 2003; Plack *et al.*, 2006), or one forward and one backward masker (Oxenham and Moore, 1994, 1995). Despite some attempts to distinguish psychophysically between the adaptation and persistence hypotheses (e.g. Oxenham, 2001), no convincing evidence has yet emerged to strongly support one theory over the other.

2.3.5 **Temporal effects in simultaneous masking**

Overshoot

Under certain conditions, the threshold for a brief tonal signal is higher when the signal is presented at the onset of a longer simultaneous masker than when it is presented after a brief delay, or when it is presented in a continuous masker. This elevated threshold at masker onset has been referred to as 'overshoot' (Zwicker, 1965) or simply the 'temporal effect' (Strickland, 2004). Under 'ideal' overshoot conditions, the effect can be as large as 15 dB, but is typically quite variable across subjects and depends crucially on parameters such as signal frequency, level, and masker spectral content. In general, high signal frequencies yield more overshoot than low frequencies (Zwicker, 1965), mid-level maskers produce more overshoot than either low- or high-level maskers (Bacon 1990), and masker frequencies away from, and particularly above, the signal frequency seem to be most responsible for the effect (Schmidt and Zwicker, 1991). Despite numerous studies on its effects, there is no consensus as to the mechanisms underlying overshoot. Aspirin use (which is known to affect outer hair cell function) and cochlear hearing loss both lead to a reduction in the effect, suggesting a peripheral origin (McFadden and Champlin, 1990; Bacon and Takahashi, 1992). It has also been suggested that the efferent system may play a role (Schmidt and Zwicker, 1991; von Klitzing and Kohlrausch, 1994; Strickland, 2001, 2008), and more 'central' mechanisms, such as selective attention, have also been implicated (Scharf *et al.*, 2008).

Masking period patterns

The detection of a signal in the presence of a masker can be substantially improved when the masker's envelope fluctuates over time. This is mainly because envelope fluctuations provide an opportunity for detecting brief glimpses of the signal during the dips in the masker envelope. Since most real-life stimuli have dynamically varying envelopes, the question arises as to how fast the fluctuations must be before we are unable to take advantage of the local temporal dips in the masker. One way to address this question is by comparing thresholds for detection of a tone that continues throughout a noise masker for conditions where the masker is unmodulated in one case and sinusoidally amplitude modulated at different rates in another case (Zwicker and Schorn, 1982; Bacon and Lee, 1997; Bacon *et al.*, 1997). As the modulation rate increases, the difference becomes smaller and disappears when listeners are unable to take advantage of the dips in the masker. Another way to assess the ability to use the dips to detect the signal is by measuring masking period patterns (Zwicker, 1976*a,b*, 1986). A masking period pattern is a plot of masked threshold for a short signal as a function of its temporal position within a period of the masker envelope. Some studies focused on only two points of the masking period pattern: the threshold measured for the signal positioned at the peak and the threshold measured for the signal centred in the trough of the masker (Zwicker and Schorn, 1982; Nelson and Swain, 1996). The ability to use information in the trough of the modulated masker was estimated by taking the difference

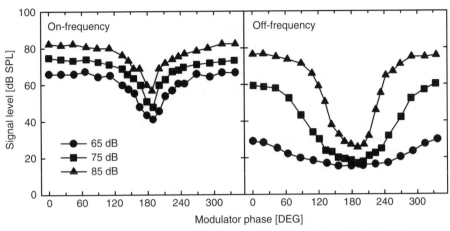

Fig. 2.3 Masking period patterns measured in a listener with normal hearing, for a 6-kHz probe presented at different temporal positions during a modulation cycle of a sinusoidally amplitude modulated masker. Data for different masker levels, 65, 75, and 85 dB SPL are shown by different symbols. The left panel shows data for a 6-kHz carrier (on-frequency masker) and the right panel shows data for a 3-kHz carrier (off-frequency masker). Data replotted from Wojtczak et al. (2001).

between the two thresholds. This measure is very similar to the difference between thresholds for a long-duration signal measured in an unmodulated and modulated masker. However, for a given rate of modulation, that difference depends on whether the masker frequency is the same or different than the frequency of the signal (Zwicker, 1976c). A masker with a frequency about an octave below the signal leads to substantially greater peak–trough differences between the masked thresholds. More detailed sampling of a masking period pattern measured with on- and off-frequency maskers in the study by Wojtczak et al. (2001) revealed that masking period patterns measured with the off-frequency maskers exhibit not only deeper but also much longer troughs than the masking patterns measured with the on-frequency modulated masker. Figure 2.3 shows an example of data from their study for a normal-hearing listener. The difference between on- and off-frequency masking period patterns diminishes in listeners with cochlear hearing loss. Wojtczak et al. demonstrated that the different shapes of masking period patterns could be predicted, assuming a linear (level-invariant) sliding temporal integrator operating on a compressive transform of the squared instantaneous envelope of the on-frequency masker and a linear transform of the squared envelope of the off-frequency masker. Overall, masking period patterns show that fluctuating maskers with frequency components below the frequency of the signal provide a much better opportunity for listening in the dips than maskers with the same rate and depth of envelope fluctuations but with components at or near the signal frequency. This is because at the CF equal to the signal frequency, the internal representation of the off-frequency fluctuating maskers exhibits relatively deeper and longer dips.

Masker phase effects

Changing the phase relationships of the harmonics within a harmonic tone complex can have a dramatic effect on the shape of the waveform, going from something approaching a pulse train when all the components have the same starting phase to a much 'flatter' temporal envelope, when the same components are shifted in phase to minimize envelope fluctuations (Schroeder, 1970). A twist to the story is that the auditory filters have their own phase and amplitude response, which alters the phase relationships of the components, meaning that the temporal envelope of a waveform could, in principle, be quite different after auditory filtering than before. Such effects were illustrated by Kohlrausch and Sander (1995), who showed that rising linear frequency sweeps (with negative phase curvature) produced much flatter masking period patterns and more masking overall than falling linear frequency sweeps (with positive phase curvature) with the same power spectrum and same temporal envelope. Their explanation was that the positive phase curvature of the stimulus 'cancelled out' the inherent negative phase curvature of the auditory filters to produce a waveform (after filtering) that was highly temporally modulated. For the stimulus with the negative phase curvature, the auditory filters simply made the phase curvature even more negative, which had less effect on the temporal envelope of the waveform.

Oxenham and Dau (2001) extended this idea by measuring detection thresholds for tonal signals in maskers with a wide range of different phase curvatures. They reasoned that the lowest thresholds would be obtained for the conditions in which the masker temporal envelope was the most modulated, which would be expected to occur when all the components had the same starting phase (i.e. zero phase curvature) after cochlear filtering. By repeating the measurements over signal frequencies ranging from 125 to 8000 Hz, they were able to derive estimates of the phase curvature of the human auditory filters that were in reasonable agreement with physiological estimates from the cochleae of other species (Shera, 2001a,b).

2.4 Psychophysical measures of frequency selectivity

Masking has been studied in its own right, but has primarily been used as a tool to uncover certain properties of the auditory system. Perhaps most commonly, masking has been used to probe the frequency selectivity of the human auditory system. Dating back to the first quantitative studies in psychoacoustics, scientists have observed that the ability of a sound to mask another is dependent on the spectral content of the two sounds as well as their relative levels (Wegel and Lane, 1924). From these early studies also came the idea that the patterns of masking reflected the patterns of activity set up within the inner ear—hence the term 'excitation pattern', which is still in common use today. The history of masking studies since the early 20th century has been one of continual efforts to refine the techniques, to reduce potential artefacts, and to come as close as possible to results that provide us with accurate estimates of peripheral auditory frequency selectivity.

2.4.1 Masking patterns and excitation patterns

The early studies of auditory masking typically involved a narrowband masker—either a tone or a narrow band of noise—and a tonal signal, the threshold of which was measured at numerous frequencies below, at, and above the frequency of the masker (Wegel and Lane, 1924; Egan and Hake, 1950). The function that relates signal level at threshold to signal frequency is termed the 'masking pattern'. At face value, masking patterns can be used to predict whether a given sound will be detected in the presence of another: if all the frequency components of the target are lower in level than the masking pattern of the masker, it is likely that the target will not be detected. In fact, predictions of masking patterns along these lines have been implemented in low-bit-rate audio coding techniques, such as those used in MP3 players, in order to determine how much noise or distortion can be tolerated in a recording before the degradation becomes audible.

Taken literally, the masking pattern can be treated as a substitute for the activity produced by the masker at that particular frequency. In this way, the masking pattern can be interpreted as an 'excitation pattern'—the pattern of activity as a function of place along the BM (Zwicker, 1970). However, equating masking patterns with excitation patterns has some potential pitfalls. First, as mentioned above, masking is not necessarily excitatory but in some cases can have a substantial

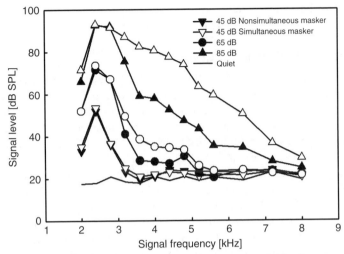

Fig. 2.4 Masking patterns from an individual subject (Oxenham, unpublished), measured using a narrowband masker centred at 2.4 kHz in simultaneous masking (open symbols) and non-simultaneous masking (filled symbols). Different types of symbols correspond to different levels of the masker: 45 dB SPL (inverted triangles), 65 dB SPL (circles), and 85 dB SPL (triangles).

suppressive component. In other words, the masked threshold measured in an experiment reflects not only the excitation of the masker along the BM, but also its suppressive effects on the signal. This is illustrated in Fig. 2.4, which shows a masking pattern produced by a narrow band of noise centred at 2.4 kHz, which was either a simultaneous masker (open symbols) or a non-simultaneous masker (filled symbols) at three different masker levels (45, 65, and 85 dB SPL) and in quiet.

The signal was a brief tone burst (10-ms total duration, gated on and off with 5-ms ramps). At the lower masker level of 45 dB SPL, both the simultaneous and non-simultaneous masking patterns look comparable; however, at the higher masker level of 85 dB SPL, the two patterns diverge, particularly at signal frequencies well above those of the masker. The difference has been explained in terms of suppression affecting simultaneous masking but not non-simultaneous masking. Thus, the non-simultaneous masking patterns might be a better reflection of the underlying masker excitation, particularly at high masker levels. However, even with suppression taken into account, masking patterns may not necessarily provide an accurate reflection of excitation. For instance, because the response to a signal is compressive, a given difference in excitation level between two points along the BM may be reflected in a larger change of signal level at threshold. If the compression ratio of the BM is 5:1, then a 5-dB difference in excitation level would be reflected by a 25-dB change in signal level at threshold. Another potential complication in interpreting masking patterns is termed 'off-frequency listening'.

Off-frequency listening is a construct of psychophysicists to describe how a signal might be most detectable in the auditory periphery not at the place with a CF corresponding to the signal frequency (as is assumed by the excitation pattern interpretation of masking patterns) but at a place with a CF higher or lower than the signal. Consider, for instance, the situation where a signal is below the masker in frequency. It might be that the excitation produced by the signal is greatest, relative to that produced by the masker, at a place further away from the signal frequency. In addition, it may be possible to combine information across multiple places where the signal-to-masker ratio is favourable. Thus, the possibility of off-frequency listening makes it more difficult to relate psychophysical masking patterns to the possible underlying patterns of BM and neural excitation (Johnson-Davies and Patterson, 1979; O'Loughlin and Moore, 1981*a*).

2.4.2 Psychophysical tuning curves

Psychophysical tuning curves (PTCs) are the closest that behavioural experiments can come to the neural tuning curves that are obtained by plotting iso-response curves for single auditory nerve fibres (see Section 2.2.1 above). The paradigm involves taking a low-level tonal signal at, say, 10-dB sensation level (SL, i.e. 10 dB above the threshold in quiet) and determining what level a masking tone (or narrowband noise) must be in order to mask the tone, as a function of the masker's centre frequency. An example of a PTC is given in Fig. 2.5.

Although the general pattern of results found in PTC studies are in good qualitative agreement with studies of neural tuning curves, some difficulties with the procedure remain. First, off-frequency listening is a potential issue, although it can be addressed by adding a low-level noise to restrict the degree to which it can be used (Johnson-Davies and Patterson, 1979; O'Loughlin and Moore, 1981*a,b*). Second, if PTCs are measured in simultaneous masking, suppression effects can play a role, resulting in wider estimated bandwidths, although this can be mitigated by measuring PTCs in forward masking (Moore, 1978; Vogten, 1978). Third, even in forward masking, detection cues can vary depending on the frequency relationship between the masker and signal. For instance, particularly in forward masking, when the masker and signal are at the same or very similar frequencies, the signal may be mistaken for a continuation of the masker (described as a 'confusion' effect), leading to artefactually low masker levels at threshold (Moore and Glasberg, 1985; Neff, 1985), and hence an artificially sharp PTC, particularly around the tip. Also, in simultaneous masking, care must be taken to avoid the detection of beating cues when the masker and signal are close, but not equal, in frequency. Nevertheless, when forward masking is used, and care is taken to avoid potential confusion effects, it may be that PTCs provide the most accurate reflection of cochlear tuning, as would be measured by neural tuning curves in the auditory nerve (e.g. Yasin and Plack, 2003).

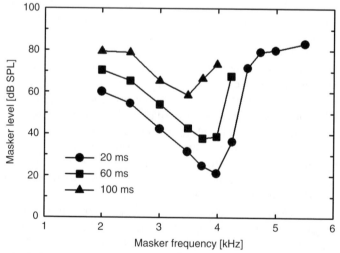

Fig. 2.5 Psychophysical tuning curves measured in forward masking for a 4-kHz signal, at different masker-signal delays: 20 ms (circles), 60 ms (squares), and 100 ms (triangles). Data replotted from Yasin and Plack (2003).

2.4.3 Notched noise methods

The notched noise method overcomes some of the problems of PTCs and masking patterns, first by using noise maskers, which avoid issues of potential confusion and beating, second by using masker noise bands both below and above the signal frequency, to restrict the possibility of off-frequency listening (Patterson, 1976). Along with most other methods, the notched noise method makes certain assumptions about how the signal is detected. The first assumption is that the auditory system can be modelled in terms of a bank of overlapping linear bandpass filters—the so-called 'auditory filters'. The second assumption is that the signal is detected at the output of the auditory filter with the highest signal-to-masker ratio. The third is that the signal is detected when the signal-to-masker ratio equals or exceeds a certain value, which remains constant across different conditions. The fourth assumption is that masking is purely excitatory and is determined solely by the masker power falling within the passband of the auditory filter. These assumptions are also built into the some of the first attempts to define human frequency analysis in terms of the 'critical band' and the power spectrum model of masking (Fletcher, 1940); see Moore (1995) for a more detailed exposition of Fletcher's technique. Although all these assumptions can be questioned, or even shown to be false (such as the assumption of excitatory masking), they have nevertheless provided a powerful analysis tool for understanding many of the phenomena associated with masking and frequency selectivity.

The concept behind the original notched noise technique is illustrated in Fig. 2.6. Essentially, a spectral notch is introduced into an otherwise broadband masker, and signal thresholds are measured as a function of the spectral notch width and its position. On an intuitive level, the more rapid the decline in signal threshold as the notch width is increased, the sharper the filter must be. However, in order to derive quantitative conclusions regarding its slopes and bandwidth, certain assumptions must be made regarding the underlying shape of auditory filter. The notched noise method is probably the most popular method by which to define human frequency selectivity and has been used to form the basis of the more recent models of excitation patterns, masking and loudness in both normal (Moore *et al.*, 1997) and impaired (Moore *et al.*, 1999) hearing.

It has long been known that frequency selectivity becomes poorer, with broader PTCs and masking patterns, as stimulus level increases (Egan and Hake, 1950; Nelson and Freyman, 1984).

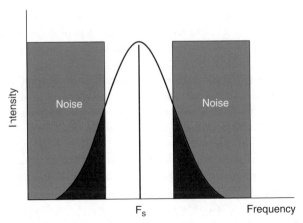

Fig. 2.6 A schematic illustration of the notched noise technique for deriving the shape of the auditory filter centred at frequency F_s. Dark blue areas represent total power of the notched noise at the output of the filter.

The fact the filters change shape with level violates the assumption of filter linearity; however, this has usually been dealt with by assuming that the filter is quasi-linear and constant in shape over a restricted level range. Even then, the question arises as to how level is defined, whether it should be defined as the masker spectrum level, as was done in the early notched noise studies (Patterson, 1976; Glasberg and Moore, 1990) or, as is more often done today, in terms of the signal level at threshold (Rosen and Baker, 1994; Rosen et al., 1998; Oxenham and Shera, 2003; Oxenham and Simonson, 2006). This question is addressed further below (Section 2.6.1).

Studies using the notched noise method have resulted in estimates of filter bandwidth that are roughly consistent with the estimates from other methods. The most widely used unit of the estimated filter bandwidth today is that proposed by Glasberg and Moore (1990), which has become known as the ERB (equivalent rectangular bandwidth), ERB_N (to denote that these are specific values of ERB), or CAM (after the fact that it was derived in Cambridge, England) scale. According to this scale, the filter's ERB (in Hz) at a given centre frequency (F in kHz) at medium sounds levels is given as:

$$ERB = 24.7(4.37F + 1) \qquad (2.1)$$

This equation results in bandwidths that are roughly proportional to the filter centre frequency at frequencies above about 1 kHz, with a tendency to become narrower (in a relative sense) as frequency increases. For instance, the predicted ERB at 1 kHz is about 130 Hz (or 13% of the CF) and the predicted ERB at 10 kHz is about 1100 Hz (11% of the CF). At lower CFs, the bandwidth as a proportion of CF increases, so that at 100 Hz, the ERB is about 35 Hz, or 35% of the CF.

As with masking patterns and PTCs, notched noise filter shapes derived using forward masking are typically narrower than those derived using simultaneous masking, presumably because those using forward masking are not influenced by the additional effects of suppression (Moore and Glasberg, 1981; Glasberg and Moore, 1982; Oxenham and Shera, 2003; Oxenham and Simonson, 2006). Furthermore, some recent studies have suggested that the ERBs at very low signal levels become narrower with increasing CF at a faster rate than is suggested by eqn 2.1 above. For instance, Oxenham and Shera (2003) provide the following equation relating Q_{ERB} (the 'quality factor' of a filter, defined as CF/ERB) derived in forward masking to CF (F in kHz):

$$Q_{ERB} = 11F^{0.27} \qquad (2.2)$$

To provide some direct comparisons, the ERB for a CF of 1 kHz using this equation is 91 Hz, and the ERB for a CF of 10 kHz is 490 Hz. Thus, the estimated bandwidths are considerably narrower than those derived from Glasberg and Moore's (1990) equation, particularly at high frequencies.

Which equation is more appropriate or accurate will depend on the application. The measurements of Oxenham and Shera (2003) are valid using forward masking at very low signal levels—just 10 dB above absolute threshold. The data used by Glasberg and Moore (1990) were obtained at moderate levels (the notched noise had a spectrum level of about 30 dB, or a level per ERB of about 51 dB SPL) using a simultaneous masker. Thus, in terms of predicting masking in everyday situations, where simultaneous masking dominates, it is likely that the equation of Glasberg and Moore is more relevant. Furthermore, the equation of Glasberg and Moore provides a convenient rule of thumb whereby the filter ERB is between 10 and 15% of the CF for frequencies above about 500 Hz. However, for comparative purposes, the equation of Oxenham and Shera may provide a more precise match to the situations typically used to define frequency selectivity physiologically in animal auditory nerve studies and in human and animal studies using otoacoustic emissions (see Section 2.4.5 below).

2.4.4 **Hearing out partials**

The complex tones that we encounter in everyday life, such as voiced speech sounds and notes from musical instruments, comprise a series of sinusoids, often with frequencies at integer multiples of the fundamental frequency (F0). Such sounds are usually heard as a single auditory object (like a single violin note) with a pitch corresponding to the F0. However, as was already noted by Ohm (1843) and Helmholtz (1863), it is possible to 'hear out' some of the individual harmonics or partials within each complex with practice or if attention is drawn to them in some way. The limits on our ability to hear out individual partials are also a reflection of frequency selectivity: if selectivity is poor, then neighbouring partials will not be resolved and it will not be possible to hear out their individual frequencies.

Some of the earliest systematic studies of the resolution of individual partials within a harmonic complex were undertaken by Plomp (1964a) and Plomp and Mimpen (1968). They concluded that only the first 5–7 harmonics of a complex could be heard out, and that the results were basically consistent with the concept of the critical band, such that only components that were separated by more than a critical band could be heard out individually. The results were strengthened by a forward masking experiment, using a complex tone with a 500-Hz F0 as the masker and a signal that varied in frequency (Plomp, 1964a). The results showed distinct peaks in the forward masking pattern of the complex tone corresponding to the first 5 harmonics, again suggesting that at least the first 5 harmonics were spectrally resolved.

Moore and Ohgushi (1993) and Moore *et al.* (2006) assessed the audibility of partials within inharmonic complexes, where the partials were spaced equally according to the ERB_N scale of Glasberg and Moore (1990) rather than the linear scale of harmonic tones. The results from both studies were again basically in line with expectations based on frequency selectivity, in that partials were not well heard out if the spacing between them was less than 1 ERB_N. Two other findings are of note: first, outer partials (the lowest or highest in a complex) were more readily heard out than the others, and second, higher frequency partials were heard out less well than lower frequency partials, despite the fact that the component spacing should have ensured equal resolvability according to the auditory filters. The second finding may indicate a role for the temporal coding of individual partials, via phase-locking in the auditory nerve (Rose *et al.*, 1967). Phase-locking in all mammals so far investigated degrades at higher frequencies, somewhere between 1 and 4 kHz, depending on the species and the measure used. If phase-locking is important for hearing out harmonics, the degradation in phase-locking at high frequencies may explain why performance worsened at high partial frequencies. The first finding of superior performance for the outer components is in line with many other studies finding an 'edge effect' for stimuli with abrupt spectral transitions; such findings can be explained either spectrally—in terms of spectral enhancement of edges, which could occur through BM suppression and later neural lateral inhibition networks (e.g. Shamma, 1985)—or in terms of phase-locking, with more neurons phase-locking to the outer components than to any others (Moore and Ohgushi, 1993).

Despite the approximate correspondence between the ability to hear out partials and the band widths of the auditory filters measured in other ways, some issues make a straightforward interpretation of the results problematic. First, as mentioned, effects related to the coding of temporal fine structure may play a role. Second, the ability to hear out partials seems to depend not just on frequency selectivity but also on factors such as attention and musical training (Soderquist, 1970; Fine and Moore, 1993), suggesting a role for 'higher level' perceptual segregation as well as peripheral frequency selectivity. Bernstein and Oxenham (2003) avoided some of the issues relating to selective attention and perceptual segregation by gating the 'target' harmonic partial on and off twice during each presentation of the otherwise continuous complex. The rationale was to draw attention to the correct harmonic. Because asynchronous gating does not lead to changes in detection threshold in notched noise experiments, it is unlikely to affect the underlying (peripheral) frequency selectivity of the auditory system; on the other hand, it does make it easier for trained and untrained listeners to 'focus' on the target frequency and perceptually segregate it more successfully from the other partials. Bernstein and Oxenham (2003) found that when the complexes were presented in random phase (the phase of each harmonic was selected at random on each presentation), listeners were typically able to reliably hear out the first 10 harmonics of complexes with F0s of 100 and 200 Hz. The limit of 10 harmonics corresponds well with findings from pitch perception studies that suggest that the strong pitch salience associated with low-order resolved harmonics is no longer found if no harmonics below about the 10th are presented (Houtsma and Smurzynski, 1990; Shackleton and Carlyon, 1994; Bernstein and Oxenham, 2003). A recent study by Hartmann and Goupell (2006) found that the limit for hearing out gated harmonics could be as high as the 20th harmonic when the target harmonic was gated on and off very slowly, and when the harmonics were presented in certain phase relationships. This again suggests a role for temporal coding, in which certain phase relationships may result in an enhanced representation of certain harmonics, even when they are almost certainly spectrally unresolved. In summary, although results from hearing out partials can be explained, at least in part, in terms of frequency selectivity, other factors, including the temporal coding of partials and musical training, may influence the outcomes.

2.4.5 Relations between behavioural and physiological estimates of frequency selectivity

Given the difficulty in obtaining physiological data about cochlear tuning from humans, and the challenges associated with obtaining behavioural data from other animals, it is perhaps not surprising that relatively few studies have attempted to directly compare cochlear and behavioural (whole-system) measures of frequency selectivity in the same species. Many of the effects of frequency selectivity and masking that are found in human psychoacoustic studies can be explained in terms of phenomena that are observed in the cochlear responses of other mammals, and it seems reasonable to assume that the same processes occur in human cochleae. However, because we still have no safe method of observing human cochlear activity directly, we must still rely on indirect methods involving behavioural studies and, more recently, non-invasive physiological measures, such as otoacoustic emissions and evoked potentials.

Evans and colleagues have investigated frequency selectivity in the guinea-pig using both physiological and behavioural paradigms (Evans *et al.* 1992; Evans, 2001). They derived ERB estimates from auditory nerve fibre responses in anesthetized guinea-pigs and compared them to behavioural measures, using both the notched noise method and a comb-filtered (or rippled) noise method, where simultaneous masked thresholds of a pure tone are measured at the spectral peak and spectral valley of spectrally rippled noise as a function of the ripple density. All three measures (one physiological and two behavioural) resulted in very similar estimates of filter bandwidth (Evans, 2001), providing strong support for the idea that the frequency selectivity of the auditory system is determined in large part by cochlear mechanisms.

More recently, attempts have been made to derive indirect measures of cochlear frequency selectivity in humans, using otoacoustic emissions. One such attempt included a direct comparison with psychoacoustic measures in the same human subjects for frequencies between 1 and 8 kHz (Shera *et al.* 2002). The psychoacoustic measure was based on the notched noise method, but used a fixed low-level signal in a forward masking paradigm in order to provide as close a comparison as possible to cochlear tuning at low levels, without the potentially confounding effects of suppression. The physiological measure involved stimulus-frequency otoacoustic emissions (SFOAEs), which can be measured using a probe microphone in the ear canal. Details of these emissions, along with the assumptions and calculations needed to convert the measurements into estimates of cochlear tuning can be found elsewhere (Shera and Guinan, 2003). The outcome was that the inverse of the latency of the SFOAEs could be related to estimates of cochlear tuning by a constant factor, and that the changes in inferred cochlear bandwidth with CF varied in a way that was very similar for both the behavioural and emissions data. Furthermore, a comparison of emissions data from humans, cats, and guinea-pigs with auditory nerve data from cats and guinea-pigs, and notched noise data from humans, led to the conclusion that human cochlear tuning may be sharper than that found in cats and guinea-pigs at a given CF by about a factor of two.

Ruggero and Temchin (2005) have questioned the conclusion that humans have sharper cochlear tuning than other mammals. In particular, they argue that animal studies have shown that forward masking produces estimates of tuning that are artificially sharp, and support this claim by citing earlier studies that measured forward-masked psychophysical tuning curves in animals (McGee *et al.*, 1976; Kuhn and Saunders, 1980; Serafin *et al.*, 1982) and found bandwidth estimates that were sharper than the neural tuning curves in the same species. Unfortunately, the comparison is not valid, because all the animal studies carried out so far have used pure-tone forward masked tuning curves, which are known to lead to biased estimates of tuning, due to factors such as off-frequency listening and 'confusion', as discussed above in Section 2.4.2. To date, no one has measured frequency selectivity behaviourally in animals using notched noise in a forward masking paradigm, as was done by Shera *et al.* (2002). If humans do indeed have sharper tuning than other (non-primate) mammals, then one would expect filter bandwidth estimates obtained using forward-masking notched noise to be broader than those found in humans, and to match up with auditory nerve measurements in the same species. For the time being, therefore, the important issue of across-species differences in cochlear tuning remains controversial.

2.5 Psychophysical methods for estimating cochlear gain and compression

Psychophysical measures of frequency selectivity may provide us with a window into human cochlear function, which cannot be gained by direct physiological measures of the live human cochlea. Another measure of cochlear function is the input–output function. The input–output function provides an estimate of cochlear gain and cochlear compression. Both these BM response characteristics are important for perception, as a loss of gain and compression may account for a number of the difficulties faced by hearing-impaired listeners; see Oxenham and Bacon (2003) and Zeng and Djalilian (Chapter 14, this volume). As with frequency selectivity, there is no way to directly observe the input–output function of the human BM, but a number of indirect psychophysical measures have been derived. This section outlines the various methods, their underlying assumptions, and their conclusions. In all these cases non-simultaneous masking has been used to avoid the potentially confounding effects of suppression. Despite the different techniques, and their different underlying assumptions, the methods described below have yielded estimates of BM compression and gain that are reasonably consistent with each other, and with direct physiological measurements in other species.

2.5.1 Growth of masking (GOM)

One property of the BM response is the linear response to tones well below the CF of the place of measurement (see Section 2.2.2 above). This property has been used in psychoacoustic studies to compare growth of masking by an on-frequency forward masker to that by an off-frequency

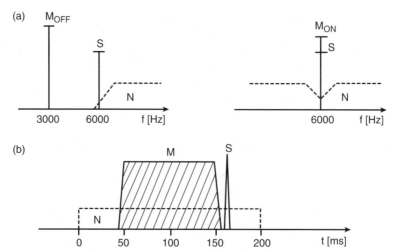

Fig. 2.7 A schematic illustration of the stimuli used to derive the BM response from growth of masking (GOM): (a) spectral representation of the signal (S), off-frequency masker (M_{OFF}; left-hand side) and on-frequency masker (M_{ON}; right-hand side) (N; noise). The dashed lines represent the spectral envelopes of the background noise used to limit off-frequency listening. (b) The time course of the stimuli.

forward masker—one that is well below the signal in frequency. The main assumptions here are that (1) the response to the off-frequency masker at the BM place responding best to the signal is linear, and (2) the signal level at threshold represents the same degree of masker excitation at the place with a CF corresponding to signal frequency, regardless of what the masker frequency is. Using these assumptions, Oxenham and Plack (1997) provided an estimate of BM non-linearity in humans by comparing the growth of forward masking for on- and off-frequency forward maskers. In their study, the signal frequency was 6 kHz and the two masker frequencies were 6 kHz (on-frequency masker) and 3 kHz (off-frequency masker). To produce forward masking over a sufficiently large range of levels of the off-frequency masker, they used a very short signal (4 ms, 2-ms ramps and no steady-state) directly following the masker offset.

Figure 2.7 illustrates the spectra of the stimuli (Fig. 2.7(a)) and the time course in the observation interval that contained the signal (Fig. 2.7(b)). To eliminate the possibility of off-frequency listening, they added a notched-noise (or a high-pass noise in the off-frequency masking condition) that started 50 ms before the onset of the masker and was terminated 50 ms after the offset of the signal. The left panel of Fig. 2.8 shows average masker levels at threshold plotted as a function of signal level, for three normal-hearing listeners tested in the study by Oxenham and Plack. The dashed line has a slope of 1. Data for the on-frequency masker fall very close to that line, whereas data for the off-frequency masker can be represented by a function with a much shallower slope. The slope for the on-frequency masker may be close to unity because the signal and the masker are at similar levels and undergo similar compression. Consequently, every change in signal level requires a similar change in masker level to maintain a constant criterion increase in excitation, and thus to maintain masked threshold across signal levels. For the off-frequency masker, the response on the BM at the signal-frequency place grows roughly linearly, whereas the response to the signal is compressed. This implies that every change in signal level should require a much smaller change in masker level to maintain masked threshold. This is reflected by the shallow slope of the function showing off-frequency masker levels at threshold in Fig. 2.8. Assuming that the response to the off-frequency masker is linear, the slope of the off-frequency masking

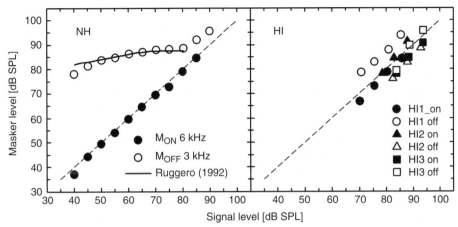

Fig. 2.8 Growth-of-masking data averaged across three normal hearing listeners (left panel) for the on-frequency masker (filled symbols) and the off-frequency masker (open symbols). The solid line represents the animal basilar-membrane response replotted from Ruggero (1992) for comparison. Data from three hearing-impaired listeners are shown in the right panel. The dashed lines in both panels have a slope of 1. Data replotted from Oxenham and Plack (1997).

function reflects the rate of growth of BM response to the signal. In other words, the slope of the off-frequency masking function represents the amount of compression at the CF equal to the signal frequency. Oxenham and Plack (1997) reported that the estimated amount of compression in a healthy human cochlea at high frequencies is 0.16 dB/dB. Their result agrees well with compression estimates from direct physiological measurements of BM vibration in animals (e.g. Ruggero, 1992), as shown by the solid line in Fig. 2.8. Data from three listeners with moderate-to-severe hearing loss in the same study showed slopes that were similar for both on- and off-frequency maskers, and were close to unity (right panel in Fig. 2.8), consistent with the physiological results, which show that the BM response in a damaged cochlea is linear. Overall, therefore, the results suggested that it may be possible to provide indirect estimates of BM compression using psychophysical techniques.

2.5.2 **Temporal masking curves (TMCs)**

The GOM method involved measuring levels of forward maskers needed to just mask a signal at a range of signal levels, at a fixed delay between the masker offset and the signal onset. As the signal level increases, the signal stimulates a larger area on the BM. This creates a possibility that as the signal level increases, the signal can be detected over a broader range of places along the BM, and not necessarily just at the place with a CF corresponding to the signal frequency. Oxenham and Plack (1997) avoided off-frequency listening by using a low-level background noise. However, choosing the appropriate level and spectral content of the noise can be a challenging task, especially for hearing-impaired listeners. Nelson *et al.* (2001) demonstrated that compression can be substantially underestimated due to off-frequency listening in the absence of such a noise, and proposed another method that eliminates the problems associated with off-frequency listening without necessitating the use of a notched noise. Instead of measuring masker levels needed to mask the signal at different levels, Nelson *et al.* kept the signal fixed at a level of just 10 dB SL. Masker levels needed to mask the signal were measured as a function of the delay between the masker and the signal. The constant and low level of the signal means that off-frequency listening is much less of a concern.

As the delay between a forward masker and a signal increases, the masker level must be increased to maintain masked threshold. The changes in masker level have to be such that they produce increases in the BM response to the masker that will compensate for the recovery from the forward masking. A plot of the masker level needed for threshold as a function of the masker-signal delay represents a temporal masking curve (TMC). If the BM response to the masker is linear at the signal frequency (the presumed CF) place, as is assumed for masker frequencies about an octave or more below the signal frequency, the TMC for the off-frequency masker (or off-frequency TMC) directly reflects the rate of recovery from forward masking. In contrast, because the on-frequency masker is subject to compression at the place with a CF corresponding to the signal frequency, the on-frequency TMC represents changes in masker level with increasing delay that are necessary to overcome both recovery from forward masking *and* compression. This leads to a steeper TMC for the on-frequency than for the off-frequency masker. Moreover, since the rate of recovery from forward masking is assumed to be independent of the masker frequency (Nelson and Pavlov, 1989), the difference between the slopes of the two TMCs is attributed solely to the difference between the amounts of compression of the BM responses to the two maskers. The left panel of Fig. 2.9 shows an example of data from one normal-hearing listener in the study by Nelson *et al.* (2001). The data for their off-frequency masker (500 Hz, open circles) show increases in masker level needed to overcome recovery from forward masking. The data were approximated by a straight line and used as a linear reference for deriving the BM input–output function. The filled symbols show changes in level that were needed to just mask the signal for the 1012-Hz on-frequency masker, which produced the greatest estimate of compression. The function is relatively shallow at low masker levels (short delays) but the slope becomes very steep once masker level reaches the range of medium levels (at medium delays), indicating strong compression of the masker response. For the highest levels, the slope becomes essentially parallel to the off-frequency TMC, which suggests lack of compression at high levels. Comparing the on- and off-frequency temporal masking curves allows for a derivation of the presumed shape of the BM response function, which in turn allows for estimation of the cochlear gain and compression. It should be noted that the fixed low signal level ensures that the position and extent of the BM

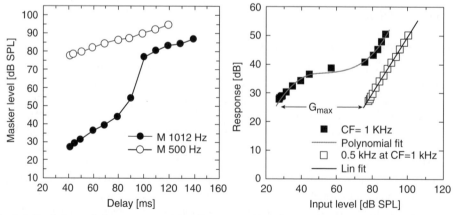

Fig. 2.9 The left panel shows temporal masking curves (TMCs) measured in a normal-hearing listener for a 1012-Hz masker (on-frequency; filled symbols) and a 500-Hz masker (off-frequency; open symbols). The right panel shows the derived BM response functions for the on-frequency masker (filled squares) and the off-frequency masker (open squares). The grey solid line represents the third-order polynomial fit to the data. Data replotted from Nelson *et al.* (2001).

stimulation produced by the signal remains constant for all data points (masker levels), thus ensuring that the derived BM response function is for the signal-frequency place.

By assuming that the forward masking effect itself is the same for both on- and off-frequency maskers, and by assuming that the BM response to the off-frequency masker is linear, it is possible to derive an estimate of on-frequency input–output function simply by plotting the off-frequency masker level at threshold (y-axis) against the on-frequency masker level at threshold (x-axis) for each masker-signal delay. This is because the BM response to the on- and off-frequency masker at threshold is assumed to be the same for any given signal delay. Thus, if the response to the off-frequency masker (y-axis) is linear, then any increase in the off-frequency masker level with increases in on-frequency masker level will reflect the effects of compression on the on-frequency masker. For instance, if a 10-dB increase in on-frequency masker level leads to a 2-dB increase in off-frequency masker level for the same change in signal delay, this implies a 5:1 compression ratio, or an exponent of 0.2.

The right panel of Fig. 2.9 shows an input–output function obtained from the temporal masking curves (TMCs) by Nelson *et al.* (2001). The derived function has a steeper segment at low levels, reflecting roughly linear response growth at low sensation levels. As the level increases the slope becomes very shallow consistent with the notion that cochlear gain decreases with increasing level thereby causing compressive response growth. At high levels, the BM response becomes linear. The three-segment function, i.e. linear at low levels, compressive at mid levels, and linear at high levels, is typically observed in humans with normal hearing, although not all listeners exhibit the linear segment at high levels (Plack *et al.*, 2004; Rosengard *et al.*, 2005).

The data from measured TMCs have been analysed in different ways, depending on the specific goals of the study in question. For instance, Nelson *et al.* (2001) estimated local compression exponents by fitting a third-order polynomial to the derived BM response function. The derivative of the fitted polynomial represented the local slope of the BM response as a function of level. The minimum of the derivative function represented the maximum amount of compression (i.e. the minimum compression exponent). To provide a more 'global' estimate of compression over a range of medium sound levels, it is possible to fit a straight line over a limited range of levels, while fitting line segments with other slopes (sometimes fixed at 1) to the lowest and highest levels, where the response is often found to be more linear (Lopez-Poveda *et al.*, 2003; Plack *et al.*, 2004).

Maximum cochlear gain can be estimated from the horizontal shift between the low-level linear portion of the BM response to the on-frequency masker and the response to the off-frequency masker at the signal-frequency place (see the right panel in Fig. 2.9). The linear response growth at low levels reflects a constant value of the cochlear gain, and thus the gain is likely at its maximum over that range of levels. The BM response becomes compressive when the cochlear gain decreases with increasing level. The gain can be also estimated from the vertical distance between the data points on the on- and off-frequency TMCs, for the shortest masker-signal delay. The distance represents a difference between on- and off-frequency masker levels that produce the same excitation on the BM at the signal-frequency place. Assuming that cochlear gain is applied only to the on-frequency masker and not to the off-frequency masker, the difference between the levels needed to produce the same excitation reflects the cochlear gain in dB. It should be noted that passive processing on the BM exhibits some (albeit relatively broad) frequency selectivity and thus, the off-frequency masker is attenuated by the passive filter tuned to the signal (and on-frequency masker) frequency. Consequently, the actual cochlear gain is probably less than that estimated from the TMCs or the horizontal distance between the BM responses to the on- and off-frequency maskers.

2.5.3 **Additivity of non-simultaneous masking**

Measures of the BM response function using the method based on growth of forward masking and the method based on TMCs rely on an assumption that the rate of decay of forward masking does not depend on the masker frequency. Although intuitively appealing, this assumption is hard to verify physiologically because the nature and the origin of forward masking have not yet been established with certainty. An alternative method, using additivity of non-simultaneous masking, eliminates the need for that assumption by using only on-frequency maskers. On the other hand, an additional assumption, that the effects of individual maskers add linearly, is required. This 'linear summation' assumption has some support from earlier (Penner and Shiffrin, 1980) and more recent (Plack *et al.*, 2006, 2007) studies using either a forward and a backward masker, or a combination of two non-overlapping forward maskers.

The basic idea behind this approach is that 'internal' effect produced by combining two equally effective maskers will be twice the effect produced by either masker alone. If the signal intensity is processed linearly by the system, then a doubling in masker effectiveness can be countered by a 3-dB increase in signal level (i.e. a doubling in signal intensity). On the other hand, if the signal is compressed with a compression ratio of 2:1 (i.e. a compression exponent of 0.5), then the signal level will need to be increased by 6 dB to counteract the doubling in masker effectiveness. Thus, the increase in signal threshold when the two maskers are combined can provide an estimate of compression.

Oxenham and Moore (1995) combined pairs of equally effective forward and backward broad-band noise maskers in three normal-hearing and three hearing-impaired listeners. For the normal-hearing listeners, masked thresholds in the presence of two equally effective maskers were typically between 10 and 20 dB higher than the thresholds in either masker alone. In contrast, for the hearing-impaired listeners, who all had hearing losses of around 60 dB at the test frequency, thresholds increased by only about 3 dB on average. The results are consistent with the idea that a loss of compression with hearing loss leads to additivity that is linear with respect to intensity. For the normal-hearing listeners, the estimated compression exponent was around 0.2 (implying a compression ratio of 5:1), which is in broad agreement with the other psychoacoustic estimates of compression.

More recently, two studies estimated compression from additivity of the effects of two equally effective forward maskers (Plack and O'Hanlon, 2003; Plack *et al.*, 2006), and came to similar conclusions with respect to the maximum amount of compression in normal-hearing listeners. Plack *et al.* (2006) used a similar experimental paradigm but instead of using two equally effective maskers, the masker that was second in the sequence (M2) was presented at different levels around its masked threshold by the preceding masker (M1). A brief 4-kHz tone was used as the signal. Detection of the signal was measured for each masker presented alone and for the two maskers combined. When the signal level fell into a range of compressive BM responses, masker M2 produced additional masking even when it was presented at a level below its masked threshold, in line with the predictions of a model based on compression followed by linear temporal summation. The overall compression exponent of 0.21 derived from the Plack *et al.* (2006) study is again in good agreement with estimates of compression from other psychophysical studies.

2.5.4 **Estimating compression at different frequencies or CFs**

The most reliable data we have on BM motion come predominantly from the basal end of the cochlea, which for technical reasons is easier to access than medial or apical regions. The sparse data available from the apical (low-frequency) end of the cochlea suggest that there may be less compression than at high frequencies, and that the compression is less frequency-specific, so that the response to tones well below the CF is still compressive (e.g. Rhode and Cooper, 1996). The notion that compression is less frequency-specific at low CFs is supported by psychophysical studies using the TMC technique, which have shown that the on- and off-frequency TMCs become more similar at low signal frequencies (Lopez-Poveda *et al.*, 2003; Plack and Drga, 2003). However, the other physiological finding, that compression is reduced overall at low CFs, has not been supported by psychophysical studies, which have so far suggested that compression exponents are similar at both low and high CFs, using both TMC (Lopez-Poveda *et al.*, 2003; Plack and Drga, 2003) and masking additivity (Plack and O'Hanlon, 2003) techniques.

It is not clear what accounts for the discrepancy between the direct physiological measurements and indirect psychophysical estimates. It may be that there are differences between species, or it may also be that some of the assumptions made in the psychophysical derivations are not valid. A final possibility suggested by Rhode and Cooper (1996) is that their measurements of compression from the apical end of the cochlea might have been affected by changes in the cochlear mechanics introduced by manipulations necessary to access and then place reflective beads at the apical end of the BM.

2.6 Models of psychophysical frequency selectivity

Cochlear filtering is probably the best understood part of the processing that occurs within the auditory system. Furthermore, as discussed above, there are many psychophysical correlates of the neuromechanical phenomena observed in the cochlea. Finally, all sounds must pass through the cochlea before being processed by higher stages of the auditory system. For all these reasons, cochlear filtering, and auditory frequency selectivity in general, lends itself to computational modelling. Such models can help us gain a better understanding of how the system functions, but they can also be of practical value in many applications, such as the front-end of an automatic speech recognition system, or as part of a system that predicts the audibility of coding artefacts in digital audio applications, such as MP3 players. This section provides a brief overview of some of the methods that have been used to provide us with a quantitative understanding of frequency selectivity, ranging from the early purely spectral linear models to more recent non-linear time-domain models.

2.6.1 Variants of power spectrum model

One of the first models used to describe frequency selectivity based on psychophysical masking data was proposed by Fletcher (1940). Fletcher measured the detection of a tone in the presence of a bandpass noise that was centred around the tone frequency, as a function of the bandwidth of the noise. The spectrum level of the noise was kept constant as the bandwidth was increased, so that the overall power of the noise doubled for every doubling in noise bandwidth. When the band was very narrow, the noise produced relatively little masking. Increasing the bandwidth led to an increase in masked threshold because the overall level of the masker increased. However, once the noise extended over a range of frequencies that exceeded a certain bandwidth, the amount of masking of the tone remained the same even as the bandwidth increased. Fletcher termed the narrowest bandwidth at which masking no longer increased the 'critical band', and concluded that the critical band defined the range of frequencies that excite the signal-frequency place on the BM, and are thus capable of masking the signal. Noise components outside of the critical band do not excite the signal-frequency place and therefore do not mask the signal. The size of the critical band was thus the first estimate of the auditory filter bandwidth. The main underlying assumptions of the model are that: (1) the filters overlap so that there is always a filter centred on the signal frequency; (2) the filters can be approximated as symmetric around the centre frequency and rectangular in shape; (3) the filters are linear; (4) the detection of the signal is based only on overall power within the filter and occurs when the signal-to-masker ratio exceeds a certain threshold value. Certainly the last three assumptions are not true, but in some situations may be a reasonable approximation. In fact, many of the models used to predict masking today are basically refinements of Fletcher's original power spectrum model.

One such refinement was proposed by Patterson (1976) in the form of the notched noise method, as described in Section 2.4.3. Patterson noted that the area around the tip of the filter was well approximated by a Gaussian curve, which he fitted to the measured masked threshold. However, the skirts of the Gaussian-shaped filter fell off more rapidly than the masked thresholds and consequently, the tails of the filter were not accurately represented by the Gaussian curve. To remedy this, Patterson et al. (1982) proposed an alternative function. They found that a better fit was obtained when each side of the derived auditory filter was represented by a sum of two rounded-exponential (roex) functions:

$$W(g) = (1-w)(1+pg)\exp(-pg) + w(1+tg)\exp(-tg) \qquad (2.3)$$

where $g = \dfrac{|f - f_c|}{f_c}$ represents the normalized frequency deviation from the centre frequency of the filter, p determines the slope around the tip of the filter (the main passband), t determines the slope of the tail of the filter, and w is the point where the tail begins to dominate over the tip. Masked thresholds measured with notched noise placed asymmetrically about the centre frequency revealed that the filter has a shallower slope on the lower frequency side, especially for higher stimulus levels. To accommodate the asymmetry of the filters, the values of parameters p and t have been allowed to differ, for the lower and the upper side of the filter (e.g. Glasberg et al., 1984).

Later studies incorporated the level-dependence in the shape of the auditory filter by assuming filters that could be considered linear at any given sound level, but the parameters of which varied as a function of the sound input level (Glasberg and Moore, 1990) or filter output level (Rosen and Baker, 1994). Rosen et al. (1998) demonstrated that a roex function with parameters depending on the signal level consistently produces a better fit to notched-noise masking data than the same function with parameters depending on the masker level. Thus, they concluded that the shape of the auditory filter is controlled by the output rather than the input level. Consequently, they argued that to derive a filter shape at a given level from masking by a notched noise, masked thresholds should be measured with the signal level fixed and the masker level varied to find threshold. An example of filters derived with the fixed-level signal is shown in Fig. 2.10. The filter's bandwidth increases with increasing level due to a decreased gain of the tip filter relative to that of the tail filter.

Another step taken by Rosen et al. (1998) was to link the shape of the psychophysically derived filters to the underlying cochlear mechanisms of compression and gain, by explicitly changing the gain of the filter tip (the on-frequency response), while assuming a linear response in the filter tail (the off-frequency response). A similar approach was adopted by Glasberg and Moore (2000), who described the lower side of the filter by a sum of a tip filter with a level-dependent gain representing the operation of the cochlear amplifier at the signal-frequency place and a tail filter representing passive processing (related to hydromechanical properties) in the cochlea. The upper side was described by a single roex function

$$W(g) = (1 + p_u g)\exp(-p_u g) \qquad (2.4)$$

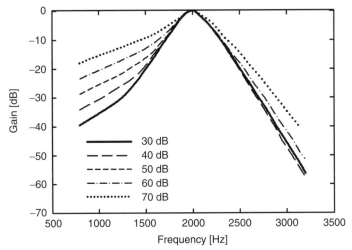

Fig. 2.10 Auditory filter shapes derived using the notched-noise technique, for signal levels between 30 and 70 dB SPL. Data replotted from Rosen *et al.* (1998).

where g is the normalized frequency deviation from the centre of the filter, and p_u describes the slope of the upper skirt of the filter. The lower side of the filter was described by:

$$W(g) = [G(1 + p_l g) \exp(-p_l g) + (1 + tg) \exp(-tg)]/(G + 1) \qquad (2.5)$$

where G represents gain as a function of level and thus, the gain of the tip relative to the gain of the tail filter. The gain function of level is chosen to provide best fit to the data. All the free parameters of the roex functions were optimized assuming a constant signal-to-noise power ratio at the output of the filter.

Despite the more recent refinements to the power spectrum model, it remains a frequency-domain representation that does not take into account non-linear interactions, such as suppression, or temporal factors, such as envelope fluctuations, which can also play an important role in auditory perception. For this reason, power spectrum models do not lend themselves to applications that require time as well as frequency analysis, such as automatic speech recognition. The following section reviews some recent attempts to provide time-domain models of frequency selectivity that maintain the attractive properties of the frequency-domain filters, while also allowing more realistic non-linear behaviour, as well as temporal analysis of the signals.

2.6.2 **Time-domain filters**

Attempts to characterize the time-domain response of the auditory filters were made by de Boer and colleagues (de Boer and Kuyper, 1968; de Boer and de Jongh, 1978), using the so-called 'reverse correlation' (or revcor) method to derive the impulse responses of auditory nerve fibres from their response to white noise (for a review, see Eggermont *et al.*, 1983). It was found that the responses could be quite well approximated by a mathematical function that has come to be known as the 'gammatone function' (Aertsen and Johannesma, 1980; de Boer and Kruidenier, 1990). Patterson *et al.* (1995) published an application of the gammatone filter bank in conjunction with other 'modules' of auditory processing to form a general platform for quantitative modelling of auditory perceptual phenomena. The impulse response of the gammatone filter is defined as:

$$g(t) = at^{n-1} \exp(-2\pi b ERB(f_c)t) \cos(2\pi f_c t + \Phi) \qquad (2.6)$$

where f_c is the centre frequency of the filter, ERB (f_c) is the equivalent rectangular bandwidth of the filter, and a, b, n, and Φ are parameters. The gammatone filters have been widely used in psychophysical, as well as physiological, models of auditory processing (Meddis *et al.*, 2001; Zhang *et al.*, 2001; Chi *et al.*, 2005). The gammatone filter in its original form is linear and so suffers from the same shortcomings as spectral-domain representations that are linear and level-invariant. A more recent variation, which incorporates level dependencies, was introduced by Irino and Patterson (1997), who modified the time-domain characteristic of a gammatone filter by introducing an additional parameter that produces a frequency glide in the impulse response. The impulse response of the new filter is represented by:

$$g(t) = at^{n-1} \exp(-2\pi b ERB(f_r)t)\cos(2\pi f_r t + c \ln t + \Phi) \qquad (2.7)$$

where c is the additional level-dependent parameter, f_r is the centre frequency of the filter that varies predominantly with the value of c (parameters b and n can also produce a slight shift in the centre frequency), and the remaining parameters are the same as in eqn 2.6. The term $c \ln t$ introduces a frequency glide in the impulse response—hence the name 'gammachirp'. The gammachirp filter possesses many properties of a realistic auditory filter. Its spectral shape is asymmetric with the lower side becoming shallower as the input level increases. The ERB of the gammachirp filter increases with increasing level. The tip of the filter changes its position, which allows for including the well-established peak shift in the BM response with increasing level (e.g. Ruggero *et al.*, 1997). The frequency glide in the impulse response is also supported by some physiological evidence (Carney *et al.*, 1999; Shera, 2001*a*), as well as being consistent in principle with psychophysical studies of auditory phase responses (Oxenham and Dau, 2001). Irino and Patterson (1997) showed that the gammachirp filter and a six-parameter roex filter provide equally good fits to the notched-noise masking data, with the former having an advantage by offering a well-defined impulse response with a realistic frequency glide. For a more recent exposition of the gammachirp filter, see Unoki *et al.* (2006).

2.7 Across channel processing and comodulation masking release

2.7.1 Listening across channels

Much of the work discussed in this chapter relates masking and frequency selectivity by assuming that the signal is detected by means of an increase in the output of one auditory filter. It is as if the auditory system can focus in on one auditory filter (one place on the BM, or one subset of auditory nerve fibres) to the exclusion of everything else. This is clearly not how perception works in any general sense. Most sounds in the environment have their energy spread over a wide range of frequencies in a dynamically varying way, and our ability to identify and distinguish them relies on broadband and temporally sensitive analysis. As a simple example, consider the sound of a train 100 m away. It may have the same energy in the auditory filter centred at 1000 Hz as a flute being played 1 m away, but most people will have no trouble distinguishing the two sounds. Similarly, a train only 10 m away will still be recognized as a train even though the overall level is now higher than before. Clearly some form of across-channel 'profile analysis' is needed to distinguish between sounds with different frequency spectra (Green, 1988) see Chapter 3.

One aspect of many environmental sounds, including speech, is that there are significant correlations in the patterns of amplitude variations in different frequency channels. It has been hypothesized that the auditory system makes use of these when segregating sounds from different sources (Nelken *et al.*, 1999). A laboratory demonstration of this effect has been termed 'comodulation masking release' or CMR (Hall *et al.* 1984). The initial demonstration of CMR involved detecting a tone in a band of noise that was centred on the frequency of the tone. Thresholds for the tone were measured for a number of different masker bandwidths, with the masker spectrum level (level per unit Hz) remaining constant, meaning that the masker intensity doubled for every doubling in masker bandwidth. As was found with earlier band-widening experiments (Fletcher, 1940; Bos and de Boer, 1966), thresholds initially increased with increasing masker bandwidth and then remained constant at bandwidths where the additional masker energy is no longer thought to fall within the bandwidth of the auditory filter centred at the signal frequency. The novel condition involved multiplying the unfiltered noise masker by a low-frequency noise (lowpass-filtered at 50 Hz) to produce a noise waveform that had coherent amplitude fluctuations across frequency. As with the original noise, thresholds initially increased with increasing comodulated masker bandwidth; however, thresholds then started to decrease as the masker bandwidth was increased beyond the assumed bandwidth of the auditory filter. The standard explanation is that the auditory system is able to compare the time-varying outputs of the auditory filters, and to detect the presence of the signal better, either by comparing patterns of temporal modulations across channels (Richards, 1987) or by using the channels in which the masker is dominant to determine when the short-term masker level is low to improve the detectability of the signal (Buus, 1985). In other words, as one might expect, the auditory system is able to perform a form of spectrotemporal analysis, and not just independent analyses in individual spectral channels, to detect and identify acoustic events.

2.7.2 Within- and across-channel mechanisms in CMR

Soon after the initial report of CMR (Hall *et al.*, 1984), researchers began to question whether it was a 'true' across-channel effect, or an effect that could be explained simply by changes in the waveform at the output of a single auditory filter. Various ways to distinguish between these two possibilities have been attempted. For instance, instead of using a single masker band that varied in bandwidth, researchers have used multiple narrow bands of noise, the one centred on the signal frequency being the masker and others being termed the 'flankers'. In this way, the frequency spacing between the masker and the flankers can be varied, which in turn influences the extent to which potential within-channel cues are available. For instance, Schooneveldt and Moore (1987, 1989) found a release from masking with comodulated flanking bands, even when all the bands fell within the bandwidth of a single auditory filter, meaning that the benefit was unlikely to be due to a comparison of outputs from different frequency bands. On the other hand, some CMR is found even when the spacing between the masker and flankers is so large as to make peripheral interaction between them very unlikely. Another way to vary the amount of information available within single peripheral channels is to present the masker and flankers to opposite ears (Schooneveldt and Moore, 1987). In all these cases, some CMR remains when peripheral interactions between the masker and flankers are minimized; however, the overall release tends to be less than 10 dB.

To quantify the amount of within-channel information available in the original CMR paradigm, Verhey *et al.* (1999) used a single-channel model of auditory processing, including peripheral stages (filtering, compression, and neural adaptation) along with a modulation filterbank (see Verhey, Chapter 5, this volume) to simulate the results of an experiment similar to that of Hall *et al.* (1984). They were able to produce fairly accurate simulations using the output of just a single auditory filter, suggesting that across-channel processing is not necessary to account for the original CMR results. This does not, of course, imply that across-channel processing cannot be involved in these experiments. Similarly, the fact that CMR is reduced when the flanking bands are very remote from the masker band (or in the opposite ear) does not necessarily imply within-channel processing is involved when the bands are spaced more closely together. It could simply be that across-channel comparison mechanisms work most efficiently for bands that are close in frequency (and in the same ear). In fact, it becomes rather difficult to separate within- and across-channel contributions in a satisfactory way.

2.7.3 Perceptual organization and CMR

Recent attempts to explain CMR in terms of the underlying physiology have concentrated on brainstem mechanisms of lateral inhibition (e.g. Pressnitzer *et al.*, 2001; Verhey *et al.*, 2003; Neuert *et al.*, 2004), suggesting a fairly low-level 'automatic' processing of CMR-like effects. On the other hand, a number of psychoacoustic studies have shown that CMR seems to be susceptible to certain constraints of auditory perceptual organization. For instance, Grose and Hall (1993) found that CMR was almost entirely eliminated when the masker band and the flanking bands were gated on at different times. Asynchronous gating typically leads to a perceptual segregation of the sounds in question (Bregman, 1990), suggesting that CMR may only occur if the masking band and flankers are perceived as belonging to a single perceptual object. The masking band has also been perceptually segregated from the flanking bands by inducing auditory streams comprising only the flanking bands. Repeating sequences of flanking bands that either precede (Grose and Hall, 1993) or follow (Dau *et al.*, 2009) the masker–flanker combination lead to the percept of a stream of flanking bands and an isolated masker band. In these cases, CMR can also be either reduced (Grose and Hall, 1993) or completely eliminated (Dau *et al.*, 2009). The fact that stimulus manipulations that affect perceptual grouping can influence CMR suggests a high-level (cortical?) locus for the effect.

2.8 Informational masking

In the previous section we reviewed evidence that masker energy remote from the signal can under certain circumstances *enhance* signal detection. In contrast, the wide range of phenomena that share the name 'informational masking' have one property in common: masker energy remote from the signal in time and/or frequency can significantly *impair* signal detection or discrimination. Informational masking as a term came into use in the 1970s in a series of studies by Watson and colleagues (e.g. Watson and Kelly, 1978). The basic finding is that subjects' ability to discriminate small changes in the frequency of a given tone, or to even detect a tone, is severely impaired if the tone is embedded in a sequence of unpredictable, random-frequency 'masker' tones. Similarly, Neff and Green (1987) found that the ability to detect a signal tone was diminished when the signal was presented simultaneously with other tones that varied in frequency randomly from presentation to presentation, to the extent that detection threshold could be elevated by as much as 30–40 dB. Because none of the masking tones were close to the target in frequency, and so fell outside the passband of the auditory filter centred at the signal frequency, such masking cannot be explained simply in terms of peripheral excitation or suppression.

Initial explanations of the effect focused on the unpredictability or uncertainty surrounding the masker tones (e.g. Lutfi, 1993). Since then, attention has also been paid to the similarity between the masker and signal, and the difficulty associated with perceptually segregating the masker from the signal (Durlach *et al.*, 2003*a*, *b*; Kidd *et al.*, 2003). Selective attention and analytic listening abilities also appear to play a role, in the sense that good performance in an informational masking task depends on being able to selectively attend to the temporal position and/or spectral or spatial position of the signal. For instance, musicians have been found to be generally much less susceptible to informational masking than people with no musical training (Oxenham *et al.*, 2003).

Finally, informational masking can be greatly reduced by making the signal 'stand out' in some way from the masker by, for instance, gating it on after and off before the onset and offset of the maskers, respectively (Neff, 1995) (for a recent review of informational masking with non-speech sounds, see Watson, 2005).

The concepts of informational masking do not only apply to pure-tone signals. In fact, some of the earliest examples of what would now be termed informational masking related to speech perception (e.g. Carhart *et al.*, 1969). The extent to which speech understanding in the background of interfering speech, or other fluctuating complex maskers, can be attributed to factors other than 'energetic masking' (i.e. audibility as predicted, for instance, from excitation patterns), has become a major topic of research in normal hearing (Freyman *et al.*, 1999; Brungart, 2001), impaired hearing (Jin and Nelson, 2006), and hearing with a cochlear implant (Stickney *et al.*, 2004). Used in the context of speech, the term informational masking generally refers to the potential confusion of the target speech with aspects of the masking sounds. As with tonal informational masking, manipulations that make the target and the masker less perceptually similar, along dimensions such as voice pitch, vocal tract length, and perceived spatial location, typically lead to large reductions in masking (Freyman *et al.*, 1999; Darwin *et al.*, 2003).

Informational masking as a concept has become something of dustbin for any form of masking or interference that cannot be explained by interactions within the cochlea ('energetic masking'). It is clear to most researchers, however, that a number of different mechanisms must be involved. Despite this realization (or perhaps because of it) there have been few attempts to determine the underlying neural bases of informational masking. Because of the presumably important role of attention in many of the paradigms, informational masking does not lend itself to traditional auditory physiological studies involving anesthetized animals. Even with awake animals, it would not be trivial to train them to detect signals in an informational masking paradigm. To our knowledge, only one imaging study has attempted to find neural correlates of informational masking in the human auditory pathways. Using MEG, Gutschalk *et al.* (2008) found that the steady-state response (SSR) to tones was the same whether or not listeners detected them in an informational masking paradigm. Because the SSR is thought to be an early (primary) cortical response, the fact that no correlate of informational masking was found here suggests that informational masking is not a product of brainstem processing. In contrast, a strong correlate of informational masking was found in an evoked cortical response with a latency of about 150 ms, which was localized to auditory cortex: here, strong responses were found to detected tones, whereas no measurable response was found to tones that were undetected. Based on these data, it seems that correlates of informational masking can be found in auditory cortex but not earlier. However, the neural mechanisms responsible for informational masking remain a matter of speculation.

2.9 Summary

Frequency selectivity—our ability to 'hear out' sounds of different frequencies within a complex mixture—involves perhaps the most important organizational principle within the auditory system. Frequency selectivity is established within the cochlea, via the frequency-to-place mapping that occurs along the basilar membrane, and is maintained throughout the auditory pathways to the auditory cortex. Studies in animals and humans have typically found that the frequency selectivity established in the cochlea is accurately reflected by behavioural measures. This somewhat remarkable fact suggests that the cochlea defines and limits our ability to separate components of different frequencies, and that no dramatic sharpening or broadening of frequency tuning occurs between the auditory periphery and the central auditory system.

Masking is an everyday phenomenon in our acoustic environment, where loud sounds regularly obscure quieter ones. Over a century of research on masking has established that masking depends not only on relative (and absolute) intensity, but also on the frequency content of the masker and the signal. In fact, masking has been the primary tool with which the limits of frequency selectivity have been probed behaviourally. Methods for estimating frequency selectivity have been refined over the years, and our understanding of the mechanisms of masking, and the limitations of the various masking techniques, has progressed. Nevertheless, the answers to some of the most fundamental questions—the relationship between cochlear tuning in humans and in other species, the neural bases of non-simultaneous masking, and the influence of 'top-down' efferent control on cochlear responses and perceptual frequency selectivity—remain controversial or unknown.

References

Aertsen, A. M. and Johannesma, P. M. (1980). Spectro-temporal receptive fields of auditory neurons in the grassfrog. I. Characterization of tonal and natural stimuli. *Biological Cybernetics* 382:23–34.

Bacon, S. P. (1990). Effect of masker level on overshoot. *Journal of the Acoustical Society of America* 88:698–702.

Bacon, S. P. and Lee, J. (1997). The modulated–unmodulated difference: Effects of signal frequency and masker modulation depth. *Journal of the Acoustical Society of America* 101:3617–24.

Bacon, S. P. and Takahashi, G. A. (1992). Overshoot in normal-hearing and hearing-impaired subjects. *Journal of the Acoustical Society of America* 91:2865–71.

Bacon, S. P., Lee, J., Peterson, D. N., and Rainey, D. (1997). Masking by modulated and unmodulated noise: Effects of bandwidth, modulation rate, signal frequency, and masker level. *Journal of the Acoustical Society of America* 101:1600–10.

Bernstein, J. G. and Oxenham, A. J. (2003). Pitch discrimination of diotic and dichotic tone complexes: Harmonic resolvability or harmonic number? *Journal of the Acoustical Society of America* 113:3323–34.

Bos, C. E. and de Boer, E. (1966). Masking and discrimination. *Journal of the Acoustical Society of America* 39:708–15.

Bregman, A. S. (1990). *Auditory Scene Analysis: The Perceptual Organisation of Sound.* Cambridge, MA: MIT Press.

Brungart, D. S. (2001). Informational and energetic masking effects in the perception of two simultaneous talkers. *Journal of the Acoustical Society of America* 109:1101–09.

Buus, S. (1985). Release from masking caused by envelope fluctuations. *Journal of the Acoustical Society of America* 78:1958–65.

Cai, Y. and Geisler, D. (1996). Suppression in auditory-nerve fibers of cats using low-side suppressors. III. Model results. *Hearing Research* 96:126–40.

Carhart, R., Tillman, T., and Greetis, R. (1969). Perceptual masking in multiple sound backgrounds. *Journal of the Acoustical Society of America* 45:694–703.

Carlyon, R. P. (1988). The development and decline of forward masking. *Hearing Research* 32:65–80.

Carney, L. H., McDuffy, M. J., and Shekhter, I. (1999). Frequency glides in the impulse responses of auditory-nerve fibers. *Journal of the Acoustical Society of America* 105:2384–91.

Chi, T., Ru, P., and Shamma, S. A. (2005). Multiresolution spectrotemporal analysis of complex sounds. *Journal of the Acoustical Society of America* 118:887–906.

Dallos, P., Zheng, J., and Cheatham, M. A. (2006). Prestin and the cochlear amplifier. *Journal of Physiology* 576:37–42.

Darwin, C. J., Brungart, D. S., and Simpson, B. D. (2003). Effects of fundamental frequency and vocal-tract length changes on attention to one of two simultaneous talkers. *Journal of the Acoustical Society of America* 114:2913–22.

Dau, T., Püschel, D., and Kohlrausch, A. (1996a). A quantitative model of the 'effective' signal processing in the auditory system. I. Model structure. *Journal of the Acoustical Society of America* **99**:3615–22.

Dau, T., Püschel, D., and Kohlrausch, A. (1996b). A quantitative model of the 'effective' signal processing in the auditory system. II. Simulations and measurements. *Journal of the Acoustical Society of America* **99**:3623–31.

Dau, T., Ewert, S., and Oxenham, A. J. (2009). Auditory stream formation affects comodulation masking release retroactively. *Journal of the Acoustical Society of America* **125**: 2182–8.

de Boer, E. and de Jongh, H. R. (1978). On cochlear encoding: potentialities and limitations of the reverse-correlation technique. *Journal of the Acoustical Society of America* **63**: 115–35.

de Boer, E. and Kruidenier, C. (1990). On ringing limits of the auditory periphery. *Biological Cybernetics* **63**:433–42.

de Boer, R. and Kuyper, P. (1968). Triggered correlation. *IEEE Transactions on Bio-medical Engineering* **15**:169–79.

Delgutte, B. (1990). Physiological mechanisms of psychophysical masking: Observations from auditory-nerve fibers. *Journal of the Acoustical Society of America* **87**:791–809.

Duifhuis, H. (1973). Consequences of peripheral frequency selectivity for nonsimultaneous masking. *Journal of the Acoustical Society of America* **54**:1471–88.

Durlach, N. I., Mason, C. R., Shinn-Cunningham, B. G., Arbogast, T. L., Colburn, H. S., and Kidd, G., Jr. (2003a). Informational masking: counteracting the effects of stimulus uncertainty by decreasing target-masker similarity. *Journal of the Acoustical Society of America* **114**:368–79.

Durlach, N. I., Mason, C. R., Kidd, G., Jr, Arbogast, T. L., Colburn, H. S., and Shinn-Cunningham, B. G. (2003b). Note on informational masking. *Journal of the Acoustical Society of America* **113**:2984–7.

Egan, J. P. and Hake, H. W. (1950). On the masking pattern of a simple auditory stimulus. *Journal of the Acoustical Society of America* **22**:622–30.

Eggermont, J. J., Johannesma, P. M., and Aertsen, A. M. (1983). Reverse-correlation methods in auditory research. *Quarterly Review of Biophysics* **16**:341–414.

Evans, E. F. (2001). Latest comparisons between physiological and behavioural frequency selectivity. In *Physiological and Psychophysical Bases of Auditory Function* (ed. J. Breebaart, A. J. M. Houtsma, A. Kohlrausch, V. F. Prijs, and R. Schoonhoven), pp. 382–87. Maastricht: Shaker.

Evans, E. F., Pratt, S. R., Spenner, H., and Cooper, N. P. (1992). Comparisons of physiological and behavioural properties: Auditory frequency selectivity. In *Auditory Physiology and Perception* (ed. Y. Cazals, K. Horner, and L. Demany), pp. 159–69. Oxford: Pergamon.

Fine, P. A. and Moore, B. C. J. (1993). Frequency analysis and musical ability. *Music Perception* **11**:39–53.

Fletcher, H. (1940). Auditory patterns. *Reviews of Modern Physics* **12**:47–65.

Freyman, R. L., Helfer, K. S., McCall, D. D., and Clifton, R. K. (1999). The role of perceived spatial separation in the unmasking of speech. *Journal of the Acoustical Society of America* **106**:3578–88.

Geisler, C. D. and Nuttall, A. L. (1997). Two-tone suppression of basilar membrane vibrations in the base of the guinea pig cochlea using 'low-side' suppressors. *Journal of the Acoustical Society of America* **102**:430–40.

Glasberg, B. R. and Moore, B. C. J. (1982). Auditory filter shapes in forward masking as a function of level. *Journal of the Acoustical Society of America* **71**:946–9.

Glasberg, B. R. and Moore, B. C. J. (1990). Derivation of auditory filter shapes from notched-noise data. *Hearing Research* **47**:103–8.

Glasberg, B. R. and Moore, B. C. J. (2000). Frequency selectivity as a function of level and frequency measured with uniformly exciting notched noise. *Journal of the Acoustical Society of America* **108**:2318–28.

Glasberg, B. R., Moore, B. C. J., Patterson, R. D., and Nimmo-Smith, I. (1984). Dynamic range and asymmetry of the auditory filter. *Journal of the Acoustical Society of America* **76**:419–27.

Gorga, M. P., Stelmachowicz, P. G., Abbas, P. J., and Small, A. M. J. (1980). Some observations on simultaneous and nonsimultaneous masking. *Journal of the Acoustical Society of America* **67**:1821–2.

Green, D. M. (1988) *Profile Analysis*. Oxford: Oxford University Press.

Green, D. M. and Swets, J. A. (1966) *Signal Detection Theory and Psychophysics*. New York: Krieger.

Grose, J. H. and Hall, J. W. (1993). Comodulation masking release: Is comodulation sufficient? *Journal of the Acoustical Society of America* **93**:2896–902.

Gutschalk, A., Micheyl, C., and Oxenham, A. J. (2008). Neural correlates of auditory perceptual awareness under informational masking. *PLoS Biology* **10**:1156–65.

Hall, J. W., Haggard, M. P., and Fernandes, M. A. (1984). Detection in noise by spectro-temporal pattern analysis. *Journal of the Acoustical Society of America* **76**:50–6.

Hartmann, W. M. and Goupell, M. J. (2006). Enhancing and unmasking the harmonics of a complex tone. *Journal of the Acoustical Society of America* **120**:2142–57.

Hellman, R. P. (1972). Asymmetry of masking between noise and tone. *Perception and Psychophysics* **11**:241–6.

Helmholtz, H. L. F. v. (1863). *Die Lehre von den Tonempfindungen als physiologische Grundlage für die Theorie der Musik* (1st edn). Braunschweig: F.Vieweg.

Houtgast, T. (1972). Psychophysical evidence for lateral inhibition in hearing. *Journal of the Acoustical Society of America* **51**:1885–94.

Houtgast, T. (1974). Lateral suppression and loudness reduction of a tone in noise. *Acustica* **30**:214–21.

Houtsma, A. J. M. and Smurzynski, J. (1990). Pitch identification and discrimination for complex tones with many harmonics. *Journal of the Acoustical Society of America* **87**:304–10.

Irino, T. and Patterson, R. D. (1997). A time-domain, level-dependent auditory filter: The gammachirp. *Journal of the Acoustical Society of America* **101**:412–19.

Jin, S. H. and Nelson, P. B. (2006). Speech perception in gated noise: The effects of temporal resolution. *Journal of the Acoustical Society of America* **119**:3097–108.

Johnson-Davies, D. and Patterson, R. D. (1979). Psychophysical tuning curves: Restricting the listening band to the signal region. *Journal of the Acoustical Society of America* **65**:765–70.

Kiang, NY-S., Watanabe, T., Thomas, E. C., and Clark, L. F. (1965). *Discharge Patterns of Single Fibres in the Cat's Auditory Nerve*. Cambridge, Mass.: MIT Press.

Kidd, G., Jr, Mason, C. R., and Richards, V. M. (2003). Multiple bursts, multiple looks, and stream coherence in the release from informational masking. *Journal of the Acoustical Society of America* **114**:2835–45.

Kohlrausch, A. and Sander, A. (1995). Phase effects in masking related to dispersion in the inner ear. II. Masking period patterns of short targets. *Journal of the Acoustical Society of America* **97**:1817–29.

Kohlrausch, A., Fassel, R., van der Heijden, M., et al. (1997). Detection of tones in low-noise noise: Further evidence for the role of envelope fluctuations. *Acta Acustica* **83**:659–69.

Kuhn, A. and Saunders, J. C. (1980). Psychophysical tuning curves in the parakeet: A comparison between simultaneous and forward masking procedures. *Journal of the Acoustical Society of America* **68**:1892–4.

Levitt, H. (1971). Transformed up-down methods in psychoacoustics. *Journal of the Acoustical Society of America* **49**:467–77.

Lopez-Poveda, E. A., Plack, C. J., and Meddis, R. (2003). Cochlear nonlinearity between 500 and 8000Hz in listeners with normal hearing. *Journal of the Acoustical Society of America* **113**:951–60.

Lutfi, R. A. (1993). A model of auditory pattern analysis based on component-relative-entropy. *Journal of the Acoustical Society of America* **94**:748–58.

McFadden, D. and Champlin, C. A. (1990). Reductions in overshoot during aspirin use. *Journal of the Acoustical Society of America* **87**:2634–42.

McGee, T., Ryan, A., and Dallos, P. (1976). Psychophysical tuning curves of chinchillas. *Journal of the Acoustical Society of America* **60**:1146–50.

Macmillan, N. A. and Creelman, C. D. (2004). *Detection Theory: A User's Guide* (2nd edn). Mahwah, NJ: Lawrence Erlbaum Associates.

Martin, P., Mehta, A. D., and Hudspeth, A. J. (2000). Negative hair-bundle stiffness betrays a mechanism for mechanical amplification by the hair cell. *Proceedings of the National Academy of Sciences USA* **97**:12026–31.

Meddis, R., O'Mard, L. P., and Lopez-Poveda, E. A. (2001). A computational algorithm for computing nonlinear auditory frequency selectivity. *Journal of the Acoustical Society of America* **109**:2852–61.

Micheyl, C., Bernstein, J. G., and Oxenham, A. J. (2006). Detection and F0 discrimination of harmonic complex tones in the presence of competing tones or noise. *Journal of the Acoustical Society of America* **120**:1493–505.

Moore, B. C. J. (1978). Psychophysical tuning curves measured in simultaneous and forward masking. *Journal of the Acoustical Society of America* **63**:524–32.

Moore, B. C. J. (1995). Frequency analysis and masking. In *Handbook of Perception and Cognition*, Vol. 6: Hearing (ed. B. C. J. Moore), pp. 161–205. Orlando, Fl: Academic Press.

Moore, B. C. J. and Glasberg, B. R. (1981). Auditory filter shapes derived in simultaneous and forward masking. *Journal of the Acoustical Society of America* **70**:1003–14.

Moore, B. C. J. and Glasberg, B. R. (1985). The danger of using narrowband noise maskers to measure suppression. *Journal of the Acoustical Society of America* **77**:2137–41.

Moore, B. C. J. and Ohgushi, K. (1993). Audibility of partials in inharmonic complex tones. *Journal of the Acoustical Society of America* **93**:452–61.

Moore, B. C. J. and Vickers, D. A. (1997). The role of spread of excitation and suppression in simultaneous masking. *Journal of the Acoustical Society of America* **102**:2284–90.

Moore, B. C. J., Glasberg, B. R., Plack, C. J., and Biswas, A. K. (1988). The shape of the ear's temporal window. *Journal of the Acoustical Society of America* **83**:1102–16.

Moore, B. C. J., Glasberg, B. R., and Baer, T. (1997). A model for the prediction of thresholds, loudness, and partial loudness. *Journal of the Audio Engineering Society* **45**:224–40.

Moore, B. C. J., Glasberg, B. R., and Vickers, D. A. (1999). Further evaluation of a model of loudness perception applied to cochlear hearing loss. *Journal of the Acoustical Society of America* **106**:898–907.

Moore, B. C. J., Glasberg, B. R., Low, K. E., Cope, T., and Cope, W. (2006). Effects of level and frequency on the audibility of partials in inharmonic complex tones. *Journal of the Acoustical Society of America* **120**:934–44.

Neff, D. L. (1985). Stimulus parameters governing confusion effects in forward masking. *Journal of the Acoustical Society of America* **78**:1966–76.

Neff, D. L. (1995). Signal properties that reduce masking by simultaneous, random-frequency maskers. *Journal of the Acoustical Society of America* **98**:1909–20.

Neff, D. L. and Green, D. M. (1987). Masking produced by spectral uncertainty with multi-component maskers. *Perception and Psychophysics* **41**:409–15.

Nelken, I., Rotman, Y., and Bar Yosef, O. (1999). Responses of auditory-cortex neurons to structural features of natural sounds. *Nature* **397**:154–7.

Nelson, D. A. and Freyman, R. L. (1984). Broadened forward-masked tuning curves from intense masking tones: delay-time and probe level manipulations. *Journal of the Acoustical Society of America* **75**:1570–7.

Nelson, D. A. and Pavlov, R. (1989). Auditory time constants for off-frequency forward masking in normal-hearing and hearing-impaired listeners. *Journal of Speech and Hearing Research* **32**:298–306.

Nelson, D. A. and Swain, A. C. (1996). Temporal resolution within the upper accessory excitation. *Acustica/Acta Acustica* **82**:328–34.

Nelson, D. A., Schroder, A. C., and Wojtczak, M. (2001). A new procedure for measuring peripheral compression in normal-hearing and hearing-impaired listeners. *Journal of the Acoustical Society of America* **110**:2045–64.

Neuert, V., Verhey, J. L., and Winter, I. M. (2004). Responses of dorsal cochlear nucleus neurons to signals in the presence of modulated maskers. *Journal of Neuroscience* 24:5789–97.

Ohm, G. S. (1843). Über die Definition des Tones, nebst daran geknüpfter Theorie der Sirene und ähnlicher tonbildender Vorrichtungen. *Annalen der Physik und Chemie* 59:513–65.

O'Loughlin, B. J. and Moore, B. C. J. (1981a). Off-frequency listening: Effects on psychoacoustical tuning curves obtained in simultaneous and forward masking. *Journal of the Acoustical Society of America* 69:1119–25.

O'Loughlin, B. J. and Moore, B. C. J. (1981b). Improving psychoacoustical tuning curves. *Hearing Research* 5:343–6.

Oxenham, A. J. (2001). Forward masking: Adaptation or integration? *Journal of the Acoustical Society of America* 109:732–41.

Oxenham, A. J. and Bacon, S. P. (2003). Cochlear compression: Perceptual measures and implications for normal and impaired hearing. *Ear and Hearing* 24:352–66.

Oxenham, A. J. and Dau, T. (2001). Towards a measure of auditory-filter phase response. *Journal of the Acoustical Society of America* 110:3169–78.

Oxenham, A. J. and Moore, B. C. J. (1994). Modeling the additivity of nonsimultaneous masking. *Hearing Research* 80:105–18.

Oxenham, A. J. and Moore, B. C. J. (1995). Additivity of masking in normally hearing and hearing-impaired subjects. *Journal of the Acoustical Society of America* 98:1921–34.

Oxenham, A. J. and Plack, C. J. (1997). A behavioral measure of basilar-membrane nonlinearity in listeners with normal and impaired hearing. *Journal of the Acoustical Society of America* 101:3666–75.

Oxenham, A. J. and Plack, C. J. (1998). Suppression and the upward spread of masking. *Journal of the Acoustical Society of America* 104:3500–10.

Oxenham, A. J. and Shera, C. A. (2003). Estimates of human cochlear tuning at low levels using forward and simultaneous masking. *Journal of the Association for Research in Otolaryngology* 4:541–54.

Oxenham, A. J. and Simonson, A. M. (2006). Level dependence of auditory filters in nonsimultaneous masking as a function of frequency. *Journal of the Acoustical Society of America* 119:444–53.

Oxenham, A. J., Fligor, B. J., Mason, C. R., and Kidd, G., Jr. (2003). Informational masking and musical training. *Journal of the Acoustical Society of America* 114:1543–9.

Patterson, R. D. (1974). Auditory filter shape. *Journal of the Acoustical Society of America* 55:802–9.

Patterson, R. D. (1976). Auditory filter shapes derived with noise stimuli. *Journal of the Acoustical Society of America* 59:640–54.

Patterson, R. D. and Moore, B. C. J. (1986). Auditory filters and excitation patterns as representations of frequency resolution. In *Frequency Selectivity in Hearing* (ed. B. C. J. Moore), pp. 123–77. London: Academic.

Patterson, R. D., Nimmo-Smith, I., Weber, D. L., and Milroy, R. (1982). The deterioration of hearing with age: Frequency selectivity, the critical ratio, the audiogram, and speech threshold. *Journal of the Acoustical Society of America* 72:1788–803.

Patterson, R. D., Allerhand, M. H., and Giguere, C. (1995). Time-domain modelling of peripheral auditory processing: A modular architecture and a software platform. *Journal of the Acoustical Society of America* 98:1890–4.

Penner, M. J. and Shiffrin, R. M. (1980). Nonlinearities in the coding of intensity within the context of a temporal summation model. *Journal of the Acoustical Society of America* 67:617–27.

Plack, C. J. and Drga, V. (2003). Psychophysical evidence for auditory compression at low characteristic frequencies. *Journal of the Acoustical Society of America* 113:1574–86.

Plack, C. J. and O'Hanlon, C. G. (2003). Forward masking additivity and auditory compression at low and high frequencies. *Journal of the Association for Research in Otolaryngology* 4:405–15.

Plack, C. J. and Moore, B. C. J. (1990). Temporal window shape as a function of frequency and level. *Journal of the Acoustical Society of America* 87:2178–87.

Plack, C. J. and Oxenham, A. J. (1998). Basilar-membrane nonlinearity and the growth of forward masking. *Journal of the Acoustical Society of America* **103**:1598–608.

Plack, C. J., Drga, V., and Lopez-Poveda, E. A. (2004). Inferred basilar-membrane response functions for listeners with mild to moderate sensorineural hearing loss. *Journal of the Acoustical Society of America* **115**:1684–95.

Plack, C. J., Oxenham, A. J., and Drga, V. (2006). Masking by inaudible sounds and the linearity of temporal summation. *Journal of Neuroscience* **26**:8767–73.

Plack, C. J., Carcagno, S., and Oxenham, A. J. (2007). A further test of the linearity of temporal summation in forward masking. *Journal of the Acoustical Society of America* **122**:1880–3.

Plomp, R. (1964a). The ear as a frequency analyzer. *Journal of the Acoustical Society of America* **36**:1628–36.

Plomp, R. (1964b). The rate of decay of auditory sensation. *Journal of the Acoustical Society of America* **36**:277–82.

Plomp, R. and Mimpen, A. M. (1968). The ear as a frequency analyzer II. *Journal of the Acoustical Society of America* **43**:764–7.

Pressnitzer, D., Meddis, R., Delahaye, R., and Winter, I. M. (2001). Physiological correlates of comodulation masking release in the mammalian ventral cochlear nucleus. *Journal of Neuroscience* **21**:6377–86.

Recanzone, G. H. (2000). Response profiles of auditory cortical neurons to tones and noise in behaving macaque monkeys. *Hearing Research* **150**:104–18.

Relkin, E. M. and Turner, C. W. (1988). A reexamination of forward masking in the auditory nerve. *Journal of the Acoustical Society of America* **84**:584–91.

Rhode, W. S. (1971). Observations of the vibration of the basilar membrane in squirrel monkeys using the Mössbauer technique. *Journal of the Acoustical Society of America* **49**:1218–31.

Rhode, W. S. (2007). Basilar membrane mechanics in the 6–9kHz region of sensitive chinchilla cochleae. *Journal of the Acoustical Society of America* **121**:2792–804.

Rhode, W. S. and Cooper, N. P. (1996). Nonlinear mechanics in the apical turn of the chinchilla cochlea in vivo. *Auditory Neuroscience* **3**:101–21.

Richards, V. M. (1987). Monaural envelope correlation perception. *Journal of the Acoustical Society of America* **82**:1621–30.

Richards, V. M. (1992). The detectability of a tone added to narrow bands of equal-energy noise. *Journal of the Acoustical Society of America* **91**:3424–35.

Richards, V. M. (2002). Varying feedback to evaluate detection strategies: the detection of a tone added to noise. *Journal of the Association for Research in Otolaryngology* **3**:209–21.

Richards, V. M. and Nekrich, R. D. (1993). The incorporation of level and level-invariant cues for the detection of a tone added to noise. *Journal of the Acoustical Society of America* **94**:2560–74.

Rose, J. E., Brugge, J. F., Anderson, D. J., and Hind, J. E. (1967). Phase-locked response to low-frequency tones in single auditory nerve fibers of the squirrel monkey. *Journal of Neurophysiology* **30**:769–93.

Rose, J. E., Brugge, J. F., Anderson, D. J., and Hind, J. E. (1968). Patterns of activity in single auditory nerve fibres of the squirrel monkey. In: *Hearing Mechanisms in Vertebrates* (ed. A. V. Sd, Reuck, J. Knight), pp. 144–57. London: Churchill.

Rosen, S. and Baker, R. J. (1994). Characterising auditory filter nonlinearity. *Hearing Research* **73**:231–43.

Rosen, S., Baker, R. J., and Darling, A. (1998). Auditory filter nonlinearity at 2kHz in normal hearing listeners. *Journal of the Acoustical Society of America* **103**:2539–50.

Rosengard, P. S., Oxenham, A. J., and Braida, L. D. (2005). Comparing different estimates of cochlear compression in listeners with normal and impaired hearing. *Journal of the Acoustical Society of America* **117**:3028–41.

Ruggero, M. A. (1992). Responses to sound of the basilar membrane of the mammalian cochlea. *Current Opinion in Neurobiology* **2**:449–56.

Ruggero, M. A. and Temchin, A. N. (2005). Unexceptional sharpness of frequency tuning in the human cochlea. *Proceedings of the National Academy of Sciences USA* **102**:18614–19.

Ruggero, M. A., Rich, N. C., Recio, A., Narayan, S. S., and Robles, L. (1997). Basilar-membrane responses to tones at the base of the chinchilla cochlea. *Journal of the Acoustical Society of America* **101**:2151–63.

Ruggero, M. A., Narayan, S. S., Temchin, A. N., and Recio, A. (2000). Mechanical bases of frequency tuning and neural excitation at the base of the cochlea: Comparison of basilar-membrane vibrations and auditory-nerve-fiber responses in chinchilla. *Proceedings of the National Academy of Sciences USA* **97**:11744–50.

Sachs, M. B. and Kiang, N. Y. S. (1968). Two-tone inhibition in auditory nerve fibers. *Journal of the Acoustical Society of America* **43**:1120–8.

Scharf, B. (1970). Critical bands. In *Foundations of Modern Auditory Theory* (ed. J. V. Tobias). New York: Academic.

Scharf, B., Reeves, A., and Giovanetti, H. (2008). The role of attention in overshoot: Frequency certainty versus uncertainty. *Journal of the Acoustical Society of America* **123**:1555–61.

Schmidt, S. and Zwicker, E. (1991). The effect of masker spectral asymmetry on overshoot in simultaneous masking. *Journal of the Acoustical Society of America* **89**:1324–30.

Schooneveldt, G. P. and Moore, B. C. J. (1987). Comodulation masking release (CMR): Effects of signal frequency, flanking-band frequency, masker bandwidth, flanking-band level, and monotic versus dichotic presentation of the flanking band. *Journal of the Acoustical Society of America* **82**:1944–56.

Schooneveldt, G. P. and Moore, B. C. J. (1989). Comodulation masking release (CMR) as a function of masker bandwidth, modulator bandwidth and signal duration. *Journal of the Acoustical Society of America* **85**:273–81.

Schroeder, M. R. (1970). Synthesis of low peak-factor signals and binary sequences with low autocorrelation. *IEEE Transactions on Information Theory* **16**:85–9.

Sellick, P. M., Patuzzi, R., and Johnstone, B. M. (1982). Measurement of basilar membrane motion in the guinea pig using the Mössbauer technique. *Journal of the Acoustical Society of America* **72**:131–41.

Serafin, J. V., Moody, D. B., and Stebbins, W. C. (1982). Frequency selectivity of the monkey's auditory system: psychophysical tuning curves. *Journal of the Acoustical Society of America* **71**:1513–18.

Shackleton, T. M. and Carlyon, R. P. (1994). The role of resolved and unresolved harmonics in pitch perception and frequency modulation discrimination. *Journal of the Acoustical Society of America* **95**:3529–40.

Shamma, S. A. (1985). Speech processing in the auditory system, II: Lateral inhibition and the central processing of speech evoked activity in the auditory nerve. *Journal of the Acoustical Society of America* **78**:1622–32.

Shannon, R. V. (1976). Two-tone unmasking and suppression in a forward masking situation. *Journal of the Acoustical Society of America* **59**:1460–70.

Shera, C. A. (2001a). Frequency glides in click responses of the basilar membrane and auditory nerve: Their scaling behavior and origin in traveling-wave dispersion. *Journal of the Acoustical Society of America* **109**:2023–34.

Shera, C. A. (2001b). Intensity invariance of fine time structure in basilar-membrane click response: Implications for cochlear mechanics. *Journal of the Acoustical Society of America* **110**:332–48.

Shera, C. A. and Guinan, J. J., Jr. (2003). Stimulus-frequency-emission group delay: a test of coherent reflection filtering and a window on cochlear tuning. *Journal of the Acoustical Society of America* **113**:2762–72.

Shera, C. A., Guinan, J. J., and Oxenham, A. J. (2002). Revised estimates of human cochlear tuning from otoacoustic and behavioral measurements. *Proceedings of the National Academy of Sciences USA* **99**:3318–23.

Smith, R. L. (1977). Short-term adaptation in single auditory nerve fibers: Some poststimulatory effects. *Journal of Neurophysiology* **40**:1098–112.

Smith, R. L. (1979). Adaptation, saturation, and physiological masking in single auditory-nerve fibers. *Journal of the Acoustical Society of America* 65:166–78.

Soderquist, D. R. (1970). Frequency analysis and the critical band. *Psychonomic Science* 21:117–19.

Stickney, G. S., Zeng, F. G., Litovsky, R., and Assmann, P. (2004). Cochlear implant speech recognition with speech maskers. *Journal of the Acoustical Society of America* 116:1081–91.

Strickland, E. A. (2001). The relationship between frequency selectivity and overshoot. *Journal of the Acoustical Society of America* 109:2062–73.

Strickland, E. A. (2004). The temporal effect with notched-noise maskers: analysis in terms of input-output functions. *Journal of the Acoustical Society of America* 115:2234–45.

Strickland, E. A. (2008). The relationship between precursor level and the temporal effect. *Journal of the Acoustical Society of America* 123:946–54.

Treurniet, W. C. and Boucher, D. R. (2001). A masking level difference due to harmonicity. *Journal of the Acoustical Society of America* 109:306–20.

Unoki, M., Irino, T., Glasberg, B., Moore, B. C., and Patterson, R. D. (2006). Comparison of the roex and gammachirp filters as representations of the auditory filter. *Journal of the Acoustical Society of America* 120:1474–92.

Verhey, J. L., Dau, T., and Kollmeier, B. (1999). Within-channel cues in comodulation masking release (CMR): Experiments and model predictions using a modulation-filterbank model. *Journal of the Acoustical Society of America* 106:2733–45.

Verhey, J. L., Pressnitzer, D., and Winter, I. M. (2003). The psychophysics and physiology of comodulation masking release. *Experimental Brain Research* 153:405–17.

Vogten, L. L. M. (1978). Low-level pure-tone masking: A comparison of 'tuning curves' obtained with simultaneous and forward masking. *Journal of the Acoustical Society of America* 63:1520–7.

von Békésy, G. (1960). *Experiments in Hearing*. New York: McGraw-Hill.

von Klitzing, R. and Kohlrausch, A. (1994). Effect of masker level on overshoot in running- and frozen-noise maskers. *Journal of the Acoustical Society of America* 95:2192–201.

Warren, R. M., Obusek, C. J., and Ackroff, J. M. (1972). Auditory induction: perceptual synthesis of absent sounds. *Science* 176:1149–51.

Watson, C. S. (2005). Some comments on informational masking. *Acta Acustica united with Acustica* 91:502–12.

Watson, C. S. and Kelly, W. J. (1978). Informational masking in auditory patterns. *Journal of the Acoustical Society of America* 64:S39.

Wegel, R. L. and Lane, C. E. (1924). The auditory masking of one sound by another and its probable relation to the dynamics of the inner ear. *Physical Review* 23:266–85.

Wojtczak, M., Schroder, A. C., Kong, Y. Y., and Nelson, D. A. (2001). The effect of basilar-membrane nonlinearity on the shapes of masking period patterns in normal and impaired hearing. *Journal of the Acoustical Society of America* 109:1571–86.

Yasin, I. and Plack, C. J. (2003). The effects of a high-frequency suppressor on tuning curves and derived basilar-membrane response functions. *Journal of the Acoustical Society of America* 114:322–32.

Zhang, X., Heinz, M. G., Bruce, I. C., and Carney, L. H. (2001). A phenomenological model for the responses of auditory-nerve fibers: I. Nonlinear tuning with compression and suppression. *Journal of the Acoustical Society of America* 109:648–70.

Zwicker, E. (1965). Temporal effects in simultaneous masking by white-noise bursts. *Journal of the Acoustical Society of America* 37:653–63.

Zwicker, E. (1970). Masking and psychological excitation as consequences of the ear's frequency analysis. In *Frequency Analysis and Periodicity Detection in Hearing* (ed. R. Plomp, G. F. Smoorenburg), pp. 376–94. Leiden: Sijthoff.

Zwicker, E. (1976a). Masking period patterns of harmonic complex tones. *Journal of the Acoustical Society of America* 60:429–39.

Zwicker, E. (1976b). Psychoacoustic equivalent of period histograms (in memoriam Dr. Russel Pfeiffer). *Journal of the Acoustical Society of America* 59:166–75.

Zwicker, E. (1976c). Masking period patterns of amplitude modulated pure tones. *Acustica* 36:113–20.

Zwicker, E. (1986). Das Zeitauflosungsvermogen des Gehors—Eine zweckmassige Messmethode im Hinblick auf die Sprachverstandlichkeit. *Audiological Acoustics* 25:170–84.

Zwicker, E. and Schorn, K. (1982). Temporal resolution in hard-of-hearing patients. *Audiology* 21:474–92.

Zwislocki, J. J. and Relkin, E. M. (2001). On a psychophysical transformed-rule up and down method converging on a 75% level of correct responses. *Proceedings of the National Academy of Sciences USA* 98:4811–14.

Chapter 3

Loudness and intensity coding

Michael Epstein and Jeremy Marozeau

3.1 Introduction

3.1.1 Definition of loudness

Loudness is the primary perceptual correlate of physical sound intensity or strength, often described as the characteristic of sound ranging from very soft to very loud. Loudness is often mistakenly used in non-scientific discussions to refer to the physical volume or the physical intensity of a sound, but proper usage refers only to perception. A number of other physical sound parameters also affect loudness, including frequency, duration, spectrum, bandwidth, and context. The perception of loudness also depends on the individual characteristics of the listener, particularly the integrity of the auditory system. Even within a normal population, loudness can vary from person to person.

Despite the fact that loudness has been studied formally for close to 150 years, there is still substantial scientific discourse and debate regarding not only the complexities of the neural coding of intensity and loudness, but also even the most basic measurements of the perceptions of a simple sound, such as a pure tone. Much like Newtonian laws remained a standard in physics until they were replaced by Einstein's relativity, the forefathers of loudness put forth simple and elegant models that gave us great insight into perception, but could not explain all the phenomena later discovered. Currently, more and more complex models are being developed to include the loudnesses of complex or mixed sounds, the summation of sounds across the two ears, context effects, and the effects of the many aetiologic causes of hearing impairment.

The purpose of this chapter is to provide a brief, but thorough overview of how loudness is measured, how it is affected by physical parameters, and how intensity is coded in the auditory system. It will also provide a historical overview of loudness modelling and examine how context and impairment can affect our perception of loudness.

3.1.2 Intensity, level, and the dynamic range of hearing

Perhaps the most remarkable characteristic of the auditory system is the dynamic range of hearing. Average, normal-hearing humans are capable of detecting sounds that are presented at 0 dB SPL and are generally able to tolerate sounds, at least brief ones, as high as about 120 dB SPL. That means that the auditory system is capable of handling sound intensities that are 10^{12} times as large as the minimum detectable intensity. It is an extraordinarily impressive system that can detect the sounds of a mosquito beating its wings 1 m away and still withstand the blast of a nearby thunderclap.

Dynamic ranges are significantly smaller for most common audio systems. Audiotape is capable of approximately a 65-dB dynamic range without significant distortion. This is equivalent to a maximum intensity that is on the order of 10^6 times the minimum intensity. Compact discs are capable of producing a 96-dB dynamic range or a maximum intensity that is on the order of 10^9 times the minimum intensity.

3.1.3 Loudness units

Because loudness is primarily correlated with sound intensity, loudness is most often displayed or described as a function of physical sound intensity or pressure. This typically results in plots of loudness on a logarithmic scale as a function of sound level in dB SPL. Loudness is also sometimes expressed as a function of dB HL (hearing level) or dB SL (sensation level), variations of the dB SPL scale that are shifted by average (dB HL) or individual (dB SL) audibility threshold data as a function of the frequency of the stimuli.

Loudness itself is sometimes mathematically expressed in one of two distinct units, both of which are based on 1-kHz reference tones. The loudness level in phons refers to the level of an equally loud 1-kHz tone in dB SPL presented to both ears of a listener in a free field with frontal incidence (Fletcher and Munson, 1933). For example, if the loudness of a sound were equal to the loudness of a 1-kHz tone at 60 dB SPL, that sound would have a loudness level of 60 phons. By definition, the loudness level of any 1-kHz tone in phons is simply equal to its level in dB SPL.

The sone is a relative loudness unit referenced to a 1-kHz tone at 40 dB SPL, presented to a listener in a free field, by assigning a loudness of 1 sone for that stimulus (Stevens, 1936). If a sound is twice as loud as a 1-kHz tone at 40 dB SPL, then its loudness is 2 sones. If a sound is half as loud, its loudness is 0.5 sones. Therefore, any audible sound must have a loudness in sones that is non-zero and positive.

3.2 Representing and measuring loudness

By definition, there is no objective way to directly measure any psychological phenomenon. Because loudness is a purely perceptual characteristic, its measurement requires subjective reporting of the sensation by a listener. A good loudness measurement technique should provide a repeatable, reliable, and precise description of the perception of loudness while removing possible experimental biases that could affect the outcome. A number of different methodologies have been used, each with its own advantages and disadvantages.

3.2.1 Category scaling

The categorical scaling of loudness is perhaps the most intuitive approach to making subjective judgments of sound. In a category-scaling procedure, listeners are asked to select a category that best describes the loudness of a sound. Category labels may vary somewhat from study-to-study, but typically are similar to: not heard, very soft, soft, comfortable, loud, very loud, and too loud.

Recent advancements in categorical scaling include the use of a greater number of categories, adaptive procedures, and mathematical modelling to generate loudness functions (Keidser et al., 1999; Brand and Hohmann, 2002). Because of the general ease of use of category scaling, it has been used in the clinical assessment of loudness for rapid hearing-aid fitting (Kiessling et al., 1996). However, some studies have indicated that category scaling generally cannot provide valuable information for hearing-aid fitting (Elberling, 1999).

3.2.2 Magnitude estimation and production

In magnitude estimation, proposed for use with auditory stimuli by Stevens (1956), listeners are asked to assign any positive number that represents the loudness of a presented sound. These assignments are allowed to include decimal and fractional numbers. Listeners are typically instructed or assumed to assign numbers within a ratio scale. That is, if a sound were twice as loud as another sound, that sound would be assigned a number with twice the value of the other sound. These estimates expose the relationships among all presented sounds within an experiment (Stevens, 1975).

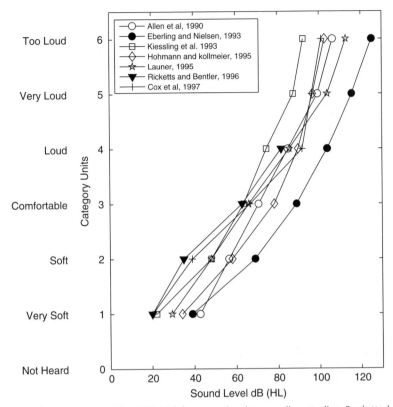

Fig. 3.1 Categories versus sound level (dB HL) for seven loudness scaling studies. Replotted summary of data from Elberling (1999).

Magnitude estimation may also be performed with a standard. In such a paradigm, the listener is presented with a reference sound that is assigned to a specific reference number. The listener is then asked to assign numbers to subsequent sounds such that ratios are maintained. If a sound were half as loud as the reference sound, it would be assigned a number that is half of the reference number. If a sound were twice as loud as the reference sound, it would be assigned a number that is twice the reference number.

Some researchers have suggested that there are a number of biases present in magnitude estimation (see Poulton, 1989 for review). To a degree, these biases may be resolved by counterbalancing with the opposing task, i.e. magnitude production. In this task, a listener is given a number and asked to adjust the level of a sound such that the loudness matches that number (Hellman, 1981). Typically, results from magnitude estimation and magnitude production from the same listener might be averaged together to determine a final estimate of loudness.

A number of researchers have also shown that magnitude estimation is a useful tool for assessing group mean loudness, but is less suitable for individual assessments due to variability (Green and Luce, 1974; Epstein and Florentine, 2006). This limitation makes it an uncommon tool for loudness assessment in clinical hearing-aid fitting scenarios.

3.2.3 Cross-modality matching

Cross-modality matching is a general description of a procedure in which two different modalities of perception are matched together. In fact, magnitude estimation is technically a form of cross-modality matching in which the perception of loudness is matched with the perception of the magnitude of a number. Cross-modality matching procedures used for loudness most often use line length (Teghtsoonian and Teghtsoonian, 1983), but other modalities have been used to match features of sounds, including the brightness of a light and tactile vibration. In theory, there is no particular limitation to the selection of a modality for comparison. However, when multiple modalities are compared, a mathematical transformation must be determined in order to equate the measurements with a more direct technique. Cross-modal matches between line length and loudness are most common because they have been found to be consistent with magnitude estimation results in both normal-hearing and hearing-impaired listeners (Hellman and Meiselman, 1988; Hellman, 1999).

3.2.4 Loudness matching

Another approach for determining information about the loudness of sound is to equate the loudness of one sound with the loudness of another. This is particularly useful for comparing the loudnesses of sounds with different physical parameters such as frequency (Fletcher and Steinberg, 1924), duration (Florentine et al., 1996), spectrum (Leibold et al., 2007), or bandwidth (Zwicker et al., 1957), as well as combinations of those parameters (Anweiler and Verhey, 2006). Loudness matching is also the fundamental basis of the phon scale of loudness. Listeners are typically presented with two sounds and are asked to adjust the level of one of the sounds to find the point of subjective equality in which the loudnesses of the two sounds are equal. Most experimenters counterbalance loudness matches by then reversing the roles of the fixed and variable sounds and averaging between these two conditions.

3.2.5 Other correlates of loudness

In addition to measuring loudness subjectively, a number of objective experimental techniques have been examined as possible correlates of loudness. Correlates of loudness that require less active participation or cognitive activity from the listener may be more suitable for rapid, objective clinical assessments of loudness, particularly in young children or cognitively impaired adults.

Reaction time

Measurements of simple reaction time, the speed at which a listener provides a response to a sound, correlate with loudness, with louder sounds yielding faster reaction times. In other words, reaction time is inversely correlated with loudness. In a typical reaction-time task, listeners are presented with sounds and asked to press a trigger immediately upon hearing the sound. In particular, this technique has been used to examine loudness near threshold, which is typically difficult with magnitude estimation (see Wagner et al., 2004 for a review). There may be some limitations to the use of reaction time to derive loudness information as some listeners have shown frequency dependence.

Basilar-membrane velocity

The basilar membrane is a membrane running through the centre of the cochlea and the location on which sound is transduced from physical vibration to neural activity. The relationship between sound intensity and basilar-membrane motion has been measured in animals using laser Doppler velocimetry (Nuttall et al., 1991). Buus and Florentine (2001) plotted human loudness functions modeled from temporal integration data and spectral summation data with basilar-membrane velocity measures made in a chinchilla (Ruggero et al., 1997). They demonstrated that loudness was approximately a linear function of basilar-membrane velocity squared. Other psychoacoustical measurements associated with basilar-membrane compression also correspond well with loudness

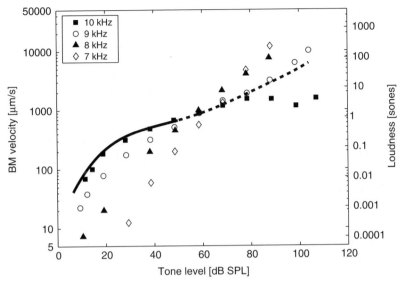

Fig. 3.2 Human loudness functions derived using two psychoacoustical methods plotted with basilar-membrane velocity measured in a chinchilla at a 10-kHz characteristic frequency location. The loudness data matches the basilar-membrane response to a tone close to characteristic frequency if it is assumed that loudness is linearly related to the square of basilar-membrane velocity. Responses at the same location to tones at lower frequencies are also shown for response comparison. Replotted from Buus and Florentine (2001).

growth functions (Oxenham and Plack, 1997). This indicates that, at least for pure tones, loudness is closely associated with the intensity of physical vibrations on the basilar membrane (Fig. 3.2). This, of course, is not of direct practical clinical use, but does provide insight into the process of sound transduction and processing within the auditory system.

Auditory brainstem response

The auditory brainstem response (ABR) is an objective neurological measure of the evoked potential that results from auditory stimulation. A number of researchers have examined the relationship between the ABR and loudness (Howe and Decker, 1984; Serpanos *et al.*, 1997). These studies have primarily monitored the most common ABR landmark used for the clinical testing of auditory-system integrity, Wave V latency. Wave V latency decreases with increasing intensity and, much like reaction time, has a strong inverse correlation with loudness. However, Wave V latency asymptotes at a relatively low intensity, while loudness continues to grow with increasing intensity. It is possible to estimate the basilar-membrane response function by measuring the effects of an on- and off-frequency forward masker on Wave V latency (Krishnan and Plack, 2009), and this may provide a better estimate of loudness.

Pratt and Sohmer (1977) hypothesized that, rather than examining Wave V latency, the first few components, approximately waves I+II of the ABR, are better suited for finding a correlate of loudness. Physiologically, it is likely that the early components of the ABR result from electrical activity within the cochlea itself as well as the first and second order neurons in the auditory nerve.

Otoacoustic emissions

Otoacoustic emissions, low-level sound by-products of the active mechanism of the auditory system, have been recently examined as a possible correlate of loudness after some suggestion that they might reflect basilar-membrane non-linearity. Acoustic recordings of otoacoustic emissions are typically made by inserting a microphone into the ear canal.

A number of researchers have measured distortion-product otoacoustic emissions, which result from the interaction of two stimuli presented simultaneously, in both normal-hearing and hearing-impaired listeners (Neely *et al.*, 2003; Muller and Janssen, 2004). It has been generally found that distortion-product otoacoustic emissions exhibit many of the characteristics of loudness and basilar-membrane compression. Transient-evoked otoacoustic emissions, acoustic responses of the ear made after short stimuli are presented, have also been measured as a function of level and shown to correlate well with loudness functions estimated using a number of psychoacoustical tasks for normal-hearing listeners (Epstein and Florentine, 2005*a*).

3.3 **Parametric effects**

Loudness depends primarily on sound intensity, however two sounds with the same intensity can be perceived with different loudnesses. This results from the effects of other parameters that can influence the loudness of a sound. This section will review the relationships between loudness and several physical parameters of sound.

3.3.1 **Level**

Intensity is the primary physical parameter that influences loudness. This effect is the most intuitive parametric adjustment of loudness and can easily be experienced by turning the volume knob on a radio up or down. The study of loudness began with an examination of the relationship between intensity and loudness, typically referred to as a 'loudness function'.

Figure 3.3 reviews a number of experiments measuring the relationship between intensity and loudness using both magnitude estimation and doubling or halving of loudness (Hellman and Zwislocki, 1963). This figure shows the average estimate of loudness on a logarithmic scale as a function of sound level in dB SL. Note that loudness and level have a monotonic relationship (i.e. an increase in level will always be perceived as an increase in loudness). However, this relationship is not linear. If the intensity of a sound is doubled (3-dB increase), its loudness will not be perceived as doubled. The slope of the loudness curve is steepest at low levels and decreases at moderate levels. This implies that the same change in level will be perceived as a greater change in loudness at low levels than at moderate levels.

At moderate levels, the logarithm of loudness is classically modeled as proportional to the level. The slope of this line indicates that it is necessary to raise the level approximately 10 dB in order to double loudness. The shape of the loudness function is approximately independent of the duration (Epstein and Florentine, 2005*b*) and the presentation mode, binaural vs. monaural (Marozeau *et al.*, 2006), but it does depend somewhat on spectral content (Scharf, 1959) and frequency (Hellman *et al.*, 2001).

3.3.2 **Frequency/equal-loudness contours**

In addition to being dependent on intensity, loudness is dependent on frequency. In typical experiments to examine this effect, listeners are asked to adjust the level of a tone to match the loudness of a 1-kHz tone. The experiment is repeated many times with the frequency of the adjusted tone varied and the 1-kHz reference tone kept fixed in frequency. Additionally, the level of the 1-kHz tone is changed from condition to condition to obtain a series of functions showing equally loud tones of different frequencies using a particular level 1-kHz tone as reference. Each of these functions is called an equal-loudness contour. Figure 3.4 shows a series of equal-loudness contours for different levels of the 1-kHz reference tone.

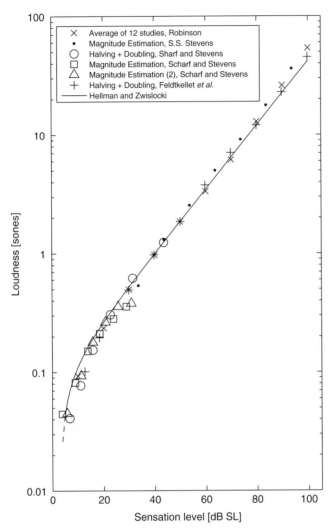

Fig. 3.3 Loudness as a function of dB SL from a number of studies. Replotted from Hellman and Zwislocki (1963).

Along each contour line, the tones are perceived as equally loud. For example, a 125-Hz tone at 44 dB SPL has the same loudness as a 500-Hz tone at 23 dB SPL. These contours also illustrate the loudness level of a variety of sounds in phons, as the loudness level is equal to the level of the equally loud 1-kHz tone.

Hearing threshold is represented as a dashed line in the equal-loudness contour because some studies have showed that the loudness at threshold varies and that equal detectability does not imply equal loudness level (Buus and Florentine, 2002). However, it seems that there is some relationship between threshold microvariations, relatively large threshold differences for relatively small differences in frequency, and loudness at higher levels (Mauermann *et al.*, 2004).

For low-frequency sounds, the contour lines are closer together as level increases than they are for moderate frequencies. This implies that loudness grows faster with changes in level for low-frequency sounds. For example, the loudness of a 31.5-Hz tone increases from 20 phons to 90 phons with less than a 40-dB increase in level (from 76 to 115 dB SPL). Therefore, for a 31.5-Hz tone, a 40-dB dynamic range will span the same range of loudnesses as a 70-dB dynamic range for a 1-kHz tone.

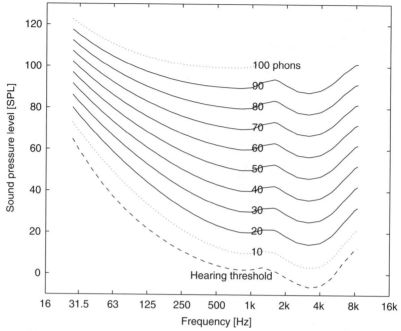

Fig. 3.4 Equal-loudness contours. Replotted from Suzuki and Takeshima (2004).

3.3.3 Duration

The duration of a signal also has an effect on its loudness. For sounds shorter than about 500 ms to 1 s, the loudness of the sound will increase with increasing duration. This phenomenon, the summing of sound energy over time, is known as 'temporal integration' (see Chapter 5). The effects of duration are typically measured using a loudness-matching procedure similar to that used to measure equal-loudness contours. Listeners are asked to match the loudness of two sounds with different durations by adjusting the level of one until the two sounds are equally loud. Instead of varying frequency, as in the equal-loudness contour measurements, the duration of the sound is varied. Figure 3.5 shows the levels of equally loud 1-kHz tones with different durations for a range of levels from threshold to 95 dB SPL. The figure shows the level of the tone such that it is equally loud to a 640-ms tone at the indicated level as a function of the duration of the tone.

Each of these lines then represents an equal-loudness contour with respect to duration. For all levels, shorter sounds need to be more intense to be as loud as longer sounds.

It is notable that the amount of temporal integration, that is the difference in level between equally loud short and long sounds, is dependent on level (Florentine *et al.*, 1996). While for the 35-dB 640-ms tone, there is approximately a 22 dB difference between the long tone and an equally loud 5-ms tone; for the 95-dB 640-ms tone, there is approximately a 12 dB difference between the long tone and an equally loud 5-ms tone. Because the loudness function is approximately the same shape for sounds of all durations (Epstein and Florentine, 2005*b*), this variation in the amount of temporal integration as a function of level also indicates that the slope of the loudness function must be shallower at moderate levels than at low and high levels (Buus *et al.*, 1997).

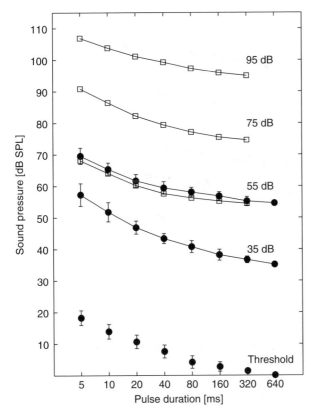

Fig. 3.5 An illustration of temporal integration of loudness. Equal-loudness functions for 1-kHz tones with a series of fixed levels (ranging from threshold to 95 dB SPL) and varied durations (ranging from 5 to 640 ms). Replotted from Poulsen (1981).

3.3.4 Bandwidth

Loudness also increases with increasing bandwidth. This phenomenon is known as 'spectral summation'. As with previously discussed experiments to examine parametric effects, spectral summation of loudness is typically measured using loudness matching. Typically, listeners are asked to adjust the level of a 1-kHz tone to match the loudness of a noise geometrically centred at 1 kHz with a constant overall level as a function of the bandwidth of the noise.

Figure 3.6 shows the results of this experiment. The figure shows the level to which the reference tone is set at the point of subjective loudness equality as a function of the bandwidth of the signal. Each curve shows the influence of bandwidth for a specific level of noise. As the bandwidth widens beyond shorter bandwidths, loudness increases, except at 20 phons. The bandwidth at which summation begins is known as the 'critical bandwidth'. The maximum amount of spectral summation depends on level (Scharf, 1997) and duration (Verhey and Kollmeier, 2002), and the effect can be as large as 18 dB in very specific scenarios (Zwicker and Fastl, 1990).

3.3.5 Binaural summation

A sound presented monaurally, through one headphone, will sound softer than the same sound presented binaurally, through a pair of headphones. Generally, it has been assumed that the loudness ratio between a binaural sound and a monaural sound is equal to two (see Hellman, 1991 for a review). That means that sounds presented to both ears would be twice as loud as the same

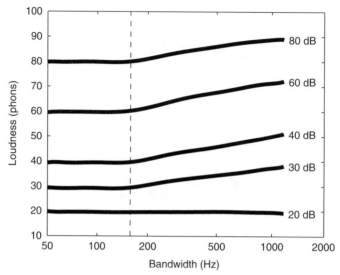

Fig. 3.6 Spectral summation of loudness. Loudness level of band-filtered white noise as a function of bandwidth. Dashed line indicates the location of the critical band. Replotted from Scharf (1997).

sounds presented to one ear. However, some studies have suggested a lower binaural-to-monaural loudness ratio, between 1.5 and 1.7, and that the ratio is constant and independent of level (see Marozeau *et al.*, 2006 for a review).

3.4 **Intensity coding**

The auditory system is capable of coding a tremendous range of physical intensities and identifying relatively small differential intensities. This section will outline the perceptual and physiological effects of intensity variations.

3.4.1 **Intensity discrimination and Weber's law**

The smallest intensity change that is detectable is often called the 'just noticeable difference', JND, or 'difference limen'. This can be measured using a number of different experimental paradigms, most of which involve a two (or more) -interval task in which the listener chooses the sound with a greater intensity. These paradigms include direct comparison of two sound bursts to determine which one has a higher intensity, identification of an amplitude modulated sound, and detection of a brief increment in a longer, continuous background sound. Each of these test paradigms results in somewhat different values for the JND, but the trends of the results are the same.

Weber's law states that the JND is a constant proportion of the intensity of the sound. In other words, some constant K exists such that K is equal to the detectable change in intensity, ΔI, divided by the pedestal intensity of the sound, I. This is known as the Weber fraction:

$$K = \Delta I / I \text{ or in dB} = 10 \log_{10} \left(\Delta I / I \right) \tag{3.1}$$

The Weber fraction indicates the proportion of change that is required for detection. The constant proportion for detectability can be experienced in everyday situations. If a jar contains 100 marbles, it would be difficult to distinguish that jar from an identical jar containing one fewer marble. However, if the jar contains five marbles, it would be quite easy to distinguish it from a similar jar containing four marbles. In each case, the same number of marbles has been removed

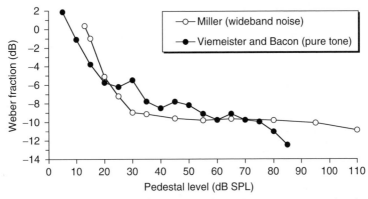

Fig. 3.7 Intensity discrimination for a wideband noise and for a 1 kHz pure tone, as a function of level. In both experiments listeners were required to detect a brief increment in a continuous sound. Data are from Miller (1947) and Viemeister and Bacon (1988). Reprinted from Plack (2005), p. 122, with permission.

(i.e. the change in intensity, ΔI, is the same, but the ratio of change to pedestal intensity is not). Weber's law indicates that 20 marbles would need to be removed from the jar with 100 marbles to create the same effect:

$$\text{Weber fraction, constant } K = \Delta I / I = (\text{for jar 1}) \ 20/100 = (\text{for jar 2}) \ 1/5 \qquad (3.2)$$

To determine the level difference in decibels between two just discriminable sounds, ΔL, for a particular pedestal intensity, I:

$$\Delta L = 10 \log_{10} (I + \Delta I) - 10 \log_{10} (I) = 10 \log_{10} \left[(I + \Delta I)/I \right] \qquad (3.3)$$

Where ΔI = IK
Therefore:

$$\Delta L = 10 \log_{10} \left[(I + IK)/I \right] = 10 \log_{10} (1 + K) \qquad (3.4)$$

The value of K at higher levels is approximately 0.1 or −10 dB, which corresponds to a ΔL, of about 0.4 dB. That is, listeners can detect changes in level of about 0.4 dB. Figure 3.7 shows the Weber fraction as a function of the level of the pedestal. For wideband sounds (such as a noise with a flat spectrum) Weber's law holds well from about 30 to 110 dB SPL, but the Weber fraction is greater at low levels (Miller, 1947). For pure tones and other narrowband sounds, however, the Weber fraction decreases with level. This phenomenon is known as the near miss to Weber's law (McGill and Goldberg, 1968).

3.4.2 Excitation

The basilar membrane, the vibration of which activates the neural portion of the auditory system, is tonotopically organized. That is, it vibrates in a particular location for a stimulus of a particular frequency. Responses to high-frequency sounds occur near the base of the cochlea and responses to low-frequency sounds occur at the apex of the cochlea. When a tone is presented, vibration peaks at the location specifically tuned to that frequency. Additionally, nearby regions also vibrate. At low levels, the vibration spreads approximately equally toward the apex and the base. At higher levels, the vibrations spread more toward the base than the apex. This is known as the upward spread of excitation. In fact, the upward skirt of the excitation grows linearly with level, while the peak of excitation grows compressively (see Chapter 2).

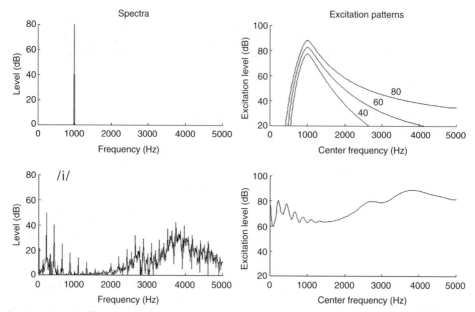

Fig. 3.8 Spectra (left) and excitation patterns (right) for a 1-kHz pure tone (top) and the vowel /i/ (bottom). Excitation patterns for the pure tone were calculated at three levels, 40, 60, and 80 dB SPL. Only the 80 dB SPL tone is shown in the spectrum. Reprinted from Plack (2005), p. 108, with permission.

Figure 3.8 shows the shapes of the excitation of the basilar membrane for 1-kHz pure tones at several levels as a function of frequency. As level increases, there is little change in the amount of excitation that spreads toward low frequencies. In contrast, as level increases, the spread toward higher frequencies increases rapidly.

The near miss to Weber's law can be explained by the additional information provided by the skirt excitation at high levels. In an experiment performed by Moore and Raab (1974), a masking noise with a band notch, designed to only mask skirt excitation, presented during a JND experiment resulted in only a small decrease in performance that only occurred at high levels. This change in performance eliminated the near miss to Weber's law. This is also consistent with the findings of Florentine *et al.* (1987). They found that high-frequency tones do not exhibit the near miss, probably because there is no room in the cochlea for excitation to spread toward higher frequencies.

3.4.3 Neural intensity coding (dynamic range problem)

Auditory nerve fibres increase their firing rate as the intensity of a sound increases. Rate-level functions show the number of times a nerve fibre activates, on average, per second for a given stimulus. These functions show that the vast majority of auditory nerve fibres tend to saturate (i.e. reach maximum firing rate) within only a 30–60 dB dynamic range. Because the auditory system as a whole is capable of processing a dynamic range of 120 dB, some mechanism other than general firing rate of the neurons must account for this ability. It is not yet well understood how this dynamic-range problem is overcome by the system.

One mechanism that may contribute to the wide dynamic range of the system is the spread of excitation, which increases the number of neurons involved in coding the sound and includes neurons from the skirts of the excitation pattern that receive less excitation and are therefore not saturated. Another is phase locking (see Volume 1, Chapter 9), for which the synchrony of firing to the waveform of the stimulus becomes greater as level increases. Despite these contributions, when both of these cues are eliminated by masking and using high frequencies to eliminate phase-locking cues (Carlyon and Moore, 1984), the auditory system is still capable of quite good intensity discrimination, so these cues cannot explain psychophysical performance on their own. It is also possible that the small proportion of fibres with wide dynamic ranges are sufficient to account for the wide dynamic range and acute intensity discrimination seen in the auditory system (for reviews, see Viemeister, 1988; Plack, 2005).

In general, the relationship between neural coding and intensity discrimination is not well understood. One example is the expectation that rapidity of onset of an increment in a continuous sound would improve the detection of that increment. This would be expected because rapid onsets result in strong transient responses in the auditory nerve and elsewhere in the auditory system (see Volume 2, Chapter 6). However, Plack *et al.* (2006) found that increment detection was not altered by changing the slope of the onset ramp on the increment. All these findings indicate that there may be variations in the function of specific fibres, and that the information in these fibres is integrated in a form that is far more complex than simply energy summation.

3.4.4 Profile analysis

Profile analysis experiments demonstrate further that the complexities of neural coding go far beyond the use of firing rate or firing population. Profile analysis occurs in the auditory system when comparisons are made between two sounds with different spectral envelopes. Typically, experimental comparisons are made between multitone complexes in two presentation intervals. In one interval, all the tones in the multitone complex are presented at the same level (flat spectrum). In the other interval, one of the tones (target tone) is presented at a higher level than all the other tones (bumped spectrum). Listeners are asked to identify the interval containing the bumped-spectrum sound. In order to prevent listeners from simply comparing the loudnesses of the target tone in the two intervals, the level of the entire complex is varied randomly in each interval. Therefore, the bumped-spectrum sound is higher in level than the flat-spectrum sound only 50% of the time. In the experiment, the level of the target tone is varied in the bumped spectrum to find the smallest detectable bump. Even when the overall levels of the sounds are varied within a 40-dB range, listeners are able to identify bumps of only a few dB. It has been hypothesized that this ability is closely related to the spectral analysis used in speech perception, and demonstrates that auditory intensity analysis does not occur solely on a frequency-by-frequency basis (for a review see Green, 1988).

3.5 Models of loudness

Loudness is assessed by asking listeners to make judgments of their perception of sound using psychoacoustic methods. Although individual variations exist, there has been a continuing search to develop a mathematical model of loudness such that, given the physical parameters of a particular sound, one could predict the loudness of that sound for a particular listener and listening condition. Originally, loudness models predicted loudness from only intensity. Newer models grow more and more complex and attempt to incorporate many physical parameters as well as the interactions between those parameters.

3.5.1 Pure-tone loudness model

The simplest loudness model predicts the loudness of a pure tone from the intensity of that tone. However, even these simple models, which originated almost 150 years ago, are still being revised to improve accuracy today.

Logarithmic function

Fechner (1860) was the first to propose a loudness model based on a logarithmic relationship between intensity and loudness. This relationship is a natural evolution of Weber's law, which, as described in Section 3.4.1, states that the minimum amount of intensity increase ΔI needed to induce a perceptible loudness difference is a constant proportion of intensity:

$$K = \Delta I / I \text{ or } \Delta I = KI \tag{3.5}$$

According to Fechner, every ΔI can be associated with an increase on the perceptual (or sensation) scale, ΔS, corresponding to the smallest perceptible sensation increase, and that each sensation increase would be identical in magnitude. That is, for each detectable intensity increase, sensation would change the same amount. Figure 3.9, which shows the sensation of the sound as a function of intensity, illustrates this relationship.

Each vertical dashed line represents one ΔI and each horizontal dashed line represents one ΔS. For convenience, a stimulus with an intensity of one has been set to a sensation of one. Starting with that first reference point, one can add a new point with an intensity of $I+KI$ (for which I is equal to the present value of one) and a sensation of $S+\Delta S$, for which $S=1$. The next point is added at intensity $(1+(K\times 1))+K\times(1+(K\times 1))$, which is equal to the previous intensity, $(1+(K\times 1))$, plus ΔI, which equals K times the previous intensity. This simplifies to $1+2K+K^2$ or $(1+K)^2$. The sensation for this intensity is equal to $1+2\times\Delta S$. The next point would have an intensity of $I+KI=(1+K)^2 + K(1+K)^2 = 1+2K+K^2 + K+2K^2+K^3 = K^3+3K^2+K+1 = (1+K)^3$ and a sensation of $1+3\times\Delta S$. Therefore, the nth point would be equal to $[(1+K)^n, 1+n\times\Delta S]$. The function is logarithmic and the sensation S due to a stimulus with an intensity I can be predicted by $M\log_{10}(I/I_o)$; where M and I_o are constants. Based on this type of logarithmic relationship, sound level in dB SPL $[10\log_{10}(I/I_o)]$ is commonly used as the model parameter for which to evaluate the loudness of a sound. This model does not predict loudness correctly as it has been shown that equal JNDs do not correspond to equal loudness increments (Harper and Stevens, 1948).

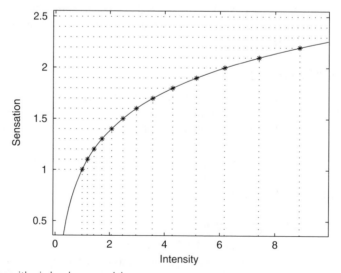

Fig. 3.9 The logarithmic loudness model.

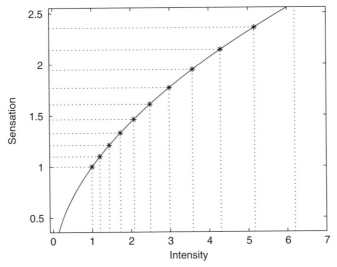

Fig. 3.10 The power function loudness model.

Power function

Another loudness model based on Weber's law is the power function, which can be derived by assuming that Weber's law also holds true for sensation. That is, for a constant, T:

$$\Delta S = TS \tag{3.6}$$

as proposed by Bretano (Stevens, 1961). Figure 3.10 illustrates this relationship. Again, an intensity of 1 is defined to evoke a sensation of magnitude 1. The next noticeable intensity will be equal to $1+K$, corresponding to a sensation $1+T$. Then an intensity of $(1+K)^2$ will evoke a sensation of $(1+T)^2$. Therefore, an intensity equal to $(1+K)^n$ will evoke a sensation equal to $(1+T)^n$. The general form of this relationship can be described by a power function:

$$S = MI^a \tag{3.7}$$

where M and a are constants.

Referring back to Fig. 3.3, intensity and loudness are both plotted on logarithmic scales (dB SL is proportional to the logarithm of intensity). The results show that, for levels above 40 dB SPL, the logarithm of loudness is approximately proportional to the logarithm of the intensity (dB SPL). This relationship is predicted by the power function: $\log(S) = a\log(I) + a\log(M)$. The slope of the function in this study (Hellman and Zwislocki, 1963), which is the exponent a, is equal to 0.26 (0.54 when measured as a function of pressure rather than intensity, as pressure is proportional to intensity squared). Most early examinations of the power function determined a slope close to 0.3 (Hellman, 1991).

Modern views on classical models

Recently, studies have suggested that the power law is a fairly good descriptor for loudness growth, but that it does not accommodate all local variations. Florentine and Epstein (2006) summarizes these variations and they have synthesized them into the form of a modified function, known as an 'inflected exponential function' (INEX). These variations result from two primary deviations from the power function. At low levels, the slope is close to 1, and then the slope gradually declines as level increases until it reaches a minimum slope at moderate levels, in the 40–60 dB

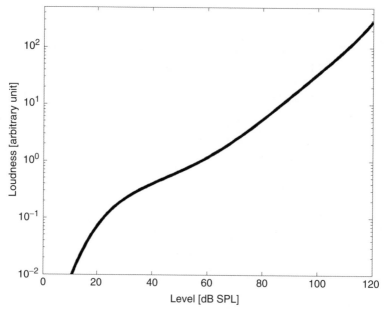

Fig. 3.11 The inflected exponential (INEX) loudness function.

SPL range. At these levels, the slope of the loudness function must be shallower than the standard power function slope of 0.3 in order to explain temporal integration and loudness summation data. At higher levels, the slope gradually increases, but does not reach 1. To account for these variations in the loudness function, the INEX function replaces the constant slope of the power function model with a continuous polynomial such that the slope is allowed to vary slowly with level.

Figure 3.11 shows a model INEX function for an average of normal-hearing listeners. For this data set, the INEX is modelled as:

$$\log_{10}(S) = 1.7058 \times 10^{-9} L^5 - 6.587 \times 10^{-7} L^4 + 9.7515 \times 10^{-5} L^3 - 6.6964 \times 10^{-3} L^2$$
$$+ 0.2367 L - 3.4831 \tag{3.8}$$

where S is the sensation and L is the level in dB SPL. In fact, these parameters typically vary somewhat from listener to listener, but the general form is roughly the same.

Although the differences between the INEX and the power function are relatively subtle, the INEX's modifications to the power function provide a better description and predictor for loudness data gathered across a wide range of levels than the original power function.

3.5.2 Models of complex sounds

The basic loudness functions are sufficient for modelling the relationship between loudness and intensity for pure tones, but do not account for variations in loudness caused by other physical parameters, listening conditions, or listener impairments. As a result, more advanced models of loudness have been developed for a variety of predictive and informative purposes.

Sound pressure level weighting

The loudness of sounds varies with changes in frequency, so it is not surprising that for wideband signals that contain energy at many frequencies, overall loudness is not equally dependent on each frequency. Perhaps the most common field examining this problem is hearing conservation. Conservationists want to predict the potential hazard of a particular sound. In order to do this, they typically weight sound such that the frequencies that result in the most auditory system activity are given more weight than those that create less activity in the system. The typical weighting systems are A-, B-, and C-weighting. Each weighting is based on sound sensitivity at a particular sound pressure level determined using the equal-loudness contours described in Section 3.3.2. A-weighting uses a 40 dB SPL reference, B-weighting uses a 70 dB SPL reference, and C-weighting uses a 100 dB SPL reference. Sounds weighted using these references are given levels in units of dB A, dB B and dB C, respectively. Effectively, the sound is filtered using the inverse of the loudness contour, so that frequency regions that contribute less to loudness are attenuated. These are, however, rough approximations and do not guarantee that loudness is properly balanced across frequency. It is possible to generate sounds with the same level in dB A that have distinctly different loudnesses (Zwicker and Fastl, 1990). The way loudness increases with bandwidth, particularly the critical bandwidth, is not taken into consideration in any of these weightings.

Complex loudness model

The current ANSI standard (ANSI, 2007) is a five-stage predictor of loudness for a variety of sounds. The model accepts the power spectrum of the signal as input and outputs a prediction of loudness. The five stages of the model are:

1 *Transmission through the outer ear*: The transmission of a sound based on its power spectrum depends on how the sound is delivered to the ear. Primarily, sounds are presented via sound fields or headphones. Each presentation mode modifies the sound by attenuating or amplifying certain frequencies. Regardless of presentation mode, the ear canal and tympanic membrane resonances are included in this power spectrum alteration. Provided that the sound is not presented via headphones, the resonances of the room, head, body, and pinna shape will also alter the characteristics of the sound. The effects of all these external processes are modelled in this stage by applying a filter to the power spectrum to characterize the listening condition.

2 *Transmission through the middle ear*: The principal role of the middle ear is to match the impedance between the air of the outside world and ear canal and the lymphic fluid of the inner ear. This system does not have a flat frequency response and, therefore, the amount of acoustic energy transmitted to the inner ear depends on the frequency of the signal. Again, a filter is used to model the middle ear response.

3 *Transformation of the spectrum to excitation pattern*: Once transmitted to the inner ear, sound vibrations travel along the basilar membrane, which is organized tonotopically. That is, each part of the basilar membrane responds best to a different frequency. A bank of band-pass filters models this stage, with each filter representing the frequency selectivity at a specific place on the basilar membrane. The shapes of these filters were selected using data gathered from notched-noise experiments, a paradigm designed to examine frequency-specific listening (see Chapter 2).

4 *Transformation of excitation pattern to specific loudness*: Specific loudness is roughly like a loudness density. Psychoacoustical experiments have shown that the magnitude of the excitation on the basilar membrane is not linearly related to the acoustic power. Specifically, changes in basilar-membrane vibration do not occur proportionally to level changes, as the system is compressive at moderate levels. The behaviour is modelled in this stage by applying a non-linear, compressive, monotonic function to the excitation pattern to transform it into specific loudness.

5 *Transformation from specific loudness to overall loudness*. Finally, the overall loudness of the sound is obtained by integrating the specific loudnesses across the whole basilar membrane.

The ANSI standard also calls for a doubling of the loudness if the sound is presented binaurally. As discussed in Section 3.3.5 and specifically suggested for the ANSI loudness model by Moore and Glasberg (2007), less than perfect summation serves as a better predictor of binaural loudness.

This standard is also only valid for steady sounds heard by normal-hearing listeners. Variations of the model have been presented to predict loudnesses for time-varying sound (Glasberg and Moore, 2002) and for listeners with hearing impairment (Moore and Glasberg, 2004).

3.6 **Context effects**

Although all the presented loudness models compute loudness *a priori*, the loudness of a sound can be substantially affected by the sounds that precede it, both immediately and from relatively long periods prior.

3.6.1 **Masking**

The loudness of sound can be reduced if other competing sounds are presented simultaneously. This phenomenon is known as 'partial masking' (Scharf, 1964, 1971; Pavel and Inverson, 1981). Partial masking is primarily believed to result from overlapping excitation patterns. The loudness of a sound is characterized not only by the activity it causes on the basilar membrane at the place tuned to the frequency of the sound, but also the regions activated by the spread of excitation. Therefore, if two sounds are presented simultaneously, it is possible that the sounds may have some overlap in excitation. If the excitation of one sound is so strong that the excitation of the second sound is completely covered by it, the first sound becomes inaudible. This is known simply as 'masking'. If only some portion of the excitation of the second sound is covered by the excitation of the first sound, the second sound may be audible, but its loudness is reduced. This is known as 'partial masking'.

In fact, this masking effect can also occur when the masking sound is not presented at the same time as the masked sound. This is known as 'non-simultaneous masking' (see Chapter 2). When the masker precedes the target sound by a small amount of time, typically less than 100 ms, the detectability of the target sound may decrease. This is known as 'forward masking'. This effect increases as the masker and target move closer together in time. The amount of forward masking depends on the temporal proximity of the masker and target as well as the relationship between their levels. Backward masking, the opposite effect in which a masker is presented after a target, results in a very weak effect and only occurs under specific conditions.

3.6.2 **Loudness adaptation**

Loudness adaptation is the decrease in loudness of a sound presented continuously over an extended period. Loudness adaptation occurs only for sounds presented below about 30 dB SL, with high-frequency tones adapting more than low-frequency tones. In fact, it is possible for continuous tones at high frequencies and low levels to become completely inaudible over time. However, it is important to note that adaptation occurs only for continuous, constant sounds and if the sound is amplitude-modulated sufficiently, the effect disappears (see Scharf, 1983 for a review).

3.6.3 **Loudness fatigue/temporary threshold shift**

Exposure to very high-level sounds, particularly for an extended period, may cause a reduction in sensitivity to intensity. This is known as 'loudness fatigue' or specifically, in the case of threshold, 'temporary threshold shift'. This effect can last from minutes to days and is often a result of noise exposures like gunfire (Bapat and Tolley, 2007) or loud music (Sadhra *et al.*, 2002). Temporary threshold shift is known to increase rapidly with increases in exposure level and exposure time. Hirsh and Ward (1952) observed that after just 3 minutes of exposure to a 120 dB SPL 500-Hz tone, a maximum temporary threshold shift of about 20 dB occurred 2 minutes after the tone ended. The maximum shift also tends to occur for sounds around 4 Hz, even when exposure occurs at lower frequencies. Recovery from a 3-minute exposure took somewhat over 10 minutes. Sometimes, sound exposure can result in longer term temporary effects. Rabinowitz (2000) discusses a case of a young girl who attended a rock concert the night before auditory evaluation. She showed a temporary 30-dB hearing loss at 4 kHz, which returned to normal after several days.

It is not clear that loudness fatigues by the same amount as threshold shifts. In fact, Botte *et al.* (1993) hypothesized that loudness fatigue and temporary threshold shift result from two different, but correlated mechanisms. Regardless when a temporary threshold shift occurs, loudness fatigue is typically also present.

3.6.4 Loudness enhancement/decrement

Loudness enhancement is a context effect in which the loudness of a sound (target) is increased by a higher level sound that immediately precedes it (much like a forward masker). The forward masker and target must be presented at similar frequencies and the forward masker must be presented less than 500 ms prior to the target in order for the effect to occur. This is different than the partial masking effect discussed in Section 3.6.1, as that effect primarily results from maskers that are lower in frequency than the target sounds.

Conversely, loudness decrement is a context effect in which the loudness of the target is decreased by a lower level forward masker that immediately precedes it. The relationship between the levels of the forward masker and the target affects the quantity of enhancement and decrement with maximal changes in loudness around 20 phons (see Oberfeld, 2007 for a review). Additionally, there is some debate regarding the degree to which loudness enhancement and decrement are intertwined with induced loudness reduction (Scharf *et al.*, 2002; Oberfeld, 2007).

3.6.5 Induced loudness reduction

Induced loudness reduction is a phenomenon by which the loudness of a sound is reduced when it is preceded by one or more higher intensity sounds presented at a nearby frequency, anywhere from several hundred milliseconds to several minutes prior. While loudness adaptation and fatigue may affect the loudness of all levels of sound equally, induced loudness reduction tends to primarily reduce the loudnesses of sounds at moderate levels. This phenomenon is one likely cause of discrepancies between estimates of loudness performed by listeners at the beginning of an experiment, when a listener has little prior sound exposure, and at the end of an experiment, after the listener is exposed to a wide range of sound levels (see Epstein, 2007 for a review). In fact, because only moderate levels are affected, induced loudness reduction can alter the entire shape of a loudness curve, when plotted as a function of level.

3.7 Hearing-impaired listeners

Chapter 14 examines the details of many aspects of auditory perception for hearing-impaired listeners. Here, a brief review of loudness for these listeners is presented.

3.7.1 Impaired loudness models

Hearing-impaired listeners (HILs) with sensorineural hearing have a reduced dynamic range. That is, the difference between the highest tolerable sound level and the lowest detectable sound level is less than for normal-hearing listeners (NHLs). This primarily results from the fact that HILs have elevated thresholds and cannot detect low-level sounds. Despite threshold elevation, most HILs experience the same tolerability at high levels as NHLs. Therefore, the loudness function must be different for HILs than for NHLs. Two models have been proposed that can explain the reduction of dynamic range.

Recruitment

The primary assumption for the recruitment model is that loudness at threshold is the same for both HILs and NHLs. If loudness at threshold for a HIL is the same as for a NHL, then loudness functions must grow more steeply for HILs than NHLs in order for loudness to catch up at high levels.

Softness imperception

The primary assumption for the softness imperception model is that loudness at threshold is not the same for the HILs and NHLs. Softness imperception is based on the ideas that the loudness at threshold is higher for a HIL than for a NHL and the loudness function shows little-to-no compression at moderate levels, but otherwise is not steeper than the loudness function seen for NHLs.

Comparison

The recruitment model has traditionally been accepted as the foundation for algorithms used in hearing aids to adapt gain as function of level. Although softness imperception is a more recent concept and is less commonly implemented in hearing aid fits, many fitting procedures include gating such that low-level sounds are not amplified into the audible range. This fitting is compatible with the idea that low-level sounds amplified to audibility may be disconcertingly loud for HILs.

There is still significant debate regarding these two models (Florentine *et al.*, 2004; Moore, 2004) and some evidence supports the idea that some HILs exhibit recruitment, some exhibit softness imperception, and some exhibit an intermediate behaviour (see Marozeau and Florentine, 2007 for a review).

Figure 3.12 shows a variety of loudness models including: the power function (dashed) and INEX (star) for NHLs, and the recruitment (circle) and softness imperception (square) models for HILs. Note that the loudness function for HILs begins at a higher level because the listener has an elevated threshold. In the case of the recruitment HIL, loudness at threshold is the same as it is for a NHL and the function is steeper so that it can catch up in loudness. For the HIL with softness imperception, loudness at threshold is elevated. Although the function is never steeper than the maximum INEX steepness, this listener does not exhibit compression at moderate levels, so the function approaches the INEX loudness function at high levels. Around 80 dB SPL, all the functions show close to the same loudness and slope. If a listener exhibited a loudness function that exceeded normal loudness at high levels, this listener would be said to have hyperacusis.

3.7.2 **Hyperacusis**

Hyperacusis is an abnormal sensitivity to loudness. While it is typical for impaired listeners to have a reduced dynamic range of hearing resulting from elevations of their threshold, these impaired listeners typically have approximately the same sensitivity to high-level sounds as normal-hearing listeners. That is, their maximum tolerable level remains about 120 dB SPL. Those who experience hyperacusis have a reduction in tolerable sound level. Some listeners may experience discomfort for sounds as low in level as 65 dB SPL. Additionally, many of these

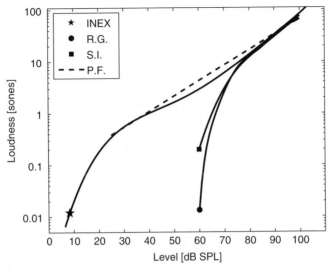

Fig. 3.12 A comparison of the power function (PF), INEX, rapid-growth recruitment (RG), and softness imperception (SI) loudness functions. Reprinted from Marozeau and Florentine (2007), with permission.

listeners also cope with elevated thresholds, so they may experience a substantially truncated dynamic range of hearing. Relatively little is know about the causes of hyperacusis, but it is often associated with traumatic noise exposure, tinnitus, drug reaction, neurological disease, or head injury (Katzenell and Segal, 2001; Nelson and Chen, 2004).

3.8 Conclusions

Perhaps the greatest limitation present in hearing aids and auditory prostheses is the inability to replicate the functions of the auditory system responsible for helping to provide the tremendous dynamic range of hearing as well as remarkable acuity within that range. Despite many years of scientific study, there is still much to ascertain about the processes used to encode the intensities of basic and complex sounds into both loudness and envelope-shape information. Models of loudness and intensity coding have gone from simple predictors relying on a single sound parameter to multistage processes based on many physical parameters of sound as well as the anatomy and physiology of the auditory system. Future mathematical models will perhaps incorporate more about the experience of listening: the context of sound, the syntax of sound, and the meaning of sound, as well as the condition of the listener: awareness, attention, and impairment aetiology. Despite nearly 150 years of study, the field of loudness still holds many mysteries.

References

Allen, J. B., Hall, J. L., and Seng, P. S. (1990). Loudness growth in 1/2-octave bands (LGOB)—a procedure for the assessment of loudness. *Journal of the Acoustical Society of America* **88**:745–53.

ANSI (2007). American National Standard Procedure for the Computation of Loudness of Steady Sounds. *ANSI* S3.4.

Anweiler, A. K. and Verhey, J. L. (2006). Spectral loudness summation for short and long signals as a function of level. *Journal of the Acoustical Society of America* **119**:2919–28.

Bapat, U. and Tolley, N. (2007). Temporary threshold shift due to recreational firearm use. *Journal of Laryngology and Otology* **121**:927–31.

Botte, M. C., Charron, S., and Bouayad, H. (1993). Temporary threshold and loudness shifts: frequency patterns and correlations. *Journal of the Acoustical Society of America* 93:1524–34.

Brand, T. and Hohmann, V. (2002). An adaptive procedure for categorical loudness scaling. *Journal of the Acoustical Society of America* 112:1597–604.

Buus, S. and Florentine, M. (2001). Modifications to the power function for loudness. In *Fechner Day 2001* (ed. E. Sommerfeld, R. Kompass, and T. Lachmann). Berlin: Pabst.

Buus, S. and Florentine, M. (2002). Growth of loudness in listeners with cochlear hearing losses: Recruitment reconsidered. *Journal of the Association for Research in Otolaryngology* 3:120–39.

Buus, S., Florentine, M., and Poulsen, T. (1997). Temporal integration of loudness, loudness discrimination, and the form of the loudness function. *Journal of the Acoustical Society of America* 101:669–80.

Carlyon, R. P. and Moore, B. C. J. (1984). Intensity discrimination: a severe departure from Weber's Law, *Journal of the Acoustical Society of America* 76:1369–76.

Cox, R. M., Alexander, G. C., Taylor, I. M., and Gray, G. A. (1997). The contour test of loudness perception. *Ear and Hearing* 18:388–400.

Elberling, C. (1999). Loudness scaling revisited. *Journal of the American Academy of Audiology* 10:248–60.

Elberling, C. and Nielsen, C. (1993). The dynamics of speech and the auditory dynamic range in sensorineural hearing impairment. In *Recent Developments in Hearing Instrument Technology; Proceedings of the 15th Danavox Symposium* (ed. J. Beilin and G. R. Jensen), pp. 99–133. Copenhagen: Stougard Jensen.

Epstein, M. (2007). An introduction to induced loudness reduction. *Journal of the Acoustical Society of America* 122:EL74–80.

Epstein, M. and Florentine, M. (2005a). Inferring basilar-membrane motion from tone-burst otoacoustic emissions and psychoacoustic measurements. *Journal of the Acoustical Society of America* 117:263–74.

Epstein, M. and Florentine, M. (2005b). A test of the Equal-Loudness-Ratio hypothesis using cross-modality matching functions. *Journal of the Acoustical Society of America* 118:907–13.

Epstein, M. and Florentine, M. (2006). Loudness of brief tones measured by magnitude estimation and loudness matching. *Journal of the Acoustical Society of America* 119:1943–5.

Fechner, G. T. (1860). *Elemente der Psychophysik*. Leipzig: Breitkopf und Heitel.

Feldtkeller, R., Zwicker, E., and Port, E. (1959). Lautstärke, erhältnislautheit und Summenlautheit. *Frequenz* 13:108–17.

Fletcher, H. and Munson, W. A. (1933). Loudness, its definition, measurement and calculation. *Journal of the Acoustical Society of America* 5:82–108.

Fletcher, H. and Steinberg, J. C. (1924). The dependence of the loudness of a complex sound upon the energy in the various frequency regions of the sound. *Physical Review* 24:306–17.

Florentine, M. and Epstein, M. (2006). To honor Stevens and repeal his law (for the auditory system). In *Fechner Day* (ed. D. E. Kornbrot, R. M. Msetfi, and A. W. MacRae). St. Albans, England: International Society for Psychophysics.

Florentine, M., Buus, S., and Mason, C. R. (1987). Level discrimination as a function of level for tones from 0.25 to 16 kHz. *Journal of the Acoustical Society of America* 81:1528–41.

Florentine, M., Buus, S., and Poulsen, T. (1996). Temporal integration of loudness as a function of level. *Journal of the Acoustical Society of America* 99:1633–44.

Florentine, M., Buus, S., and Rosenberg, M. (2004). Reaction-time data support the existence of softness imperception in cochlear hearing loss. In *Auditory Signal Processing: Physiology, Psychoacoustics, and Models* (ed. D. Pressnitzer, A. de Cheveigné, S. McAdams, and L. Collet). New York: Springer-Verlag.

Glasberg, B. R. and Moore, B. C. (2002). A model of loudness applicable to time-varying sounds. *Journal of the Audio Engineering Society* 50:331–42.

Green, D. M. (1988). *Profile Analysis*. Oxford: Oxford University Press.

Green, D. M. and Luce, R. D. (1974). Variability of magnitude estimates: A timing theory analysis. *Perception and Psychophysics* 15:291–300.

Harper, R. S. and Stevens, S. S. (1948). A psychological scale of weight and a formula for its derivation. *American Journal of Psychology* **61**:343–51.

Hellman, R. P. (1981). Stability of individual loudness functions obtained by magnitude estimation and production. *Perception and Psychophysics* **29**:63–70.

Hellman, R. P. (1991). Loudness scaling by magnitude scaling: Implications for intensity coding. In *Ratio Scaling of Psychological Magnitude: In Honor of the Memory of S. S. Stevens* (ed. G. A. Gescheider and S. J. Bolanowski). Hillsdale, NJ: Erlbaum.

Hellman, R. P. (1999). Cross-modality matching: A tool for measuring loudness in sensorineural impairment. *Ear and Hearing* **20**:193–213.

Hellman, R. P. and Meiselman, C. H. (1988). Prediction of individual loudness exponents from cross-modality matching. *Journal of Speech and Hearing Research* **31**:605–15.

Hellman, R. P. and Zwislocki, J. J. (1963). Monaural loudness function at 1000 cps and interaural summation. *Journal of the Acoustical Society of America* **35**:856–65.

Hellman, R. P., Takeshima, H., Suzuki, Y., Ozawa, K., and Sone, T. (2001). Determination of equal-loudness relations at high frequencies. In *Fechner Day 2001* (ed. E. Sommerfeld, R. Kompass, and T. Lachmann). Berlin: Pabst.

Hirsh, I. J. and Ward, W. D. (1952). Recovery of the auditory threshold after strong acoustic stimulation. *Journal of the Acoustical Society of America* **24**:131–41.

Hohmann, V. and Kollmeier, B. (1995). Weiterentwicklung und klinischer Einsatz der Hörfeldskalierung [Further development and use of hearing field scaling in clinics]. *Audiologische Akustik* **34**:48–59.

Howe, S. W. and Decker, T. N. (1984). Monaural and binaural auditory brainstem responses in relation to the psychophysical loudness growth function. *Journal of the Acoustical Society of America* **76**:787–93.

Katzenell, U. and Segal, S. (2001). Hyperacusis: review and clinical guidelines, *Otology and Neurotology* **22**:321–6; discussion 326–7.

Keidser, G., Seymour, J., Dillon, H., Grant, F., and Byrne, D. (1999). An efficient, adaptive method of measuring loudness growth functions. *Scandinavian Audiology* **28**:3–14.

Kiessling, J., Steffens, T., and Wagner, I. (1993). On the clinical applicability of loudness scaling. *Audiologische Akustik* **32**:100–15. [In German.]

Kiessling, J., Schubert, M., and Archut, A. (1996). Adaptive fitting of hearing instruments by category loudness scaling (ScalAdapt). *Scandinavian Audiology* **25**:153–60.

Krishnan, A. and Plack, C. J. (2009). Auditory brainstem correlates of basilar membrane nonlinearity in humans. *Audiology and Neuro-otology* **14**:88–97.

Launer, S. (1995). Loudness perception in listeners with sensorineural hearing impairment. Doctoral thesis, University of Oldenburg, Germany.

Leibold, L. J., Tan, H., Khaddam, S., and Jesteadt, W. (2007). Contributions of individual components to the overall loudness of a multitone complex. *Journal of the Acoustical Society of America* **121**:2822–31.

McGill, W. J. and Goldberg, J. P. (1968). A study of the near-miss involving Weber's law and pure-tone intensity discrimination. *Perception and Psychophysics* **4**:105–9.

Marozeau, J. and Florentine, M. (2007). Loudness growth in individual listeners with hearing losses: A review. *Journal of the Acoustical Society of America* **122**:EL81–87.

Marozeau, J., Epstein, M., Florentine, M., and Daley, B. (2006). A test of the binaural equal-loudness-ratio hypothesis for tones. *Journal of the Acoustical Society of America* **120**:3870–7.

Mauermann, M., Long, G. R., and Kollmeier, B. (2004). Fine structure of hearing threshold and loudness perception. *Journal of the Acoustical Society of America* **116**:1066–80.

Miller, G. A. (1947). Sensitivity to changes in the intensity of white noise and its relation to masking and loudness. *Journal of the Acoustical Society of America* **19**:609–19.

Moore, B. C. (2004). Testing the concept of softness imperception: loudness near threshold for hearing-impaired ears. *Journal of the Acoustical Society of America* **115**:3103–11.

Moore, B. C. J. and Glasberg, B. R. (2004). A revised model of loudness perception applied to cochlear hearing loss. *Hearing Research* **188**:70–88.

Moore, B. C. J. and Glasberg, B. R. (2007). Modeling binaural loudness. *Journal of the Acoustical Society of America* **121**:1604–12.

Moore, B. C. J. and Raab, D. H. (1974). Pure-tone intensity discrimination: some experiments relating to the near-miss to Weber's law. *Journal of the Acoustical Society of America* **55**:1049–54.

Muller, J. and Janssen, T. (2004). Similarity in loudness and distortion product otoacoustic emission input/output functions: implications for an objective hearing aid adjustment. *Journal of the Acoustical Society of America* **115**:3081–91.

Neely, S. T., Gorga, M. P., and Dorn, P. A. (2003). Cochlear compression estimates from measurements of distortion-product otoacoustic emissions. *Journal of the Acoustical Society of America* **114**:1499–507.

Nelson, J. J. and Chen, K. (2004). The relationship of tinnitus, hyperacusis, and hearing loss. *Ear, Nose, and Throat Journal* **83**:472–6.

Nuttall, A. L., Dolan, D. F., and Avinash, G. (1991). Laser Doppler velocimetry of basilar membrane vibration. *Hearing Research* **51**:203–13.

Oberfeld, D. (2007). Loudness changes induced by a proximal sound: Loudness enhancement, loudness recalibration, or both? *Journal of the Acoustical Society of America* **121**:2137–48.

Oxenham, A. J. and Plack, C. J. (1997). A behavioral measure of basilar-membrane nonlinearity in listeners with normal and impaired hearing. *Journal of the Acoustical Society of America* **101**:3666–75.

Pavel, M. and Inverson, G. J. (1981). Invariant characteristics of partial masking: implications for mathematical models. *Journal of the Acoustical Society of America* **69**:1126–31.

Plack, C. J. (2005). *The Sense of Hearing*. Mahwah, NJ: Erlbaum.

Plack, C. J., Gallun, F. J., Hafter, E. R., and Raimond, A. (2006). The detection of increments and decrements is not facilitated by abrupt onsets or offsets. *Journal of the Acoustical Society of America* **119**:3950–9.

Poulsen, T. (1981). Loudness of tone pulses in a free field. *Journal of the Acoustical Society of America* **69**:1786–90.

Poulton, E. C. (1989). *Bias in Quantifying Judgments*. Hillsdale, NJ: Erlbaum.

Pratt, H. and Sohmer, H. (1977). Correlations between psychophysical magnitude estimates and simultaneously obtained auditory nerve, brain stem and cortical responses to click stimuli in man. *Electroencephalography and Clinical Neurophysiology* **43**:802–12.

Rabinowitz, P. M. (2000). Noise-induced hearing loss. *American Family Physician* **61**:2749–56; 2759–60.

Ricketts, T. A. and Bentler, R. A. (1996). The effect of test signal type and bandwidth on the categorical scaling of loudness. *Journal of the Acoustical Society of America* **99**:2281–7.

Robinson, D. W. (1957). The subjective loudness scale. *Acustica* **7**:217–33.

Ruggero, M. A., Rich, N. C., Recio, A., Narayan, S. S., and Robles, L. (1997). Basilar-membrane responses to tones at the base of the chinchilla cochlea. *Journal of the Acoustical Society of America* **101**:2151–63.

Sadhra, S., Jackson, C. A., Ryder, T., and Brown, M. J. (2002). Noise exposure and hearing loss among student employees working in university entertainment venues, *Annals of Occupational Hygiene* **46**:455–63.

Scharf, B. (1959). Critical bands and the loudness of complex sounds near threshold. *Journal of the Acoustical Society of America* **33**:365–70.

Scharf, B. (1964). Partial masking. *Acustica* **14**:17–23.

Scharf, B. (1971). Patterns of partial masking. In *Proceedings of the 7th International Congress on Acoustics*, pp. 461–4. Budapest.

Scharf, B. (1983). Loudness adaptation. In *Hearing Research and Theory*, Vol. 2 (ed. J. V. Tobias and E. D. Schubert). New York: Academic.

Scharf, B. (1997). Loudness. In *Encyclopedia of Acoustics*, Vol. 3 (ed. M. J. Crocker). New York: Wiley.

Scharf, B. and Stevens, J. C. (1961). The form of the loudness function near threshold. In *Proceedings of the Third International Congress on Acoustics, Stuttgart, September 1959* (ed. L. Cremer). Amsterdam: Elsevier Publishing Company.

Scharf, B., Buus, S., and Nieder, B. (2002). Loudness enhancement: induced loudness reduction in disguise? *Journal of the Acoustical Society of America* 112:807–10.

Serpanos, Y. C., O'Malley, H., and Gravel, J. S. (1997). The relationship between loudness intensity functions and the click-ABR wave V latency. *Ear and Hearing* 18:409–19.

Stevens, S. S. (1936). A scale for the measurement of a psychological magnitude: loudness. *Psychological Review* 43:405–16.

Stevens, S. S. (1955). The measurement of loudness. *Journal of the Acoustical Society of America* 27:815–27.

Stevens, S. S. (1956). The direct estimation of sensory magnitudes-loudness. *American Journal of Psychology* 69:1–25.

Stevens, S. S. (1961). To honor Fechner and repeal his law. *Science* 13:80–6.

Stevens, S. S. (1975). *Psychophysics: Introduction to its Perceptual, Neural, and Social Prospects*. New York: Wiley.

Suzuki, Y. and Takeshima, H. (2004). Equal-loudness-level contours for pure tones. *Journal of the Acoustical Society of America* 116:918–33.

Teghtsoonian, M. and Teghtsoonian, R. (1983). Consistency of individual exponents in cross-modal matching. *Perception and Psychophysics* 33:203–14.

Verhey, J. and Kollmeier, B. (2002). Spectral loudness summation as a function of duration. *Journal of the Acoustical Society of America* 111:1349–58.

Viemeister, N. F. (1988). Intensity coding and the dynamic range problem, *Hearing Research* 34:267–74.

Viemeister, N. F. and Bacon, S. P. (1988). Intensity discrimination, increment detection, and magnitude estimation for 1-kHz tones. *Journal of the Acoustical Society of America* 84:172–8.

Wagner, E., Florentine, M., Buus, S., and McCormack, J. (2004). Spectral loudness summation and simple reaction time. *Journal of the Acoustical Society of America* 116:1681–6.

Zwicker, E. and Fastl, H. (1990). *Psychoacoustics–Facts and Models*. Berlin: Springer-Verlag.

Zwicker, E., Flottorp, G., and Stevens, S. S. (1957). Critical band width in loudness summation. *Journal of the Acoustical Society of America* 29:548–57.

Chapter 4

Pitch perception

Alain de Cheveigné

4.1 Introduction

Pitch is the stuff of which music is made. Melody, harmony, and tonality are either built upon pitch, or else they depend upon similar properties of the physical stimulus. In speech, pitch is a vector of prosody, and for tonal languages it also carries syllabic information. Pitch (or its physical correlate, periodicity) is important to perceptually segregate competing sound sources. Pitch and harmony have fascinated thinkers since antiquity and, for many early authors, to explain pitch amounted to explaining auditory perception.

For the psychoacoustician, pitch is the perceptual correlate of fundamental frequency (F0), that is, the rate at which a periodic waveform repeats itself. A periodic sound produces a pitch that depends on the period $T = 1/F0$: the shorter the period, the higher the pitch. The quantitative relation between period of vibration and notes of the musical scale was established early in the 17th century by Mersenne and Galileo (see de Cheveigné (2005) for a review). Recent work has been invested in mapping out the properties and limits of pitch perception (Plack and Oxenham, 2005), and probing the mechanisms by which the pitch percept emerges within the auditory system (Winter, 2005).

Stimuli may differ in amplitude, duration, spatial position, and spectral content, and nevertheless evoke the same pitch. Pitch is a many-to-one mapping from a high dimensional set of sounds to a percept that is unidimensional (in first approximation). Thus, a trained listener may accurately match a piano note to a pure tone, to a complex tone with high-order partials, or to an exotic binaural stimulus that sounds like a featureless 'shhhh' when listened to with one ear, but is distinctly pitch-like when listening with both ears (Cramer and Huggins, 1958). Pitch is the abstract quality common to these sounds. To understand pitch perception, we must explain not only our exquisite sensitivity to small changes along the physical dimension of period (or fundamental frequency), but also our ability to ignore enormous differences along other dimensions.

It is customary in psychoacoustics to distinguish *pure tones*, with a sinusoidal waveform and a single-component spectrum, from *complex tones* with a waveform that is arbitrarily shaped but nevertheless periodic, and a spectrum with multiple components that are harmonically related (i.e. all multiples of the same F0). Much past research on pitch has focused on pure tones under the belief that the percept that they evoke is somehow 'elementary'. Here we treat the pure tone as one among the many stimuli that may evoke a pitch. Some examples of pitch-evoking stimuli are illustrated in Fig. 4.1.

4.2 What is pitch?

In 1960 the American Standards Association defined pitch as 'that attribute of auditory sensation in terms of which sounds may be ordered on a musical scale' (ASA, 1960), a definition that suggests a percept with extent along a linear perceptual dimension. The concept of 'dimension' carries the idea that diverse sounds may map to the same point along this dimension. Indeed, notes

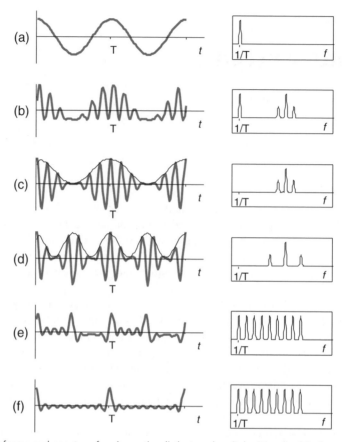

Fig. 4.1 Waveforms and spectra of various stimuli that evoke pitch. Stimuli with the same period tend to evoke the same pitch despite their different amplitude, duration, spectra, or spatial characteristics. (a) Pure tone; (b) complex tone made up of the fundamental and three higher harmonics; (c) same, without the fundamental; (d) same, with partials spaced by twice the F0; (e) complex made up of 9 partials in alternating sine/cosine phase; (f) same, in cosine phase. The stimuli in (c) and (d) can be described as the result of modulating a carrier of frequency $f = 7/T$ by a more slowly varying *temporal envelope* (thin line). The frequency of the temporal envelope is equal to the spacing of the partials, whereas the fundamental frequency $F0 = 1/T$ is equal to the largest common divisor of the partial frequencies. For some stimuli, pitch may follow the period of the temporal envelope, rather than the true fundamental, i.e. tones as in (d) (and also (e)) may sound an octave higher than expected based on their F0. In the spectral domain, the *spectral envelope* is a smooth function of frequency that describes the amplitude of the partials. The spectral envelope mainly determines the timbre.

produced on different instruments may have distinct timbres but the same pitch. A more recent version of the standard (ANSI, 1994) added that pitches are ordered from *low to high*, suggesting a vertical orientation for this dimension. Whether this orientation is universal or cultural is a matter of debate (e.g. Rusconi *et al.*, 2006), but in our culture it fits the vertical axis of a musical score or a spectrogram.

In music, pitch usually varies over time. Every new note of a melody evokes a percept that depends to some extent on the physical characteristics of that note, but also on the note that precedes it.

Indeed, it may seem that our perception of melodic pitch is determined by *intervals* between notes rather than, or in addition to, the notes themselves. More generally, the musical effect of each new note depends strongly on its context (Bigand and Tillmann, 2005), a property that is not quite captured by the ANSI definitions, or indeed, by most psychoacoustic accounts of pitch.

To a first approximation, equal *ratios* of frequency produce pitch steps of equal salience, as if pitch were a logarithmic function of frequency. However, the relation between notes on the scale is also governed by complex rules of harmony, also not captured by the standard definition of pitch. For example, notes an octave apart are perceptually similar, and in some cases interchangeable. They are said to share the same *chroma*. Chroma is an equivalence relation: multiple notes map to the same chroma. The similarity between two notes depends in part on their proximity along a logarithmic frequency scale, and in part on their chroma.

To capture this property, more complex geometrical models of pitch have been proposed, such as a helix with a linear axis that fits the standard 'low-to-high' dimension of pitch height, and a circular dimension of chroma (Bachem, 1950; Ueda and Ohgushi, 1987; Giangrande *et al.*, 2003). Yet more complex structures such as toroids have been proposed to incorporate additional tonal relations such as fifths (Shepard, 1982). However it has been argued that they may reflect less the perceptual structure of pitch than the harmonic spectra of most European instrumental sounds (Burns, 1981; Sethares, 1997). In any case, the fixed nodes of such a structure cannot capture the dynamic effects noted earlier, such as determined by the order in which two notes appear (Giangrande *et al.*, 2003; Bigand and Tillmann, 2005).

A fascinating aspect of pitch perception is inter-individual variability. Discrimination thresholds vary between individuals over several orders of magnitude. Thresholds improve considerably with training (Demany and Semal 2002; Micheyl *et al.*, 2006a), and thus experience may account for some differences between listeners. Genetic factors may also contribute (Drayna *et al.*, 2001; Douglas and Bilkey 2007), and there are hints that the phenomenology of pitch may actually differ among people. For example, Semal and Demany (2006) found that most subjects can judge the direction of a pitch change (high to low or vice versa) as soon as it is detectable, but other subjects found it impossible to say which note is higher, for a pitch difference that they nevertheless could detect with ease.

Absolute pitch is the relatively rare capability to assign labels to pitches regardless of context (Ward 1999; Zatorre, 2003; Levitin and Rogers 2005; Hsieh and Saberi 2007). Most listeners possess instead *relative pitch*, the ability to judge the pitch of a note relative to a preceding note. This question is interesting because the two forms of pitch imply rather different mechanisms. For example, most models of pitch easily account for absolute pitch but not relative pitch. Something else is required for relative pitch, and as both types of pitch exist, the brain must be capable of both.

To summarize, pitch is a very important aspect of sound perception. We can discriminate exquisitely small differences in pitch, while ignoring salient differences along other perceptual dimensions. Pitch has more to it than the simple, one-dimensional construct assumed by psychophysics, and yet we have few models to account for these complexities. That so much is yet unknown about pitch is sobering for those of us who have been working on it for years, and exhilarating for whoever sets out to search for more: there's lots more to discover!

4.3 **The limits of pitch**

Periodic stimuli evoke pitch over a very wide range of their parameters: F0, amplitude, duration, spectral envelope, etc. Pitch is exquisitely sensitive to the first parameter (F0), and yet remarkably *stable* over large variations of the others, variations that themselves may produce salient changes in loudness, subjective duration, or timbre. Stimuli that are only approximately periodic may also evoke a pitch (inharmonic complexes, stimuli in noise), and the same may occur for stimuli that are, strictly speaking, not periodic at all, such as amplitude-modulated noise or binaurally correlated noise. Conversely, a periodic stimulus may fail to evoke a pitch if its parameters fall outside certain bounds that delimit the *region of existence* of pitch.

Musical pitch arises if the F0 is within a range of about 30 Hz to 5000 Hz. At the lower end of the scale, Pressnitzer *et al.*, (2001) found that subjects failed to detect a one-semitone mistuning in a four-note chromatic melody if its lowest note fell below 30 Hz (33 ms). Periodicity can be detected, and the period discriminated, for longer periods up to several seconds, but the percept is not 'musical' and discrimination thresholds are large (Warren *et al.*, 1980; Kaernbach, 1993). Thresholds improve by an order of magnitude as F0 increases from 16 Hz to 64 Hz (Krumbholz *et al.*, 2000). At the other end of the scale, stimuli lose their musical properties beyond about 5 kHz (Bachem, 1948; Semal and Demany, 1990). The limit is rather sharp (subjects report a 'highest musical note') but it is subject- (and even ear-) dependent. Burns (1983) nevertheless found that some subjects performed above chance on musical tasks at frequencies of 10 kHz or beyond.

Difference limens for pure tones (expressed as a proportional change in frequency) are smallest at around 1–2 kHz (about 0.2% for good subjects) but they increase abruptly as frequency exceeds 4 kHz (Moore, 1973) (see Fig. 4.2). The interval from 30 Hz to 4000 Hz spans about seven octaves and includes the range of most musical instruments.

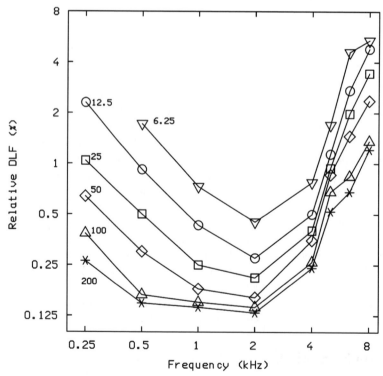

Fig. 4.2 Frequency difference limens (smallest detectable relative frequency difference) for pure tones. Each curve is for a different stimulus duration (in ms). Discrimination is best for frequencies near 2 kHz and degrades rapidly above 4 kHz. Discrimination is better for longer durations. From Moore (1973) with permission.

Pitch changes remarkably little with level. The frequency of a pure tone can be discriminated, presumably on the basis of pitch, as soon as it is detectable (Pollack, 1947; Cardozo, 1974; Gockel et al., 2006). Indeed, pitch may be the cue that allows us to detect a tone in noise (Moore, 1981; Carney et al., 2002). Frequency discrimination is less good at low levels (e.g. Wier et al., 1977) or high levels (e.g. Bernstein and Oxenham, 2006), but the value of the pitch changes with level by at most a few percent for pure tones, and even less for complex tones (Hartmann, 1997). This is remarkable in the face of the strong level-dependency of several physiological responses to sound that have been considered as candidate substrates for pitch perception (Winter, 2005).

Frequency discrimination is possible for stimuli as short as one or two cycles (Mark and Rattay, 1990), although at such short durations it is uncertain whether discrimination is based on pitch or timbre changes (Hartmann et al., 1985). A clear tonal percept requires a longer stimulus (Mark and Rattay, 1990; Robinson and Patterson, 1995). For very short stimuli, the value of the pitch may differ according to the duration, or the shape of the temporal envelope, but the differences are no more than a few percent (Hartmann, 1978; Hartmann et al., 1985). As stimuli are made longer, frequency discrimination becomes more accurate (Moore, 1973; White and Plack, 2003; Gockel et al., 2007; Hsieh and Saberi, 2007) (Fig. 4.2).

For stimuli with only low-order harmonics, differences in their relative phase are imperceptible, as stated by Ohm's acoustic law. With higher harmonics (closer spaced relative to their frequencies), phase may affect the *timbre* of the stimulus, but usually not the value of its pitch. Phase may, however, affect the *salience* of the pitch, and it may also change the relative weight of competing pitch candidates in stimuli with ambiguous pitch. For example, the pitch of a stimulus with closely spaced partials may be one octave higher if phases alternate between sine and cosine (as illustrated in Fig. 4.1(e)), than if they are all sine or all cosine (as illustrated in Fig. 4.1(f)). In a few rare situations one may observe small phase-dependent shifts of the value of the pitch (Plomp, 1967b; Pressnitzer et al., 2002).

Pitch is evoked by many periodic stimuli, with very different spectra, but not all: some periodic stimuli evoke a pitch that is weak or absent. The stimulus parameter space has many dimensions, and therefore it is not straightforward to map the limits of the existence region. Roughly speaking, a complex tone may fail to evoke a pitch if: (1) its period is too long (Pressnitzer et al., 2001), or (2) the *rank* of its lowest harmonic is too high, or (3), the *frequency* of its lowest harmonic is too high. These limits depend somewhat on the total number of harmonics within the stimulus: they are narrower for two adjacent harmonics (Smoorenburg, 1970) than for three harmonics (Ritsma, 1962, 1963) or more. There are also interactions between parameters, for example musical pitch extends to a lower F0 (30 Hz) for a wideband stimulus than for a 3200-Hz, high-pass stimulus (270 Hz) (Fig. 4.3) (Pressnitzer et al., 2001).

Tones with the same period but different spectral envelopes usually evoke the same pitch, despite large timbre differences. It is nevertheless more difficult to match the pitches of stimuli that occupy distinct rather than overlapping spectral regions (Micheyl and Oxenham, 2004). Such is notably the case when a pure tone is matched to a complex tone (Moore et al., 1992). This difficulty might be due to perceptual interference from the salient difference in timbre, or it might result from the lack of overlap within an internal tonotopically organized representation of stimuli, or both.

For wideband stimuli, with partials spread over a wide frequency range, the various spectral regions carry unequal weight. One way to reveal this is to mistune the frequency of one partial of the complex and observe the shift in the overall pitch. This effect is appreciable only if the partial falls within the *dominant region*. The extent of this region depends on the F0: below 50 Hz partials beyond the 6th are dominant (Moore et al., 2007), above 1400 Hz the fundamental is dominant, and in the intermediate range the dominant partials are usually between 2 and 6 but with considerable interindividual differences (Plomp, 1967a; Moore et al., 1985b).

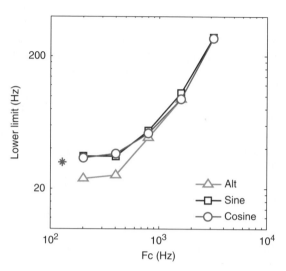

Fig. 4.3 The lower limit of melodic pitch as a function of the frequency of the lowest partial (Fc) and for different phase relationships: sine, cosine, and alternating sine and cosine (alt). The asterisk is for wideband cosine phase stimuli (click trains). Mean of three subjects. Replotted from Pressnitzer *et al.* (2001).

Pitch may be evoked by stimuli that are only imperfectly periodic such as 'iterated rippled noise', IRN. IRN is obtained by delaying a segment of white noise repeatedly, and adding together the delayed and non-delayed waveforms (Yost, 1996; Hartmann, 1997—Chapter 15). Pitch may also arise with stimuli that are, strictly speaking, aperiodic such as amplitude-modulated white noise (Burns and Viemeister, 1976). It is as if the auditory system searches for the best periodic approximation to the stimulus, according to some metric that tolerates various forms of mismatch. The same stimulus might allow multiple matches, in which case its pitch may be ambiguous. For example, a complex tone with a narrow spectral peak or 'formant' (Fig. 4.1(c)) may evoke a pitch that fits that peak. This high pitch, corresponding to the formant, may compete with the low pitch corresponding to the F0, particularly if the F0 is relatively low and constant, and the frequency of the spectral peak varies. This effect is exploited in overtone singing (Bloothooft *et al.*, 1992).

To summarize, pitch may be evoked by a very wide range of stimuli. Pitch depends mainly on the period (1/F0) and is remarkably insensitive to changes along other stimulus dimensions that provoke salient changes in qualities other than pitch. A very wide range of different stimuli map to the same pitch. This is possibly the hardest to explain: how does the auditory system perform tasks that require accurate discrimination using pitch, while ignoring the very salient effects of differences along other stimulus dimensions? Pitch theories need to explain both the accuracy and the constancy of pitch perception.

4.4 **The pure tone**

Much of the psychoacoustics of pitch has been established using pure-tone stimuli with sinusoidal waveforms (Fig. 4.1(a)). A pure tone evokes a pitch similar to other periodic stimuli of the same period (e.g. Fig. 4.1(b–f)). However, two things make pure tones 'special', and set them apart from stimuli with complex spectra. The first is their special status for the physics and mathematics of sounds. The second is that a pure tone produces essentially the same shape of vibration at every point of the cochlea, albeit with different amplitude and phase.

Sinusoids (more precisely: complex exponentials) are eigenvectors of linear transforms. This means that a pure tone remains a pure tone after propagation through air, reflection from obstacles, or mechanical transmission within the ear. The amplitude and phase of the waveform may be affected by the filtering involved, but it retains a sinusoidal shape, and its frequency remains the same. Furthermore, according to Fourier's theorem any waveform may be decomposed into a sum of such sinusoids. Sinusoids are not the only functions to allow such a decomposition, but their mathematical properties make them a good basis of 'elementary waveforms' from which other waveforms can be built.

It is tempting to assume that, just like a complex stimulus is a sum of sinusoids, the percept that it evokes too is the sum of *elementary percepts* evoked by its sinusoidal components. If this were the case psychophysics would be very much simplified indeed: we would only need to study effects of pure tones to predict the effect of a stimulus of arbitrary complexity. To some extent, psychoacoustics has progressed on the basis of this assumption, witness the large proportion of studies involving pure tones. The idea was inspired by the intense development of harmonic analysis between the 17th and 19th centuries that culminated in Fourier's theorem, that Ohm (1843) and Helmholtz (1877) extended to the sensory domain (de Cheveigné, 2005; Darrigol, 2007). The same idea is embodied in the 'virtual pitch' theory of Terhardt (1974, 1979), according to which the pitch of a complex tone is composed from 'spectral pitches' evoked by its partials.

Unfortunately, there is little to support this idea. Introspection tells us that the percept evoked by a complex tone differs radically from the percepts evoked by its sinusoidal parts in isolation. It requires some faith to believe that one is *composed* of the others. True, we can sometimes focus our attention and 'hear out' an individual partial, but this requires skill and training, and it succeeds only in particular situations. The issue of hearing out multiple pitches is addressed in Section 4.6.

Anticipating that discussion, note that a complex tone causes different parts of the cochlea to vibrate with different waveforms depending on which stimulus components are reinforced by cochlear filtering (see Fig. 4.4 in Section 4.7 below). In particular, some channels may respond mostly to a single resolved partial (e.g. 3rd harmonic in Fig. 4.4). If we suppose that attention can be focused on that subset of cochlear channels, it may be possible to hear out the partial as originally reported by Mersenne (1636), or instead possibly a 'residue' of unresolved partials described by Schouten (1940). In the case of a pure tone, however, all parts of the cochlea respond with the same waveform, so attending to a subset of channels should not produce a different percept. Pure tones are 'pure' in the sense that they cannot be partitioned in this way, not in the sense that the percepts that they evoke compose those of complex sounds. Studies that use pure-tone stimuli are informative for those particular stimuli, and by extension for the wider class of periodic stimuli that they belong to, but they do not really probe the 'elements' of the perception of sound.

The value of the pitch of an arbitrary stimulus has been defined as the frequency of the pure tone to which it can be matched (Hartmann, 1997). This provides a convenient means to quantify pitch. However, the pitch of a pure tone varies with sound level and across ears (Burns, 1982), at low frequencies a pure tone must have a high amplitude to compensate for the high-pass characteristics of the middle ear (this may introduce distortion products), and for F0s below 2 kHz frequency discrimination is less accurate for pure than for complex tones (Henning and Grosberg, 1968). The presence of noise induces pitch shifts that tend to be larger for pure tones than complex tones (Houtsma, 1981). For all these reasons, it would make sense to replace the pure-tone standard by a complex tone standard, for example a click train.

Studies that use only pure tones do not probe the property of invariance across stimuli with different spectral content. This is a concern for physiological and brain imaging studies, as it may be uncertain that a response reflects pitch rather than some other correlate of stimulus manipulation.

To summarize, pure-tone stimuli are illustrative of a wider class of pitch-evoking stimuli, but there is little reason to think that the percept evoked by a complex sound is *composed* of the percepts evoked by each of its sinusoidal components. Studies that aim to establish that a response reflects pitch need to use a wider range of stimuli.

4.5 **The missing fundamental**

Rarely has a paradox provoked such a long-lasting and heated debate. The pitch evoked by a pure tone remains the same if we add additional tones with frequencies that are integer multiples of that of the original pure tone (harmonics). It also does not change if we then remove the original pure tone (the fundamental): this is the 'paradox' of the missing fundamental. At issue is whether, and how, a periodic tone that lacks a sinusoidal component at its F0 can evoke a pitch. Concerning the stimulus itself there is no paradox: Fourier's theorem states that a periodic waveform is composed of sinusoids with frequencies that are integer multiples of F0, but it does not say that they must *all* be present. Compare, for example, the waveforms of Fig. 4.1(b) and Fig. 4.1(c): both are clearly periodic. Concerning the percept, the paradox vanishes if one accepts that pitch is associated with the *periodicity* of the stimulus. The paradox appears only if we insist that pitch requires the presence of a sinusoidal fundamental component.

The psychophysics is quite clear: the presence of a fundamental component is not required for pitch. This was established already in the 19th century by Seebeck, who synthesized stimuli where the fundamental was weak or absent (de Boer, 1976; Turner, 1977). It was confirmed by Schouten (1938) who addressed the issue of a possible distortion product (created within the apparatus or within the ear) by adding to the stimulus a sinusoidal component with carefully controlled amplitude and phase to cancel any remaining energy at the F0. Licklider (1954) corroborated his conclusion by adding low-pass noise to mask any distortion products, and this has since been replicated in hundreds of studies. There is little support for Ohm's dogma, according to which pitch requires a sinusoidal component at the fundamental.

In spite of all this evidence, there is a reluctance to abandon this idea. The observation of fundamental components in the analysis of physiological recordings (where they arise naturally as the result of non-linearities), or the demonstration that relatively high-amplitude distortion products may arise in the ear (Pressnitzer and Patterson, 2001), keep alive the suspicion that the fundamental might sneak into the ear unnoticed. However the most potent reason to retain Helmholtz's picture of the ear as a Fourier analyzer is that it is too attractive to abandon. The missing fundamental will be with us for some time.

4.6 **Hearing out pitch**

We are adept at *hearing out* sounds, for example a faint voice among the sounds of a forest, or the melodic line of an instrument within the orchestra. We usually study pitch in relation to the acoustic waveform, but in real life it often emerges from a fraction of the stimulus, the rest constituting a masker to be ignored. The masker itself may include one or more pitch-evoking sources, as in music when several instruments play at the same time. In order to hear each pitch, the ear must overcome masking from the energy of the competing sounds ('energetic masking'), and also ignore the percepts that those sounds evoke ('informational masking'). This is an example of the process of Auditory Scene Analysis (Bregman, 1990) by which we parse an acoustic scene and attend to its parts. There are large interindividual differences in the susceptibility to informational masking, musicians being more adept at focusing on a frequency range than non-musicians (Oxenham *et al.*, 2003).

Despite its obvious musical relevance, the psychoacoustics of competing pitches is surprisingly sparse (Beerends and Houtsma, 1989; Carlyon, 1996a; Assmann and Paschall, 1998; Micheyl *et al.*, 2006b). If several partials of a tone dominate part of the spectrum, such that they are resolved by at least some cochlear channels, the ear may be able to focus on that tone and ignore the others. For example, in polyphonic music, the spectrotemporal envelope of one voice may have 'windows' of low energy within which the other voices may be glimpsed in this way. However, experiments have shown that concurrent tone pairs that overlap in both frequency and time may also evoke salient pitches, as long as their partials are sufficiently spaced to be *resolvable* by coch-lear filtering (Carlyon, 1996a; Micheyl *et al.*, 2006b). In contrast, if two tones contain only unre-solved partials, mixing them gives rise to a noise-like sound or 'crackle' (Carlyon, 1996a) unless one is stronger than the other, in which case only one pitch is heard (Micheyl *et al.*, 2006b). The concept of resolvability is discussed in more detail in Section 4.7. In summary, it is often possible to hear out a pitch from a background of interfering sounds, some of which may themselves evoke a pitch.

Pitch is nevertheless degraded by sounds presented simultaneously, or even sequentially in close temporal proximity. Presenting temporal 'fringes' before or after a stimulus degrades dis-crimination (Carlyon, 1996b; Micheyl and Carlyon, 1998), apparently because information from the fringes leaks into the integration window that sums pitch information over time. Likewise, a distractor tone presented simultaneously in a remote frequency region produces what is known as 'pitch discrimination interference' (Gockel *et al.*, 2004; Micheyl and Oxenham, 2007). The degree of interference depends on both *spectral proximity* and *pitch similarity*, suggesting that interference may occur at two stages: within a tonotopically organized, low-level representation of the signal, and within a higher level representation of pitch (or yet higher levels such as atten-tion, etc.).

If the masker is a noise band that overlaps the target in time and frequency region, the pitch of the target may be discriminable as soon as the target is detectable (Moore and Glasberg, 1991; Gockel *et al.*, 2006; Micheyl *et al.*, 2006b). It is as if the cue for detecting the tone within noise were pitch. In contrast, if the masker is a complex tone, the detection threshold is about 15–25 dB *below* the level at which the target's pitch can be discriminated (Micheyl *et al.*, 2006b). The detec-tion cue here is more likely the disruption of the tonal percept evoked by the masker. These phe-nomena are of interest because they may shed light on how pitch is extracted and represented within the auditory system.

Perhaps the earliest report of multiple pitches within the same sound is that of Mersenne (1636), who heard, within the sound of a plucked string, 'at least five sounds' corresponding to the fundamental and first few harmonics. Hearing out partials requires concentration and train-ing: Sauveur (1701) recommended listening at night, while Helmholtz (1877) relied on special resonators that he designed to enhance the partials. The task is easier for harmonics of low rather than high rank. Estimates of the highest audible partial vary according to the method employed, ranging from the 5th to 8th (Plomp, 1964) or the 9th to 11th (Bernstein and Oxenham, 2003). They are roughly consistent with the hypothesis that a partial may be heard out if the distance from its closest neighbor is greater than about 1.25 ERB (Moore and Ohgushi, 1993; Moore *et al.*, 2006) (the equivalent rectangular bandwidth, ERB, is a measure of cochlear filter width, Moore and Glasberg, 1983). Hearing out partials is easier for tones of long rather than short duration (Gockel *et al.*, 2007). It is also easier if the partial is mistuned from the harmonic series, or amplitude-modulated, or turned on later than the rest of the complex tone (Peters *et al.*, 1983; Moore *et al.*, 1985a; Hartmann and Doty, 1996; Bernstein and Oxenham, 2003; Hartmann and Goupell, 2006).

Although partials of a complex may be heard out with effort and attention, they are rarely sali-ent spontaneously unless enhanced by some spectral or temporal irregularity (Bernstein and Oxenham, 2003; Hartmann and Goupell, 2006). Listeners differ in their propensity to listen to a complex tone as a whole ('synthetic listening') or as composed of parts ('analytic listening') (Smoorenburg, 1970; Laguitton *et al.*, 1998). Audibility of partials inspired the doctrine accord-ing to which the percept of a complex tone is composed of the percepts of its partials, but an alternative interpretation is that the ear, being adept at hearing out weak sounds within a background, can sometimes perform this feat with the partials that compose a complex tone.

4.7 **Resolvability**

An important concept, already mentioned, is *resolvability*, the ability of cochlear filtering to isolate individual partials of a complex sound. A partial is resolved if it is sufficiently remote in frequency from other partials so that it dominates the response of at least some cochlear filters. By extension, a complex stimulus is said to be 'resolved' if it contains at least some resolved partials (and 'unresolved' if it contains none). Figure 4.4 illustrates the concept for a 30-component complex tone with a 100 Hz fundamental. Each of the lowest 3–5 partials dominates the output of a few filters, near the apex of the cochlea. The output of these filters is quasi-sinusoidal at the frequency of the partial (Fig. 4.4, bottom left): these partials are resolved. Partials of higher rank are less well isolated: the best filter contains a large proportion of power from other components, and the output waveform is more strongly modulated and less sinusoidal (Fig. 4.4, bottom right). Partials such as these are unresolved. As an aside, we note that the uppermost partial is comparatively well isolated, which might account for the relatively salient pitch of the highest partial of such a complex (Moore *et al.*, 2006).

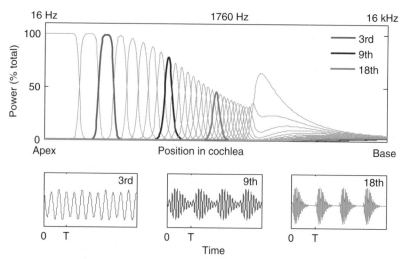

Fig. 4.4 Resolvability of harmonics of a complex tone. Top: percentage of power for each harmonic of a 30-component complex tone at the output of cochlear filters, plotted as a function of their position along the cochlea. The apex of the cochlea is tuned to low frequencies (left) and the base to high frequencies (right). Bottom: waveforms at the output of filters tuned to the 3rd harmonic, 9th harmonic, and 18th harmonic. Each of the lower harmonics is isolated within a set of filters near the apex of the cochlea (left of upper plot). The output of these filters is quasi-sinusoidal (bottom left): the lower harmonics are 'resolved'. Each of the higher harmonics excites a narrower range of filters (middle and right of upper plot). Outputs of these filters are 'pulsatile', indicating that the filters respond to more than one harmonic: higher harmonics are 'unresolved'. The cochlea is modeled here as a bank of linear 4th-order gammatone filters uniformly spaced in terms of equivalent rectangular bandwidth (ERB; Moore and Glasberg, 1983), which is roughly equivalent to uniform spacing along the cochlea.

Resolvability determines, in part, whether partials of a complex tone can be 'heard out'. It also seems to play a role in the pitch of the complex as a whole: stimuli with one or more resolved partials tend to have a strong pitch, while those with only unresolved partials have a weak pitch. This is puzzling because unresolved partials produce beats along the basilar membrane at the F0, and one might expect this to be a clear cue to pitch. Instead, partials of low rank dominate the pitch of a complex. For example, mistuning those partials affects the pitch of the complex (Plomp, 1967a; Moore *et al.*, 1985b), and F0 discrimination thresholds are an order of magnitude smaller if the stimulus contain partials below about the 10th (Fig. 4.5) (Houtsma and Smurzynksi, 1990; Shackleton and Carlyon, 1994; Plack and Carlyon, 1995; Bernstein and Oxenham, 2003) than if it does not. Accurate discrimination requires longer stimuli for unresolved than resolved partials (White and Plack, 2003). The ability to hear the pitches of concurrent complex tones is limited to tones with resolved partials: mixtures of unresolved tones evoke a crackling sound (Carlyon, 1996a). All these phenomena hint at a role for resolvability in pitch.

The contrast between performance for resolved- and unresolved-partial stimuli has led to the hypothesis that their pitches are processed by different mechanisms: *pattern matching* for resolved, and *autocorrelation* for unresolved (see Section 4.9). This necessarily implies also a third mechanism to translate between the two. Indeed, degraded performance in comparing pitch between resolved and unresolved stimuli has been taken as evidence of a translation cost between pitch mechanisms (Carlyon and Shackleton, 1994).

However, several results do not fit with this interpretation: (1) Moore *et al.* (2007) found for F0s of 35 and 50 Hz that partials with ranks greater than 6 (presumably *unresolved* at those F0s)

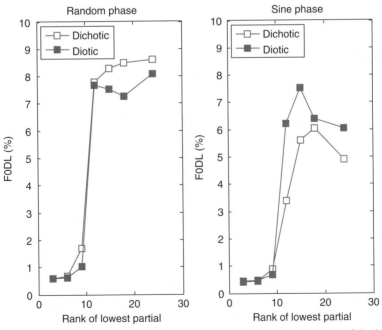

Fig. 4.5 F0 difference limens for a 200-Hz complex tone as a function of the rank of the lowest partial. Phases were either random (left) or sine (right). In the 'diotic' condition (full markers) all partials were presented to both ears. In the 'dichotic' condition (open markers) partials of odd rank were presented to one ear, and partials of even rank to the other ear. Average of four subjects, replotted from Bernstein and Oxenham (2003).

dominated the pitch of the complex. This suggests that dominance may depend on a factor other than resolvability. (2) The lower limit of melodic pitch does not coincide with the limit of resolvability: tones that lack any resolved partial may nevertheless evoke a pitch that supports melody (Pressnitzer et al., 2001). (3) Bernstein and Oxenham (2003, 2008) found that the deterioration of discrimination thresholds beyond the 10th partial occurred regardless of whether all partials were presented to the same ear (in which case they were too closely spaced to be resolved) or else partials of even and odd rank were distributed to opposite ears (in which case their spacing is doubled, so that partials up to the 20th should be resolved according to their criteria) (Fig. 4.5). Peripheral resolvability is therefore not the factor that determines accurate pitch. (4) It was said earlier that complex tones that are mixed together each evoke a pitch only if they contain resolved partials. However, the meaning of 'resolved' in that context applied to the complex tones *in isolation*, before mixing. Obviously after mixing, the partials may no longer be resolved. The pitches may nevertheless be salient, so resolvability of partials *within the stimulus* is not crucial (Micheyl et al., 2006b). (5) Finally, Micheyl and Oxenham (2004) reexamined the issue of a putative translation cost between distinct pitch mechanisms for resolved and unresolved stimuli, and concluded that there is none (see also Gockel et al., 2004 and Micheyl and Oxenham, 2005). All these results suggest that peripheral resolvability *per se* is not what determines the salience of the pitch of a complex tone.

To summarize, stimuli with partials of low rank may evoke a pitch that is more salient and accurately discriminable than stimuli that only contain partials of high rank. This is often attributed to differences in resolvability of partials within the complex tones, but this interpretation does not fit some aspects of the data, and other interpretations have been proposed, such as that the duration of internal delays varies according to cochlear filter characteristic frequency (Moore, 1982; Bernstein and Oxenham, 2005; de Cheveigné and Pressnitzer, 2006). The debate is of importance to decide which strategies are used to hear pitch (Section 4.9).

4.8 **Binaural pitch**

Our ears sample the acoustic field in two points, and this helps us to localize sounds and make sense of complex acoustic scenes. Certain pitch phenomena require binaural interaction, and binaural hearing and pitch may actually have something in common. Both seem to be based on temporal cues analyzed within the brain, and two influential models of sound localization (Jeffress, 1948) and pitch (Licklider, 1951) both postulate neural processing based on time delays and coincidence counting. Experimentally, binaural stimulation adds a degree of freedom that may help us locate the site of pitch extraction within the brain.

Fascinating among auditory phenomena is *Huggins pitch*, which arises while listening with two ears to a binaural stimulus that sounds like noise when listened to with either ear alone (Cramer and Huggins, 1958; Culling, 1999). Huggins pitch is one of several binaurally created pitch phenomena (see Culling et al., 1998 for a review). The stimulus consists of white noise that is identical at the two ears except for a narrow frequency region for which noise is decorrelated between the two ears (for example, the noise in one ear may undergo a phase transition of 2π over this frequency region) (Fig. 4.6). The percept resembles that of a narrowly filtered band of noise, embedded within a wideband noise background. Relatively faint, it nevertheless supports accurate matching (Hartmann, 1993). It becomes stronger if multiple transitions occur at frequencies that follow a harmonic series, forming a 'Huggins complex tone' (Bilsen, 1976). Huggins pitch supports melody (Akeroyd et al., 2001), and streaming effects similar to those produced by pure tones (Akeroyd et al., 2005). Huggins pitch necessarily arises from the interaction of neural patterns from the two ears, and this puts a constraint on the locus of pitch extraction (see Section 4.10 below).

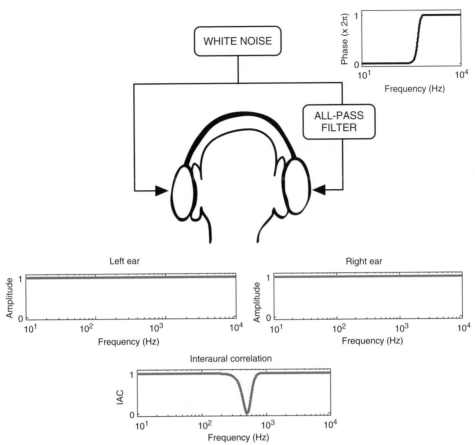

Fig. 4.6 Huggins pitch is obtained by presenting white noise to both ears. The noises at both ears are identical apart from a narrow phase transition created by an all-pass filter in the pathway to one ear. Interaural correlation is high, except at the frequency of the phase transition. The pitch matches this frequency.

Houtsma and Goldstein (1972) presented musically trained subjects with pairs of partials that formed 'complex tones' with an F0 determined by the largest common divisor of their frequencies. They successfully performed an interval recognition task, showing that they could hear a low pitch related to this F0, regardless of whether the partials were sent both to the same or to different ears. This is a second example of central formation of pitch from information from both ears. Listening to either ear alone, one hears only a single partial and not the low pitch.

Binaural interactions can create pitch, but they can also weaken it. In a study mentioned earlier (Section 4.7), Bernstein and Oxenham (2003) found that F0 discrimination thresholds of complex tones increased by an order of magnitude when the rank of the lowest harmonic was increased from the 9th to the 12th (Fig. 4.5). Interestingly, the same occurred when all harmonics went to both ears (diotic condition), or even and odd harmonics to opposite ears (dichotic condition). A complex with even harmonics of F0 starting from the 12th is identical to a complex with all harmonics of 2 F0 starting from the 6th. Listening to that ear alone should therefore give a *low* threshold. The fact that thresholds were instead high implies that the subjects could not shut off the contribution of the other ear. Surprisingly, the additional information from the odd harmonics within the other ear was deleterious rather than useful.

With a slightly different paradigm, in which stimuli were sent to the same ear within blocks, rather than to opposite ears on each trial as in their previous study, Bernstein and Oxenham (2008) did find a benefit of binaural presentation, but still not as great as if the ear receiving the odd harmonics could be ignored. Gockel *et al.* (2005) found that a mistuned partial presented contralaterally to the rest of a complex affected the low pitch, but less than when presented to the same ear. Similarly, Gockel *et al.* (1999) found that the interference produced by 'fringes' that preceded or followed a complex tone was reduced, but not abolished, by contralateral presentation.

Interestingly, the spatial percept also appears to be affected by interactions with pitch. Huggins pitch is hard to localize (Akeroyd and Summerfield, 2000). In the well-known 'octave illusion', Deutsch (1974) found that, when tones of 400 and 800 Hz were presented in alternation such that one ear received the lower when the other received the higher, subjects reported two tones pulsing, the lower tone at one ear and the higher at the other ear. The side that heard the higher tone depended on the subject's handedness, and was subject to spontaneous reversals. Interactions between pitch and spatial hearing might arise if they shared physiological substrates (see Section 4.10).

4.9 **How do we perceive pitch?**

How we perceive pitch has been a matter of intense debate for many years (see de Cheveigné, 2005 for a review). It is not yet resolved, and so there is no authoritative explanation of how pitch emerges within the auditory system. The best that we can do is to try to understand the positions in this debate. Two properties need explaining: (1) the *sensitivity* of pitch to small changes in F0, and (2) the relative *invariance* of pitch to large changes in other stimulus parameters. The second property is less often considered, but it is just as important as the first.

According to the *place* hypothesis (Helmholtz, 1877), pitch is determined from the position of maximum excitation along the basilar membrane, within the cochlea. This hypothesis is attractive because it readily accounts for sensitivity: a change in F0 is necessarily accompanied by spectral differences that the excitation pattern should—cochlear frequency resolution permitting—reveal. However, the place hypothesis has a harder time accounting for invariance of pitch across stimuli with different spectra, for example the fact that a pure tone and complex tone can evoke the same pitch.

A pure tone evokes a localized peak of excitation along the basilar membrane, and its frequency could conceivably be discriminated on the basis of this cue, or other cues such as changes along the flanks of the peak of excitation as it shifts with frequency. There are some issues with this idea: excitation patterns measured physiologically are rather broad. They tend to broaden and shift with increasing intensity, without commensurable changes in pitch or discrimination acuity (Chatterjee and Zwislocki, 1997). The parameter dependence of pure-tone pitch discrimination does not fit what is expected of an excitation pattern-based cue (e.g. Moore, 1973, Moore and Sek, 1995, 1998). These and other considerations argue against the place hypothesis, even in the case of pure-tone pitch, except for relatively high frequencies (above about 5 kHz). However, the main problem is that the place hypothesis fails to explain how pure and complex tones might have the same pitch. A complex tone typically evokes multiple peaks, one for each resolved partial (or group of unresolved partials), so the hypothesis needs amending to address this situation. The solution proposed by Ohm (1843) and Helmholtz (1877) was to assume that the pitch of the complex is determined by the peak associated with its *fundamental* partial. That solution floundered on the missing-fundamental phenomenon mentioned previously.

According to the *time* hypothesis, pitch is derived from the periodic pattern of the acoustic waveform, transduced by the cochlea into a pattern of nerve pulses that is processed by the brain. The appeal of this hypothesis is that pitch maps more directly to the stimulus period than to spectral features such as the—possibly missing—fundamental. However, the hypothesis is also incomplete: we still need to explain how the ear reliably extracts one pulse per period, how the pulses are transmitted to the brain, and how the brain counts them. The second point was once contentious because nerve fibers cannot transmit spikes at rates beyond a few hundred spikes per second. This issue was resolved by Wever and Bray (1930) who pointed out that higher rates can be transmitted collectively by groups of fibers. Today it is accepted that periodicities may be coded by the instantaneous probability of spikes within groups of auditory nerve fibers (up to about 5 kHz in cat, Johnson, 1980).

The main difficulty with the time hypothesis is that it is not easy to extract one pulse per period, in a way that is reliable and fully general. If we were dealing only with pure tones, then we could postulate some mechanism that triggers a pulse on a peak, or a zero-crossing of the waveform. However, complex tones often have several peaks and/or zero-crossings per period. Furthermore, the position and number of such cues is highly phase-dependent, which is hard to reconcile with the largely phase-independent nature of pitch (Wightman, 1973a). In their simplest form, place and time hypotheses both have insurmountable difficulties in accounting for pitch. Both explain sensitivity to variations in period, but not invariance across stimuli with same period. The debate has now shifted to two newer models, *pattern matching* and *autocorrelation*.

According to the pattern-matching hypothesis, pitch is associated with the harmonic pattern of the partials. The ear is assumed to contain a dictionary of *harmonic templates*, against which the incoming patterns of frequencies are compared. The template that best matches the pattern indicates the pitch. Pattern matching was proposed by de Boer in his thesis (1956) and later promoted by Wightman (1973b), Goldstein (1973), and Terhardt (1974); but the seeds of the idea were already in Helmholtz's concept of *unconscious inference*, according to which perception proceeds by matching internal models against incoming sensory evidence. Helmholz, himself in turn borrowed it from Alhazen who had formulated it in the 11th century (Hatfield, 2002).

Pattern matching allows the place hypothesis to be salvaged by assuming that individual partials (not just the fundamental) give rise to local peaks in excitation along the basilar membrane. For that reason it is sometimes equated with the 'place' hypothesis. However, pattern matching is also compatible with the time hypothesis, if one supposes that frequencies of individual partials are extracted from the temporal patterns that they produce locally at different points along the basilar membrane (supposing that they are resolved). The pattern-matching mechanism ensures invariance across stimuli of differing spectra (but the same F0), and in particular it solves the 'paradox' of the missing fundamental. For example, a set of partials at, 200, 300, and 400 Hz would trigger the same harmonic template as a 100-Hz pure tone, or any other complex of same period.

The pattern-matching hypothesis works if enough partials are resolved so as to constrain the choice of template (Section 4.7). However, pitch is also known to arise for stimuli for which there are no resolved partials. Pattern matching cannot account for such a pitch. This would bring us to discard the hypothesis, if it were not for three conjectures that might save it. The first is that human cochlear frequency resolution might somehow be finer than usually assumed (e.g. Oxenham and Shera, 2003). The second is that stimuli with non-resolved partials might produce distortion products that are resolvable. The third is that pattern matching might coexist with some other mechanism (see below).

The *autocorrelation* hypothesis differs from the time hypothesis in that it does not require spikes to be triggered at a well-defined position within the period. Rather, the periodic neural pattern is processed by coincidence-detector neurons that calculate the equivalent of an autocorrelation function (Licklider, 1951, 1959; Meddis and Hewitt, 1991a,b; Cariani and Delgutte, 1996a,b). The spike trains are delayed within the brain by various time lags (using neural delay lines) and combined or correlated with the original. When the lag is equal to the time delay between spikes the correlation is high and outputs of the coincidence detectors tuned to that lag are strong. Spike trains in each frequency channel are processed independently and the results combined into an aggregate pattern (Fig. 4.7). In response to a periodic tone, a ridge appears in the pattern at a lag equal to the period, and this is the cue to pitch. This cue appears for stimuli with *unresolved* partials because the partials beat together at the fundamental (Fig. 4.7, right column). It also appears for stimuli with only *resolved* partials (which produce no beating at the fundamental period in any peripheral channel). This happens because all partials are multiples of the same F0, and therefore share a common period multiple equal to 1/F0 (Fig. 4.7, middle column).

The autocorrelation process is insensitive to phase, and this addresses the objection against time models mentioned earlier. Phase sensitivity may nevertheless arise from non-linearities in its

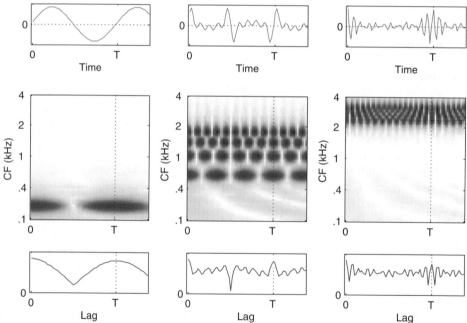

Fig. 4.7 Autocorrelation model of pitch. Top: acoustic waveforms, middle: array of autocorrelation functions (ACFs); bottom: summary autocorrelation functions (SACFs). Stimuli were: 200-Hz pure tone (left column), 200-Hz complex tone with partials 3, 5, 7, 9 (central column), and, 200-Hz complex tone with partials 12, 13, 14, 15, 16 (right column). For the central column, I chose a complex tone with well-spaced partials to illustrate the point that salient within-channel F0 cues are not necessary to produce a salient F0 cue in the overall pattern (middle row) or summary (bottom row). The autocorrelation model was modeled with a linear gammatone filterbank followed by half-wave rectification, calculation of a running autocorrelation function, cubic root compression, and summation over filter channels. The cue to pitch is the position of a ridge across channels in the ACF pattern (middle) or a peak in the SACF (bottom).

physiological implementation, see Section 4.10. Coincidence detection is plausible in terms of known physiology, but the hypothesis also requires *neural delays* of up to about 30 ms (to cover the range of musical pitch down to 30 Hz). There is little direct evidence for neural delays that long (Winter, 2005, but see de Cheveigné and Pressnitzer, 2006). Autocorrelation is theoretically related to pattern matching (de Cheveigné, 2005), and indeed it could be proposed that autocorrelation is the way pattern matching is implemented in the brain: the two hypotheses are not mutually exclusive.

An argument sometimes made against autocorrelation is that it works too well: it predicts that pitch should be equally salient for stimuli with resolved and unresolved partials, whereas we saw that such is not the case. This led to the *multiple-mechanism hypothesis*, already mentioned in Section 4.7, according to which pattern matching explains the strong pitch of stimuli with resolved harmonics, and autocorrelation the weaker pitch of stimuli with only unresolved harmonics (or electrical stimulation in cochlear implantees). The alternative to two mechanisms is that a *unitary model* can account for all aspects of pitch (Meddis and Hewitt, 1991a,b; Meddis and O'Mard, 1997). This debate is fueled by recent work on the psychophysics of resolved vs. unresolved stimuli (Section 4.7).

In addition to these main theories (place, time, pattern matching, autocorrelation), there are many variants such as the strobed temporal integration model of Patterson *et al.*, (1992) or the cancellation model of de Cheveigné (1998). They address the two main aspects of pitch mentioned at the beginning of this section: (1) sensitivity of pitch to F0; (2) invariance across stimuli with the same F0. Other aspects that also need explaining are: (3) how we perceive pitch in the presence of other sounds; (4) musical properties such as harmony; and (5) the detailed aspects of pitch reported in the psychophysics literature. We are unfortunately rather far from a complete answer to the question 'How do we perceive pitch?'.

4.10 **The physiological basis of pitch perception**

Sound entering the ear is transduced within the cochlea into neural patterns that are processed at several stages within the brainstem, thalamus, and cortex. Each of these stages could be involved in pitch perception, either as processing stage or as a relay of relevant information.

The cochlea is sometimes likened to a 'spectrum analyzer' that transforms the sound waveform into a spectrum coded as a profile of discharge rate across the auditory nerve. However, the auditory system also has access to the temporal patterns (so-called *fine structure*) at the output of each filter, and one could propose instead that the role of the cochlea is to transduce acoustic vibrations into temporal patterns of neural firing. According to this hypothesis, the role of cochlear selectivity would be to improve the quality of transduction and assist scene analysis (de Cheveigné, 2001). These two views (spectrum analyzer vs. frequency-selective transducer) map to the 'place' and 'time' hypotheses. How do they fit with what we now know about cochlear filter properties?

Our knowledge is inferred mainly from psychophysical studies in humans (Patterson, 1976; Glasberg and Moore, 2000) and measurements from the basilar membrane or the auditory nerve in animals (Ruggero, 1992; Robles and Ruggero, 2001; Cedolin and Delgutte, 2005). The results are roughly consistent across species (Ruggero and Temchin, 2005), but there are wide differences in estimates of cochlear filter bandwidth depending on the technique used. For example, bandwidths measured psychophysically (in humans) in forward-masking experiments are narrower than those measured with simultaneous masking by a factor of up to two (Oxenham and Shera, 2003). Likewise, auditory nerve fiber tuning curves measured with pure tones are considerably narrower than transfer functions estimated by the reverse correlation technique using noise stimuli (Carney and Yin, 1988). This is a problem for our purpose, because the plausibility of different hypotheses depends crucially on the available selectivity.

We can attempt to make sense of these conflicting estimates by recalling that cochlear filtering involves a non-linear active process. In response to a weak *isolated pure tone* at the best frequency of the measurement site, the gain of the cochlear amplifier is large. The gain decreases as the level of the tone increases, implying a concomitant reduction in selectivity (Robles and Ruggero, 2001). The gain also decreases if a second, off-frequency pure tone is added to the on-frequency probe, a phenomenon known as 'two-tone suppression' (Ruggero *et al.*, 1992; Jülicher *et al.*, 2001). Thus, pure-tone tuning curves may reflect a sharp selectivity that is available only for isolated pure tones at threshold, and not for more complex stimuli. This would explain the much wider estimates obtained with reverse correlation using wide-band noise stimuli, and also possibly the discrepancy between psychophysical estimates of selectivity from simultaneous and forward masking (Oxenham and Shera, 2003). When speaking of cochlear selectivity as applies to pitch, we must be careful to distinguish between the case of isolated pure tones and that of individual partials of complex tones. Selectivity is less good for the latter.

How does this relate to our different pitch theories? The *place* hypothesis assumes a peak of excitation along the basilar membrane. This is plausible for pure tones at low levels, but at higher levels the peak becomes broader and tends to shift towards a lower frequency place. By contrast, the pitch is rather stable with increasing intensity. For complex tones, it is unlikely that accurate estimates of the frequencies of individual partials, required by the pattern-matching hypothesis, can be derived from peaks in a rate–place representation (but see Cedolin and Delgutte, 2005). They could, however, be derived from *temporal cues*, supposing that each partial is resolved at some point along the basilar membrane so that its periodicity can be measured without interference from its neighbors (Section 4.7, see also Fig. 4.7 middle column). It has also been suggested that the *phase* characteristics of the cochlear filter may contribute to the estimation of the frequencies of individual partials (Shamma and Klein, 2000). Cochlear selectivity is not essential for the *time* and *autocorrelation* hypotheses, but it may facilitate hearing out the pitch of a sound in the presence of competing sounds by improving the signal-to-noise ratio within individual channels (de Cheveigné, 2001). To summarize, cochlear frequency analysis certainly plays an important role in pitch perception, but there is little support for the idea that pitch is derived from peaks in a place–rate representation.

At each point along the basilar membrane, the acoustic stimulus gives rise to vibrations that are transduced into a pattern of firing ('spikes') within the auditory nerve. The occurrence of each spike is random, but the *instantaneous probability* of occurrence is not: it follows roughly the half-wave rectified waveform of the mechanical vibration at each locus of transduction. The shape of that vibration reflects the stimulus (spectrum, amplitude), but also the filtering and non-linear properties of the cochlea. For a periodic stimulus, the overall discharge pattern is periodic in terms of instantaneous probability.

For a *pure tone*, basilar membrane vibration is sinusoidal, narrowly localized for a low-amplitude tone, and more spread out for a louder tone. The phase of vibration varies along the basilar membrane, slowly from stapes to just before the locus of maximal sensitivity, and more rapidly thereafter. Thus, there is a phase shift across the population of fibers that respond to a pure tone. The pitch of a pure tone could be derived by measuring the period of the discharge probability, or by locating the point of most rapid phase transition (this is a 'time'-based version of the place hypothesis) (Shamma and Klein, 2000).

For a *complex tone*, there are three cases of interest. A locus that responds to a partial of low rank may vibrate sinusoidally at that partial's frequency (Fig. 4.4 bottom left). A locus that responds to a *combination tone* produced by cochlear distortion may likewise vibrate sinusoidally at the frequency of that combination tone. Other loci, which respond to multiple partials, may vibrate with a complex waveform with an envelope period equal to the fundamental (Fig. 4.4, bottom, middle, and right panels). Thus there are multiple temporal cues within the discharge pattern of auditory nerve fibers that could support the pitch of a complex tone.

Phase-locking of spike trains to the stimulus decreases as stimulus frequency is raised, and is no longer measurable beyond about 5 kHz in cats (Johnson, 1980). The limit is lower in guinea-pigs (Palmer and Russell, 1986), higher in the barn owl (9 kHz; Köppl, 1997), and unknown in humans (Fig. 4.8). A small synchronization index does not necessarily imply that all temporal information

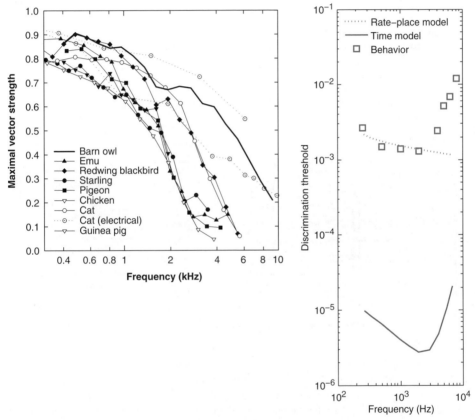

Fig. 4.8 The synchronization index (or vector strength) is used as a measure of quality of the temporal information carried by auditory nerve fiber discharge patterns. It is plotted here as a function of stimulus frequency for several species (reproduced from Köppl, 1997, with permission). A higher value indicates a better representation of a pure tone of that frequency. Data labeled 'electric' are for electric stimulation of the auditory nerve (see Köppl, 1997, for references). Right: human pure-tone frequency discrimination thresholds (symbols) and predictions by a place-rate model (dashed line) and a temporal model fit to cat synchronization data (full line), replotted from Heinz *et al.* (2001). Loss of synchrony at high frequencies produces a degradation of predicted thresholds that parallels that observed behaviorally in humans. However, the predicted thresholds are two orders of magnitude too good: to account for this discrepancy would require the additional assumption of a uniformly inefficient processing of temporal information. The place-rate model does not predict higher thresholds at high frequencies.

is lost: a modeling study based on Johnson's cat data found that residual temporal information might be useful up to 10 kHz (Heinz *et al.*, 2001). As one proceeds to higher relays within the auditory system, synchrony is limited to yet lower frequencies.

Where are temporal cues processed? Obviously this can only occur at a level within the nervous system where they are accurately represented. Auditory nerve fibers terminate within the cochlear nucleus, and from there they are relayed to a series of nuclei within the brainstem and midbrain, that themselves project to the auditory thalamus and cortex. Specializations for time are observed at several levels. For example, within the cochlear nucleus (CN), bushy cells are fed from auditory nerve fibers via large synapses, so that their activity resembles that of their afferents with little loss of temporal accuracy (so-called 'primary-like' response). Other cells (stellate-D and octopus)

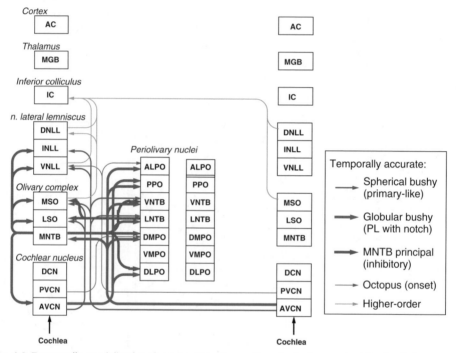

Fig. 4.9 Temporally specialized pathways within the auditory brainstem and midbrain. Spike patterns from the cochlea are relayed by several types of cell within the cochlear nucleus (CN): globular bushy (thick red) and spherical bushy (medium red), with firing patterns similar to auditory nerve fibers. Globular bushy cells feed principal cells of MNTB and LNTB that drive temporally accurate inhibitory pathways (blue). Octopus cells (thin red) have a temporally accurate onset response. Not shown on this schema, certain multipolar (stellate) cells within AVCN have a temporally accurate onset response (onset-C). Only pathways that feed nuclei on one side of the head are shown here (the same pathways exist on both sides). Pitch extraction could, in principle, occur at any level that receives accurate temporal information. Abbreviations: AC, auditory cortex; MGB, medial geniculate body; IC, inferior colliculus; DNLL, INLL, VNLL, dorsal, intermediate, and ventral nuclei of the lateral lemniscus; MSO, LSO, medial and lateral superior olive; MNTB, VNTB, LNTB, medial, ventral, and lateral nuclei of the trapezoid body; ALPO, PPO, DMPO, VMPO, DLPO, anterolateral, posterior, dorsomedial, ventromedial, and dorsolateral periolivary nuclei; DCN, PVCN, AVCN, dorsal, posteroventral, and anteroventral cochlear nuclei. From Schwartz, (1992); Helfert and Aschoff, (1997); Thompson and Schofield, (2000).

discharge accurately on the onset of a stimulus, or at each period of wideband stimuli such as click trains. These cells project to multiple nuclei within the superior olivary complex (SOC) and lateral lemniscus (LL) (Fig. 4.9).

Spherical bushy cells within the CN project bilaterally to the medial superior olive (MSO) and ipsilaterally to the lateral superior olive (LSO), as well as to other nuclei of the SOC and LL. Globular bushy cells within the CN project to the contralateral medial nucleus of the trapezoid body (MNTB) via secure synapses that ensure spikes are relayed reliably and with low jitter. In turn, MNTB neurons, which are inhibitory, project to ipsilateral LSO and other nuclei within the SOC and to the ventral nucleus of the lateral lemniscus (VNLL), which also receives input from octopus cells of the CN via large synapses. Octopus cell projections to the VNLL are numerous in humans (Adams, 1997). All these nuclei, and others within the brainstem, receive input from temporally specialized CN cells (Thompson and Schofield, 2000). Some of these nuclei, such as MSO, MNTB, and LSO, are thought to subserve binaural processing, but this does not preclude them from other tasks that involve temporally accurate patterns, such as pitch processing. Ascending projections from these nuclei mostly terminate in the inferior colliculus (IC) (Ehret, 1997).

Cells within IC and beyond synchronize to stimulus periodicities of at most a few hundred Hertz (Liu et al., 2005). Therefore it is likely that fast temporal processing is performed at a lower level: *subcollicular* nuclei are potential substrates for the signal processing operations required by pitch.

Tonotopically organized fields exist at all levels up to the thalamus and cortex, reflecting orderly projections from the cochlea, but I argued earlier that pitch is unlikely to emerge from a place–rate representation. Neural activity follows stimulus periodicity up to at most 1000 Hz in the IC, 1200 Hz in the thalamus or 250 Hz in the cortex (Liu et al., 2005; Wallace et al., 2007). However, most neurons have cutoffs well below these limits, and furthermore these ranges cover only part of the range of pitch periodicities. Relaying and processing temporally accurate spike trains entails a cost (in terms of specialized circuitry and metabolism), and it is likely that pitch processing occurs at an early level, possibly as early as the dendritic fields of CN neurons that receive input from the auditory nerve. However, the existence of Huggins pitch suggests a locus beyond the level of binaural interaction.

On the assumption that pattern matching is a 'high-order' operation, it is sometimes proposed that pattern matching is performed by secondary auditory cortical fields operating on the output of a tonotopically organized primary cortical field. It is more likely that cortical responses elaborate (and possibly recapitulate) pitch-relevant features (or conjunctions of features) extracted at subcortical levels.

It is frustrating that little direct evidence has been found for any particular locus, or model. Signatures of a pitch extractor, expected from pattern matching and autocorrelation alike, are (1) sensitivity to changes in F0, and (2) invariance across other stimulus dimensions. The first property is readily observed, but alone it is not sufficient to signal pitch. Evidence for a cortical 'pitch centre' has been reported based on cortical recordings in animal or brain imaging in humans (Patterson et al., 2002; Bendor and Wang, 2006), but methodological issues complicate the interpretation of experimental results (McAlpine, 2004; Hall and Plack, 2008; Nelken et al., 2008). A recent report describes single unit responses from presurgical recordings from electrodes implanted in the brains of epileptic patients. Tuning to pure tones (embedded within 3-tone random chords) was extremely narrow, limited only by the resolution of stimulus sampling (1/18th of an octave) (Bitterman et al., 2008). The protocol did not test invariance, and thus we cannot exclude that those responses merely reflect a remarkably selective tonotopy, but the sharp frequency resolution is evocative of a sensitivity to pitch.

Physiologists have obviously looked hard for proof of the various pitch theories mentioned earlier, such as Shamma and Klein's (2000) pattern matching model, Licklider's autocorrelation model (Licklider, 1951; Meddis and Hewitt, 1991a), or de Cheveigné's (1998) cancellation model. Direct evidence is still lacking, although most of the ingredients (lateral inhibition, within- and cross-channel coincidence, inhibition, etc.) are ubiquitous. Autocorrelation and cancellation models require delays of up to about 30 ms to accommodate a lower limit of pitch of 30 Hz (Pressnitzer et al., 2001). Evidence for appropriate delays is fragmentary (Behrend et al., 2002; Nayagam et al., 2005), although it has been suggested that delays might arise indirectly from cross-channel interaction (de Cheveigné and Pressnitzer, 2006). Numerous cells have been found to be sensitive to stimulus features relevant for pitch, but they are usually also sensitive to irrelevant features, or otherwise disorderly, making them hard to relate to known models. For example, onset cells within the cochlear nucleus fire accurately to each period of certain stimuli (Winter, 2005), but their phase sensitivity makes them poor candidates for pitch. Winter et al. (2001) and Wiegrebe and Meddis (2004) proposed that arrays of periodicity-tuned chopper cells in the cochlear nucleus are 'read out' by coincidence cells in IC. However, the best frequencies of those cells cover a limited range (100–500 Hz) and their properties are level-dependent at low levels (Winter, 2005).

Physiological correlates of pitch processing might escape observation, for example because they are technically hard to measure. It also could be that we *have* observed the correlates of pitch processing, but that they follow a principle that we do not understand. Or it might be the case that pitch is a human trait which is *not* shared by animal models. For example, the selectivity of single neuron responses observed by Bitterman et al. (2008) within human auditory cortex is not often reported in animal models.

To summarize, the auditory system is equipped with much neural circuitry to process spectral and temporal features relevant for pitch, but exactly where and how this occurs is still a mystery. The answer may come from progress in recording and imaging techniques in animal models and humans, or it may come from theoretical and modeling efforts to make sense of data that are already available.

4.11 Methods and tools for the study of pitch

Students of pitch are sometimes dismayed, on reading a paper, to find so much devoted to arcane issues of methodology. It is worth understanding what these issues are, if only to filter them out and focus more easily on pitch. It is also important to be able to judge, based on its methodology, whether a study is credible or not.

Introspection once was our only tool to probe the perceptual reality of pitch. Its drawback is that introspection cannot be communicated reliably. Without an external reference to calibrate what one hears, and compare it with others, the researcher is vulnerable to his or her subjectivity, and disagreements are hard to resolve. Psychophysics provides tools to insure that perceptual phenomena are real and general, and codified in a form that can be shared. Careful control of stimuli and design of task ensure that the quantity probed in the experiment is that intended by the experimenter. Objective procedures and signal detection theory (Green and Swets, 1974) allow the performance limits of a subject to be factored from the effects of response bias and criteria. Statistical tests protect us from over-interpreting random quirks in the data, and they can also give some indication about whether patterns observed reflect the idiosyncrasies of the subjects used in the experiment, or instead are of wider validity. These tools help produce results that are reproducible and credible. The downside is that the task (remembering instructions, pushing buttons, etc.) and stimulus repetition may interfere with the process of perception. Phenomena that do not fit the requirements of these tools may be overlooked.

Psychophysics allows strong inferences to be drawn on mechanisms within the brain, but it is no substitute for direct observation of neural activity. The most detailed observations are made in animal models using invasive techniques, such as the recording of the electrical activity of single or multiple neural units in response to the kind of stimuli that would produce pitch in humans. Other techniques involve measuring local field potentials or optical correlates of neural activity. With a background of knowledge of the brain from a variety of techniques, physiology in animal models gives us the most detailed picture of the neural processes that could be involved in pitch processing (Cariani and Delgutte, 1996*a,b*; Tramo *et al.*, 2005; Winter, 2005). An obvious drawback is that animals may differ from us in some important way in their experience of pitch, or in their processing of pitch-evoking sounds, or both. It is hard to do psychoacoustics in animals (see Chapter 7, this volume) and impossible to get them to describe what they heard, so we cannot be sure whether an observed response reflects pitch.

Brain imaging allows observation of brain activity in the species that interests us most: our own. *Structural* magnetic resonance imaging (MRI) has found correlations between the size of anatomical structures and pitch-related abilities (Gaser and Schlaug, 2003; Schneider *et al.*, 2005). *Functional* magnetic resonance imaging (fMRI) and positron emission tomography (PET) have been used to investigate pitch-related activity within the brain (Griffiths *et al.*, 1998; Patterson *et al.*, 2002; Warren *et al.*, 2003; Griffiths, 2005). Evidence has been found for a 'pitch centre' in lateral or anterolateral Heschl's gyrus (Patterson *et al.*, 2002; Penagos *et al.*, 2004), but this result has recently been questioned (Hall and Plack, 2008). The spatial resolution of fMRI (on the order of 1 cm) allows gross localization of neural activity, but its limited temporal resolution (about 10 s) constrains conclusions concerning the sequence of neural events (Griffiths, 2005).

Electroencephalography (EEG) and magneto-encephalography (MEG) offer better temporal resolution than fMRI, on the order of 1 ms. The onset response to periodic tones (pure or complex) includes a component (N100m) with a latency close to 100 ms that varies systematically with the period (Forss *et al.*, 1993; Stufflebeam *et al.*, 1998; Crottaz-Herbette and Ragot, 2000; Roberts *et al.*, 2000; Lütkenhöner *et al.*, 2001; Seither-Preisler *et al.*, 2006). However, similar onset responses occur for sounds that do not evoke pitch. It is thus imprudent to claim that N100m latency 'codes' pitch, or any other stimulus parameter or qualia. Presenting the pitch-evoking stimulus preceded by a noise-like waveform with similar spectral envelope allows a 'pitch onset response' (POR) to be separated from the generic onset response (Krumbholz *et al.*, 2003; Gutschalk *et al.*, 2004). POR latency and amplitude vary with stimulus period and degree of periodicity, suggesting a pitch-specific response. However, similar responses were observed for transitions between stimuli that differ in regularity but do not evoke a pitch (Chait *et al.*, 2007, 2008). MEG claims relatively good spatial resolution, and has been used to find evidence for a 'tonotopic' or 'periodotopic' organization of human auditory cortex (Romani *et al.*, 1982; Pantev *et al.*, 1988; Langner *et al.*, 1997). Results of different studies are unfortunately contradictory. Localization of sources is highly dependent on a single-dipole model that is not sufficiently accurate to allow such fine-grained conclusions (Lütkenhöner, 2003; Lütkenhöner *et al.*, 2003).

In summary, despite their considerable popularity and authority, non-invasive brain imaging techniques offer only limited insight into pitch perception mechanisms. Issues are limited spatial or temporal resolution, high levels of noise and variability in measured responses, bias towards structures and phenomena that are easy to image, the uncertain relation between the quantities measured (BOLD in fMRI, currents in dendrites of large populations of pyramidal neurons for

MEG and EEG) and relevant activity within the brain, and the need for sophisticated models and statistical procedures to make sense of the data.

Invasive recording techniques potentially provide a more detailed picture of human brain activity (Liégeois-Chauvel *et al.*, 1994; Lachaux *et al.*, 2003; Bitterman, 2008; Schnupp and King, 2008; Schönweiser and Zatorre, 2008). As part of presurgical protocol in epileptic patients, arrays of subdural electrodes are placed on the surface of the cortex (similar to EEG but without the deleterious effect of the high-impedance skull), or depth electrodes are inserted to record both local field potentials and individual neural units within the brain. Proximity to structures of interest, and favorable signal-to-noise ratio, give them an advantage over non-invasive recording techniques, at the expense of severe constraints on the availability of patients and the sampling of brain areas of interest. In common with brain imaging, invasive recording techniques offer only a sparse sampling of the complex activity within the brain.

Models and theories are important tools, indispensable to guide the design of experiments, and stitch their fragmentary results together into a picture that 'makes sense' to our understanding. Models of pitch are reviewed by de Cheveigné (2005). Special mention must be made of software models that allow complex experimental data to be compiled and confronted against theoretical hypotheses. A promising new trend is the use of theoretical neuroscience and machine-learning techniques to bridge the gap between experimental data and high-level functions involving cognition and action. Unfortunately it may be difficult for the student of pitch to judge the validity of theories that require mathematical sophistication, or that are embodied by the lines of a computer program. Modeling, to be useful, requires care paid to specification (*what* does the model do?) and pedagogy (*how* does it work?).

Applications, such as automatic speech recognition, music processing, or sensory prostheses, obviously benefit from our understanding of hearing. They also contribute to understanding in an important way: by testing the validity of our hypotheses in the context of 'real world' tasks.

As mentioned earlier, the arcane methodological details of many studies on pitch may disorient the reader interested in pitch. Complex-tone stimuli are often presented without their fundamental component. Originally the aim was to probe effects beyond those expected from a classic 'place' explanation, an aim that makes sense within the context of the 'missing fundamental' debate (Section 4.5). That debate has subsided, but excluding the fundamental component is still useful in physiological studies to distinguish between the selectivity to pure-tone frequency that is ubiquitous in the auditory system, and sensitivity to pitch. Complex tones may also be stripped of additional low-order harmonics (e.g. below the 10th). The aim here is to remove resolved partials so that the stimuli offer only 'temporal' cues, as opposed to spectral cues usable by a pattern-matching mechanism. This precaution is relevant in the context of the 'resolvability' debate (Section 4.7).

Without additional precautions, these efforts may be compromised by non-linear distortion products that arise within the cochlea. For example, *difference tones* produced by pairs of partials $(f2-f1$, where f1 and f2 are partial frequencies) may introduce components at the fundamental and low harmonics (Pressnitzer and Patterson, 2001). Likewise, *cubic difference tones* $(2f1-f2)$ may introduce components just below the lowest harmonic of a set of high-frequency partials. To mask these distortion products, that behave like rogue stimulus components, noise is added in the frequency region where they occur. The noise may be white (flat spectrum), or pink (power varies as 1/f), or adjusted for uniform masking or for equal thresholds in each cochlear channel (threshold-equalized noise, TEN, Moore, 2000). The aim in each case is to mask the distortion products while minimizing any deleterious effect on the stimulus itself.

Stimulus manipulations designed to affect pitch might also affect other perceptual dimensions. To rule out the possibility that a subject uses, for example, a change in loudness instead of pitch as a cue for a task, the stimulus level may be *roved* between trials. Likewise, a change in F0 may produce physiological responses unrelated to pitch in physiological or brain imaging experiments, and therefore characterizing a genuine pitch effect may require testing over a range of pitch-producing stimuli (Hall and Plack, 2008).

In summary, we have many tools at our disposal to explore pitch. Each has 'blind spots' that we must understand, and that we may compensate for to some degree by combining them. Advances in tools and methods may induce major leaps in our understanding, as argued earlier by von Békésy and Rosenblith (1948). In particular, progress in the resolution and signal-to-noise ratio of recording and imaging techniques, coupled with careful use of standard behavioral techniques, might lead to a quantum leap in understanding pitch.

4.12 **Conclusions**

Pitch is an important quality of sound, the focus of intense inquiry and investigation since antiquity. Pitch is basic to two forms of behavior specific to humans: speech and music. Pitch is usually understood as a one-dimensional percept determined by the period of the stimulus (or its inverse, F0), and insensitive to changes along other stimulus dimensions. However, its complex role within music involves harmonic and melodic effects that go beyond this simple one-dimensional model.

There is still debate as to where, and how, pitch is extracted within the auditory system. Helmholtz's influential idea that pitch is determined by the locus of maximal vibration within the cochlea is no longer accepted. Rather, it is more likely that pitch is extracted within the auditory nervous system on the basis of temporal patterns transduced from acoustic vibrations within the cochlea. The site of pitch extraction is unknown, but probably relatively peripheral within the lower auditory brainstem or midbrain where temporally accurate neural information is available. Multiple neural substrates appear to be specialized for time, but the shape of many of their responses to sound are complex and difficult to relate to existing models of pitch.

According to the pattern-matching hypothesis, the frequencies of individual partials are estimated and matched against a set of internal harmonic templates. Partial frequencies could be estimated from neural temporal patterns within neural channels within which they are isolated by cochlear filtering, and possibly also from temporal patterns between those channels. As such, pitch perception might be dependent on both the selectivity and the phase properties of a healthy cochlea. According to the autocorrelation hypothesis, the period is instead determined directly from the temporal pattern of nerve activity transduced by the cochlea, by a neural circuit involving an array of delays (or one tunable delay) and coincidence-detecting neurons. According to that hypothesis, cochlear selectivity would not be directly involved in period estimation, but it might be useful to isolate sources within noise and facilitate perception of their pitch. Alternatively, cochlear mechanics might contribute to create the necessary delays, which would then also depend on the healthy condition of the cochlea. Physiological and psychophysical investigations have failed to rule decisively in favor of either hypothesis, and it may be the case that pitch is extracted according to a mechanism that is yet to be discovered.

Investigation tools for pitch include psychophysics, electrophysiology in animal models, brain imaging in humans, and theoretical and engineering approaches to solve similar problems in artificial systems. The study of pitch requires special care paid to methodological questions (e.g. combination tones), that sometimes obscure the pitch-related issues and make the literature hard to read for the newcomer. Once these issues are understood, pitch unfolds itself as a fascinating field where there is still much to be learned.

Acknowledgements

Part of this chapter was written during a scholarship at St John's College, Cambridge, at the invitation of Ian Winter. Thanks to Chris Plack, Maria Chait, Bill Hartmann, Jennifer Linden, Mark Sayles, Marion Cousineau, Shihab Shamma, Laurent Demany, Brian Moore, Andrew Oxenham, and Adrian Fourcin for comments on previous drafts.

References

Adams, J. C. (1997). Projections from octopus cells of the posteroventral cochlear nucleus to the ventral nucleus of the lateral lemniscus in cat and human. *Auditory Neuroscience* 3:335–50.

Akeroyd, M. A. and Summerfield, A. Q. (2000). The lateralization of simple dichotic pitches. *Journal of the Acoustical Society of America* 108:316–34.

Akeroyd, M. A., Moore, B. C. J., and Moore, G. A. (2001). Melody recognition using three types of dichotic-pitch stimulus. *Journal of the Acoustical Society of America* 110:1498–504.

Akeroyd, M. A., Carlyon, R. P., and Deeks, J. M. (2005). Can dichotic pitches form two streams? *Journal of the Acoustical Society of America* 118:977–81.

ANSI (1994). *ANSI S1.1–1994. American National Standard Acoustical Terminology.* New York: American National Standards Institute.

ASA (1960). *Acoustical Terminology SI, 1–1960.* New York: American Standards Association.

Assmann, P. F. and Paschall, D. D. (1998). Pitches of concurrent vowels. *Journal of the Acoustical Society of America* 103:1150–60.

Bachem, A. (1948). Chroma fixation at the ends of the musical frequency scale. *Journal of the Acoustical Society of America* 20:704–5.

Bachem, A. (1950). Tone height and tone chroma as two different pitch qualities. *Acta Psychologica* 7: 80–8.

Beerends, J. G. and Houtsma, A. J. M. (1989). Pitch identification of simultaneous diotic and dichotic two-tone complexes. *Journal of the Acoustical Society of America* 85:813–19.

Behrend, O., Brand, A., Kapfer, C., and Grothe, B. (2002). Auditory response properties in the superior paraolivary nucleus of the gerbil. *Journal of Neurophysiology* 87:2915–28.

Bendor, D. and Wang, X. (2006). Cortical representations of pitch in monkeys and humans. *Current Opinion in Neurobiology* 16:391–9.

Bernstein, J. G. W. and Oxenham, A. J. (2003). Pitch discrimination of diotic and dichotic tone complexes: Harmonic resolvability or harmonic number? *Journal of the Acoustical Society of America* 113:3323–34.

Bernstein, J. G. W. and Oxenham, A. J. (2005). An autocorrelation model with place dependence to account for the effect of harmonic number on fundamental frequency discrimination. *Journal of the Acoustical Society of America* 117:3816–31.

Bernstein, J. G. W. and Oxenham, A. J. (2006). The relationship between frequency selectivity and pitch discrimination: effects of stimulus level. *Journal of the Acoustical Society of America* 120:3912–28.

Bernstein, J. G. W. and Oxenham A. J. (2008). Harmonic segregation through mistuning can improve fundamental frequency discrimination. *Journal of the Acoustical Society of America* 124:1653–67.

Bigand, E. and Tillmann, B. (2005). Effect of context on the perception of pitch structures. In *Pitch—Neural Coding and Perception* (ed. C. J. Plack, A. Oxenham, R. R. Fay, and A. N. Popper), pp. 306–51. New York: Springer.

Bilsen, F. A. (1976). Pronounced binaural pitch phenomenon. *Journal of the Acoustical Society of America* 59:467–8.

Bitterman, Y., Mukamel, R., Malach, R., Fried, I., and Nelken, I. (2008). Ultra-fine frequency tuning revealed in single neurons of human auditory cortex. *Nature* 451:197–201.

Bloothooft, G., Bringmann, E., van Cappellen, M., van Luipen, J. B., and Thomassen, K. P. (1992). Acoustics and perception of overtone singing. *Journal of the Acoustical Society of America* 92:1827–36.

Bregman, A. S. (1990). *Auditory Scene Analysis.* Cambridge, Mass: MIT Press.

Burns, E. M. and Viemeister, N. (1976). Nonspectral pitch. *Journal of the Acoustical Society of America* 60:863–9.

Burns, E. M. (1981). Circularity in relative pitch judgments for inharmonic complex tones: the Shepard demonstration revisited, again. *Perception and Psychophysics* 30:467–72.

Burns, E. M. (1982). Pure-tone pitch anomalies. I. Pitch-intensity effects and diplacusis in normal ears. *Journal of the Acoustical Society of America* 72:1394–402.

Burns, E. M. (1983). Pitch of sinusoids and complex tones above 10 kHz. In *Hearing—Physiological Bases and Psychophysics* (ed. R. Klinke and W. M. Hartmann), pp. 327–33. Berlin: Springer-Verlag.

Cardozo, B. L. (1974). Some notes on frequency discrimination and masking. *Acustica* 31:330–6.

Cariani, P. A. and Delgutte, B. (1996a). Neural correlates of the pitch of complex tones. I. Pitch and pitch salience. *Journal of Neurophysiology* 76:1698–716.

Cariani, P. A. and Delgutte, B. (1996b). Neural correlates of the pitch of complex tones. II. Pitch shift, pitch ambiguity, phase-invariance, pitch circularity, rate-pitch and the dominance region for pitch. *Journal of Neurophysiology* 76:1717–34.

Carlyon, R. P. (1996a). Encoding the fundamental frequency of a complex tone in the presence of a spectrally overlapping masker. *Journal of the Acoustical Society of America* 99:517–24.

Carlyon, R. P. (1996b). Masker asynchrony impairs the fundamental-frequency discrimination of unresolved harmonics. *Journal of the Acoustical Society of America* 99:525–33.

Carlyon, R. P. and Shackleton, T. M. (1994). Comparing the fundamental frequencies of resolved and unresolved harmonics: evidence for two pitch mechanisms? *Journal of the Acoustical Society of America* 95:3541–54.

Carney, H. and Yin, T. C. T. (1988). Temporal coding of resonances by low-frequency auditory nerve fibers: single fiber responses and a population model. *Journal of Neurophysiology* 60:1653–77.

Carney, L. H., Heinz, M. G., Evilsizer, M. E., Gilkey, R. H., and Colburn, H. S. (2002). Auditory phase opponency: a temporal model for masked detection at low frequencies. *Acta Acustica United with Acustica* 88:334–47.

Cedolin, L. and Delgutte, B. (2005). Pitch of complex tones: rate-place and interspike interval representations in the auditory nerve. *Journal of Neurophysiology* 94:347–62.

Chait, M., Poeppel, D., de Cheveigné, A., and Simon, J. Z. (2007). Processing asymmetry of transitions between order and disorder in human auditory cortex. *Journal of Neuroscience* 27:5207–14.

Chait, M., Poeppel, D., and Simon, J. Z. (2008). Auditory temporal edge detection in human auditory cortex. *Brain Research* 1213:78–90.

Cramer, E. M. and Huggins, W. H. (1958). Creation of pitch through binaural interaction. *Journal of the Acoustical Society of America* 30:413–17.

Crottaz-Herbette, S. and Ragot, R. (2000). Perception of complex sounds: N1 latency codes pitch and topography codes spectra. *Clinical Neurophysiology* 111:1759–66.

Chatterjee, M. and Zwislocki, J. J. (1997). Cochlear mechanisms of frequency and intensity coding. I. The place code for pitch. *Hearing Research* 111:65–75.

Cramer, E. M. and Huggins, W. H. (1958). Creation of pitch through binaural interaction. *Journal of the Acoustical Society of America* 30:413–17.

Culling, J., Summerfield, A. Q., and Marshall, D. H. (1998). Dichotic pitches as illusions of binaural unmasking. I. Huggins pitch and the binaural edge pitch. *Journal of the Acoustical Society of America* 103:3509–26.

Culling, J. (1999). The existence region of Huggins pitch. *Hearing Research* 127:143–8.

Darrigol, O. (2007). The acoustic origins of harmonic analysis. *Archive for History of Exact Sciences* 61: 343–424.

de Boer, E. (1956). On the 'residue' in hearing. Unpublished thesis, University of Amsterdam.

de Boer, E. (1976). On the residue and auditory pitch perception. In *Handbook of Sensory Physiology*, Vol. V–3 (ed. W. D. Keidel and W. D. Neff), pp. 479–583. Berlin: Springer-Verlag.

de Cheveigné, A. (1998). Cancellation model of pitch perception. *Journal of the Acoustical Society of America* **103**:1261–71.

de Cheveigné, A. (2001). The auditory system as a separation machine. In *Physiological and Psychophysical Bases of Auditory Function* (ed. J. Breebaart, A. J. M. Houtsma, A. Kohlrausch, V. F. Prijs, and R. Schoonhoven), pp. 453–60. Maastricht, The Netherlands: Shaker Publishing BV.

de Cheveigné, A. (2005). Pitch perception models. In *Pitch—Neural Coding and Perception* (ed. C. J. Plack, A. J. Oxenham, R. R. Fay, and A. N. Popper), pp. 169–233. New York: Springer.

de Cheveigné, A. and Pressnitzer, D. (2006). The case of the missing delay lines: synthetic delays obtained by cross-channel phase interaction. *Journal of the Acoustical Society of America* **119**:3908–18.

Demany, L. and Semal, C. (2002). Learning to perceive pitch differences. *Journal of the Acoustical Society of America* **111**:1377–88.

Deutsch, D. (1974). An auditory illusion. *Nature* **251**:307–9.

Douglas, K. M. and Bilkey, D. K. (2007). Amusia is associated with deficits in spatial processing. *Nature Neuroscience* **10**:915–21.

Drayna, D., Manichaikul, A., de Lange, M., Sneider, H., and Spector, T. (2001). Genetic correlates of musical pitch recognition in humans. *Science* **291**:1969–72.

Ehret, G. (1997). The auditory midbrain, a shunting yard of acoustical information processing. In *The Central Auditory System* (ed. G. Ehret and R. Romand), pp. 259–316. New York: Oxford University Press.

Forss, N., Mäkelä, J. P., McEvoy, L., and Hari, R. (1993). Temporal integration and oscillatory responses of the auditory cortex revealed by evoked magnetic fields to click trains. *Hearing Research* **68**:89–96.

Gaser, C. and Schlaug, G. (2003). Brain structures differ between musicians and non-musicians. *Journal of Neuroscience* **23**:9240–5.

Giangrande, J., Tuller, B., and Kelso, J. (2003). Perceptual dynamics of circular pitch. *Music Perception* **20**:241–62.

Glasberg, B. R. and Moore, B. C. J. (2000). Frequency selectivity as a function of level and frequency measured with uniformly exciting notched noise. *Journal of the Acoustical Society of America* **108**: 2318–28.

Gockel, H., Carlyon, R. P., and Micheyl, C. (1999). Context dependence of fundamental-frequency discrimination: lateralized temporal fringes. *Journal of the Acoustical Society of America* **106**:3553–63.

Gockel, H., Carlyon, R. P., and Plack, C. J. (2004). Across-frequency interference in fundamental frequency discrimination: questioning evidence for two pitch mechanisms. *Journal of the Acoustical Society of America* **116**:1092–104.

Gockel, H., Carlyon, R. P., and Plack, C. J. (2005). Dominance region for pitch: effects of duration and dichotic presentation. *Journal of the Acoustical Society of America* **117**:1326–36.

Gockel, H., Moore, B. C. J., Plack, C. J., and Carlyon, R. (2006). Effect of noise on the detectability and fundamental frequency discrimination of complex tones. *Journal of the Acoustical Society of America* **120**:957–65.

Gockel, H., Moore, B. C. J., Carlyon, R. P., and Plack, C. J. (2007). Effect of duration on the frequency discrimination of individual partials in a complex tone and on the discrimination of fundamental frequency. *Journal of the Acoustical Society of America* **121**:373–82.

Goldstein, J. L. (1973). An optimum processor theory for the central formation of the pitch of complex tones. *Journal of the Acoustical Society of America* **54**:1496–516.

Green, D. M. and Swets, J. (1974). *Signal Detection Theory and Psychophysics*. New York: Krieger.

Griffiths, T. D. (2005). Functional imaging of pitch processing. In *Pitch—Neural Coding and Perception* (ed. C. J. Plack, A. J. Oxenham, R. R. Fay, and A. N. Popper), pp. 147–68. New York: Springer.

Griffiths, T. D., Buchel, C., Frackowiak, R. S., and Patterson, R. D. (1998). Analysis of temporal structure in sound by the human brain. *Nature Neuroscience* **4**:633–7.

Gutschalk, A., Patterson, R. D., Scherg, M., Uppenkamp, S. and Rupp, A. (2004). Temporal dynamics of pitch in auditory cortex. *NeuroImage* **22**:755–66.

Hall, D. and Plack, C. J. (2008). Pitch processing sites in the human auditory brain. *Cerebral Cortex* **19**:576–85.

Hartmann, W. M. (1978). The effect of amplitude envelope on the pitch of sine wave tones. *Journal of the Acoustical Society of America* **63**:1105–13.

Hartmann, W. M. (1993). On the origin of the enlarged melodic octave. *Journal of the Acoustical Society of America* **93**:3400–9.

Hartmann, W. M. (1997). *Signals, Sound, and Sensation*. Woodbury, NY: AIP Press.

Hartmann, W. M. and Doty, S. L. (1996). On the pitches of the components of a complex tone. *Journal of the Acoustical Society of America* **99**:567–78.

Hartmann, W. M. and Goupell, M. J. (2006). Enhancing and unmasking the harmonics of a complex tone. *Journal of the Acoustical Society of America* **120**:2142–57.

Hartmann, W. M., Rakerd, B., and Packard, T. N. (1985). On measuring the frequency-difference limen for short tones. *Perception and Psychophysics* **38**:199–207.

Hatfield, G. (2002). Perception as unconscious inference. In *Perception and the Physical World: Psychological and Philosophical Issues in Perception* (ed. D. Heyer and R. Mausfeld), pp. 115–43. New York: John Wiley and Sons.

Heinz, M. G., Colburn, H. S., and Carney, L. H. (2001). Evaluating auditory performance limits: I. One-parameter discrimination using a computational model for the auditory nerve. *Neural Computation* **13**:2273–316.

Helfert, R. H. and Aschoff, A. (1997). Superior olivary complex and nuclei of the lateral lemniscus. In *The Central Auditory System* (ed. G. Ehret and R. Romand), pp. 193–258. New York: Oxford University Press.

Helmholtz, H. von (1877). *On the Sensations of Tone* (English translation A. J. Ellis, 1st edn, 1885; 2nd edn, 1954). New York: Dover.

Henning, G. B. and Grosberg, S. L. (1968). Effect of harmonic components on frequency discrimination. *Journal of the Acoustical Society of America* **44**:1386–9.

Houtsma, A. J. M. (1981). Noise-induced shifts in the pitch of pure and complex tones. *Journal of the Acoustical Society of America* **70**:1661–8.

Houtsma, A. J. M. and Goldstein, J. L. (1972). The central origin of the pitch of complex tones. Evidence from musical interval recognition. *Journal of the Acoustical Society of America* **51**:520–9.

Houtsma, A. J. M. and Smurzynski, J. (1990). Pitch identification and discrimination for complex tones with many harmonics. *Journal of the Acoustical Society of America* **87**:304–10.

Hsieh, I. H. and Saberi, K. (2007). Temporal integration in absolute identification of musical pitch. *Hearing Research* **233**:108–16.

Jeffress, L. A. (1948). A place theory of sound localization. *Journal of Comparative and Physiological Psychology* **41**:35–9.

Johnson, D. H. (1980). The relationship between spike rate and synchrony in responses of auditory-nerve fibers to single tones. *Journal of the Acoustical Society of America* **68**:1115–22.

Jülicher, F., Andor, D., and Duke, T. (2001). Physical basis of two-tone interference in hearing. *Proceedings of the National Academy of Sciences USA* **98**:9080–5.

Kaernbach, C. (1993). Temporal and spectral basis of the features perceived in repeated noise. *Journal of the Acoustical Society of America* **94**:91–7.

Köppl, C. (1997). Phase locking to high frequencies in the auditory nerve and cochlear nucleus magnocellularis of the barn owl *Tyto alba. Journal of Neuroscience* **17**:3312–21.

Krumbholz, K., Patterson, R. D., and Pressnitzer, D. (2000). The lower limit of pitch as determined by rate discrimination. *Journal of the Acoustical Society of America* **108**:1170–80.

Krumbholz, K., Patterson, R. D., Seither-Preisler, A., Lammertmann, C., and Lütkenhöner, B. (2003). Neuromagnetic evidence for a pitch processing center in Heschls gyrus. *Cerebral Cortex* **13**:765–72.

Lachaux, J. P., Rudrauf, D., and Kahane, P. (2003). Intracranial EEG and human brain mapping. *Journal of Physiology, Paris* **97**:613–28.

Laguitton, V., Demany, L., Semal, C., and Liégeois-Chauvel, C. (1998). Pitch perception: a difference between right- and left-handed listeners. *Neuropsychologia* **36**:201–7.

Langner, G., Sams, M., Heil, P., and Schultze, H. (1997). Frequency and periodicity are represented in orthogonal maps in the human auditory cortex: evidence from magnetoencephalography. *Journal of Comparative Physiology, A* **181**:665–76.

Levitin, D. J. and Rogers, S. E. (2005). Absolute pitch: perception, coding, and controversies. *Trends in Cognitive Sciences* **9**:26–33.

Licklider, J. C. R. (1951). A duplex theory of pitch perception *Experientia* **7**:128–34. [Reproduced in Schubert, E. D. (1979). Psychological acoustics. In *Benchmark Papers in Acoustics*, Vol. 13, pp. 155–60. Stroudsburg, PA: Dowden, Hutchinson & Ross, Inc.]

Licklider, J. C. R. (1954). Periodicity pitch and place pitch. *Journal of the Acoustical Society of America* **26**:945. [Abstract]

Licklider, J. C. R. (1959). Three auditory theories. In: *Psychology, a Study of a Science* (ed. S. Koch), pp. 41–144. New York: McGraw–Hill.

Liégeois-Chauvel, C., Musolino, A., Badier, J. M., Marquis, P., and Chauvel, P. (1994). Evoked potentials recorded from the auditory cortex in man: evaluation and topography of the middle latency components. *Electroencephalography and Clinical Neurophysiology* **92**:204–14.

Liu, L.-F., Palmer, A. R., and Wallace, M. N. (2005). Phase-locked responses to pure tones in the inferior colliculus. *Journal of Neurophysiology* **95**:1926–35.

Lütkenhöner, B. (2003). Single-dipole analyses of the N100m are not suitable for characterizing the cortical representation of pitch. *Audiology and Neuro-otology* **8**:222–3.

Lütkenhöner, B., Lammertmann, C., and Knecht, S. (2001). Latency of auditory evoked field deflection N100m ruled by pitch or spectrum. *Audiology and Neuro-otology* **6**:263–78.

Lütkenhöner, B., Krumbholz, K., and Seither-Preisler, A. (2003). Studies of tonotopy based on wave N100 of the auditory field are problematic. *NeuroImage*, **19**:935–49.

McAlpine, D. (2004). Neural sensitivity to periodicity in the inferior colliculus: evidence for the role of cochlear distortions. *Journal of Neurophysiology* **92**:1295–311.

Mark, H. E. and Rattay, F. (1990). Frequency discrimination of single-, double- and triple-cycle sinusoidal acoustic signals. *Journal of the Acoustical Society of America* **88**:560–3.

Meddis, R. and Hewitt, M. J. (1991a). Virtual pitch and phase sensitivity of a computer model of the auditory periphery. I: Pitch identification. *Journal of the Acoustical Society of America* **89**:2866–82.

Meddis, R. and Hewitt, M. J. (1991b). Virtual pitch and phase sensitivity of a computer model of the auditory periphery. II: Phase sensitivity. *Journal of the Acoustical Society of America* **89**:2883–94.

Meddis, R. and OMard, L. (1997). A unitary model of pitch perception. *Journal of the Acoustical Society of America* **102**:1811–20.

Mersenne, M. (1636). *Harmonie Universelle*. Paris: Cramoisy (reprinted, 1975, Paris: Editions du CNRS).

Micheyl, C. and Carlyon, R. P. (1998). Effects of temporal fringes on fundamental-frequency discrimination. *Journal of the Acoustical Society of America* **104**:3006–18.

Micheyl, C. and Oxenham, A. J. (2004). Sequential F0 comparisons between resolved and unresolved harmonics: No evidence for translation noise between two pitch mechanisms. *Journal of the Acoustical Society of America* **116**:3038–50.

Micheyl, C. and Oxenham, A. J. (2005). Comparing F0 discrimination in sequential and simultaneous conditions. *Journal of the Acoustical Society of America* **118**:41–4.

Micheyl, C. and Oxenham, A. (2007). Across-frequency pitch discrimination interference between complex tones containing resolved harmonics. *Journal of the Acoustical Society of America* **121**:1621–31.

Micheyl, C., Delhommeau, K., Perrot, X., and Oxenham, A. (2006a). Influence of musical and psychoacoustical training on pitch discrimination. *Hearing Research* **219**:36–47.

Micheyl, C., Bernstein, J. G., and Oxenham, A. (2006*b*). Detection and F0 discrimination of harmonic complex tones in the presence of competing tones or noise. *Journal of the Acoustical Society of America* **120**:1493–505.

Moore, B. C. J. (1973). Frequency difference limens for short-duration tones. *Journal of the Acoustical Society of America* **54**:610–19.

Moore, B. C. J. (1981). Relation between pitch shifts and MMF shifts in forward masking. *Journal of the Acoustical Society of America* **69**:594–7.

Moore, B. C. J. (1982, 2003). *An Introduction to the Psychology of Hearing*. London: Academic Press.

Moore, B. C. J. (2000). A test for the diagnosis of dead regions in the cochlea. *British Journal of Audiology* **34**:205–24.

Moore, B. C. J. and Glasberg, B. R. (1983). Suggested formulae for calculating auditory-filter bandwidths and excitation patterns. *Journal of the Acoustical Society of America* **74**:750–3.

Moore, B. C. J. and Glasberg, B. R. (1991). Effects of signal-to-noise ratio on the frequency discrimination of complex tones with overlapping and nonoverlapping harmonics. *Journal of the Acoustical Society of America* **89**:1888. [Abstract]

Moore, B. C. J. and Ohgushi, K. (1993). Audibility of partials in inharmonic complex tones. *Journal of the Acoustical Society of America* **93**:452–61.

Moore, B. C. J. and Sek, A. (1995). Effects of carrier frequency, modulation rate, and modulation waveform on the detection of modulation and the discrimination of modulation type (amplitude modulation versus frequency modulation). *Journal of the Acoustical Society of America* **97**:2468–78.

Moore, B. C. J. and Sek, A. (1998). Discrimination of frequency glides with superimposed random glides in level. *Journal of the Acoustical Society of America* **104**:411–21.

Moore, B. C. J., Peters, R. W., and Glasberg, B. R. (1985*a*). Thresholds for the detection of inharmonicity in complex tones. *Journal of the Acoustical Society of America* **77**:1861–7.

Moore, B. C. J., Peters, R. W., and Glasberg, B. R. (1985*b*). Relative dominance of individual partials in determining the pitch of complex tones. *Journal of the Acoustical Society of America* **77**:1853–60.

Moore, B. C. J., Glasberg, B. R., and Proctor, G. M. (1992). Accuracy of pitch matching for pure tones with overlapping or nonoverlapping harmonics. *Journal of the Acoustical Society of America* **91**:3443–50.

Moore, B. C. J., Glasberg, B. R., Low, K. E., Cope, T., and Cope, W. (2006). Effects of level and frequency on the audibility of partials in inharmonic complex tones. *Journal of the Acoustical Society of America* **120**:934–44.

Moore, B. C. J., Glasberg, B., Aberkane, I., and Pinker, S. (2007). Dominance region at low frequencies: implications for pitch theories, *Journal of the Acoustical Society of America* **121**:3091–2. [Abstract]

Nayagam, D. A. X., Clarey, J. C., and Paolini, A. G. (2005). Powerful, onset inhibition in the ventral nucleus of the lateral lemniscus. *Journal of Neurophysiology* **94**:1651–4.

Nelken, I., Bizley, J. K., Nodal, F. R., Ahmed, B., King, A. J. and J. W. S. (2008). Responses of auditory cortex to complex stimuli: functional organization revealed using intrinsic optical signals. *Journal of Neurophysiology* **91**:1928–41.

Ohm, G. S. (1843). On the definition of a tone with the associated theory of the siren and similar sound producing devices. *Poggendorfs Annalen der Physik und Chemie* **59**:497ff. [Translated and reprinted in Lindsay (1973). *Acoustics: Historical and Philosophical Development*, pp. 242–7. Stroudsburg, PA: Dowden, Hutchinson and Ross].

Oxenham, A. and Shera, C. A. (2003). Estimates of human cochlear tuning at low levels using forward and simultaneous masking. *Journal of the Association for Research in Otolaryngology* **4**:541–54.

Oxenham, A., Fligor, B. J., Mason, R., and Kidd, G. J. (2003). Informational masking and musical training. *Journal of the Acoustical Society of America* **114**:1543–9.

Palmer, A. and Russell, C. (1986). Phase-locking in the cochlear nerve of the guinea-pig and its relation to the receptor potential of inner hair-cells. *Hearing Research* **24**:1–15.

Pantev, C., Hoke, M., Lehnertz, K., Lutkenhoner, B., Anogianakis, G., and Wittkowski, W. (1988). Tonotopic organization of the human auditory cortex revealed by transient auditory evoked magnetic fields. *Electroencephalography and Clinical Neurophysiology* **69**:160–70.

Patterson, R. D. (1976). Auditory filter shapes derived with noise stimuli. *Journal of the Acoustical Society of America* **59**:640–54.

Patterson, R. D., Robinson, K., Holdsworth, J., McKeown, D., Zhang, C., and Allerhand, M. (1992). Complex sounds and auditory images. In *Auditory Physiology and Perception* (ed. Y. Cazals, K. Horner, and L. Demany), pp. 429–46. Oxford: Pergamon Press.

Patterson, R. D., Uppenkamp, S., Johnsrude, I. S., and Griffiths, T. D. (2002). The processing of temporal pitch and melody information in auditory cortex. *Neuron* **36**:767–76.

Penagos, H., Melcher, J. R., and Oxenham, A. J. (2004). A neural representation of pitch salience in nonprimary human auditory cortex revealed with functional magnetic resonance imaging. *Journal of Neuroscience* **24**:6810–15.

Peters, R. W., Moore, B. C. J., and Glasberg, B. R. (1983). Pitch of components of complex tones. *Journal of the Acoustical Society of America* **73**:924–9.

Plack, C. J. and Carlyon, R. P. (1995). Differences in frequency modulation detection and fundamental frequency discrimination between complex tones consisting of resolved and unresolved harmonics. *Journal of the Acoustical Society of America* **98**:1355–64.

Plack, C. J. and Oxenham, A. J. (2005). The psychophysics of pitch. In *Pitch—Neural Coding and Perception* (ed. C. J. Plack, A. J. Oxenham, R. R. Fay, and A. N. Popper), pp. 1–6. New York: Springer.

Plomp, R. (1964). The ear as a frequency analyzer. *Journal of the Acoustical Society of America* **36**:1628–36.

Plomp, R. (1967a). Pitch of complex tones. *Journal of the Acoustical Society of America* **41**:1526–33.

Plomp, R. (1967b). Beats of mistuned consonances. *Journal of the Acoustical Society of America* **42**:462–74.

Pollack, I. (1947). The atonal interval. *Journal of the Acoustical Society of America* **20**:146–8.

Pressnitzer, D. and Patterson, R. D. (2001). Distortion products and the pitch of harmonic complex tones. In *Physiological and Psychophysical Bases of Auditory Function* (ed. D. J. Breebaart, A. J. M. Houtsma, A. Kohlrausch, V. F. Prijs, and R. Schoonhoven), pp. 97–104. Maastricht: Shaker.

Pressnitzer, D., Patterson, R. D., and Krumbholz, K. (2001). The lower limit of melodic pitch. *Journal of the Acoustical Society of America* **109**:2074–84.

Pressnitzer, D., Winter, I. M., and de Cheveigné, A. (2002). Perceptual pitch shift for sounds with similar waveform autocorrelation. *Acoustic Research Letters Online* **3**:1–6.

Ritsma, R. J. (1962). Existence region of the tonal residue, I. *Journal of the Acoustical Society of America* **34**:1224–9.

Ritsma, R. J. (1963). Existence region of the tonal residue, II. *Journal of the Acoustical Society of America* **35**:1241–5.

Roberts, T. P. L., Ferrari, P., Stufflebeam, S. M., Steven, M., and Poeppel, D. (2000). Latency of the auditory evoked neuromagnetic field components: stimulus dependence and insights toward perception. *Journal of Clinical Neurophysiology* **17**:114–29.

Robinson, K. and Patterson, R. D. (1995). The stimulus duration required to identify vowels, their octave, and their pitch chroma. *Journal of the Acoustical Society of America* **98**:1858–65.

Robles, L. and Ruggero, M. A. (2001). Mechanics of the mammalian cochlea. *Physiological reviews* **81**: 1305–52.

Romani, G. L., Williamson, S. J., and Kaufman, L. (1982). Tonotopic organization of the human auditory cortex. *Science* **216**:1339–40.

Ruggero, M. A. (1992). Physiology of the auditory nerve. In *The Mammalian Auditory Pathway: Neurophysiology* (ed. A. N. Popper and R. R. Fay), pp. 34–93. New York: Springer-Verlag.

Ruggero, M. A. and Temchin, A. N. (2005). Unexceptional sharpness of frequency tuning in the human cochlea. *Proceedings of the National Academy of Sciences USA* **102**:18614–19.

Ruggero, M. A., Robles, L., and Rich, N. C. (1992). Two-tone suppression in the basilar membrane of the cochlea: mechanical basis of auditory-nerve rate suppression. *Journal of Neurophysiology* **68**:1087–99.

Rusconi, E., Kwan, B., Giordano, B. L., Umiltà, C., and Butterworth, B. (2006). Spatial representation of pitch height: the SMARC effect. *Cognition* **99**:113–29.

Sauveur, J. (1701). Système général des intervalles du son. *Mémoires de l'Académie Royale des Sciences* 279–300; 347–54. [Transl. by R. B. Lindsay as 'General system of sound intervals and its application to sounds of all systems and all musical instruments'; and reprinted in *Acoustics: Historical and Philosophical Development*, pp. 88–94. Stroudsburg, PA: Dowden, Hutchinson and Ross.]

Schneider, P., Sluming, V., Roberts, N., Scherg, M., Goebel, R., Specht, H. J., Dosch, H. G., Bleek, S., Stippich, C., and Rupp, A. (2005). Structural and functional asymmetry of lateral Heschls gyrus reflects pitch perception preference. *Nature Neuroscience* **8**:1241–7.

Schnupp, J. W. H. and King, A. J. (2008). Auditory neuroscience: neuronal sensitivity in humans. *Current Biology* **18**:R382–5.

Schönwieser, M. and Zatorre, R. J. (2008). Depth electrode recordings show double dissociation between pitch processing in lateral Heschl's gyrus and sound onset processing in medial Heschls gyrus. *Experimental Brain Research* **187**:97–105.

Schouten, J. F. (1938). The perception of subjective tones. *Proceedings of the Koninklijke Akademie van Wetenschappen te Amsterdam* **41**:1086–94. [Reprinted in Schubert (1979). Psychological acoustics. In *Benchmark Papers in Acoustics*, Vol. 13, pp. 146–54. Stroudsburg, PA: Dowden, Hutchinson & Ross, Inc.]

Schouten, J. F. (1940). The residue, a new component in subjective sound analysis. *Proceedings of the Koninklijke Akademie van Wetenschappen te Amsterdam* **43**:356–65.

Schwartz, I. R. (1992). The superior olivary complex and lateral lemniscal nuclei. In *The Mammalian Auditory Pathway: Neuroanatomy* (ed. D. B. Webster, A. N. Popper, and R. R. Fay), pp. 117–67. New York: Springer-Verlag.

Seither-Preisler, A., Patterson, R. D., Krumbholz, K., Seither, S., and Lutkenhoner, B. (2006). Evidence of pitch processing in the N100m component of the auditory evoked field. *Hearing Research* **213**:88–98.

Semal, C. and Demany, L. (1990). The upper limit of musical pitch. *Music Perception* **8**:165–76.

Semal, C. and Demany, L. (2006). Individual differences in the sensitivity to pitch direction. *Journal of the Acoustical Society of America* **120**:3907–15.

Sethares, W. A. (1997). *Tuning, Timbre, Spectrum, Scale*. London: Springer-Verlag.

Shackleton, T. M. and Carlyon, R. P. (1994). The role of resolved and unresolved harmonics in pitch perception and frequency modulation discrimination. *Journal of the Acoustical Society of America* **95**:3529–40.

Shamma, S. and Klein, D. (2000). The case of the missing pitch templates: how harmonic templates emerge in the early auditory system. *Journal of the Acoustical Society of America* **107**:2631–44.

Shepard, R. N. (1982). Structural representations of musical pitch. In *The Psychology of Music* (ed. D. Deutsh), pp. 343–90. Orlando, FL: Academic Press.

Smoorenburg, G. F. (1970). Pitch perception of two-frequency stimuli. *Journal of the Acoustical Society of America* **48**:924–42.

Stufflebeam, S. M., Poeppel, D., Rowley, H. A., and Roberts, P. L. (1998). Peri-threshold encoding of stimulus frequency and intensity in the M100 latency. *Neuroreport* **9**:91–4.

Terhardt, E. (1974). Pitch, consonance and harmony. *Journal of the Acoustical Society of America* **55**:1061–9.

Terhardt, E. (1979). Calculating virtual pitch. *Hearing Research* **1**:155–82.

Thompson, A. M. and Schofield, B. R. (2000). Afferent projections of the superior olivary complex. *Microscopy Research and Technique* **51**:330–54.

Tramo, M. J., Cariani, P., Koh, C. K., Makris, N., and Braida, L. D. (2005). Neurophysiology and neuroanatomy of pitch perception: auditory cortex. *Annals of the New York Academy of Science* **1060**:148–74.

Turner, R. S. (1977). The Ohm–Seebeck dispute, Hermann von Helmholtz, and the origins of physiological acoustics. *British Journal for the History of Science* **10**:1–24.

Ueda, K. and Ohgushi, K. (1987). Perceptual components of pitch: spatial representation using a multidimensional scaling technique. *Journal of the Acoustical Society of America* **82**: 1193–200.

von Békésy, G. and Rosenblith, W. A. (1948). The early history of hearing—observations and theories. *Journal of the Acoustical Society of America* 20:727–48.

Wallace, M. N., Anderson, L. A., and Palmer, A. R. (2007). Phase-locked responses to pure tones in the auditory thalamus. *Journal of Neurophysiology* 98:1941–52.

Ward, W. D. (1999). Absolute pitch. In *The Psychology of Music* (ed. D. Deutsch), pp. 265–98. Orlando, FL: Academic Press.

Warren, R. M., Bashford, J. A., and Wrightson, J. M. (1980). Infrapitch echo. *Journal of the Acoustical Society of America* 65:1301–5.

Warren, J. D., Uppenkamp, S., Patterson, R. D., and Griffiths, T. D. (2003). Separating pitch chroma and pitch height in the human brain. *Proceedings of the National Academy of Sciences USA* 100:10038–42.

Wever, E. G. and Bray, C. W. (1930). The nature of acoustic response: the relation between sound frequency and frequency of impulses in the auditory nerve. *Journal of Experimental Psychology* 13: 373–87.

White, L. J. and Plack, C. J. (2003). Factors affecting the duration effect in pitch perception for unresolved complex tones. *Journal of the Acoustical Society of America* 114:3309–16.

Wiegrebe, L. and Meddis, R. (2004). The representation of periodic sounds in simulated sustained chopper units of the ventral cochlear nucleus. *Journal of the Acoustical Society of America* 115:1207–18.

Wier, C. C., Jesteadt, W., and Green, D. M. (1977). Frequency discrimination as a function of frequency and sensation level. *Journal of the Acoustical Society of America* 61:178–84.

Wightman, F. L. (1973a). Pitch and stimulus fine structure. *Journal of the Acoustical Society of America* 54:397–406.

Wightman, F. L. (1973b). The pattern-transformation model of pitch. *Journal of the Acoustical Society of America* 54:407–16.

Winter, I. M. (2005). The neurophysiology of pitch. In *Pitch—Neural Coding and Perception* (ed. C. J. Plack, A. J. Oxenham, R. R. Fay, and A. N. Popper), pp. 99–146. New York: Springer.

Winter, I. M., Wiegrebe, L., and Patterson, R. D. (2001). The temporal representation of the delay of iterated rippled noise in the ventral cochlear nucleus of the guinea-pig. *Journal of Physiology* 537: 553–66.

Yost, W. A. (1996). Pitch strength of iterated rippled noise. *Journal of the Acoustical Society of America* 100:3329–35.

Zatorre, R. J. (2003). Absolute pitch: a model for understanding the influence of genes and development on neural and cognitive function. *Nature Neuroscience* 6:692–5.

Chapter 5

Temporal resolution and temporal integration

Jesko L. Verhey

5.1 Introduction

Sound waves are longitudinal waves in a medium—usually air—where the pressure varies periodically around the mean pressure of the medium. It is common to distinguish between rapid pressure changes, referred to as 'fine structure', and slower overall changes of the amplitude of the pressure fluctuations. These slower changes are usually characterized by means of the temporal envelope or instantaneous intensity of the sound wave. Many natural sounds, including speech, show envelope fluctuations over time, and it is generally assumed that the auditory system makes use of this information to identify sounds and to separate sounds from different sound sources (Nelken *et al.*, 1999).

The auditory system has only a limited ability to follow the time-varying envelope. This limited acuity in the perception of envelope fluctuations is commonly referred to as 'temporal resolution'. A summary of different measures of temporal resolution is given in Section 5.2. This section provides a slightly broader view of temporal resolution by briefly discussing a study on pitch and one on binaural perception. In those experiments the performance is presumably limited by temporal resolution in the fine structure and not the envelope. Sections 5.3 and 5.5 describe two different approaches to characterizing temporal resolution in more detail, namely non-simultaneous masking experiments and the perception of periodic envelope fluctuations. Section 5.4 briefly describes physiological constraints of temporal resolution.

The second topic of this chapter—temporal integration—is mainly discussed in Sections 5.6 and 5.7. Note, however, that the temporal-window model described in Section 5.3 also uses temporal integration to describe non-simultaneous masking. Section 5.6 describes the classical approach to temporal integration, i.e. an increase in auditory sensitivity as the duration of the sound is increased. Section 5.7 provides a different view on temporal integration describing the theory of multiple looks. A summary of the chapter is given in Section 5.8.

5.2 Measures of temporal resolution

As in the frequency domain (see Chapter 2), the auditory system also has a limited resolution in the time domain. Several different experiments have been proposed to measure the temporal resolution of the auditory system.

One possibility is to measure the sensitivity to short temporal gaps in a signal (e.g. Moore *et al.*, 1993). The smallest detectable gap is in the range from 2 to 20 ms and depends on the level and spectral properties of the signal (e.g. Fitzgibbons, 1983; Moore *et al.*, 1993). A similar time constant can be observed in a forward-masking paradigm, where a short signal is presented after the offset of a masker. Forward masking persists for about 50–200 ms (Duifhuis, 1973; Zwicker, 1984), which corresponds to an exponential integrator time constant of about 10 ms if peripheral compression is taken into account (Plack and Moore, 1990; see also Penner, 1978). More details about non-simultaneous masking and the time constants derived from the data can be found in Section 5.3.

The perception of level fluctuations (modulations) is another possibility to assess the temporal resolution of the auditory system. There are several time constants that can be derived from modulation data. For example, a change in the phase of modulation is inaudible if the modulation frequency exceeds about 32 Hz (Sheft and Yost, 2007). From this frequency f a time constant τ of a leaky integrator (see Section 5.6) can be derived using the following equation:

$$\tau = \frac{1}{2 \cdot \pi \cdot f}$$

(5.1)

Thus, for the data on the sensitivity of the modulation phase the time constant is about 5 ms. The time constant is a factor of two to three smaller if data on modulation detection is used. Finally, modulation-masking data provides a whole set of time constants if the modulation frequency selectivity at different modulation frequencies is transformed into time constants for temporal resolution. More details about modulation perception and the time constants derived from the data can be found in Section 5.5.

Data on binaural localization by interaural time differences show that differences in arrival times of the order of 10 μs are distinguishable (Henning, 1974), i.e. on a much shorter time scale than the time constants described so far. There are also monaural experiments involving iterated rippled noise (IRN) and inter-pulse gaps showing similar thresholds in temporal resolution (Leshowitz, 1971; Krumbholz et al., 2003). In contrast, binaural gap detection data and data on changes of interaural correlation indicate a time constant in the range of 100 ms (Akeroyd and Summerfield, 1999; Boehnke et al., 2002). This is comparable to the time constants' data that were proposed in the context of monaural temporal integration (see Section 5.6). Some loudness studies on temporal integration even indicate a temporal integration of up to 10 s (Ogura et al., 1991). At this time scale, memory effects are likely to play a role. For example, the overall loudness of sounds with a duration of several seconds seems to be dominated by loud events (percentile loudness; Zwicker and Fastl, 1999) and to be higher if the signal level is higher at the end of the signal (Susini et al., 2002). Limitations in the auditory memory may also be found on a shorter time scale, as briefly discussed in Section 5.7.

In summary, temporal resolution and temporal integration cannot be quantified with a single time constant. The time constant strongly depends on the experimental paradigm and ranges from a few microseconds to 100 ms or more.

5.3 Non-simultaneous masking and the temporal window

The temporal window was developed to account for masking data where the masker and the signal are presented non-simultaneously (e.g. Plack and Moore, 1990). There are two basic non-simultaneous masking conditions: forward masking and backward masking (see also Chapter 2).

5.3.1 Forward masking

When a short signal tone pulse is presented shortly after a noise or tone masker, the threshold for detecting the signal is raised above that in quiet. The smaller the duration of the gap between the masker and the signal, the higher is the threshold. This phenomenon is termed 'forward masking' or 'post masking' and refers to the fact that a masker affects the signal threshold when they are presented in a non-simultaneous, consecutive manner. A typical example of a threshold curve in a forward-masking paradigm is shown in Fig. 5.1 (data taken from Dau et al., 1996). The signal

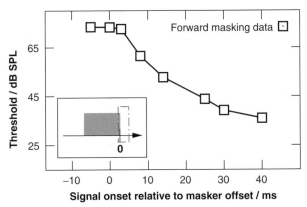

Fig. 5.1 Forward-masking data taken from Dau *et al.* (1996). Mean masked thresholds in dB SPL for three listeners are shown as a function of the signal onset relative to the masker offset. The signal was a 10-ms long, 1-kHz tone pulse and the masker a broadband noise at a level of 77 dB SPL. The inset in the lower-left corner schematically shows the range of temporal positions of the signal (red box) relative to the masker (filled grey box).

was a 10-ms long, 1-kHz tone pulse. The masker was bandpass-filtered noise (20–5000 Hz) with a duration of 200 ms.

Threshold usually drops to performance in quiet when the gap is in the region of hundreds of milliseconds, i.e. outside the temporal range shown in Fig. 5.1. The shape of the forward-masking curve depends on several physical parameters of the masker and the signal. In general, the forward-masking curve is steeper for short maskers and higher masker levels (Zwicker, 1984). In addition, forward-masking thresholds for a sinusoidal signal switched on immediately after masker offset are considerably lower for broadband than for narrowband noise maskers with the same spectrum level (Dubno and Ahlstrom, 2001). This is usually interpreted as evidence for suppression. As described in Chapter 2, forward-masking paradigms are commonly used in psychoacoustics to study cochlear non-linearities, since the masker and the signal can be assumed to be processed independently on the basilar membrane. The difference in the growth of masking for on-frequency and off-frequency tonal maskers is used to assess the suppression and non-linear behaviour of the basilar membrane at the place associated with the signal frequency (Oxenham and Plack, 1997; Nelson *et al.*, 2001; Yasin and Plack, 2003). Forward masking is also influenced by more central processes. For example, if the signal is similar in quality to the masker, i.e. having a similar centre frequency and bandwidth, listeners may experience a certain temporal uncertainty about the end of the masker. In those conditions they may perceive the signal as part of the masker. The temporal uncertainty can be reduced by presenting additional sounds to serve as cues to the end of the masker (Moore and Glasberg, 1982; see also McFadden and Wright, 1987).

5.3.2 Backward masking

A masker can also raise threshold if it follows the signal. This effect is referred to as 'backward masking' or 'pre masking'. An example of backward masking data is shown in Fig. 5.2 (data taken from Dau *et al.*, 1996). As in the case of Fig. 5.1 the signal was a 10-ms tone pulse and the masker was a bandpass-filtered noise (20-5000 Hz) with a duration of 200 ms.

The figure shows the average over two of the listeners in the study by Dau *et al.* (1996) who obtained similar results. For a gap between a signal onset and masker onset of more than 20 ms the thresholds were similar to the threshold in quiet. For shorter gaps, thresholds increased as the

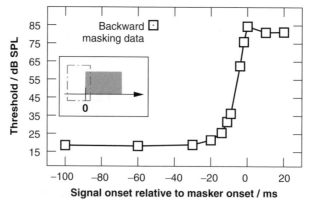

Fig. 5.2 Backward-masking data from Dau *et al.* (1996). Mean thresholds in dB SPL of a tone pulse in the presence of a noise masker averaged over the individual data of two listeners are shown. In general, the physical parameters for the signal and masker were the same as in Fig. 5.1. In contrast to the forward-masking paradigm, the signal was positioned close to the onset of the masker as indicated in the inset.

gap between signal and masker decreased. In contrast to the mean of the two listeners shown here, the third listener in the study by Dau *et al.* (1996) showed a more gradual increase in threshold as the gap between signal and masker decreased. These individual differences in backward masking are probably due to stimulus uncertainty in some listeners. As in forward-masking data, the effect of the backward masker is reduced if a cue about the temporal position of the signal is provided (Puleo and Pastore, 1980).

5.3.3 The temporal window

Backward and forward masking can be accounted for by assuming a temporal 'smoothing' device, i.e. a sliding leaky temporal integrator. The temporal integrator determines a weighted average over a certain time interval, hence the masker is assumed to be combined with the signal in the auditory system (raising signal threshold), even though the two are not physically simultaneous. Threshold is assumed to depend on the signal-to-masker intensity ratio at the output of the temporal integrator, when positioned in time to maximize that ratio. The shape of the integrator is typically determined by the threshold curves in forward- and backward-masking experiments. The shape of each of the curves can be approximated by exponential functions. A simple implementation of the temporal integrator is, thus, a pair of back-to-back exponential functions. This type of temporal integrator is referred to as 'the temporal window' (Plack and Moore, 1990).

Forward masking is presumably better described by a combination of two exponential functions (e.g. Zwicker, 1984). Thus, current temporal-window models combine more than two exponential functions (e.g. a combination of three as in Oxenham, 2001). An example of a temporal window is shown in Fig. 5.3. The window is described by the following equations:

$$W(t) = (1-w) \cdot e^{t/T_{for1}} + w \cdot e^{t/T_{for2}}, \quad t < 0,$$
$$W(t) = e^{-t/T_{back}}, \quad t \geq 0, \tag{5.2}$$

where t is time relative to the peak of the window, T_{for1} and T_{for2} are the time constants describing the decay of forward masking, w is the weighting factor determining the relative contributions of these two time constants, and T_{back} is the time constant describing the rise of backward masking.

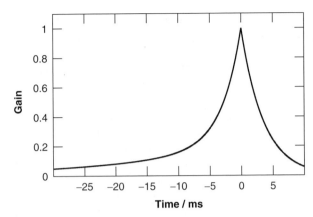

Fig. 5.3 Shape of the temporal window that was hypothesized to account for non-simultaneous masking. The parameters are taken from Oxenham (2001). For details see text.

While the early realizations of the temporal-window model integrated linear intensity (Plack and Moore, 1990), the temporal window is now usually preceded by a non-linearity simulating the compressive nature of the basilar membrane (e.g. Oxenham, 2001). This combination of non-linearity and temporal window allows the prediction of several aspects of the non-linear characteristics of non-simultaneous masking: for example, the 'excess' masking observed when a masker preceding a short signal is combined with one following the signal (e.g. Oxenham and Moore, 1994). In those conditions, thresholds are much higher than would be predicted by a linear combination of the two masking effects.

The time constants of the exponentials vary between different studies. For backward masking the time constant is about 3–5 ms. The two time constants for forward masking are about 4 and 20 ms (e.g. Oxenham, 2001). For the example shown in Fig. 5.3, the time constants were $T_{for1} = 3.1$ ms, $T_{for2} = 21.0$ ms and $T_{back} = 3.5$ ms. The weighting factor w between the two exponential functions describing forward masking was 0.206. The equivalent rectangular duration of a temporal window (i.e. the duration of a rectangular window with the same area under the curve) is typically in the range from 5 to 20 ms.

5.3.4 Persistence versus adaptation

Due to the smoothing with a temporal window the masker representation will show a slow decay of activation after masker offset. This continuing activity is commonly referred to as 'persistence'. In the light of the temporal window model this persistence is responsible for the elevated thresholds for a signal following the masker, i.e. in a forward-masking paradigm. An alternative explanation of forward masking is to assume that it results from adaptation, a decrease in activity after stimulus offset (Duifhuis, 1973; Dau et al., 1996). Neural adaptation is observed at different levels of the auditory system, starting with the auditory nerve. It is still unclear whether temporal integration or adaptation can better account for forward masking in various stimulus configurations (Oxenham, 2001; see also Chapter 2). However, recently it was shown that the mechanisms underlying forward masking in a temporal-window model and an established model using an adaptation stage (Dau et al., 1996) are very similar if the combination of the persistence or adaptation stage with the corresponding decision stage is analysed (Ewert et al., 2007).

5.4 What limits temporal resolution?

There are several physiological constraints limiting the temporal resolution of the auditory system. For example, the frequency selectivity of the auditory system can be modelled as a bank of overlapping bandpass filters. The 'ringing' (continued response after stimulus offset) of these auditory filters provides a peripheral limit to temporal resolution. Since auditory filters are narrow at low frequencies and relatively broad at high frequencies this limit depends on the carrier frequency (see Chapter 2). However, it has been shown that gap detection threshold for pure tones does not vary as a function of frequency (e.g. Shailer and Moore, 1987), except perhaps at very low frequencies, hence it is unlikely that filter ringing is the main limitation in temporal resolution.

Temporal resolution is also limited at the neural level. The first limitation is the transformation of receptor potential at the hair cell into spikes and here the absolute refractory period between two spikes. This limited encoding ability is usually incorporated in effective psychoacoustic models by filtering the envelope with a lowpass filter. The cut-off frequency is about 800 Hz. Temporal resolution is presumably further limited by central neural processes such as adaptation (see the previous section), sluggishness in synaptic transmission, or the processing of level fluctuations with modulation bandpass filters (Schreiner and Langner, 1988; for the psychoacoustics see also Section 5.5.3).

5.5 Modulation perception

A common property of many natural sounds is that their level fluctuates over time (see Section 5.1). The level fluctuations can be quantified by calculating the Hilbert envelope of a signal $s(t)$:

$$envelope(s(t)) = |s(t) - i \cdot F_{Hi}(s(t))|,$$

(5.3)

where i is the imaginary unit and $F_{Hi}(s(t))$ is the Hilbert transform of $s(t)$:

$$F_{Hi}(s(t)) = \frac{1}{\pi} \int_{-\infty}^{\infty} \frac{s(t')}{t' - t} dt'$$

(5.4)

The expression $s(t) - i \cdot F_{Hi}(s(t))$ is referred to as the 'analytic signal'. For example, the Hilbert transform of a cosine wave is a sine wave with a negative sign, and the analytical signal is an exponential function with a purely imaginary exponent. Thus, the Hilbert envelope of a cosine is constant. In contrast, noise has inherent envelope fluctuations. The fluctuations are caused by the beating of its frequency components. Since noise consists of several frequency components the envelope spectrum of noise also contains several frequency components. Thus the modulation spectrum is more complex than for a sinusoidal amplitude modulation and depends on the amplitude and phase characteristics of the frequency components of the noise. For example, for a Gaussian noise with a rectangular shape of the power spectrum, the power spectrum of the envelope is given approximately by the following equation:

$$P(f_{envelope}) \approx max\left(\pi \cdot \Delta f \cdot \rho \cdot \delta(f_{envelope}) + \frac{\pi \cdot \rho}{4 \cdot \Delta f}(\Delta f - f_{envelope}), 0 \right),$$

(5.5)

where P is the envelope power density, Δf is the carrier bandwidth, ρ is the (constant) spectral power density of the carrier, and $f_{envelope}$ indicates the envelope frequency (Lawson and Uhlenbeck, 1950, pp. 56–63; Dau et al., 1999). The envelope power spectrum of the Gaussian noise contains a dc-peak and a triangular continuous spectrum with the highest frequency equal to the carrier bandwidth.

Envelope fluctuations can be imposed on a signal by multiplying the signal with a modulator, i.e. by modulating a carrier. The most common modulator is a dc-shifted sinusoid. The dc-shift is usually larger than the amplitude of the modulation to prevent overmodulation. The resulting equation for a sinusoidal amplitude modulated signal is:

$$s(t) = c(t) \cdot (1 + m \cdot \sin(2 \cdot \pi \cdot f_m \cdot t + \phi)),$$

(5.6)

where $c(t)$ is the carrier, f_m is the modulation frequency, ϕ is the starting phase of the modulation, and m is the modulation depth. The modulation depth is usually expressed in dB as $20\log(m)$. If m is restricted to values smaller than 0 dB (100%) the modulation will add a component at the modulation frequency to the envelope spectrum of the carrier. The modulation also changes the spectrum of the sound. For a sinusoidal carrier, two sidebands are added, one on each side of the carrier frequency in the distance of the modulation frequency. For more complex carriers, the modulation adds sidebands to each frequency component of the carrier. Although one may argue that the term 'modulation' should be reserved to conditions where the experimenter modulates the signal explicitly, the terms 'modulation' and 'envelope fluctuations' are often used interchangeably.

5.5.1 Sensations associated with the perception of temporal amplitude modulations

There are two sensations associated with the perception of temporal modulations: fluctuation strength and roughness (Zwicker and Fastl, 1999). The sensation fluctuation strength implies that the listener perceives level fluctuations. Fluctuation strength is largest for 4 Hz and reaches zero at about 32 Hz. This is about the frequency where listeners are no longer able to perceive the starting phase of a modulation (Sheft and Yost, 2007). Fluctuation strength depends very little on the frequency of a sinusoidal carrier.

The sensation of roughness arises when rapid beats (at higher rates than those eliciting the sensation of fluctuation strength) are perceived as a temporal property of the sound (Zwicker and Fastl, 1999). For a carrier frequency of 1 kHz or higher, roughness perception is largest for 70 Hz. For lower carrier frequencies the modulation frequency that produces the maximum roughness decreases as the carrier frequency decreases. This decrease results presumably from the frequency selectivity of the auditory system. At a certain modulation frequency the sidebands generated by the modulation are spectrally resolved. For high modulation frequencies the sound may be perceived as a complex tone with a certain pitch and timbre. For more complex signals than amplitude modulated tones roughness also depends on the relative phase of the modulations in different frequency regions, being largest for coherent modulations across frequency (Pressnitzer and McAdams, 1999).

5.5.2 Temporal modulation transfer function

Another way of characterizing the ability of the auditory system to perceive envelope fluctuations is to measure the just-noticeable modulation depth as a function of the modulation frequency. The resulting curve is referred to as a 'temporal modulation transfer function' (TMTF; Viemeister, 1979). Figure 5.4 shows the TMTF for two common carrier types: a sine wave and a broadband noise. For the noise carrier the modulation depth at threshold is similar for low modulation frequencies up to about 100 Hz. For higher modulation frequencies the modulation depth at threshold increases as the modulation frequency increases.

To account for the data, Viemeister (1979) proposed a model that assumes a limited ability to follow amplitude modulations. The limitation was modelled as a modulation lowpass filter. The TMTF for a sinusoidal carrier is slightly different from the one for the broadband noise carrier. Beyond a certain modulation frequency the detection threshold decreases as the modulation frequency increases. This critical modulation frequency depends on the signal frequency being higher for higher carrier frequencies (Kohlrausch et al., 2000). This decrease presumably is a consequence of the resolved sidebands generated by the modulation which are used to detect the modulation. For broadband signals the sidebands are masked by the carrier and thus can not be used for modulation detection.

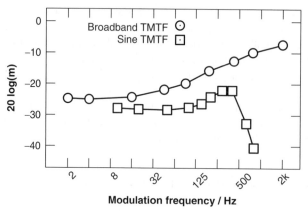

Fig. 5.4 Temporal modulation transfer functions (TMTFs) for two types of carriers: a broadband noise and a sinusoidal carrier. The data for the broadband noise carrier (circles) were taken from Viemeister (1979); the data for the 5-kHz carrier (squares) were taken from Kohlrausch *et al.* (2000). Modulation depth at threshold is plotted against modulation frequency as 20log(m).

5.5.3 Modulation masking

Apart from measuring detection of modulation in the absence of interference, modulation processing can also be studied using masking experiments. In these experiments more than one modulator is imposed on a carrier. An example of modulation masking data is shown in Fig. 5.5 (data taken from Ewert *et al.*, 2000; see also Houtgast, 1989). The target modulation frequency was 4, 16, or 64 Hz. The masker was a narrowband noise modulator with a modulation depth of −10 dB. In each on-frequency condition, the noise masker was half an octave wide. The absolute bandwidth was held constant when the masker was shifted in the range from −2 to +2 octaves relative to the target frequency. For each of the target modulation frequencies, threshold is highest for the on-frequency condition. The data indicate that the auditory system shows a frequency selectivity in the envelope-frequency domain similar to the one observed in the audio-frequency domain. The data can be accounted for by transferring the concept of the power-spectrum model proposed by Fletcher (1940) to account for masking effects in the audio-frequency domain, to the modulation-frequency domain. This modified model, known as the 'envelope-power-spectrum model' (EPSM),

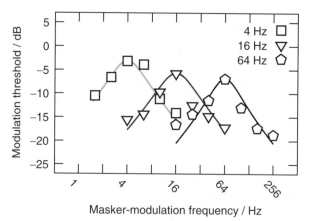

Fig. 5.5 Modulation masking data showing modulation-frequency selectivity. The data is taken from a study by Ewert *et al.* (2002). Modulation depth 20log(m) at threshold is shown for three different target modulation frequencies: 4 Hz (squares), 16 Hz (triangles), and 64 Hz (pentagrams). The masker modulation was a narrowband noise. The frequency of the sinusoidal carrier was 5.5 kHz. The solid lines indicate the bandpass filters that were fitted to the data.

assumes that the energy of the modulation masker that falls into the filter at the target modulation frequency determines threshold (Ewert and Dau, 2000). As an example, Fig. 5.5 shows the modulation filters (solid lines), which were fitted to the experimental data. The ratio of the bandwidth to the centre frequency is about one, i.e. three times less than the frequency selectivity in the audio-frequency domain (Ewert and Dau, 2000; Ewert *et al.*, 2002).

The concept of modulation filters also accounts for amplitude modulation detection for narrowband noise carriers (Dau *et al.*, 1999) where the TMTF shows a highpass or bandpass characteristic. In this case the inherent envelope fluctuations of the carrier mask the target modulation. Dau *et al.* (1999) showed that the effect of the carrier bandwidth on the modulation detection thresholds can be qualitatively predicted, i.e. by determining the portion of the inherent envelope fluctuations of the carrier within the passband of the modulation filter centred at the target modulation frequency (see also Ewert and Dau, 2000).

5.5.4 Higher order modulations

Ewert *et al.* (2002) showed that modulation masking is considerably smaller than shown in Fig. 5.5 if a sinusoidal masker modulation is used instead of a narrowband noise-masker modulation. They argued that this is due to the audibility of higher order modulation. Masker modulation and target modulation may 'beat' and thus produce audible components at the beating frequency. In agreement with this hypothesis, thresholds increased considerably if an additional masker modulation was present at the beating frequency. To characterize the beating component, Ewert *et al.* (2002) proposed to calculate the Hilbert envelope of the ac-coupled modulations and referred to this quantity as the 'venelope'. The venelope also affects the detection of a sinusoidal amplitude modulation if the target frequency is equal to the beating frequency (Moore *et al.*, 1999; Verhey *et al.*, 2003a; Füllgrabe *et al.*, 2005), indicating that venelope and envelope may be processed in a similar information channel. A sinusoidal venelope can be generated by the following equation:

$$s(t) = c(t) \cdot \left(1 + m \cdot (1 + m_{ven} \cdot \sin(2 \cdot \pi \cdot f_{ven} \cdot t + \phi_{ven})) \cdot \sin(2 \cdot \pi \cdot f_m \cdot t + \phi)\right) \tag{5.7}$$

Here the modulation depth of the modulator with a modulation frequency f_m is sinusoidally varied between $m+m_{ven}$ and $m-m_{ven}$ at the rate f_{ven}. Several studies have investigated the detection of the sinusoidal venelope, commonly referred to as the 'second-order modulation' (Tandetnik *et al.*, 2001; Uchanski *et al.*, 2006). The modulation transfer function for the second-order modulations shows a lowpass characteristic. The cut-off frequency depends on the frequency f_m of the modulator carrying the second-order modulation, being smaller for smaller f_m (Lorenzi *et al.*, 2001). Several mechanisms have been proposed to account for the perception of the venelope. The interaction between venelope and sinusoidal amplitude modulation indicates that a non-linearity introduces the venelope frequency in the envelope spectrum. The exact nature of this non-linearity is still unclear. The similarity of the detection thresholds for normal and hearing-impaired listeners (Tandetnik, *et al.*, 2001), as well as model simulations on the influence of venelope phase on the detection of sinusoidal amplitude modulation (Verhey *et al.*, 2003a), argue against a cochlear non-linearity as the main process generating a venelope component in the envelope spectrum. This suggests that retrocochlear processes generate a venelope component. In addition to non-linear mechanisms, off-frequency listening may play a role in experiments using narrowband carriers (Füllgrabe *et al.*, 2005). The detection of second-order modulation may also be partly based on the detection of temporal changes of the modulation depth in the modulation filter centred at the modulation frequency f_m carrying the second-order modulation (Milmann *et al.*, 2003; Uchanski *et al.*, 2006). So far, studies have focused their attention on first- and second-order modulations. It remains to be seen if the auditory system is sensitive to modulation of a higher order than two.

5.5.5 Modulation processing across frequency

Several psychoacoustic phenomena indicate that modulation is not processed independently in each peripheral filter. For example, modulation masking is also observed if a masker modulation is imposed on a different carrier (Yost and Sheft, 1989). This across-frequency masking is referred to as 'modulation detection interference' (MDI). The magnitude of MDI is highest if the target modulation and masker modulation are similar, further supporting the hypothesis of modulation filters analysing the incoming sound. Coherent envelope fluctuations also affect the detection of sounds in the audio-frequency domain. For example, masked thresholds for a narrow-band target signal are higher if the masker and the target have the same envelope compared to a masking situation where they have uncorrelated level fluctuations. This effect is referred to as 'comodulation detection interference' (CDD, Cohen and Schubert, 1987). A related effect is comodulation masking release (CMR; Hall *et al.*, 1984; and see Verhey *et al.*, 2003*b*, for a review). CMR describes the effect that thresholds of a sinusoidal signal are lower when the masker has coherent envelope fluctuations across frequency. Originally, CMR and CDD were discussed in the light of central auditory grouping mechanisms comparing the temporal information across different frequency channels. However, simulations with models using the information of only one peripheral filter showed that the non-linear behaviour of the basilar membrane (Borrill and Moore, 2002; Buschermöhle *et al.*, 2006; Ernst and Verhey, 2006, 2008) and modulation processing with a modulation filterbank (Verhey *et al.*, 1999; see also Piechowiak *et al.*, 2007) also contribute to the influence of comodulation on detection.

5.6 Temporal integration

5.6.1 Temporal integration as a result of leaky integration

Several experiments indicate that the auditory system integrates signal intensity over time. A typical paradigm associated with this ability is the decrease of perceived signal intensity at absolute threshold as the signal duration increases (Garner, 1947; Poulsen, 1981; for a review see Gerken *et al.*, 1990). As an example, Fig. 5.6 shows thresholds in quiet of a 1-kHz tone as a function of stimulus duration (data taken from Poulsen, 1981).

The results of experiments on temporal integration are usually modelled by assuming that the intensity or some other transformation of the signal is analysed with a leaky integrator (e.g. Plomp and Bouman, 1959; Zwislocki, 1960), effectively a longer version of the temporal window described in Section 5.3. A simple electric implementation for a leaky integrator is a resistor and

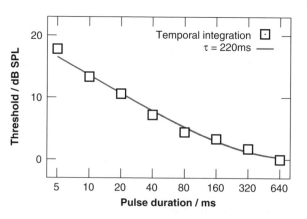

Fig. 5.6 Temporal integration data from Poulsen (1981). Symbols show absolute thresholds in quiet as a function of the duration of 1-kHz tone pulses averaged over 25 listeners. The solid grey line is the prediction of a leaky integrator using a lowpass filter with a time constant of $\tau = 220$ ms.

a capacitor in series. In this analogy the potential of the source is the intensity I of the signal, and the potential difference between the two plates of the capacitor is regarded as the strength S of an internal representation of the level which is relevant for signal detection. Mathematically, such a charging process can be described as a convolution of the incoming signal with the impulse response of the leaky integrator (see also Section 5.3.3 on the temporal-window model). For the electric circuit of resistor and capacitor, the impulse response is an exponential function. Thus, assuming that the temporal integration is comparable to a charging process of such an electric circuit, the time course of the internal representation of intensity can be written as:

$$S(t) = k \cdot \int_{-\infty}^{t} I(t') \cdot e^{-(t-t')/\tau} dt'$$

$$(5.8)$$

where $I(t)$ and $S(t)$ are the intensity and the internal representation at the time t, respectively. The parameter k is a constant of proportionality and τ is the integration time constant (i.e. the product of the resistance R and the capacitance C in the electric circuit). In contrast to the temporal window described in Section 5.3, the impulse response of this model consists of only one decaying exponential function.

It is commonly assumed that the maximum of this internal variable determines threshold. If, for simplification, it is assumed that the signal intensity is a positive constant I_T for a duration T, and zero at other times, the maximum of the internal variable is:

$$S = k \cdot I_T \cdot \left(1 - e^{-T/\tau}\right)$$

$$(5.9)$$

Assuming that the magnitude of the internal value S at threshold is the same for all durations, the following equation for the intensity at threshold for a given duration T can be derived:

$$\frac{I_T}{I_\infty} = \frac{1}{\left(1 - e^{-T/\tau}\right)}$$

$$(5.10)$$

where I_T is the intensity at threshold for the signal duration T and I_∞ is the asymptotic value for the intensity at threshold for very long signals. For a doubling of the duration one obtains:

$$\frac{I_{2T}}{I_T} = \frac{1}{\left(1 + e^{-T/\tau}\right)}$$

$$(5.11)$$

For durations considerably smaller than the time constant of the integrator, the exponential function is close to one and the ratio on the right-hand side of the equation is 0.5. Thus, the simple model predicts a 3-dB decrease in threshold as the duration is increased by a factor of two, i.e. the auditory system behaves like an energy detector. However, the data in Fig. 5.6 show a slightly steeper slope than 3 dB per doubling for very short durations, indicating that temporal integration may involve more than one time constant (Poulsen, 1981).

Temporal integration is also observed in loudness data (see Chapter 3) and in masking threshold data where the signal is masked by another signal. In masking conditions, it is generally assumed that the signal-to-masker ratio at the output of the integrator governs performance.

On average, the time constants derived from the data are similar for absolute thresholds and masked thresholds, ranging between 100 and 200 ms (Zwislocki, 1969). For the curve fitted to the data in Fig. 5.6, a time constant of $\tau = 220$ ms was used.

Temporal integration depends on the frequency characteristics of the stimulus. For sinusoidal signals, the time constant tends to decrease as the frequency increases (Plomp and Bouman, 1959). In addition, temporal integration seems to be less effective for broadband signals than for narrowband signals (van den Brink and Houtgast, 1990).

5.6.2 Temporal integration and compression

For hearing-impaired listeners, the slope of the threshold curve is smaller than for normal-hearing listeners (Florentine *et al.*, 1988; Oxenham *et al.*, 1997). The difference in slope may be a consequence of a reduced compression in hearing-impaired listeners (Carlyon *et al.*, 1990; however, see Plack and Skeels, 2007). The influence of compression on the threshold curve can be understood within the simple-leaky-integrator model described above. The influence of compression can be visualized by replacing the intensity with the compressed intensity. If the internal variable S is related to the intensity by a power law I^p then the above equation for the relation between the intensities at threshold for 2T and T becomes:

$$\frac{I_{2T}^{\,p}}{I_T^{\,p}} = \frac{1}{\left(1+e^{-T/\tau}\right)}, \quad \text{and thus:} \quad \frac{I_{2T}}{I_T} = \frac{1}{\left(1+e^{-T/\tau}\right)^{1/p}}$$

(5.12)

The above equation shows that compression changes the slope of the threshold curve by a factor of $1/p$ if plotted as level versus the log duration. Since compression implies an exponent p smaller than one, the slope is larger with compression than without compression. Data on temporal integration in loudness support the hypothesis that compression influences the magnitude of temporal integration. The level difference between equally loud signals is largest at medium levels where compression is largest and is reduced at low and high levels where the cochlea is less compressive (Florentine *et al.*, 1996; see also Chapter 3).

For signal detection the data is less clear. For example, the slope of the temporal integration curve differs only by about a factor of two between normal-hearing and hearing-impaired listeners (Florentine *et al.*, 1988; Oxenham *et al.*, 1997). This is considerably less than would be expected from a complete loss of cochlear compression. In addition, there is a large interindividual variability even between the normal-hearing listeners. The variability in the data for normal-hearing listeners may be related to the microstructure of the audiogram (Cohen, 1982).

A recent study measured compression and temporal integration within the same listeners. At absolute threshold the compression exponent is close to one (i.e. a linear growth) and seems to be similar for normal-hearing and hearing-impaired listeners (Plack and Skeels, 2007). Thus, compression may not be the main factor determining the slope of the temporal integration curve. Compression may, however, account for the apparent discrepancy between the time constants for temporal resolution and temporal integration. Penner (1978) showed that compression followed by a temporal integration stage with a short time constant of a few milliseconds can account for temporal integration in the range of hundreds of milliseconds. In contrast to the exponential impulse response described above, Penner proposed a power law with the time t as the base. The power law seems to be better suited to account for the integration of multiple bursts than the exponential function. A more physiological model was proposed by Heil and Neubauer (2003). They assumed that the internal variable relevant for test-tone integration is the integrated pressure of the signal at the level of the inner hair cells. In the light of this model the difference between normal-hearing and hearing-impaired listeners reflects a reduced sensitivity of the inner hair cells of the hearing-impaired listeners. It remains to be seen if temporal integration is governed by only one process or if a combination of several mechanisms is needed to account for all data on temporal integration (see Section 5.7).

5.7 Long integration vs. multiple looks

An alternative approach to the leaky integrator type of model described above assumes that physical integration occurs only over a limited duration of about 5–10 ms (Viemeister and Wakefield, 1991; see also Green, 1960). Instead, it is suggested that the auditory system combines information from across independent looks of short durations. This strategy is referred to as 'multiple looks'. For temporal integration it predicts a 1.5-dB decrease in threshold per doubling of sound duration if the 'looks' are independent and the information is optimally combined. Such a decrease is, for example, found for durations longer than 20 ms in hearing-impaired listeners (Oxenham et al., 1997) and for longer durations in normal-hearing listeners (Florentine et al., 1988). There is clear deviation from this slope for signals of a few milliseconds, suggesting that temporal integration may be governed by leaky integration as described in Section 5.6.1 for short durations, and multiple looks for longer durations (e.g. Oxenham et al., 1997).

Viemeister and Wakefield (1991) provided further evidence supporting the hypothesis of 'multiple looks'. They presented a masking experiment that was difficult to account for by the classical view on temporal integration. The results of their masking experiment and a schematic representation of one of their stimulus conditions are shown in Fig. 5.7. The masker was a noise with two short temporal gaps. The signal consisted of either one or two tone pulses which were positioned in the gaps of the masker. Three different temporal patterns of the masker were used: the masker intensity for the portion between the two gaps was either the same as for the rest of the stimulus or it was raised or lowered by 6 dB for a certain length of time. A schematic plot of the time course for two pulses and the masker with a higher masker intensity between the two gaps is shown in the top-right corner of Fig. 5.7. According to the temporal integration stage described in the previous section, a threshold for a pair of pulses which is lower than that for a single pulse implies that energy from both pulses is being at least partially integrated. Thus, any energy that occurs between the pulses will also be integrated. If threshold is determined by the signal energy relative to the masker energy, then the threshold for the pulse pair should depend on the masker energy between the two gaps. The data show similar thresholds for the two pulses alone and a decrease in thresholds if they are presented together. However, in contrast to the prediction of a temporal integration stage, the change in masker energy between the two gaps has a negligible

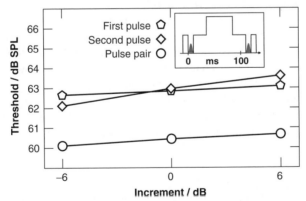

Fig. 5.7 Data supporting the 'multiple look' strategy taken from Viemeister and Wakefield (1991). Average masked thresholds for four listeners of a 1-kHz signal in the presence of a broadband masker at a spectrum level of 40 dB are shown for three different levels of the masker between two temporal gaps in the masker. The gaps were 100 ms apart from each other. The inset in the upper-right corner schematically shows the envelope of the masker for a condition where the masker level was increased by 6 dB between the two gaps (black line). Symbols indicate the three different types of signals: a single pulse positioned in the first temporal gap of the masker (pentagrams); a single pulse in the second gap (diamonds); and the two pulses (circles). The inset shows the latter signal condition, i.e. when both pulses were present (red signals).

effect on the thresholds. Viemeister and Wakefield (1991) argued that the listeners are able to selectively draw their attention to the samples ('looks') that are centred at the gaps of the masker. Such a selective attention can also be realized by a filter matched to the time course of the target signal, as shown in Dau *et al.* (1997). The spectrotemporal characteristic of such a 'look' presumably relates to the width of the auditory filters, i.e. it is slightly broader and shorter for higher frequencies than for lower frequencies (Schijndel *et al.*, 1999). The 'multiple look' strategy is also discussed in relation to the perception of sinusoidal amplitude modulations. Modulation detection thresholds and discrimination thresholds decrease as the duration is increased (Sheft and Yost, 1990; Dau *et al.*, 1997; Lee and Bacon, 1997). Some of the studies indicate that it is not the duration in milliseconds but the duration expressed as number of cycles which determines threshold (Sheft and Yost, 1990; Lee and Bacon, 1997; however. see Dau *et al.*, 1997; Ewert and Dau, 2000). On the cycle scale, performance increases for small number of cycles, in agreement with the predictions of a multiple-look strategy where it is assumed that a look is equivalent to one cycle of the modulation. In the modulation discrimination data of Lee and Bacon (1997) the multiple-look strategy overestimates the decrease in threshold for durations of more than four cycles, which may reflect memory limitations.

5.8 **Summary**

Data on temporal integration and temporal resolution reveal temporal limits of the auditory system on different time scales. While temporal integration is usually characterized by long time constants of 100 ms or more, temporal resolution data indicate considerably shorter time constants in the range of a few milliseconds. The concept of a leaky integrator following a compressive non-linearity may partly reconcile the time scales for temporal integration and temporal resolution. However, presumably more than one mechanism is involved in temporal integration, but the relative contribution of those mechanisms is still unclear. Data on the perception of periodic level fluctuations (modulations) are not in line with the concept of a leaky integration process. Instead, the data support the hypothesis that the auditory system analyses temporal level fluctuations with a bank of overlapping modulation bandpass filters. The concept is similar to the assumption of critical band filters in the audio-frequency domain. However, the tuning in the modulation-frequency domain is considerably broader than in the audio-frequency domain, which may explain why a leaky-integrator approach—the temporal window—is so successful in predicting several aspects of temporal-resolution data.

An important future challenge will be to incorporate all the different aspects of temporal resolution and temporal integration into one model. This would allow us to quantify the relative contribution of the different mechanisms underlying the data on temporal resolution and temporal integration.

References

Akeroyd, M. A. and Summerfield, A. Q. (1999). A binaural analog of gap detection. *Journal of the Acoustical Society of America* 105:2807–20.

Boehnke, S. E., Hall, S. E., and Marquardt, T. (2002). Detection of static and dynamic changes in interaural correlation. *Journal of the Acoustical Society of America* 112:1617–26.

Borrill, S. J. and Moore, B. C. J. (2002). Evidence that comodulation detection differences depend on within-channel mechanisms. *Journal of the Acoustical Society of America* 111:309–19.

Brink, W. A. C. van den and Houtgast, T. (1990). Spectro-temporal integration in signal detection. *Journal of the Acoustical Society of America* 88:1703–11.

Buschermöhle, M., Feudel, U., Klump, G. M., Beem, M. A., and Freund, J. A. (2006). Signal detection enhanced by comodulated noise. *Fluctuation and Noise Letters (FNL)* 6:L339–L347.

Carlyon, R. P., Buus, S., and Florentine, M. (1990). Temporal integration of trains of tone pulses by normal and by cochlearly impaired listeners. *Journal of the Acoustical Society of America* 87:260–8.

Cohen, M. F. (1982). Detection threshold microstructure and its effect on temporal integration data. *Journal of the Acoustical Society of America* 71:405–9.

Cohen, M. F. and Schubert, E. T. (1987). The effect of cross-spectrum correlation on the detectability of a noise band. *Journal of the Acoustical Society of America* 81:721–3.

Dau, T., Püschel, D., and Kohlrausch, A. (1996). A quantitative model of the 'effective' signal processing in the auditory system. II. Simulations and measurements. *Journal of the Acoustical Society of America* 99:3623–31.

Dau, T., Kollmeier, B., and Kohlrausch, A. (1997). Modeling auditory processing of amplitude modulation. II. Spectral and temporal integration in modulation detection. *Journal of the Acoustical Society of America* 102:2906–19.

Dau, T., Verhey, J. L., and Kohlrausch, A. (1999). Intrinsic envelope fluctuations and modulation-detection thresholds for narrowband noise carriers. *Journal of the Acoustical Society of America* 106:2752–60.

Dubno, J. R. and Ahlstrom, J. B. (2001). Forward- and simultaneous-masked thresholds in bandlimited maskers in subjects with normal hearing and cochlear hearing loss. *Journal of the Acoustical Society of America* 110:1049–57.

Duifhuis, H. (1973). Consequences of peripheral frequency selectivity for nonsimultaneous masking. *Journal of the Acoustical Society of America* 54:1471–88.

Ernst, S. M. A. and Verhey, J. L. (2006). Role of suppression and retro-cochlear processes in comodulation masking release. *Journal of the Acoustical Society of America* 120:3843–52.

Ernst, S. M. A. and Verhey, J. L. (2008). Peripheral and central aspects of auditory across-frequency processing. *Brain Research* 1220:246–55.

Ewert, S. D. and Dau, T. (2000). Characterizing frequency selectivity for envelope fluctuations. *Journal of the Acoustical Society of America* 108:1181–96.

Ewert, S. D., Verhey, J. L., and Dau, T. (2002). Spectro-temporal processing in the envelope-frequency domain. *Journal of the Acoustical Society of America* 112:2921–31.

Ewert, S., Hau, O., and Dau, T. (2007). Forward masking: temporal integration or adaptation? In *Hearing: from Sensory Processing to Perception—14th International Symposium on Hearing*, pp. 165–74. Berlin: Springer.

Fitzgibbons, P. J. (1983). Temporal gap detection in noise as a function of frequency, bandwidth and level. *Journal of the Acoustical Society of America* 74:67–72.

Fletcher, H. (1940). Auditory patterns. *Reviews of Modern Physics* 12:47–65.

Florentine, M., Fastl, H., and Buus, S. (1988). Temporal integration in normal hearing, cochlear impairment, and impairment simulated by masking. *Journal of the Acoustical Society of America* 84:195–203.

Florentine, M., Buus, S., and Poulsen, T. (1996). Temporal integration of loudness as a function of level. *Journal of the Acoustical Society of America* 99:1633–44.

Füllgrabe, C., Moore, B. C. J., Demany, L., Ewert, S. D., Sheft, S., and Lorenzi, C. (2005). Modulation masking produced by second-order modulators. *Journal of the Acoustical Society of America* 117:2158–68.

Garner, W. H. (1947). The effect of frequency spectrum on temporal integration of energy in the ear. *Journal of the Acoustical Society of America* 19:808–15.

Gerken, G. M., Bhat,V. K. H., and Hutchinson-Clutter, M. (1990). Auditory temporal integration and the power function model. *Journal of the Acoustical Society of America* 88:767–78.

Green, D. M. (1960). Auditory detection of a noise signal. *Journal of the Acoustical Society of America* 32:121–31.

Hall, J. W., Haggard, M. P., and Fernandes, M. A. (1984). Detection in noise by spectro-temporal pattern analysis. *Journal of the Acoustical Society of America* 76:50–6.

Heil, P. and Neubauer, H. (2003). A unifying basis of auditory thresholds based on temporal summation. *Proceedings of the National Academy of Sciences USA* 100:6151–6.

Henning, B. G. (1974). Detectability of interaural delay in high-frequency complex waveforms. *Journal of the Acoustical Society of America* 55:84–90.

Houtgast, T. (1989). Frequency selectivity in amplitude-modulation detection. *Journal of the Acoustical Society of America* 85:1676–80.

Kohlrausch, A., Fassel, R., and Dau, T. (2000). The influence of carrier level and frequency on modulation and beat-detection thresholds for sinusoidal carriers. *Journal of the Acoustical Society of America* 108:723–34.

Krumbholz, K., Patterson, R. D., Nobbe, A., and Fastl, H. (2003). Microsecond temporal resolution in monaural hearing without spectral cues? *Journal of the Acoustical Society of America* 113:2790–800.

Lawson, J. L. and Uhlenbeck, G. E. (1950). Threshold signals. In *Radiation Laboratory Series*, Vol. 24. Chapter 3.8, pp. 56–63 New York: McGraw-Hill.

Lee, J. and Bacon, S. P. (1997). Amplitude modulation depth discrimination of a sinusoidal carrier: Effect of stimulus duration. *Journal of the Acoustical Society of America* 101:3688–93.

Leshowitz, B. (1971). Measurement of the two-click threshold. *Journal of the Acoustical Society of America* 49:462–6.

Lorenzi, C., Soares, C., and Vonner, T. (2001). Second-order temporal modulation transfer functions. *Journal of the Acoustical Society of America* 110:1030–8.

McFadden, D. and Wright, B. A. (1987). Comodulation masking release in a forward-masking paradigm. *Journal of the Acoustical Society of America* 82:1615–20.

Millman, R. E., Green, G. G. R., Lorenzi, C., and Rees, A. (2003). Effect of a noise modulation masker on the detection of second-order amplitude modulation. *Hearing Research* 178:1–11.

Moore, B. C. J. and Glasberg, B. R. (1982). Contralateral and ipsilateral cueing in forward masking. *Journal of the Acoustical Society of America* 71:942–5.

Moore, B. C. J., Peters, R. W., and Glasberg, B. R. (1993). Detection of temporal gaps in sinusoids: Effects of frequency and level. *Journal of the Acoustical Society of America* 93:1563–70.

Moore, B. C. J., Sek, A., and Glasberg, B. R. (1999). Modulation masking produced by beating modulators. *Journal of the Acoustical Society of America* 106:908–18.

Nelken, I., Rotman, Y., and Yosef, O. B. (1999). Responses of auditory-cortex neurons to structural features of natural sounds. *Nature* 397:154–7.

Nelson, D. A., Schroder, A. C., and Wojtczak, M. (2001). A new procedure for measuring peripheral compression in normal-hearing and hearing-impaired listeners. *Journal of the Acoustical Society of America* 110:2045–64.

Ogura, Y., Suzuki, Y., and Sone, T. (1991). A temporal integration model for loudness perception of repeated impulsive sounds. *Journal of the Acoustical Society of Japan (E)* 12:1–11.

Oxenham, A. J. (2001). Forward masking: adaptation or integration? *Journal of the Acoustical Society of America* 109:732–41.

Oxenham, A. J. and Moore, B. C. J. (1994). Modeling the additivity of nonsimultaneous masking. *Hearing Research* 80:105–18.

Oxenham, A. J. and Plack, C. J. (1997). A behavioral measure of basilar-membrane nonlinearity in listeners with normal and impaired hearing. *Journal of the Acoustical Society of America* 101:3666–75.

Oxenham, A. J., Moore, B. C. J., and Vickers, D. A. (1997). Short-term temporal integration: Evidence for the influence of peripheral compression. *Journal of the Acoustical Society of America* 101:3676–87.

Penner, M. J. (1978). A power law transformation resulting in a class of short-term integrators that produce time-intensity trades for noise bursts. *Journal of the Acoustical Society of America* 63:195–201.

Piechowiak, T., Ewert, S. D., and Dau, T. (2007). Modeling comodulation masking release using an equalization-cancellation mechanism. *Journal of the Acoustical Society of America* 121:2111.

Plack, C. J. and Moore, B. C. J. (1990). Temporal window shape as a function of frequency and level. *Journal of the Acoustical Society of America* 87:2178–87.

Plack, C. J. and Skeels, V. (2007). Temporal integration and compression near absolute threshold in normal and impaired ears. *Journal of the Acoustical Society of America* 122:2236–44.

Plomp, H. and Bouman, M. A. (1959). Relation between hearing threshold and duration for tone pulses. *Journal of the Acoustical Society of America* **31**:749–57.

Poulsen, T. (1981). Loudness of tones in a free field. *Journal of the Acoustical Society of America* **69**:1786–90.

Pressnitzer, D. and McAdams, S. (1999). Summation of roughness across frequency regions. In *Temporal Processing in the Auditory System: Psychophysics, Physiology and Models of Hearing*, pp. 105–8. Singapore: World Scientific Publishing.

Puleo, J. S. and Pastore, R. E. (1980). Contralateral cueing effects in backward masking. *Journal of the Acoustical Society of America* **67**:947–51.

Schijndel, N. H. van, Houtgast, T., and Festen, J. M. (1999). Intensity discrimination of Gaussian-windowed tones: Indications for the shape of the auditory frequency-time window. *Journal of the Acoustical Society of America* **105**:3425–35.

Schreiner, C. and Langner, G. (1988). Periodicity coding in the inferior colliculus of the cat. I. Neuronal mechanism. *Journal of Neurophysiology* **60**:1799–1822.

Shailer, M. J. and Moore, B. C. J. (1987). Gap detection and the auditory filter: Phase effects using sinusoidal stimuli. *Journal of the Acoustical Society of America* **81**:1110–17.

Sheft, S. and Yost, W. (1990). Temporal integration in amplitude modulation detection. *Journal of the Acoustical Society of America* **88**:796–805.

Sheft, S. and Yost, W. (2007). Discrimination of starting phase with sinusoidal envelope modulation. *Journal of the Acoustical Society of America* **121**: EL84–EL89.

Susini, P., McAdams, S., and Smith, B. (2002). Global and continuous loudness estimation of time-varying levels. *Acustica United with Acta Acustica* **88**:536–48.

Tandetnik, S., Garnier, S., and Lorenzi, C. (2001). Measurement of first and second-order modulation detection thresholds in listeners with cochlear hearing loss. *British Journal of Audiology* **35**:355–64.

Uchanski, R. M., Moore, B. C. J., and Glasberg, B. R. (2006). Effect of modulation maskers on the detection of second-order amplitude modulation with and without notched noise. *Journal of the Acoustical Society of America* **119**:2937–46.

Verhey, J. L., Dau, T., and Kollmeier, B. (1999). Within-channel cues in comodulation masking release (CMR): Experiments and model predictions using a modulation-filterbank model. *Journal of the Acoustical Society of America* **106**:2733–45.

Verhey, J. L., Ewert, S. D., and Dau, T. (2003a). Modulation masking produced by complex tone modulators. *Journal of the Acoustical Society of America* **114**:2135–46.

Verhey, J. L., Presnitzer, D., and Winter, I. M. (2003b). The psychophysics and physiology of comodulation masking release. *Experimental Brain Research* **153**:405–17.

Viemeister, N. F. (1979). Temporal modulation transfer functions based upon modulation thresholds. *Journal of the Acoustical Society of America* **66**:1364–80.

Viemeister, N. F. and Wakefield, G. H. (1991). Temporal integration and multiple looks. *Journal of the Acoustical Society of America* **90**:858–65.

Yasin, I. and Plack, C. J. (2003). The effects of a high-frequency suppressor on tuning curves and derived basilar-membrane response functions. *Journal of the Acoustical Society of America* **114**:322–32.

Yost, W. A. and Sheft, S. (1989). Across critical band processing of amplitude modulated tones. *Journal of the Acoustical Society of America* **85**:848–57.

Zwicker, E. (1984). Dependence of post-masking on masker duration and its relation to temporal effects in loudness. *Journal of the Acoustical Society of America* **75**:219–23.

Zwicker, E. and Fastl, H. (1999). *Psychoacoustics*. Berlin: Springer.

Zwislocki, J. (1960). Theory of temporal auditory summation. *Journal of the Acoustical Society of America* **32**:1046–60.

Zwislocki, J. (1969). Temporal summation of loudness: An analysis. *Journal of the Acoustical Society of America* **46**:431–41.

Chapter 6

Spatial hearing

John F. Culling and Michael A. Akeroyd

6.1 Introduction

Spatial hearing is the capacity of the auditory system to interpret or exploit the different spatial paths by which sounds may reach the head. Using spatial hearing, the auditory system can determine the location of a sound source and/or 'unmask' sounds that would otherwise be obscured by noise. It can also orient attention towards or away from a sound source, and characterize, to some extent, the nature of the listening space. Spatial hearing is almost-entirely underpinned by 'binaural' hearing: the comparison of the signal at one ear with the signal at the other ear. In most circumstances these signals will differ. To understand why, consider a source of sound placed somewhere to the right of a listener (Fig. 6.1). The distance from the source to the left ear is further than to the right ear, so the sound arrives later at the left ear. In addition, the left ear is in the 'acoustic shadow' of the head, so the sound there is less intense at the left ear. These differences in time and level are termed, respectively, the *interaural time difference* (ITD) and *interaural level difference* (ILD). They are the basis of all binaural processing and are fundamental to nearly all spatial hearing.

6.2 Interaural time differences (ITDs)

When the source of sound is to one side, one ear is further from the source than the other, and thus receives a delayed version of the signal. The resulting ITD may be as much as 650 µs (a limit determined by the size of the head and the speed of sound) and its dependence on the direction of the source can mostly be described by simple geometry. However, the situation is complicated somewhat by an interaction of the sound with the head and torso, such that it cannot be accurately characterized as a simple time delay with a fixed value across frequency. A more accurate model of ITDs can be achieved by treating the head as a solid sphere and the ears as single points at its surface (e.g. Kuhn, 1977). Such a model correctly predicts that ITDs decline by about 30% with increasing frequency, and can give highly accurate predictions of physical measurements taken from a manikin.

Listeners are remarkably good at detecting changes in ITD: for some listeners the smallest change ('just-noticeable difference', or 'JND') in ITD that can be detected is around 10 µs (Klump and Eady, 1956). With pure-tone stimuli, the smallest JND is found for frequencies around 500–1000 Hz, yet above about 1500 Hz the JND cannot be measured. This observation should not be mistaken for evidence that listeners are insensitive at ITDs at high frequencies, however: listeners can discriminate ITDs carried by the *envelopes* of certain high-frequency sounds, such as sinusoidally amplitude-modulated tones and highpass-filtered clicks or noise. For all these sounds the JNDs are measurable, but are much larger at high frequencies than at low. There is one class of sound, 'transposed stimuli', for which the discrimination of ITDs at high frequencies can be comparable with that at low frequencies (Bernstein and Trahiotis, 2002). Transposed stimuli are

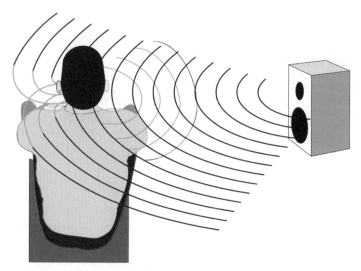

Fig. 6.1 Sound waves interacting with the head. Sound is reflected back from the surface of the head and refracts around the sides of the head, forming a complex interference pattern and differences in the intensity and arrival time of the sound at each ear.

high-frequency tones, amplitude modulated by a specially designed, low-frequency envelope (van de Par and Kohlrausch, 1997). This envelope is prepared so that the transposed tone should produce a similar temporal pattern of action potentials on the auditory nerve as a low-frequency pure tone. The success of this method suggests that the insensitivity to ITDs for *unmodulated* high-frequency pure tones may be due to the way high- and low-frequency tones are encoded on the auditory nerve. Specifically, phase-locking to the fine structure of the waveform is lost at high frequencies. Bernstein and Trahiotis (1996) have shown that a good fit to the human psycho-physical data can be produced using a model of peripheral transduction which removes this phase-locking to the fine structure using a fourth order, low-pass filter with a cut-off frequency at around 425 Hz. This cut-off frequency, which was a fitted parameter of their model, is rather low for a mammal, and so may also reflect further loss of phase-locking at later stages of processing.

With headphone-presented sounds there is no limit to the maximum value of ITD that can be delivered. Such sounds are generally heard inside the head, within which their position (on a left–right scale) is termed the 'lateralization'. For non-periodic sounds, such as noise, increases in ITD result in the lateralization staying on the *same* side of the head, at least until ITDs as large as 10 000 μs are reached (e.g. Mossop and Culling, 1998). As the ITD of noise increases up to and beyond this value, its lateralization becomes increasingly indistinct, but the correspondence of the signals at the two ears also becomes detectable as a faint pitch percept (Bilsen and Goldstein, 1974) and then as an 'infrapitch echo', which continues to be heard up to a full second of ITD (Warren *et al.*, 1981). Beyond this limit, the auditory system cannot discriminate delayed noise from independent noises at each ear. For a periodic sound, especially a pure tone, however, something different happens: the lateralization changes cyclically from one side to the other as the ITD is progressively increased. The periodicity of the sound waveform means that an ITD of 1.25 periods, or 2.25 periods, or 10.25 periods, etc., are all physically equivalent to an ITD of 0.25 periods, and so all correspond to the same lateralization.

Jeffress (1948) proposed a simple neural circuit that would allow the detection of ITDs. The circuit is based on the idea of a neural 'coincidence detector': a central neuron which receives input from both the left and right auditory nerves, and which only fires itself when *simultaneous* action potentials arrive from each. Its function is thus to compare the relative timing of the action potentials. Cells known as 'EE units', seem to have these properties. Jeffress' insight was to see that if an internal time delay was included (for instance, by the neural connection to the right ear being longer than that to the left ear) then the cell would only fire if the external ITD matched the internal delay. In this case, if the ITD favoured the right ear, then the action potentials induced by the sound on the right auditory nerve would lead those on the left. By making them travel slightly further, they can arrive at the central cell at the same time as those from the left, so giving it the simultaneous arrival of action potentials that it needs to fire. Jeffress further suggested that there would be a whole array of different coincidence detectors, each connected to the ears by axons of varying length (Fig. 6.2), so giving a 'map' of internal delay and the ability to compensate for every possible ITD that the ears may receive. The result is a spatial code for ITD: whichever central cell in the array is most active marks the ITD of the sound.

This circuit is easy to simulate in computer software and so has often formed the basis of accounts of binaural processing; indeed, it is often taken as a 'standard model' (Stern and Trahiotis, 1995, 1997). It is usual to extend the circuit to multiple frequency channels (and to assume each frequency channel is independent), in which case the activity in the complete 'map' of frequency vs. delay is called the *correlogram* (the term is a shortening of 'correlation-gram', as the coincidence operation is often implemented computationally as a cross-correlation of the left and right signals). These models have proved successful at accounting for experimental results on lateralization. They generally assume that the naturally occurring range of ITDs is fully represented (though ITDs near zero are often weighted more than those further away), but they may also

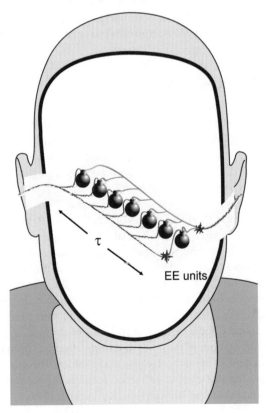

Fig. 6.2 Schematic illustration of the Jeffress model. Axonal delays are represented by burning fuses and coincidence detectors by bombs. For the analogy to work, the detonators must require ignition by two fuses at once.

EE units

assume that the array continues to much larger ITDs than could occur naturally. Recent physiological results have cast doubt on these assumptions. For instance, in guinea-pigs, the interaural delays that best excite EE units form discrete populations at ±1/8th of a period of the best frequency of the cell, regardless of whether this value is larger or smaller than the maximum ITD that can occur given the size of a guinea-pig's head (McAlpine *et al.*, 2001). This result is consistent with a 'count-comparison' model of spatial coding; that is, the ITD is represented by the relative activity of a small number of 'channels'. A more familiar example of a count-comparison code is the encoding of a wide range of colours by only three different photoreceptors in the human eye. Harper and McAlpine (2004) have suggested that this 'two-channel' encoding of ITD may always be optimal for small mammals, but only at low frequencies for humans. It is an open question as to whether the spatial map in humans is based on a two-channel code, a finely distributed array or, perhaps, an encoding that changes as a function of frequency.

There are some special sounds for which the ITD only indirectly influences the lateralization. The primary example is the 'Huggins pitch' (Cramer and Huggins, 1958). Huggins presented a white noise in stereo to listeners, through headphones. The noise was identical at the two ears except in a narrow frequency band, within which an interaural phase shift was introduced by applying an all-pass filter to the stimulus at one ear. Huggins reported that his listeners heard a faint, 600-Hz tone against the white noise, but *only* when both the left and right channels were presented: if each channel was presented in isolation, it was just heard as a white noise. Huggins did not report *where* his listeners heard the tone, but more recent studies have shown that some people hear it at the extreme left of the head, while other people hear it at the extreme right, irrespective of handedness. Moreover, the Huggins pitch has the curious property that its lateralization does not change even if exactly the same stimulus is presented but with the left and right channels of the headphones swapped. Many other 'dichotic pitches' have been discovered, similar to the Huggins pitch in that they can only be perceived on binaural presentation, but constructed in different ways (Bilsen, 1977).

6.3 Interaural level differences (ILDs)

Any large object placed in the path of a sound will cast an 'acoustic shadow'. A listener's head will also cast a shadow, with the result that the sound at the shadowed ear will be less intense than that at the other, 'illuminated', ear. This difference in level, the interaural level difference or ILD, is detectable by binaural processing and is a useful cue to the direction of some sound sources.

The dependence of ILD on source direction and frequency is far more complicated than is the case with ITDs. In general, the ILD is larger if the sound is off to one side instead of straight ahead and if the sound is of higher rather than lower frequency (in contrast to ITDs, which are *smaller* for high-frequency sounds): the largest ILDs at frequencies of 0.2, 1, 5, and 10 kHz are 3, 10, 17, and 21 dB, respectively (Shaw and Vaillancourt, 1985). The lateral angles that gave these maxima were, respectively, 90°, 60° (*and* 135°), 60°, and 105°. These angles are all roughly opposite one ear, but tend not to be *exactly* opposite. This result springs from the counterintuitive effects of a roughly spherical acoustic obstacle on the sound level at its surface; the sound is often more intense on the surface directly opposite the source than it would be if the obstacle were removed (though it is still less intense than on the side facing the source). This and other perturbations are caused by interference between sound diffracting around each side of the head, and by further interference patterns within the corrugations of the pinna and from reflections from the torso or shoulders (see Fig. 6.1). ILDs also depend upon the distance to the source. This effect is, in large part, due to the inverse-square law, but also involves diffraction around the head and is only substantial for distances less than about 0.5 m (e.g. Brungart and Rabinowitz, 1999).

A simple attenuation of the signal at one ear relative to the other (i.e. a level imbalance) is often used to create ILDs using headphones. The JND for ILD is, at best, around 0.5–1 dB, and so is slightly lower than the corresponding value for a level difference in just one ear (Hartmann and Constan, 2002), suggesting a binaural benefit to performance. In contrast to the JND for ITDs, the JND for ILD is approximately independent of frequency between 200 and 10000 Hz, although at 1000 Hz the JND is larger than at other frequencies.

Because both ITDs and ILDs induce lateralization, experimenters have been able to use one to measure the other. Usually, the experimental interest is on the ITD-induced lateralization, and so the ILD is the scale used to measure this. In this 'pointing' method, a listener is required to vary the ILD of one sound until its position matches that of the target sound, with the final ILD chosen taken as the measure of lateralization (e.g. Domnitz and Colburn, 1977). This method uses two sounds, the target given an ITD and the pointer an ILD. In another approach, one sound is used, which is given *both* an ILD and an ITD. Usually these oppose one another, with the goal of measuring the amount of ILD needed to 'trade' against a given amount of ITD, so that the sound is perceived in the centre of the head. Such experiments have shown that ITD and ILD are often equivalent, but they are not identical, as listeners sometimes report perceiving two images, one due to the applied ITD, the other to the ILD (e.g. Hafter and Carrier, 1971). Another experimental approach of opposing ITDs and ILDs is to study the weight applied to each by binaural processing. Such studies have shown that the percept of laterality is dominated by the low-frequency ITDs (e.g. Wightman and Kistler, 1992). This dominance may be attributable to the poorer encoding of ITDs at high frequency. If so, high-frequency transposed stimuli may be less dominated by low frequencies.

6.4 Sound direction

ITDs and ILDs both provide cues to whether (and to what degree) a sound comes from the left or the right: they are thus limited in the directions they can indicate. Importantly, they cannot differentiate front from back or up from down. Indeed, if the head was perfectly spherical and the pinnae were not present, discrimination of front from back or up from down would be impossible: the ITD or ILD would be zero if a source of sound was directly ahead, behind, above or below, and the ITD and ILD generated by a source at an angle of 45° to one side would be the same if that source was 45° ahead of the listener or 45° behind the listener. This perfect symmetry is not quite reached, however: the head is not a sphere, and the ears are placed slightly back from the midpoints, so introducing small acoustic differences between front and back. The presence of the shoulders results in up being different from down. The roles of these cues are relatively small, though: the pinnae contribute the most to disambiguating direction. It is because of these perturbations of level at each ear caused by the reflected sound within the pinnae (Fig. 6.3) that listeners generally have no difficulty in determining what quadrant a sound is coming from (although front–back errors can be surprisingly common). Distorting the shape of the pinna disrupts the listeners' ability to differentiate front from back or elevation. Listeners use the details of the spectral profiles created by the pinna to determine elevation, the majority of these cues coming from the shape of the concha (Lopez-Poveda and Meddis, 1996). Vertical-plane localization is less accurate than horizontal-plane localization: the best resolution for changes in vertical direction is about 4°, but it can be as little as 1° in a horizontal direction (Perrott and Saberi, 1990). Angle discrimination is best for directions directly ahead, and markedly reduces for angles opposite one of the ears, where the cues change less rapidly as a function of direction.

The overall effect of the head, shoulders, and pinnae on the ILDs, ITDs, and spectrum, can be captured by placing a microphone close to a listener's eardrums and then recording the response

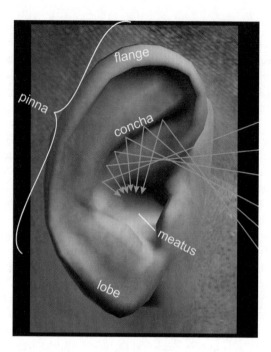

Fig. 6.3 Patterns of reflection within the human concha which depend upon the elevation of the sound source.

to an impulse presented from a loudspeaker placed in the required direction. These recordings, known as the *head-related impulse responses* (HRIRs), contain *all* the acoustic cues to sound direction (Wightman and Kistler, 2005). For instance, an impulse from the right will give a right-ear HRIR with a larger and earlier peak in its waveform than the left-ear HRIR. The Fourier transforms of these HRIRs (the head-related transfer functions or HRTFs) also display characteristic notches in the power spectrum which represent the elevation of the source. Each individual's HRIRs are idiosyncratic, a result of small differences in the physical size and shape of the head and ears (Algazi *et al.*, 2001). This means that the interpretation of spectral cues employed by each listener is somewhat different. It appears that individuals learn to decode the spectral cues associated with their own pinnae and can be confused by the cues due to someone else's pinnae, especially in front vs. back confusions or in elevation errors. The discrepancies are reduced after learning with visual or proprioceptive feedback (Zahorik *et al.*, 2006) and can also be compensated by frequency-scaling of the HRTFs (Middlebrooks, 1999).

6.5 Distance perception

As noted above, headphone-presented sounds are typically perceived inside the head, with the perceived laterality of the sound dependent upon its ITD and ILD. By default, it would seem, the distance of sounds is zero. So, before one can deal with perception of distance, one must first escape the confines of the head. This problem of the externalization of sound sources in virtual acoustics can be considered as a special case of the problem of auditory distance.

The internal perception of headphone-presented sound is, perhaps, surprising given that most sound sources are somewhere *outside*. There are, however, some circumstances in which sound emanates from within one's own head, and headphone-presented sounds may be unintentionally simulating the characteristics of these sounds. The most obvious example of internally generated sound is one's own voice, but other examples include mechanical noises when the head touches other objects, and many other sounds that we tend to ignore such as chewing and swallowing. Headphone-presented sounds can be perceived outside the head through accurate cues to virtual auditory space, through dynamic variation of these cues in accordance with head movements, and through reverberation. A common thread running through these different factors is that they are all reliable indicators that the sound is indeed outside.

In virtual acoustics (also known as constructing a 'virtual auditory space'), prerecorded left-ear and right-ear HRIRs are convolved with a target sound, such as a sentence, and presented over headphones. The listener may then perceive the sentence outside their head, in the same direction as the impulse used to record the HRIRs. If certain constraints are met then perception can be remarkably realistic: Hartmann and Wittenberg (1996) showed that the virtual source could be indistinguishable from a real one. The externalization effect produced by HRIRs is not completely understood, although if *all* the characteristics of an external sound source are accurately simulated it is perhaps not surprising that it is heard as an external sound source. Aspects of such stimuli that lead the auditory system to make the external attribution may include lawful combinations of ILD and ITD, the presence of spectral notches characteristic of particular directions, or consistency of the pinna cues with the ILD and ITD. Unfortunately, the externalization effect may break down too easily for the individual roles of these cues to be analytically investigated: the externalization of virtual sound is often reduced compared to its real equivalent, presumably due to infidelities in the required measurements, synthesis, and presentation. It also works best if the HRIRs were recorded from the listener's own ears, yet the experimental effort required to do this can be substantial, and so publicly available databases of HRIRs, recorded either on a manikin or a group of listeners, are often used instead. These usually give *some* externalization.

The illusion can be made more robust if changes in ILD, ITD, and pinna cues with head movements are included. Indeed, an additional reason for the fragile nature of externalization without head movements may be the fact that, with headphone-presented sounds, a source direction does not change when the listener's head moves. For a real sound source, the direction does change when the head moves: for instance, if a listener rotates 45° to the right, then the direction of a real stationary sound source, relative to the listener, must rotate 45° the other way. Such changes can be simulated by a system that can monitor in real-time the position of the head and then make simultaneous updates to which HRIRs are used in the synthesis. Apart from needing considerable computing resources to perform all the processing (especially given that the HRIRs must be continuously convolved with the target sound), such systems are not particularly complicated, and have been in existence for at least 15 years. The resulting source movements provide the listener with a veridical cue to an external source, because an internal source would not move relative to the head when the head is turned.

A final factor in the externalization of sound sources is reverberation (Durlach *et al.*, 1992). Simulated reverberation can create a compelling impression of an external source using relatively unsophisticated techniques. For instance, a recording made in a room from two microphones separated by 20 cm of free space (i.e. no head and consequently no acoustic shadow), will, when played back over good quality conventional headphones, create a strong sense of externalization. Again, this cue is veridical, because any internally generated sounds would have very little reverberant energy and practically all external sounds will have reflected off surrounding surfaces to some extent.

Once a sound is perceived as external, the cues to its distance include the combination of ILDs and ITDs, as well as the proportion of reverberant energy. ILDs in particular can depend on distance, as substantial ILDs at low frequency cannot occur for distances of more than 1 m or so. Brungart *et al.* (1999) showed that distance perception is considerably more accurate for sound sources within about 1 m of the listener, an effect that they attributed to the enhanced information provided by the low-frequency ILD cue. Interestingly, for such nearby sources, the ILD tends to indicate more strongly the distance of the source from the nearer ear (and thus the head) than it does the direction, while the ITD still tends to directly reflect the direction. The two cues thus provide almost independent estimates of direction and distance, rather than providing duplicate cues to direction as they do for more distant sources.

Most sources in real-world listening situations are further than 1 m away, and for these there are two other cues to distance. One results from the inverse-square law linking distance to intensity: the received intensity of the sound from a source decreases at a rate of 6 dB per doubling in distance. If the transmitted intensity is known or can be inferred or guessed, the received intensity itself determines the distance to the source. This may be the case with listening to other people talking, because the timbre of the voice will indicate to some extent the intensity of the source. For instance, quiet speech and shouting sound quite different, for reasons other than the sound level. The dependence on *doublings* of distance would suggest that a discrimination of changes in distance would follow Weber's law, giving the expectation that the ratio of the JND to the reference distance would be constant; to a first approximation, this is the case.

The other distance cue results from the reverberation and reflections of sound in a room. A room is usually so criss-crossed with rays of sound heading in different directions that the overall level of the reverberant sound throughout the room is relatively uniform, no matter how far away the source is. On the other hand, the level of the 'direct' sound (the first arriving, and the only one that has not reflected from any surface) always reduces at 6 dB per doubling, in accord with the inverse-square law. Accordingly, for a close source, the listener will receive relatively more direct sound than reverberant sound, while for a further source, the opposite will occur. The proportion of reverberant sound heard by the listener is thus a reliable index of the source's distance; the more reverberant energy, the greater the distance. Naturally, a more reverberant room will also create more reverberation, so this cue has to be calibrated against some implicit knowledge of the room. Nonetheless, the cue has been shown to be a powerful cue to distance (Bronkhorst and Houtgast, 1999), if one for which the discriminations possible are fairly coarse (Zahorik, 2002; Akeroyd *et al.*, 2007).

6.6 Spatial unmasking

When two sounds come concurrently from different directions, it is easier to detect or identify them than when they come from the same direction. This effect is generally attributed to two independent processes: 'better-ear listening' and 'binaural unmasking'.

Better-ear listening is facilitated by ILDs. If there is a masking sound placed, for example, to the left of the listener, then the masker's level at the right ear will be reduced by the acoustic shadow of the head. If there is a target sound in a different position, which is less strongly shadowed at the right ear (i.e. to the right of the listener or in front) then there will be an advantageous signal-to-noise ratio at that ear (Fig. 6.4), compared to the situation where both sources are in the same place. By attending to the right ear the listener can therefore exploit that improved signal-to-noise ratio to hear the target better. Thus, the better-ear effect is perhaps better characterized as *bilateral* listening rather than *binaural* processing.

The second process, binaural unmasking, is facilitated by ITDs. Unlike better-ear listening, it involves some processing by the auditory system in order to extract an advantage. Hirsh (1948) discovered that the detectability of a pure tone masked by noise could be improved by giving the tone a different interaural phase to the noise (Fig. 6.5). For a pure tone, an interaural phase difference (IPD) is equivalent to an ITD, so different IPDs are analogous to differences in spatial location. The reduction in masked threshold is called the *binaural masking level difference* (BMLD). For pure

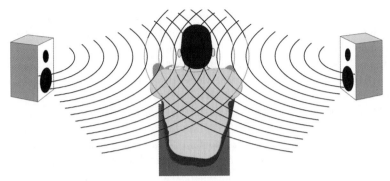

Fig. 6.4 Simultaneous sounds interacting with the head. Each sound is delayed and attenuated at the opposing ear. For simplicity, reflection and refraction (see Fig. 6.1) effects have been omitted.

tones presented over headphones in a wideband noise, four factors account for most of the variation in the magnitude of the BMLD (Durlach and Colburn, 1978). First, the BMLD is related to the phase difference between target and masker, being largest when the phase difference is 180° (or π radians). Second, the BMLD is largest (at about 15 dB) for low-frequency targets presented out-of-phase to the noise, and declines steadily with increasing frequency until it asymptotes at about 3 dB for frequencies above about 1500 Hz. Third, the BMLD depends on the interaural coherence of the masker (the maximum value of its cross-correlation); when there is a difference in interaural phase, the BMLD is largest when the coherence is 1 and smallest when it is zero. Finally, it is smaller for low masker levels, reducing to as little as about 1 dB near absolute threshold.

If a pure tone were presented from a loudspeaker in one direction and a masking noise from a loudspeaker in a different direction, it would be expected, therefore, that the detection threshold

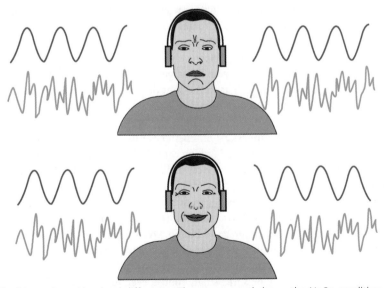

Fig. 6.5 The binaural masking level difference. The upper panel shows the NoSo condition, in which a noise and tone are both presented diotically; the frowning face indicates that the tone is difficult to detect. The lower panel shows the NoSπ condition, in which the noise is diotic, but the tone has a π-radian phase shift; the happy face indicates that the tone is easier to detect.

for the tone would be the product of both better-ear listening and binaural unmasking. However, since ILDs tend to be small at low frequencies and since binaural unmasking is less effective at high frequencies, one mechanism or the other tends to dominate the spatial unmasking effect for pure tones. The action of both mechanisms in concert consequently tends to be in the context of full spectrum target stimuli such as speech, where spatial unmasking plays a substantial role in explaining the 'cocktail-party problem' (Cherry, 1953).

Binaural unmasking also occurs for speech, giving a notable improvement in its intelligibility (Licklider, 1948). Reductions in speech reception threshold (SRT) are rather smaller than for low-frequency tone detection; Levitt and Rabiner (1967a) observed an effect of 6 dB. Levitt and Rabiner (1967b) explained this difference by appealing to theories of speech perception, such as the articulation index (Kryter, 1962), which emphasize the role of relatively high frequencies compared to those at which binaural unmasking is most effective.

The investigation of the binaural unmasking of speech has highlighted the contrast between ITD and IPD for broadband signals. Licklider's initial experiments employed IPDs to the speech or the noise. For broadband sounds, an IPD is no longer equivalent to an ITD, making such stimuli ecologically invalid; a broadband sound with an IPD has, effectively, a different ITD at each frequency, giving rise to a rather indeterminate perceived intracranial position. Remarkably, despite these manipulations being so unrealistic, they give rise to a stronger binaural unmasking effect than more realistic stimuli created using true ITDs. Culling and Summerfield (1995) suggested that the indifference of the auditory system to across-frequency differences in ITD must reflect a mechanism that operates independently in each frequency channel. The fact that perceived location of the target speech is so poorly defined in conditions that optimize binaural unmasking, has also led to an active debate over the role of spatial attention in understanding speech in noise (see Section 6.7).

In a real listening situation with target speech and interfering noise, binaural unmasking and better-ear listening have a combined effect. Using virtual acoustic techniques, Bronkhorst and Plomp (1988) analysed the individual and combined effects of these two cues in a simple listening situation. HRIRs recorded from an acoustic manikin were manipulated to separate the ILD and ITD cues and then convolved with target sentences, so putting the target voice in front of the listener but the interfering noise from a variable location. The intelligibility of the speech improved as the interfering noise was moved away from the target speech location, with the combined effect of the two cues being roughly equivalent to the sum of the effects of the two cues considered alone. When the noise came directly from the left or right, it was *better-ear* listening that provided the largest contribution.

The relative roles of binaural unmasking and better-ear listening have also been examined in more complex virtual listening situations (Culling *et al.* 2004; Hawley *et al.*, 2004). Each of these studies used up to three interfering sound sources in different spatial configurations. Hawley *et al.* sought to isolate better-ear listening effects by measuring speech intelligibility using only one ear, and inferred the effect of binaural unmasking by subtracting the spatial advantage observed with the better ear from that observed with two ears, while Culling *et al.* employed a similar virtual-acoustics technique to that of Bronkhorst and Plomp. Overall, both sets of results lead to similar conclusions: better-ear listening turns out to have a rather fragile effect, which can only lead to substantial spatial unmasking if the interfering sources are all in the same hemifield, whereas binaural unmasking turns out to be surprisingly robust, even in the most difficult condition of having *three* different sound sources spread around the listener.

Many binaural unmasking phenomena, and most dichotic pitches, can be explained by the 'Equalization–Cancellation' (E-C) model (Durlach, 1972). The model first 'equalizes' the signals at the two ears (by compensating for any ITDs), and then subtracts one from the other, so 'cancelling' as much of the masking noise as possible and giving a gain in detectability of the target. If the target is easier to detect then it can be reduced in level before reaching its threshold; this reduction is the BMLD. The model has proved remarkably influential, and the E-C principle is still used when accounting for data on the BMLD (e.g. Akeroyd, 2004). It is likely that the E-C mechanism can operate independently in each frequency channel (i.e. using different level and time compensations in the equalization stage). This allows multiple interferers to be cancelled simultaneously, so accounting for Culling *et al.*'s (2004) data on the robustness of binaural unmasking with three sound sources. It also gives an explanation of the existence of almost all of types of dichotic pitch (see Section 6.2).

The EC principle cannot, however, explain the *lateralization* of the dichotic pitches. Thus, neither the E-C model nor the Jeffress model can account for all the data: each is limited to one domain, and one is complementary to the other. It is difficult to avoid the conclusion that the binaural auditory system is also split into complementary processes. One process is optimized to detect sounds, while the other is optimized to determine where they are.

6.7 **Spatial attention and the 'cocktail party'**

Many experiments in spatial hearing have been driven by a desire to understand the 'cocktail party' problem: how can we recognize what one person is saying when there are lots of other sounds, especially from other people, happening at the same time? If asked, most people would report that they did it by concentrating (or attending) to the sound or to the direction where that sound came from. However, introspection is a notoriously unreliable guide to psychological insight. The details of how the auditory system can extract one voice from many remain elusive. In particular, it is unclear whether spatial orientation of attention is very important in the cocktail-party problem.

Cherry (1953) was the first to systematically investigate listeners' abilities to focus attention on one stream of speech while ignoring another. In his dichotic listening paradigm, target and interfering speech were either presented to the same ear, or to different ears ('dichotically') over headphones. Dichotic presentation is quite unrealistic, because diffraction will normally guarantee that both ears will receive both voices, but it has formed a valuable experimental method for researching attention in cognitive psychology. The most remarkable results from dichotic listening were found using the 'shadowing' task, in which the listener has to immediately repeat what they have heard at one ear: it was found that listeners could remember very little of any speech presented to the other, 'unattended' ear. Early theories of attention (Broadbent, 1958) consequently suggested that signals presented to unattended sensory organs were not processed at all. However, later results demonstrated that listeners can be trained to recall more, noticed stimuli that were particularly salient (such as their names or a stimulus previously associated with electric shock), and could be induced to switch attention between ears using semantic and grammatical links across the messages at each ear. These results are consistent with a less-extreme theory (Triesman, 1964), in which all signals are processed to some degree, but some are processed more than others, depending on the processing resources available: where demanding tasks, such as shadowing are used, little resources are left for the unattended ear and so only important, or particularly salient, signals on the unattended ear can be noted.

Although dichotic listening has only a limited claim to represent truly spatial attention, it may have some relevance to the process of better-ear listening, where a less complete allocation of signals to different ears is found. It should also be noted that some of the limited resources discussed by Triesman are linguistic processing resources, which could be divided during *any* competing-speech task. While these are not directly related to spatial hearing, the intrusion of linguistic information from unattended streams of speech is often interpreted as a breakdown of spatial attention.

More recent work from cognitive psychologists has been concerned with the process of allocating attention to different directions. Spence and Driver (1994) showed that listeners' reaction times to auditory stimuli are reduced if given a prior cue to the hemifield from which the sound will come. Although various discrimination tasks were improved, simple reaction times (with no decision element) were unaffected. This work demonstrates that auditory processing resources *can* be directed in a truly spatial fashion, but it does not directly address whether such spatial orientation of attention is important in the cocktail-party problem.

Culling and Summerfield (1995) considered whether sounds from a common direction are 'grouped together' and integrated into distinct 'perceptual objects', separated from sounds from different directions. This question is distinct from the process of binaural unmasking, because masking prevents signals from being detected in the first place rather than from them being organized into percepts, but both processes could potentially operate in parallel when listening to speech in noise. They used four noisebands, placed strategically at formant frequencies such that different pairs produced approximations of different whispered vowels (Fig. 6.6). Since the bands were all well separated in frequency, masking effects were minimal. When one pair of noisebands carried one ITD and the other pair an opposing ITD, Culling and Summerfield reasoned that listeners might hear one vowel on one side and a different vowel on the other. Listeners did not hear this when ITDs were used, but when the same task was presented using opposing pairs of ILDs, most listeners could hear the effect easily. Linking this observation with the fact that binaural unmasking of speech is optimal for target speech with an ambiguous location (see Section 6.6), Culling and Summerfield argued that there is little evidence that listeners make use of ITDs in order to group simultaneous sounds. Nevertheless, Culling and Summerfield speculated that ITDs might help to link together successive sounds, such as words in a sentence, in order to 'avoid mixing one discourse with that of another voice'. Darwin and Hukin (1999) proposed a formal theory of spatial attention based on these ideas, in which the formation of auditory objects occurs *prior* to the determination of sound direction. The grouping of sound elements into a single auditory object is, therefore, based on cues other than sound direction, such as common onset time and common harmonicity (e.g. Darwin and Carlyon, 1995). However, after an auditory object is formed it can still be incorporated into a stream of such objects, which together form the words

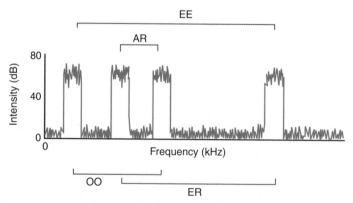

Fig. 6.6 Spectra of the whispered-vowel stimuli used by Culling and Summerfield (1995). The two different perceptual organizations of the noise bands into different vowel pairs are indicated: AR and EE or OO and ER.

of a sentence, or the notes of a melody: Darwin and Hukin proposed that sound direction is calculated prior to auditory streaming, so that it can be used in this process.

Subsequent work on the role of sound direction in the perceptual segregation of voices has concentrated on demonstrating the existence of a spatial attentional effect that is independent of binaural unmasking and better-ear listening. One method was developed by Arbogast *et al.* (2005), inspired by methods of simulating cochlear implant processing (Shannon *et al.*, 1995). They converted sentences into an array of amplitude-modulated sine waves that mirrored the modulations of corresponding frequency bands in the speech. The resulting speech is surprisingly intelligible. By generating target and interfering speech using different sets of modulated sine waves, binaural unmasking could be largely eliminated, because there was minimal spectral overlap between the two sounds. When target and interfering sentences were presented over loudspeakers, separated by 90°, the SRTs of normally hearing listeners improved by about 15 dB. This result demonstrates that listeners can use spatial attention to segregate competing messages. However, Arbogast *et al.* used an artificial sentence corpus in which only three words could vary: the Bolia *et al.* (2000) 'CRM' set uses sentences such as *'Ready Baron go to blue three now'*, *'Ready Charlie go to green one now'*. There remains some scepticism as to the importance of such mechanisms in listening to everyday sentences. For instance, Edmonds and Culling (2005) set out to test whether deliberate disruption of cues to spatial direction could interfere with performance, using sentences of less constrained form, such as *'We now have a new base for shipping'*. The disruption was attempted by dividing the speech spectrum into two bands and applying different ITDs to each band. In this way, the low frequencies of the target voice could be made to coincide in phenomenal space with the high frequencies of the masker, and vice versa. However, these 'incoherent' conditions produced SRTs that were consistently indistinguishable from coherent conditions where each voice had the same ITD at all frequencies, and which were markedly lower than a 'baseline' condition in which no ITDs were used. These results suggest that, for ITDs at least, the limits of performance with everyday sentence materials are determined by binaural unmasking, rather than by attention.

6.8 Effects of reverberation

Outside the psychoacoustic laboratory, listening often occurs in reverberant spaces. Even in the open, reflections of sound from nearby objects are a prominent feature of our normal acoustic world. These reflected copies of sound have multiple effects, which may impact on our ability to localize and identify sounds.

The effects of reverberation on sound localization are surprisingly mild, given that sound from a single source in a room will arrive at the listener from every conceivable direction (Fig. 6.7). Under most circumstances, listeners have no difficulty identifying the actual direction of the original source. This ability is known as the 'precedence effect' or the 'law of the first wavefront,' because it appears to depend upon selective processing of sound onsets (Litvosky *et al.*, 1999). Wallach *et al.* (1949) were the first to demonstrate this effect and to identify the temporal precedence of sound onsets as being critical. They presented a series of clicks to listeners from two loudspeakers in a room. They found that listeners' judgement of which loudspeaker the clicks came from was influenced only by those manipulations which affected the time of arrival of the sounds from that loudspeaker: i.e. the relative distance of the loudspeakers and the relative timing of the clicks from each.

In the laboratory, three experimental techniques have been much used to investigate the phenomena of the precedence effect. The first method is to measure 'localization dominance': two identical sounds (often clicks), the 'lead' and the 'lag,' are presented in close succession over headphones or

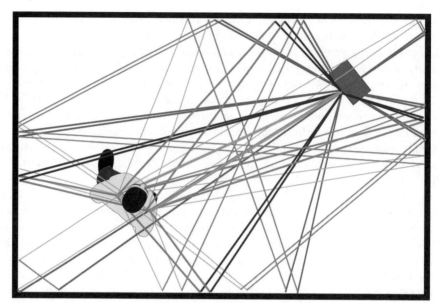

Fig. 6.7 The complex pattern of sound rays from a loudspeaker to a listener's ears. Reflected sound within a room can be modelled as sound rays, which reflect from walls like light from a mirror. The figure shows all rays travelling in the horizontal plane to each ear with up to two reflections. Direct sound is in green lines, rays reflecting once are in blue lines, and those reflecting twice are in red lines.

in an anechoic chamber (this is a simplified version of Wallach's experiment). Over headphones, the lead and lag can be set to have equal and opposite ITDs (or ILDs), but the listener hears a percept on the side indicated by the *lead*, as though the ITD information in the lag is almost completely suppressed. Shinn-Cunningham *et al.* (1993) measured the relative weighting of the lead and lag sounds by asking listeners to match the perceived laterality to that of a comparison 'pointer' stimulus containing a simple ITD. Their data indicated that the lagging sound contributed only 10–20% of the overall impression of laterality. The second method ('lag suppression') examines the contribution of the lagging sound by measuring listeners' ability to discriminate the ITD of the lagging sound itself. The asymmetry between the lead and lag can extend out to inter-click intervals to at least 10 ms, after which each contaminates equally the discrimination of the other. The third method ('fusion') examines the degree to which the lagging sound is integrated with the leading sound into a single percept. Here, listeners are required to indicate, for instance, whether they hear one or two clicks. Singular percepts occur for short inter-click intervals, but at the 'echo threshold', the second click is heard as a discrete second sound. Estimates of the echo threshold vary widely (2–50 ms) and depend on both the stimuli and the specific listening situation.

Room reverberation is often characterized by its 'reverberation time' conventionally defined as the time it takes for the reverberant energy to fall by 60 dB after the offset of a sound source. In most rooms this decay takes some time, giving a reverberant 'tail' to the end of sounds: the reverberation time can range from around half a second or less for a small room up to many seconds for a large hall. Such tails can have two effects on the perception of strongly modulated sounds such as speech. First, the sustained sound that follows the end of each energy peak tends to reduce the depth of the following energy trough, thus reducing the overall degree of amplitude modulation and filling-in any 'dips' that may be present. The reduction in amplitude modulation can have marked effects on our ability to identify sounds that are characterized by their pattern of amplitude modulation. In particular, relatively strong reverberation can detrimentally affect the perception of speech (Houtgast and Steeneken, 1985). This effect is important in the design of auditoria and classrooms in which one individual speaks to an audience. Such rooms are designed to have reflective surfaces near the source in order to project the sound to the audience, but then to absorb sound at the rear of the room to prevent this smoothing effect. Second, in a cocktail-party situation, listeners exploit the dips in the energy of an interfering voice in order to glimpse detail from a target voice (Cooke, 2006). If reverberation smoothes out the amplitude modulation of that interfering voice, this ability to 'dip listen' will be impaired.

Reverberation also has other consequences in cocktail-party situations. Plomp (1976) showed that spatial unmasking of speech in noise or cocktail-party babble can be disrupted by reverberation. This effect probably arises from separate effects upon the twin processes of better-ear listening and binaural unmasking. Better-ear listening is disrupted because the multiplicity of echoes from all directions prevent one ear from being shielded from the interfering noise, while binaural unmasking is disrupted by the fact that the reverberant energy in the room tends to have low coherence (see Section 6.6). Culling et al. (1994) found similar results using a vowel identification task, and also showed that listeners' ability to exploit fundamental frequency (F0) differences between concurrent voices could be badly affected. Although the latter effect occurred only if the fundamental frequencies of the two vowels were modulated, it should be noted that the fundamental frequency of the human voice is in a state of constant change even in the most monotonous-sounding speech. Both these results indicate that some of the auditory processes used to separate sounds will work less effectively in reverberant environments; speech intelligibility is best in un-reverberant (anechoic or 'dry') situations.

6.9 Space perception

Although reverberation can be disruptive to auditory processing, it can also be informative: echoes provide the listener with information about the structure of the listening environment. Research in this area comes from at least three perspectives. The first centres on the navigational abilities of blind people, some of whom employ self-generated sound (cane taps, footsteps, or tongue clicks) in order to hear and interpret echoes from surrounding objects. The second concerns the characterization of rooms, an area that receives particular attention in the field of music perception and concert-hall design. The third concerns the apparent display of implicit knowledge of the listening space when recognizing speech stimuli.

Blind people are known to employ acoustic cues in order to facilitate navigation (Fig. 6.8). Tests of this ability usually involve navigational tasks, such as following a wall or avoiding obstacles. Blind people have been shown to exploit the echoes from self-generated sound more efficiently than sighted individuals wearing blindfolds (e.g. Strelow and Brabyn, 1982), but it is not clear whether this ability is simply the product of practice and experience or some more fundamental difference between blind and sighted hearing. Certainly, all experiments of this type show that the capacity to navigate by echoes alone, while remarkable, is quite limited, requiring obstacles of a minimum size and resulting in much less accurate navigation than would be provided by visual cues.

A more passive exploitation of echoes occurs in the acoustic characterization of rooms. The quality of the listening environment is particularly important in auditoria and, to operate well, different functions for auditoria require different characteristics. For instance, the spoken voice requires a relatively dry room to avoid loss of intelligibility, but opera halls have always been built with much longer reverberation times than would be appropriate for speech (Beranek, 2004).

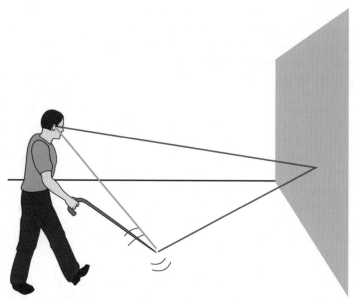

Fig. 6.8 The use of cane-tapping to navigate without vision. Sound from the cane tip reflects from nearby surfaces and interacts at the listener's ears with sound directly from the cane. This interaction causes changes in the timbre of the tapping sound depending on the distance of the wall.

In order to analyse the performance of such spaces, Jullien *et al.* (1992) used multidimensional scaling in order to investigate the perceptually salient parameters of a variety of musical auditoria. Some of the derived parameters would be familiar to architects: they include, for instance, source 'presence', 'warmth' and 'brilliance', and room 'presence', 'reverberance', and 'envelopment'. Such rich perceptual dimensions add considerably to the simple, one-parameter reverberation-time characteristic. It is thus clear that listeners are sensitive to more complex features in the pattern of reverberation a room produces, and have an aesthetic response to it, but it is less clear to what extent these parameters are informative to the listener regarding the physical structure of a listening space. Is it possible, for instance to make inferences about the shape of a room from the sound of its reverberation (Fig. 6.9)?

Listeners do display some form of passive awareness of the listening environment when listening to speech. Room reverberation can both colour and temporally smear speech, distorting its spectrum and reducing its amplitude modulation. However, a series of studies by Watkins and colleagues have shown that listeners use the spectral colouration and reverberation of the preceding and following words in order to compensate for changes in vowel spectrum and the temporal envelopes of consonants caused by reverberation of the target word (Watkins, 2005; Watkins and Makin, 2007). This ability to compensate for different transmission channels is clearly very adaptive, although the ultimate loss of intelligibility in high levels of reverberation shows that it has its limits (Houtgast and Steeneken, 1985).

6.10 **Dynamics of spatial hearing**

The binaural system has often been characterized as 'sluggish' (a term first used by Grantham and Wightman, 1978); it seems unable to follow fast dynamic fluctuations in interaural timing cues.

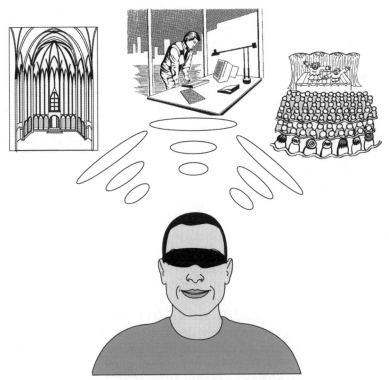

Fig. 6.9 Discriminating the sound of different rooms. Listeners can discriminate different sorts of rooms by passively listening to environmental sounds. Whether some structural discriminations can also be made is less clear.

Binaural sluggishness is manifested in both a listener's perceptions and in the detectability of sounds. An example of the former is the 'binaural beat': a pure tone (500 Hz, for example) is presented to one ear, but a different frequency pure tone (e.g. 501 Hz) is presented simultaneously to the other. This frequency difference induces a time-varying ITD (actually, it is a continuous linear change in interavral phase difference (IPD), but for a pure tone an IPD is equivalent to an ITD). A listener will perceive the tone to have a lateralized position that moves back and forth across the head at a rate equal to the difference in frequency. Note that one cannot perceive the two tones separately, as 500 Hz in one ear and 501 Hz in the other: the percept is a combined one. For frequency differences of more than about 5 Hz the sideways motion can no longer be tracked, but there is clearly some variation in lateralization; for larger frequency differences (perhaps 10–20 Hz or more), even these changes in position cannot be noticed, with the percept instead being replaced by a sensation of roughness. The inability to follow the motion at any but the slowest modulation rates is due to binaural sluggishness, although the fact that faster modulations are still audible makes it a relatively poor experimental measure of it.

Most studies of binaural sluggishness have used the size of the BMLD as the experimental measure. Grantham and Wightman (1979) measured the BMLD for a brief tone masked by noise whose interaural configuration was modulated with time. The tone was presented at a favourable part of this modulation: if the binaural system was unaffected by the rate of modulation, then the BMLD would be the usual value (some 15 dB) no matter what the rate was. Instead, they found a BMLD of about 10–12 dB at 0.5 Hz, but only some 0–3 dB at 4 Hz. A rate of 4 Hz is quite slow in comparison to the temporal resolution of monaural hearing; there is no substantial loss in the temporal resolution of monaural hearing, such as the ability to detect amplitude modulation, until the modulation rate reaches around 100 Hz, yet it was sufficient to effectively abolish the BMLD.

The reduction in BMLD with modulation rate has often been modelled by a weighted-average window, which smoothes fast changes in interaural correlation. The characteristics of this 'binaural temporal window' have been the target of many experiments, using binaural analogues of forward or backward masking, gap detection, or the notched-noise method for measuring the characteristics of the auditory filter (e.g. Kollmeier and Gilkey, 1990; Culling and Summerfield, 1998; Akeroyd and Summerfield, 1999). Although estimates of the effective duration of the window have varied widely (40–200 ms), all these estimates agree in being far longer than equivalent estimates for monaural hearing, which indicate 10–13 ms (e.g. Plack and Moore, 1990; see Chapter 5). Although the binaural-temporal window model has proved influential, and accounts for almost all the data on the effects of binaural sluggishness on the BMLD, it should be noted that it is very much a simple, 'black box', model of the phenomena, and is more of a convenient tool than a true explanation: it is unlikely that the auditory system includes a process whose *purpose* is to smooth fast changes in interaural correlations.

Attempts to measure binaural-temporal resolution using sound localization as a dependent measure have proved relatively difficult to design (Grantham and Wightman, 1978). Although, these studies have tended to indicate that processing of ITDs is also sluggish, it seems likely that it operates differently from processing of binaural detection cues to some extent. In particular, the precedence effect plays a prominent role in the temporal weighting of ITDs (Zurek, 1980; Akeroyd and Bernstein, 2001), such that ITDs presented close to the stimulus onset are weighted more strongly than ITDs embedded within a longer sound.

The precedence effect also displays temporal dynamics on a longer timescale. In the 'build-up effect', a repeated presentation of pairs of clicks leads to an increase in the threshold time gap for the perception of two separate clicks, and thus an increasing impression of a single sound from a single direction. In the 'Clifton effect' a reversal of the locations of the leading and lagging clicks 'resets' the build-up effect, temporarily restoring the perception of two separate clicks (Clifton, 1987).

6.11 **Summary**

The bilateral and binaural processes underlying spatial hearing assist in determining the direction of sound sources and the detection and identification of sound in background noise. In achieving these goals their abilities are quite remarkable: people can detect interaural time delays as short as 10 μs, effectively cancel out about 95% of low-frequency interfering noise, and suppress information about misleading echoes occurring only milliseconds after the direct sound. The auditory system can also separate the effects of room reverberation from features of a sound at its source, enabling people to make a variety of discriminations about their listening environment, and even, to some extent, to navigate around it without the aid of vision.

References

Akeroyd, M. A., Blaschke, J., Gatehouse, S. (2007). The detection of differences in the cues to distance by elderly hearing-impaired listeners. *Journal of the Acoustical Society of America* 121:1077–89.

Akeroyd, M. A. (2004). The across-frequency independence of equalization of interaural time delay in the Equalization-Cancellation model of binaural unmasking. *Journal of the Acoustical Society of America* 116:1135–48.

Akeroyd, M. A. and Bernstein, L. R. (2001). The variation across time of sensitivity to interaural disparities: Behavioral measurements and quantitative analyses. *Journal of the Acoustical Society of America* 110:2516–26.

Akeroyd, M. A. and Summerfield, A. Q. (1999). A binaural analog of gap detection. *Journal of the Acoustical Society of America* 105:2807–20.

Akeroyd, M. A. and Summerfield, A. Q. (2000). The lateralization of simple dichotic pitches. *Journal of the Acoustical Society of America* 108:316–34.

Algazi, V. R., Duda, R. O., Thompson, D. M., and Avendano, C. (2001). The CIPIC HRTF database. In *WASSAP '01: 2001 IEEE ASSP Workshop on Applications of Signal Processing to Audio and Acoustics*, Oct. 2001, Mohonk Mountain House, New Paltz, NY, pp. 99–102.

Arbogast, T. L., Mason, C. R., and Kidd, G. (2005). The effect of spatial separation on informational masking of speech in normal-hearing and hearing-impaired listeners, *Journal of the Acoustical Society of America* 117:2169–80.

Beranek, L. (2004). *Concert Halls and Opera Houses: Music, Acoustics, Architecture.* New York: Springer-Verlag.

Bernstein, L. R. and Trahiotis, C. (1996). The normalized correlation: Accounting for binaural detection across center frequency. *Journal of the Acoustical Society of America* 100:3774–84.

Bernstein, L. R. and Trahiotis, C. (2002). Enhancing sensitivity to interaural delays at high frequencies by using transposed stimuli. *Journal of the Acoustical Society of America* 112:1026–36.

Bilsen, F. A. (1977). Pitch of noise signals: Evidence for a central spectrum. *Journal of the Acoustical Society of America* 61:150–61.

Bilsen, F. A. and Goldstein, J. L. (1974). Pitch of dichotically delayed noise and its possible spectral basis. *Journal of the Acoustical Society of America* 55:292–6.

Bolia, R. S., Nelson, W. T., and Ericson M. A. (2000). A speech corpus for multitalker communications research. *Journal of the Acoustical Society of America* 107:1065–6.

Broadbent, D. E. (1958). *Perception and Communication.* Oxford: Pergamon.

Bronkhorst, A. W. and Houtgast, T. (1999). Auditory distance perception in rooms. *Nature* 397:517–20.

Bronkhorst, A. W. and Plomp, R. (1988). The effect of head-induced interaural time and level differences on speech intelligibility in noise. *Journal of the Acoustical Society of America* 83:1508–16.

Brungart, D. S. and Rabinowitz, W. M. (1999). Auditory localization of nearby sources: Head-related transfer functions. *Journal of the Acoustical Society of America* 106:1465–79.

Brungart, D. S., Rabinowitz, W. M., and Durlach, N. I. (1999). Auditory localization of nearby sources. II. Localization of a broadband source. *Journal of the Acoustical Society of America* 106:1956–68.

Cherry, E. C. (1953). Some experiments on the recognition of speech, with one and with two ears. *Journal of the Acoustical Society of America* 25:975–9.

Clifton, R. K. (1987). Breakdown of echo suppression in the precedence effect. *Journal of the Acoustical Society of America* 82:1834–35.

Cooke, M. (2006). A glimpsing model of speech perception in noise. *Journal of the Acoustical Society of America* 119:1562–73.

Cramer, E. M. and Huggins, W. H. (1958). Creation of pitch through binaural interaction. *Journal of the Acoustical Society of America* 30:413–17.

Culling, J. F., Hawley, M. L., and Litovsky, R. Y. (2004). The role of head-induced interaural time and level differences in the speech reception threshold for multiple interfering sound sources. *Journal of the Acoustical Society of America* 116:1057–65.

Culling, J. F. and Summerfield, A. Q. (1995). Perceptual separation of concurrent speech sounds: Absence of across-frequency grouping by common interaural delay. *Journal of the Acoustical Society of America* 98:785–97.

Culling, J. F. and Summerfield, A. Q. (1998). Measurements of the binaural temporal window using a detection task. *Journal of the Acoustical Society of America* 103:3540–53.

Culling, J. F., Summerfield, Q., and Marshall, D. H. (1994). Effects of simulated reverberation on the use of binaural cues and fundamental frequency differences for separating concurrent vowels. *Speech Communication* 14:71–95.

Darwin, C. J. and Carlyon, R. P. (1995). Auditory grouping. In *Hearing* (ed. B. C. J. Moore), pp. 387–424. London: Academic Press.

Darwin, C. J. and Hukin, R.W. (1999). Auditory objects of attention: The role of interaural time differences. *Journal of Experimental Psychology, Human Perception and Performance* 25:617–29.

Domnitz, R. H. and Colburn, H. S. (1977). Lateral position and interaural discrimination. *Journal of the Acoustical Society of America* 61:1586–98.

Durlach, N. I. (1972). Binaural signal detection: Equalization and Cancellation theory. In *Foundations of Modern Auditory Theory* (ed. J. V. Tobias), Vol. 2, pp. 371–462. New York: Academic Press.

Durlach, N. I. and Colburn, H. S. (1978). Binaural phenomena. In *Handbook of Perception* (ed. E. C. Carterette and M. Freidman), Vol. 4, pp. 365–466. New York: Academic Press.

Durlach, N. I., Rigopulos, A., Pang, X. D., Woods, W. S., Kulkarni, A., Colburn, H. S., and Wenzel, E. M. (1992). On the externalization of sound images. *Presence* 1:251–7.

Edmonds, B. A. and Culling, J. F. (2005). The spatial unmasking of speech: evidence for within-channel processing of interaural time delay. *Journal of the Acoustical Society of America* 117:3069–78.

Grantham, D. W. and Wightman, F. L. (1978). Detectability of varying interaural temporal differences. *Journal of the Acoustical Society of America* 63:511–23.

Grantham, D. W. and Wightman, F. L. (1979). Detectability of a pulsed tone in the presence of a masker with time-varying interaural correlation. *Journal of the Acoustical Society of America* 65:1509–17.

Hafter, E. R. and Carrier, S. C. (1971). Binaural interaction in low-frequency stimuli: The inability to trade time and intensity completely. *Journal of the Acoustical Society of America* 51:1852–62.

Harper, N. S. and McAlpine, D. (2004). Optimal neural population coding of an auditory spatial cue. *Nature* 430:682–6.

Hartmann, W. M. and Constan, Z. A. (2002). Interaural level differences and the level-meter model. *Journal of the Acoustical Society of America* 112:1037–45.

Hartmann, W. M. and Wittenberg, A. (1996). On the externalization of sound images. *Journal of the Acoustical Society of America* 99:3678–88.

Hawley, M. L., Litovsky, R. Y., and Culling, J. F. (2004). The benefit of binaural hearing in a cocktail party: Effect of location and type of interferer. *Journal of the Acoustical Society of America* 115:833–43.

Hirsh, I. J. (1948). The influence of interaural phase on interaural summation and inhibition. *Journal of the Acoustical Society of America* 20:536–44.

Houtgast, T. and Steeneken, H. J. M. (1985). A review of the MTF concept in room acoustics and its use for estimating speech intelligibility in auditoria. *Journal of the Acoustical Society of America* 77:1069–77.

Jeffress, L. A. (1948). A place theory of sound localization. *Journal of Comparative and Physiological Psychology* 41:35–9.

Jullien, J.-P. (1992). Some results on the objective and perceptual characterization of room acoustical quality in both laboratory and real environments. *Proceedings of the Institute of Acoustics*, Vol. 14.

Klump, R.G. and Eady, H. R. (1956). Some measurements of interaural time difference thresholds. *Journal of the Acoustical Society of America* 28:859–60.

Kollmeier, B. and Gilkey, R. H. (1990). Binaural forward and backward masking: Evidence for sluggishness in binaural detection. *Journal of the Acoustical Society of America* 87:1709–19.

Kryter, K. D. (1962). Methods for the calculation and use of the articulation index. *Journal of the Acoustical Society of America* 34:1689–97.

Kuhn, G. F. (1977). Model for the interaural time differences in the azimuthal plane. *Journal of the Acoustical Society of America* 82:157–67.

Levitt, H. and Rabiner, L. R. (1967a). Binaural release from masking for speech and gain in intelligibility. *Journal of the Acoustical Society of America* 42:601–8.

Levitt, H. and Rabiner, L. R. (1967*b*). Predicting binaural gain in intelligibility and release from masking for speech. *Journal of the Acoustical Society of America* **42**:820–9.

Licklider, J. C. R. (1948). The influence of interaural phase relations upon the masking of speech by white noise. *Journal of the Acoustical Society of America* **20**:150–9.

Litovsky, R. Y., Colburn, H. S., Yost, W. A., and Guzman, S. J. (1999). The precedence effect. *Journal of the Acoustical Society of America* **106**:1633–54.

Lopez-Poveda, E. A. and Meddis, R. (1996). A physical model of sound diffraction and reflections in the human concha. *Journal of the Acoustical Society of America* **100**:3248–59.

McAlpine, D., Jiang, D., and Palmer, A.R. (2001). A neural code for low-frequency sound localization in mammals. *Nature Neuroscience* **4**:396–401.

Middlebrooks, J. C. (1999). Individual differences in external-ear transfer functions reduced by scaling in frequency. *Journal of the Acoustical Society of America* **106**:1480–92.

Mossop, J. E. and Culling J. F. (1998). Lateralization of large interaural delays. *Journal of the Acoustical Society of America* **104**:1574–9.

Perrott, D. R. and Saberi, K. (1990). Minimum audible angle thresholds for sources varying in both elevation and azimuth. *Journal of the Acoustical Society of America* **87**:1728–31.

Plack, C. J. and Moore, B. C. J. (1990). Temporal window shape as a function of frequency and level. *Journal of the Acoustical Society of America* **87**:2178–87.

Plomp, R. (1976). Binaural and monaural speech intelligibility of connected discourse in reverberation as a function of azimuth of a single competing source (speech of noise). *Acustica* **34**:200–11.

Shannon, R. V., Zeng, F.-G., Wygonski, J., Kamath, V., and Ekelid, M. (1995). Speech recognition with primarily temporal cues. *Science* **270**:303–4.

Shaw, E. A. G. and Vaillancourt, M. M. (1985). Transformation of sound-pressure level from the free field to the eardrum presented in numerical form. *Journal of the Acoustical Society of America* **78**:1120–3.

Shinn-Cunningham, B. G., Zurek, P. M., and Durlach, N. I. (1993). Adjustment and discrimination measurements of the precedence effect. *Journal of the Acoustical Society of America* **93**:2923–32.

Spence, C. J. and Driver, J. (1994). Covert spatial orienting in audition—exogenous and endogenous mechanisms. *Journal of Experimental Psychology: Human Perception and Performance* **20**:555–74.

Stern, R. M. and Trahiotis, C. (1995). Models of binaural interaction. In *Hearing* (ed. B. C. J. Moore), pp. 347–86. San Diego: Academic Press.

Stern, R. M. and Trahiotis, C. (1997). Models of binaural perception. In *Binaural and Spatial Hearing in Real and Virtual Environments* (ed. R. H. Gilkey and T. R. Anderson), pp. 499–531. Mahwah, NJ: Lawrence Erlbaum Associates.

Strelow, E. R. and Brabyn, J. A. (1982). Locomotion of the blind by natural sound cues. *Perception* **11**: 635–40.

Triesman, A. M. (1964). Verbal cues, language and meaning in selective attention. *American Journal of Psychology* **77**:206–19.

van der Par, S. and Kohlrausch, A. (1997). A new approach to comparing binaural masking level differences at low and high frequencies. *Journal of the Acoustical Society of America* **101**:1671–80.

Wallach, H., Newman, E. B., and Rosenzweig, M. R. (1949). The precedence effect in sound localization. *American Journal of Psychology* **42**:315–36.

Warren, R. M. Bashford, J. A., and Wrightson, J. M. (1981). Detection of long interaural delays for broadband noise. *Journal of the Acoustical Society of America* **69**:1510–14.

Watkins, A. J. (2005). Perceptual compensation for effects of reverberation in speech identification. *Journal of the Acoustical Society of America* **118**:249–62.

Watkins, A. J. and Makin, S. J. (2007). Steady-spectrum contexts and perceptual compensation for reverberation in speech identification. *Journal of the Acoustical Society of America* **121**:257–66.

Wightman, F. L. and Kistler, D. J. (1992). The dominant role of low-frequency interaural time differences in sound localization. *Journal of the Acoustical Society of America* **91**:1648–61.

Wightman, F. and Kistler, D. (2005). Measurement and validation of human HRTFs for use in hearing research. *Acta Acustica United with Acustica* **91**:429–39.

Zahorik, P. (2002). Assessing auditory distance perception using virtual acoustics. *Journal of the Acoustical Society of America* **111**:1832–46.

Zahorik, P., Bangayan, P., Sundareswaran, V., Wang, K., and Tam C. (2006). Perceptual recalibration in human sound localization: Learning to remediate front–back reversals. *Journal of the Acoustical Society of America* **120**:343–59.

Zurek, P. M. (1980). The precedence effect and its possible role in the avoidance of interaural ambiguities. *Journal of the Acoustical Society of America* **67**:952–64.

Chapter 7

Comparative psychoacoustics

William P. Shofner and Andrew J. Niemiec

7.1 Introduction

Comparative psychoacoustics, the study of the hearing capabilities of animals using behavioral methods (Klump *et al.*, 1995), allows us a glimpse into the auditory world of another species, giving us some degree of insight into a disparate species' *Umwelt* or perceptual world (von Uexküll, 1921) and allowing us to temporarily shed our familiar anthropocentric existence. Comparative psychoacoustics is the application of behavioral techniques to the study of auditory processing in animals, and the emphasis of this approach is psychophysical, as in human studies. That is, acoustic stimuli are generally artificial and do not have any inherent behavioral importance to the animal, and it typically must be trained to make a behavioral response to the stimulus. This approach is different from an ethological approach in which animals might make a stereotypical response to a sound that is natural and thus biologically significant.

Fay (1994) has described two important goals of research in comparative psychoacoustics. One is the development of 'animal models' for human hearing. Understanding psychophysical behavior in animals is a necessary and important conceptual bridge between psychoacoustical studies in human listeners and neurophysiological experiments in animals. That is, comparing human and animal psychoacoustical data gives us some information regarding the degree to which we can rely on auditory physiological data from animals to explain human auditory behavior.

Another has been referred to by Fay as 'comparative hearing research'. This goal is to specifically study hearing in non-human animals in an effort to understand hearing as a 'general biological phenomenon'. As described by Fay (1994), results from experiments in 'animal psychoacoustics helps place human psychoacoustical data within the realms of evolutionary biology and neuroscience'. There are two general questions that can be asked with regard to an animal's perceptual world (Stebbins, 1995). The first of these, 'What are the animal's perceptual capabilities?', is the question most often addressed in comparative psychoacoustics research, primarily because the methodology to ask such as question is very well developed. Most of this chapter will revolve around this question. However, another less frequently asked question is 'What are the animal's perceptual proclivities?' That is, under naturalistic circumstances, what does an animal perceive? For example, does the animal perceive sensory illusions or aftereffects? Can animals classify and categorize stimuli, yet still discriminate among them as humans commonly do? The answer to this second question is much less clear and the methodology to address it much less advanced. For the field of comparative psychoacoustics, it remains a challenge that needs to be addressed. This chapter provides an overview of research in animal psychophysical experiments in hearing. The intent is not to provide an exhaustive survey of the literature, but to describe key findings in many different areas of research.

7.2 **Methodology**

Several methodologies are commonly used to study hearing in animals. Each of these approaches has its own strengths and weaknesses and varies in terms of the species to which it might most appropriately be applied. Because this chapter focuses primarily on hearing in birds and mammals, we will discuss the methodologies most relevant to these classes of animal: constant stimulus, tracking, and conditioned avoidance procedures. Other procedures, such as reflex modification and conditioned suppression, are also used in animal psychoacoustics; however, these are used primarily to study hearing behavior in fish, reptiles, and anurans. Although these procedures can also be applied to species higher up the evolutionary ladder, they are beyond the scope of this chapter.

7.2.1 **Training**

Constant stimulus, tracking, and conditioned avoidance procedures rely on the use of operant and classical conditioning techniques to train animals to bring about the presentation of a specific auditory stimulus, and then for them to respond appropriately in the presence of that stimulus. Typically, the animal is trained to make an 'observing response' in the absence of a stimulus and a 'reporting response' once the stimulus has been detected.

For mammals, a typical observing response consists of initiating and maintaining contact with a response manipulandum appropriate for the species under study. The reporting response usually consists of releasing the manipulandum. For small mammals such as chinchillas, the observing response typically involves a lever press while the reporting response is a lever release (Niemiec *et al.*, 1992). For larger mammals such as monkeys, contact and release with a sturdy metal cylinder is often used. The monkey's contact with the cylinder completes a circuit that sends a minute current from the cylinder through the monkey to a grounded primate restraint chair (Moody *et al.*, 1976). For birds, a series of key pecks on one LED-illuminated microswitch constitutes the observing response, while a peck on a second LED-illuminated microswitch constitutes the reporting response (Dooling and Okanoya, 1995).

The observing response serves two general purposes: (1) it indicates that the animal is prepared to participate in the testing procedure and is listening for the presentation of a stimulus; and (2) it maintains the animal in a relatively constant position within the free field, ensuring that the stimulus level does not differ greatly from trial to trial, and allows for accurate calibration of the acoustic stimulus at the position of the animal's head during stimulus presentation.

The reporting response, which requires the animal to perform a specific task to indicate stimulus detection, allows the experimenter or the apparatus controlling the testing paradigm to objectively identify and verify the animal's detection of the stimulus. Training a subject to produce consistent behavior with regard to the auditory stimulus can take several weeks. During this time, subtle adjustments may be made to the procedure in order to bring the animal's behavior under the control of the auditory stimulus.

For the remainder of our discussion of the training and testing procedure, we will describe the training of a chinchilla for the relatively simple task of threshold measurement. Similar, but not identical, training procedures for testing monkeys are also described in Moody *et al.* (1976) and Niemiec and Moody (1995). For training, and ultimately for testing, the animal is put into a cage housed within a sound-attenuating chamber. The chamber contains the testing cage, a response lever, a 20-mg food pellet dispenser for rewarding the animal, and a speaker for stimulus presentation. The speaker is placed such that it is in close proximity when the animal is operating the response lever. For example, the speaker can be suspended just above the testing cage, directly over the area the animal's head will occupy when it is manipulating the response lever. Initially, stimulus presentation and food reward should be controlled both manually and via computer, with the experimental apparatus set up such that a lever press causes the presentation of a clearly audible pure-tone stimulus while a lever release results in the cessation of the tone and the delivery of a food reward.

Generally, the training process involves some degree of food restriction for the animal so that it is motivated by the reward. The food restriction should not be severe because severe food deprivation may jeopardize the animal's health and alter its normal behavior. However, the animal should be hungry at the start of each training session and it should earn enough food during the training session so that it is relatively satiated by the session's end. One successful food restriction procedure involves determining the minimum quantity of food that will allow the animal to maintain its normal free-feed weight. Once this quantity is known, it is reduced by 25% and the animal is allowed to subsist on this reduced quantity until it reaches 85–90% of its free-feed weight. At this point, training is begun and the animal is maintained at this weight until training is complete and the animal is working consistently. Because the training phase may take several weeks/months, a small amount of food and a treat may be given after each training session to maintain the animal at 85–90% of its free-feed weight if sufficient food has not been earned during a training session. Once the animal is trained and working well, it can be allowed to slowly return to its normal free-feed weight.

Training typically begins with the shaping of the observing response, i.e. getting the chinchilla to press and hold the response lever. The trainer shapes this response by rewarding successively closer approximations of the final desired behavior with food. Initially, the trainer manually rewards the animal whenever it approaches the response lever. Once this is achieved, the food reward is withheld until the animal more closely approximates the final desired behavior, the lever press and release. Ultimately, the animal learns to press the response lever resulting in the immediate presentation of the auditory stimulus. When the chinchilla emits the reporting response by eventually releasing the response lever, the auditory stimulus shuts off and a food reward is delivered. The size of the food reward will vary with the species being trained. For a chinchilla, two 20-mg pellets per trial is an acceptable reward. Once the animal is reliably pressing and releasing the lever for food, a time window is placed on both the auditory stimulus and the release of the lever. For example, the stimulus now becomes a 1-s tone and the chinchilla must release the lever within 2 s of the tone onset to receive the food pellet reward. At the same time, the interval between the onset of the observing response and the tone presentation is gradually increased. This interval will ultimately be determined by the computer on a trial-by-trial basis and, in the final testing procedure, varies randomly from 1 to 8 s. The purpose of this 'variable hold time' is to prevent the animal from guessing when the stimulus will be presented.

Once the animal can reliably maintain the observing response for a 1–8 s hold time, 'catch trials' are inserted into the testing procedure. Catch trials monitor and control the probability that the chinchilla will make reporting responses in the absence of the test stimuli. They are identical to tone trials except that the tone is not presented. For the chinchilla, the correct behavior is to maintain the observing response throughout the duration of the catch trial, essentially reporting that no stimulus was detected on that trial. If no reporting response is emitted once the catch trial elapses, the animal is rewarded for its correct response. If the animal releases the lever during a catch trial, reporting that it heard a tone when none was presented, no reward is given, the catch trial response is noted by the computer, and the computer waits for the animal to initiate a new trial by pressing and holding the response lever. Over several sessions, the proportion of catch trials is gradually increased to 20%. Once the animal reliably reports supra-threshold tones and correctly withholds reporting responses on at least 80% of the catch trials, one of the psychophysical methods can be used to manipulate the stimulus level and measure the animal's threshold for the tone.

Some animals may have difficulty meeting the criterion of withholding responses on 80% of the catch trials and develop a propensity toward excessive guessing. An animal's willingness to guess on catch trials can be manipulated to some extent by changing the relative reward value of a catch trial in comparison to a tone trial. Normally, a reward of two 20-mg pellets is issued for each successful tone or catch trial. However, one way to curb excessive catch trial responding is to increase the value of a successful catch trial response to three pellets and to decrease the value of a successful tone trial response to one pellet. The animal will quickly discover that catch trials are worth more and will alter its responding behavior accordingly. Once the chinchilla begins to meet the criterion, the original reward structure can be reinstated.

Once an animal is under stimulus control and is responding properly to both tone trials and catch trials, its responses can also be classified into common signal detection parlance: the correct detection of a tone during a tone trial becomes a 'hit'; the non-detection of a tone during a tone trial, a 'miss'; the report that a tone was detected during a catch trial, a 'false alarm'; and the successful maintenance of an observing response through the end of a catch trial, a 'correct rejection'.

7.2.2 The method of constant stimuli

In the method of constant stimuli, several stimulus levels that bracket the animal's threshold are selected and presented multiple times. The subject's detection performance for each stimulus level is then tabulated to yield a psychometric function that describes the subject's percentage of correct detection as a function of stimulus level. The subject's absolute threshold is then estimated from the psychometric function. The definition of threshold is somewhat arbitrary, although one common definition is the stimulus level that results in 50% correct detection. Another common threshold estimation procedure that controls for the effects of response bias takes the percent correct detection midway between the catch trial response rate and 100% correct detection. Therefore, the threshold for an animal with a 10% catch trial response rate would be the stimulus level that yields 55% correct detection.

Implementation of the method of constant stimuli begins by estimating a rough threshold for the test frequency in question by presenting a supra-threshold stimulus level and decreasing the presentation level by 10 dB after each correct detection. Once the chinchilla misses a stimulus presentation, the computer chooses this missed stimulus level and five additional stimulus levels in 10-dB increments to measure the animal's psychometric function. Ideally, this yields five stimulus levels above the 50% correct point and one stimulus level below the 50% correct point on the psychometric function. The six stimulus levels are presented to the chinchilla in a random order and its detection performance for each stimulus level is tabulated. If the chinchilla's detection for the lowest stimulus level begins to exceed 50% correct, the computer removes the highest stimulus level and replaces it with one 10 dB below the current lowest stimulus level. Each stimulus level is presented several times. Once a complete set of stimulus levels have been presented at the current test frequency, the computer randomly picks a new test frequency and determines a rough threshold estimate for the new test frequency as described above. This procedure is repeated until psychometric functions have been measured for all test frequencies of interest. A 60–90-min testing session typically results in the measurement of psychometric functions for approximately nine test frequencies, allowing the measurement of a complete sensitivity function in each testing session.

A daily threshold estimate is derived from each test frequency's psychometric function. Data from testing sessions that have an overall catch trial response rate above 20% are discarded. Final threshold estimates are usually based on the average or median of several individual threshold estimates taken over several days. Often, an explicit stability criterion is used. For example, one common stability criterion requires that four out of five daily threshold estimates must fall within ± 5 dB of the median, and that there is no obvious trend towards an increase or decrease in threshold. Once these two conditions are met, the median of the five stable daily threshold estimates is taken as the final threshold. Testing continues until stable threshold estimates are measured at all test frequencies.

There are two chief advantages of the method of constant stimuli. First, because the majority of the stimulus presentations result in greater than 50% correct detection, the overall experimental task is relatively easy for the subject. The animal is not forced to make a difficult detection or discrimination on each trial, making stimulus control of the behavior easy to maintain. Second, because stimulus presentation varies over a wide range, the experimenter is able to estimate many points on the psychometric function (Levitt, 1971), making it possible to compare the data across a wider range of threshold definitions. The chief disadvantage of the method is that it is relatively inefficient, requiring many test trials in order for the experimenter to ultimately estimate a single point on the psychometric function (Levitt, 1971). The experimenter can, however, make fuller use of the resulting data by computing a linear regression over the straight portion of the psychometric function or by implementing a curve-fitting procedure.

7.2.3 Adaptive tracking

Adaptive tracking is a variation of Fechner's method of limits, and employs a one-down/one-up tracking rule in which the stimulus level is reduced following each correct detection and increased following each miss, asymptoting at the subject's 50% correct detection point on the psychometric function (Levitt, 1971). As in the method of constant stimuli, the adaptive tracking procedure uses the animal's observing and reporting responses to indicate detection or non-detection of the stimulus. The adaptive tracking procedure yields several series of ascending and descending stimulus levels based on the animal's detection performance. That is, once the animal's response to a stimulus changes from detection to non-detection or vice versa, the direction in which the stimulus level changes is reversed. Each of these 'reversals' signals the end of one series and the beginning of another.

Implementation of the adaptive tracking procedure begins with the presentation of a suprathreshold stimulus. The stimulus level is then decreased by 5 dB following each correct detection and increased by 5 dB following each miss. Reversing the direction of the stimulus level presentation continues until ten reversals take place. The first two reversals are discarded on the assumption that they will be the most variable, and the average of the remaining eight reversals are taken as the threshold estimate for the test frequency. At this point, a new test frequency is randomly selected and the computer begins tracking the subject's threshold at this new frequency. This procedure is repeated until threshold estimates are obtained for all test frequencies. A 60–90-min testing session typically results in two threshold estimates for each of the nine test frequencies. As with the method of constant stimuli, threshold testing continues until stable estimates of threshold are obtained at each test frequency.

The principal advantage of the adaptive tracking procedure is its increased efficiency over the method of constant stimuli (Levitt, 1971). Except for the small number of initial trials used to bring the stimulus level within range of the animal's threshold, only those stimulus levels needed to determine threshold are presented. There are two major factors that affect this method's efficiency: the step size used to track threshold, and the number of reversals used to define threshold. Each of these factors represents a trade-off in terms of the resulting threshold estimate. A smaller step size allows finer tracking of threshold but at the cost of increasing the number of trials per tracking run. Fewer reversals will decrease the number of trials in a tracking run but may increase the variability of the resulting threshold estimate. One successful implementation of the procedure uses a large initial step size to quickly bring the stimulus level within range of the subject's threshold. For example, after the first two reversals at the large (5 dB) step size, which will be discarded anyway, threshold is tracked using a smaller 2-dB step size.

Another possible advantage of the adaptive tracking procedure may be an increase in the reliability of the threshold estimates. Because most observations are placed near threshold, the threshold estimates may be less variable than those derived using the method of constant stimuli. On the other hand, this may be offset to some extent due to the relative difficulty of the procedure for the animal. Unlike in the method of constant stimuli, in the adaptive tracking procedure the stimulus is nearly always presented at near-threshold levels, making this procedure unsuitable for animals that do not show good stimulus control over the behavior prior to the onset of testing. Guessing can sometimes drive the stimulus level far below threshold, causing a further increase in guessing due to the animal's inability to detect the now sub-threshold stimulus. One strategy that can be employed to deal with this problem is to reduce the animal's guessing behavior by changing the reinforcement such that catch trails are more valuable than tone trials. Another further step might involve increasing the proportion of catch trials in order to give the animal additional practice with catch trials.

7.2.4 Transformed tracking

Like the one-down/one-up adaptive tracking procedure, transformed tracking is also a variation of the method of limits. Transformed tracking uses a two-down/one-up tracking rule in which the stimulus level is reduced after two correct detections in a row and increased following each miss, essentially tracking the 70.7% correct detection point on the psychometric function (Levitt, 1971). As in adaptive tracking, transformed tracking begins with the presentation of suprathreshold stimulus levels. However, the stimulus level is decreased using a 5-dB step size after two correct detections in a row and increased by 5 dB after every miss. As in adaptive tracking, after a specified number of reversals have occurred, the first two reversals are discarded and the remaining reversals are averaged to derive a threshold estimate. As before, once a threshold estimate for a given test frequency has been derived, the computer randomly chooses a new test frequency and begins tracking the subject's threshold. This continues until threshold estimates have been measured for all test frequencies. As with the previously described psychophysical methods, testing continues until stable estimates of threshold are obtained at each test frequency.

Transformed tracking is more efficient than the method of constant stimuli and the method of limits, but is less efficient than adaptive tracking. This is due to the increased number of trials required to obtain two correct detections in a row. Again, there are trade-offs associated with both the number of reversals required for a threshold estimate and the step size used to derive the threshold estimate. As described above, a compromise can be reached by reducing the step size after the first two reversals in order to more finely track threshold while reducing the number of trials for the tracking run to a minimum.

Although less efficient, transformed tracking does offer some advantages over adaptive tracking. In adaptive tracking, the stimulus is presented above and below threshold the same number of times. This makes the task difficult for the animal because it is forced to work at near-threshold levels. Transformed tracking is easier for the animal because the stimulus is presented twice as often above threshold as below threshold. This reduces the amount of guessing during a tracking run, resulting in better stimulus control over the animal's behavior, and makes it more suitable for problem animals than adaptive tracking.

Another possible advantage of transformed tracking is that the complex nature of the two-down/one-up tracking rule makes it more difficult for the animal to anticipate the next stimulus level and to adjust its responses, so that the stimulus level is easy to detect. Therefore, transformed tracking represents a good compromise between difficulty for the subject and efficiency for the experimenter, falling somewhere between the method of constant stimuli and adaptive tracking.

7.2.5 Conditioned avoidance

In the conditioned avoidance procedure an animal is trained to make continuous contact with a response manipulandum. This is typically a reward spout that dispenses food paste or water (Heffner and Heffner, 1995). An auditory 'warning' stimulus is then presented in conjunction with a mild electric shock. The mild electric shock serves as a punisher, causing the animal to break contact with the response manipulandum. After several such training trials, the animal learns to break contact with the response manipulandum whenever it detects the 'warning' stimulus, thus avoiding the mild electric shock. Breaking contact with the response manipulandum serves as an indicator that the animal detected the auditory stimulus; the stimulus level is then manipulated using a constant stimulus, tracking, or other titration procedure. 'Sham' trials are also included in the procedure to monitor the probability that the animal will respond in the absence of a warning stimulus. The general procedure consists of a series of trial blocks that end with either a 'warning' trial or a 'sham' trial. For example, the computer might decide that a given block of trials will involve six 1-s trials with a 200-ms inter-trial interval. The first five trials will consist of 'safe' trials in which no warning stimulus is presented. The response of the animal is determined by measuring contact with the response manipulandum just before the presentation of the warning stimulus (i.e. the signal) on the sixth trial and recording a response if the animal breaks contact with the manipulandum prior to the presentation of the shock. For a 'sham' trial, continued contact with the manipulandum indicates that no warning stimulus was detected. The number of trials in a block is randomly varied so that the animal cannot predict stimulus presentation based on timing cues.

7.3 Frequency selectivity

Frequency selectivity refers to the auditory system's ability to separate frequency components in a complex sound (see Chapter 2). Measures of frequency selectivity reflect how acoustic information is organized and processed with respect to frequency. Basic aspects of frequency selectivity—such as critical bands, critical ratios, and psychophysical tuning curves—have been studied in a number of mammalian and avian species. Other measures, e.g. auditory filter shapes and co-modulation masking release, have not received as much attention in species other than humans.

Critical band theory (Fletcher, 1940) was proposed to account for the results of masking experiments and is now fundamental to our understanding of frequency selectivity. Fletcher suggested that the auditory system behaves as if it consisted of a bank of bandpass filters with continuously overlapping center frequencies that serve as discrete spectral information channels. The 'critical bandwidth' is the passband width of one of these discrete information channels at a specific center frequency.

To account for the masking of tonal signals by noise, Fletcher made the simplifying assumptions that the shape of the auditory filter is rectangular and that, at threshold, the power in the tonal signal just equals the power of the noise masker falling within the critical band. The critical bandwidth (CBW) can then be estimated indirectly by computing the 'critical ratio' (CR) of the band in question. This is done by measuring the threshold for a tonal signal masked by a broadband noise and then subtracting the spectrum level of the broadband noise (in dB/Hz) from the level of the tonal signal at threshold. The CBW can then be estimated from the CR by determining the equivalent rectangular bandwidth of noise having energy equal to that of the tonal signal: $CBW\ (Hz) = 10^{(CR/10)}$. A lower CR at a given frequency indicates more efficient extraction of the signal from the masking noise, resulting in a narrower critical band.

Critical ratios have been measured in several mammalian species, including the domestic cat (Watson, 1963; Pickles, 1975; Costalupes, 1983), rhesus monkey (Clack, 1966), porpoise (Johnson, 1968; Au and Moore, 1990), seal (Terhune and Ronald, 1971, 1975; Southall *et al.*, 2000, 2003), rat (Gourevitch, 1965), mouse (Ehret, 1976), chinchilla (Miller, 1964; Seaton and Trahiotis, 1975; Niemiec *et al.*, 1992), gerbil (Kittel *et al.*, 2002), and bat (Long, 1977; Suthers and Summers, 1980). Avian species that have been tested include the blackbird and pigeon (Hienz and Sachs, 1987), the sparrow, canary, cockatiel, starling, parakeet, and zebra finch (Dooling and Saunders, 1975a; Saunders *et al.*, 1979; Dooling *et al.*, 1986; Okanoya and Dooling, 1987, 1988; Langemann *et al*, 1995; Farabaugh *et al.*, 1998), and the barn owl (Dyson *et al.*, 1998). A comprehensive summary of critical ratio data from a large number of species is available in Fay (1988); however, in general, humans, non-human primates and marine mammals have lower critical ratios than most other terrestrial mammals tested. The CRs of many species of birds fall into the same general range as those of the terrestrial mammals, with the exception of parakeets, which appear to have sharper frequency selectivity at 2–4 kHz, and blackbirds, which appear to be more variable across frequency than other bird species.

In addition to the CR, the CBW can also be measured directly by conducting a series of band-narrowing or band-widening experiments. In these experiments, the threshold for a tonal signal centered in a noise masker with constant spectrum level is measured as a function of masker bandwidth. Masked threshold for the tonal signal will increase with masker bandwidth up to the CBW, at which point the signal threshold will asymptote since frequencies outside the critical bandwidth will not contribute to masking. Human CBW estimates from band-narrowing and band-widening experiments (Egan and Hake, 1950; Schafer *et al.*, 1950; Hamilton, 1957; Zwicker *et al.*, 1957; Scharf, 1970) indicate that indirect estimates of CBW based on the CR may be of limited accuracy, primarily due to Fletcher's simplifying assumptions. However, these more direct measures are also limited, since all three techniques measure only the 'effective' bandwidth of the auditory filter and physiological studies demonstrate that the auditory filter is not rectangular. More importantly, contrary to Fletcher's second assumption, the processing efficiency of the subject is not fixed. That is, at threshold, the signal power is not equal to the noise power passing through the auditory filter. In masking experiments, human subjects need tonal signals 5–15 dB higher than the spectrum level of the masker noise at threshold, that is, the signal-to-noise ratio (E/N_0) of humans is 5–15 dB (Reed and Bilger, 1973). Other species generally show reduced processing efficiency relative to humans. For example, the E/N_0 of rats and chinchillas ranges from 25 to 40 dB (Gourevitch, 1965; Niemiec *et al.*, 1992). Canaries, finches, parakeets, sparrows, and starlings show E/N_0 values of 20–40 dB (Okanoya and Dooling, 1985, 1987, 1988), whereas the E/N_0 of blackbirds ranges from 30 to 50 dB (Hienz and Sachs, 1987).

Because the band-narrowing and band-widening approaches require additional threshold measurements at other masker bandwidths, they have been used in fewer species. However, these more direct estimates of CBW are available for the cat (Pickles, 1975, 1979), mouse (Ehret, 1976), chinchilla (Seaton and Trahiotis, 1975; Niemiec *et al.*, 1992), gerbil (Kittel *et al.*, 2002), greater horseshoe bat (Long, 1980), pig-tailed macaque (Gourevitch, 1970), dolphin (Au and Moore, 1990), seal (Southall *et al.*, 2003), parakeet (Saunders *et al.*, 1978), and starling (Langemann *et al.*, 1995).

Figure 7.1 compares typical bandwidths derived from critical ratios (CR), with typical bandwidths derived using more direct techniques (CB). The top panel contains species with hearing ranges similar to humans, whereas the bottom panel contains species with high-frequency hearing. Both panels show that the CB estimates are generally broader than the CR estimates. This was true in 34 of the 44 cases where bandwidth estimates were available at the same signal frequency. There is also considerable variability in terms of the relationship between these functions for a given species. For example, the CR and CB functions of some species including the human, cat,

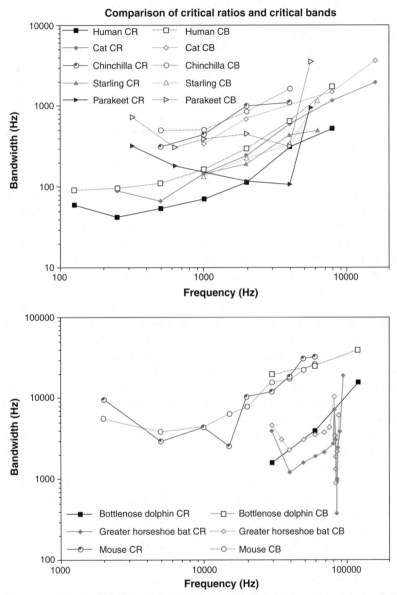

Fig. 7.1 Estimates of auditory filter bandwidth as a function of frequency derived from critical ratios (CR) and more direct techniques (CB). Top panel shows data for low-frequency hearing animals; bottom panel shows data for high-frequency hearing animals. Human CR data from Hawkins and Stevens (1950); human CB data from Zwicker *et al.* (1957); cat CB data from Pickles (1975); cat CR data are averages based on Costalupes (1983), Pickles (1975), and Watson (1963); chinchilla CR and CB data are averages based on Seaton and Trahiotis (1975) and Niemiec *et al.* (1992); starling CR and CB data from Langemann *et al.* (1995); parakeet CR data from Saunders *et al.* (1979); parakeet CB data are averages based on Saunders *et al.* (1978, 1979); bottlenose dolphin CR and CB data from Au and Moore (1990); horseshoe bat CR data from Long (1977); horseshoe bat CB data from Long (1980); mouse CR and CB data from Ehret (1976).

parakeet, dolphin, and bat are roughly parallel, while the functions of other species including the chinchilla, mouse and starling are roughly identical. These differences likely reflect species differences in processing efficiency; however, other factors such as measurement technique may also contribute to the discrepancy between the functions within a species.

Given the relative lack of a consistent relationship between CR and CB estimates across species and the fact that these techniques simply estimate the effective bandwidth of the auditory filter at some specified frequency, it makes sense to examine frequency selectivity using techniques that directly measure the shape of the auditory filter and that remove processing efficiency as a possible confound.

The psychophysical tuning curve (PTC) involves measuring the level of a pure-tone or narrow-band noise masker required to mask a pure-tone signal of fixed frequency and intensity as a function of the masker's frequency. In this paradigm, the intensity of the signal tone is typically low so that few auditory filters will be activated by the signal. Again, it is assumed that, at threshold, the masker produces a constant output from the filter in order to mask the signal. Consequently, the PTC measures the masker level needed to generate a fixed output from the auditory filter as a function of frequency. If the auditory system is assumed to be linear, the shape of the auditory filter can be obtained by inverting the PTC. However, one problem associated with using the PTC to measure auditory filter shape is off-frequency listening. Since the subject will attempt to monitor the filter that gives the best signal-to-masker ratio, it is likely the case that the subject does not monitor just one filter. When the masker frequency is below the signal frequency, the subject can improve their performance by monitoring a filter centered just above the signal frequency. Conversely, when the masker frequency is above the signal frequency, the subject can improve performance by monitoring a filter centered just below the signal frequency. In these instances, the filters centered just above or below the signal frequency give the subject a better signal-to-masker ratio than the filter centered at the signal frequency. Human studies involving off-frequency listening result in PTCs that have sharper tips than would be obtained if only one auditory filter was involved (O'Loughlin and Moore, 1981). It would not be unreasonable to expect similar results from animal subjects.

PTCs have been measured in a number of non-human species including the chinchilla (McGee et al., 1976; Ryan et al., 1979; Salvi et al., 1982a; Clark and Bohne, 1986), cat (Pickles, 1979), pig-tailed macaque (Serafin et al., 1982), patas monkey (Smith et al., 1987, 1990), and the parakeet (Saunders et al., 1978, 1979; Kuhn and Saunders, 1980). PTCs are generally measured using either a simultaneous-masking or forward-masking procedure, with the forward-masking procedure consistently providing narrower estimates of frequency selectivity than the simultaneous-masking procedure. Recently, the difference in tuning estimates resulting from these procedures has, in part, been used to argue that the auditory nerve fibers of humans are more sharply tuned than those of many non-human species (Shera et al., 2002). Ruggero and Temchin (2005), however, contend that forward-masking PTCs in several species of birds and mammals overestimate the sharpness of tuning of cochlear afferent neurons—in part due to off-frequency listening—whereas estimates from simultaneous-masking PTCs provide estimates that are closer to those derived from cochlear afferent neurons. By modeling the relationship between compound action-potential tuning curves and auditory nerve-fiber tuning curves in human and non-human species, Ruggero and Temchin argue that tuning in the human cochlea is similar to other species for which measurements are available.

Improved psychophysical procedures that allowed the estimation of auditory filter shape independent of the effects of off-frequency listening were eventually developed. Houtgast (1974, 1977) originated a technique for measuring auditory filter shape based on rippled noise-masking. Rippled noise, a complex pseudo-periodic stimulus with a cosinusoidal energy spectrum, is generated by delaying a source of white noise by some amount and adding the output of the delay to the original noise source. This results in a continuous masking noise with a cosinusoidal energy spectrum in which the spacing or density of the spectral peaks and valleys are functions of the delay. Houtgast used this attribute of rippled noise to gauge frequency selectivity by measuring threshold for a tonal signal masked by rippled noise as a function of the spectral density of the rippled noise. If masked threshold for the tonal signal corresponds to a constant signal-to-masker ratio at the output of the filter, then the change in masked threshold as a function of ripple density can be used to define a weighting function that is the shape of the auditory filter. Patterson (1976) developed a similar technique based on measuring thresholds for a tonal signal masked by noise with a bandstop or notch centered at the signal frequency. Patterson assumed a symmetrical filter shape, varied the width of the notch in the masker, and measured signal threshold as a function of masker notch width. For a signal placed symmetrically in a notched noise, the best signal-to-masker ratio is obtained with a filter centered at the signal frequency. As notch width increases, the power of the noise coming through the filter decreases, resulting in a decrease in signal threshold. If masked threshold corresponds to a constant signal-to-masker ratio at the output of the filter, then the change in masked threshold as a function of notch width shows how the area under the filter varies with notch width. Differentiating the masking function relating signal threshold to notch width gives an estimate of the auditory filter shape. The notched noise technique was eventually modified to eliminate the symmetry assumption (Patterson and Nimmo-Smith, 1980), allowing both halves of the auditory filter to be estimated independently. Both notched noise- and rippled noise-masking techniques yield auditory filters that can be approximated by a rounded exponential (ROEX) function with a rounded top and fairly steep skirts.

Halpern and Dallos (1986) were the first to use the notched noise-masking technique to measure auditory filter shape in non-humans, testing chinchillas in a forward-masking paradigm. While the data from their chinchillas yielded estimates of tuning similar to those obtained using critical ratio and more direct critical band estimation techniques, the resulting auditory filter shapes showed an unexpected dip in the region of the center frequency. These dips resulted, in part, because the animals' signal threshold did not change until the notch width increased to roughly 33% of the center frequency. This may have resulted from perceptual cueing (Terry and Moore, 1977). Perceptual cueing refers to the idea that there may be two cues available to a listener in a forward-masking experiment. In a narrow spectral gap, the listener could use the perception of a temporal change in the signal-plus-masker condition to discriminate it from the masker-alone condition. In a wider spectral gap, the listener could use the perception of a pitch difference between the signal and the masker to discriminate between the two conditions.

Niemiec et al. (1992) measured auditory filter shapes in chinchillas using both notched noise- and rippled noise-masking techniques in a simultaneous masking paradigm. Both techniques yielded similar filter shapes that were well approximated by ROEX functions. The equivalent rectangular bandwidths (ERBs) derived from the rippled noise technique were approximately 17–27% of the center frequency over the frequency range tested (500–2000 Hz). Houtgast's (1974, 1977) data showed that human ERBs were approximately 15–20% over the same frequency range. Niemiec's notched noise results yielded chinchilla ERBs ranging from approximately 8 to 19% of the center frequency over the frequency range 500–4000 Hz. Patterson's (1976) human data showed ERBs ranging from 11 to 14% over the frequency range 500–2000 Hz. Moore and Glasberg (1983) compared human ERBs estimated using both rippled noise- and notched noise-masking techniques, and found that ERBs estimated from rippled noise masking were approximately 35% greater than those estimated from notched noise masking. Niemiec et al. (1992) show similar results for chinchillas, with ERBs derived using rippled noise masking approximately 30% larger than those measured using notched noise masking.

Auditory filter shapes have also been measured in the bottlenose dolphin (Lemonds et al., 2000; Finneran et al., 2002), the white whale (Finneran et al., 2002), the guinea-pig (Evans et al., 1992),

CBA/CaJ mice (May *et al.*, 2006), and the budgerigar (Lin *et al.*, 1997). All these studies used the notched noise-masking technique, most likely due to the ease of stimulus generation and the relatively small number of threshold measurements needed in comparison to the rippled noise-masking technique, and all show that the auditory filters of animals are similar to those of humans both in terms of shape (i.e. they can be approximated by ROEX functions) and bandwidth (i.e. the ERBs of these functions range from approximately 8 to 19% of the center frequency, even for center frequencies in the ultrasonic range).

While critical band theory assumes that all auditory processing occurs within a single critical band, recent research has demonstrated that auditory information is also integrated across critical bands. Co-modulation masking release (CMR) (Hall *et al.*, 1984)—the reduced threshold for a pure-tone signal masked by a coherently modulated (co-modulated) masker in comparison to the threshold measured using a random broadband (unmodulated) masker—can be thought of as an auditory example of the Gestalt principle of organization known as 'common fate'. According to 'common fate', elements shifted together in a similar manner from a larger group tend to be grouped by themselves. The masking experiments discussed to this point use broadband noise, which by its nature is random and shows no correlation across frequency, preventing the listener from integrating information across multiple critical bands. However, if the masking noise used is non-random, with coherent amplitude or frequency fluctuations, information can potentially be integrated across critical bands, reducing the effects of masking due to the grouping that results from these cross-frequency correlations.

CMR has been measured in a small number of animal species, including the European starling (Klump and Langemann, 1995; Langemann and Klump 2001) and the gerbil (Kittel *et al.*, 2000; Klump 2001; Wagner 2002). CMR has also been measured in chinchillas; however, the results have been slightly more complicated. Niemiec *et al.* (1999) initially saw no masking release for a 1000-Hz signal tone as co-modulated noise-masker bandwidth increased from 30 to 2000 Hz; however, some masking release (4–6 dB) was seen for masker bandwidths greater than 2000 Hz (Niemiec *et al.*, 2000) and for sinusoidally amplitude-modulated masking noise (Niemiec, 2001). This may indicate that chinchillas use a different listening strategy than do other species, such as listening at the peaks of the masking waveforms rather than in the valleys. It is also possible that chinchillas adopt a broadband listening strategy in masking experiments.

7.4 Intensity discrimination and loudness perception

One of the fundamental attributes of hearing is the ability to detect changes in the level of a sound (see Chapter 3). The intensity difference limen (DL), or 'just noticeable difference', is the smallest change in sound level that can be detected by the animal, and there are three basic methods that can be used to estimate this threshold. Figure 7.2 illustrates how the stimuli might be presented to an animal based on these methods. For intensity discrimination, the standard sound is pulsed or gated continually, and the level of the signal is changed during the interval in which the animal must make a response. During the response window, the signal can alternate with the standard or the signal alone can be pulsed continually. For increment detection, the standard sound is presented continuously, and the signal is a continuous increase (or decrease) in level. For modulation detection, the standard sound is presented continuously, as in increment detection, but the signal is amplitude-modulated at a low rate. In all the above methods, the animal must detect the difference between the signal interval and the standard.

Human listeners are able to detect level changes over a wide range of sound pressure levels; that is, the dynamic range of hearing is approximately 100 dB. Figure 7.3 compares the DLs for pure tones as a function of sensation level for representative species of mammals (humans: Jesteadt *et al.*, 1977;

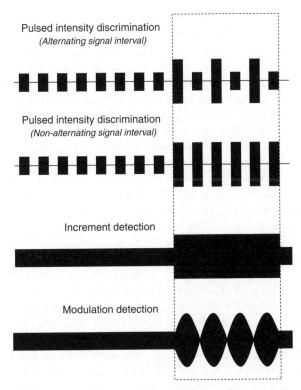

Pulsed intensity discrimination
(Alternating signal interval)

Pulsed intensity discrimination
(Non-alternating signal interval)

Increment detection

Modulation detection

Fig. 7.2 Schematic diagram showing examples of the amplitudes of the standard and signal sounds used to study intensity discrimination in animal psychophysical paradigms. The time between the dotted line indicates when the signal is presented and the time the animal has to make a response.

monkeys: Sinnott *et al.*, 1985; chinchillas: Saunders *et al.*, 1987) and birds (parakeet: Dooling and Saunders, 1975*b*; blackbirds and pigeons: Hienz *et al.*, 1980). This figure illustrates several points. First, it is clear that animals are not as sensitive as human listeners. That is, DLs for animals are higher than those obtained from human listeners. Second, the intensity discrimination thresholds for human listeners have been measured over an 80-dB dynamic range, whereas the thresholds for

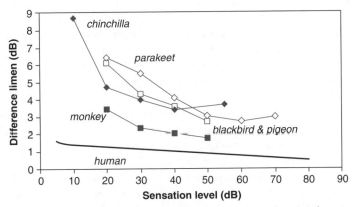

Fig. 7.3 Scatter plots showing intensity discrimination thresholds as a function for sensation level for several species of mammals. Solid line shows human thresholds (Jesteadt *et al.*, 1977); filled squares show monkey (Sinnott *et al.*, 1985); filled diamonds show chinchilla (Saunders *et al.*, 1987); open squares shows blackbird and pigeon (Hienz *et al.*, 1980); open diamonds show parakeet (Dooling and Saunders, 1975*b*).

animals have been estimated over smaller ranges. The paradox that intensity discrimination occurs over a wide range of sound levels (at least 80 dB for humans, as illustrated in Fig. 7.3) whereas the range of sound levels over which individual auditory nerve fibers can change their firing rates is smaller (approximately 30 dB), has been referred to as the 'dynamic range problem'. The animals represented in Fig. 7.3 were chosen in part because thresholds in these species were obtained over the widest range of sensational levels found in the literature. The range of sound levels over which animals can discriminate changes in pure-tone intensity is also, for the most part, larger than the dynamic range of auditory nerve fibers. Finally, if Weber's law holds for pure-tone intensity discrimination, then the DL will be constant. There is a clear decrease in DL as sensation level increases for all the species shown in Fig. 7.3, illustrating the 'near miss' to Weber's law. The DLs obtained using wideband noises are more constant over a range of sound levels than those obtained for pure tones (Clopton, 1972; Dooling and Searcy, 1981; Salvi *et al.*, 1982a; Shofner *et al.*, 1993). Moreover, similar to human listeners, thresholds decrease as the bandwidth of the noise increases (Shofner *et al.*, 1993; Shofner and Sheft, 1994).

As previously mentioned, the dynamic range of individual auditory nerve fibers is less than the range of sound levels over which animals can discriminate changes in intensity. May and McQuone (1995) examined the potential role that the olivocochlear efferent system plays in maintaining a wide dynamic range of hearing. Behavioral performance for 3-dB increases in sound level of 1-kHz and 8-kHz pure tones was measured in cats in quiet and in a background of continuous broadband noise. Performance in normal cats was then compared to performance after bilaterally sectioning at the floor of the 4th ventricle in each cat. Lesions at this location sever the projections of the medial olivocochlear pathway. There was no statistically significant difference in intensity discrimination performance after sectioning the efferent system when both 1-kHz and 8-kHz tones were presented in quiet, and there was no difference in performance for the 1-kHz tone presented in the background of broadband noise. However, there was a significant decrease in intensity discrimination performance for the 8-kHz tone in the background of broadband noise. These results suggest that the medial olivocochlear efferent system may play a role in maintaining a wide dynamic range of hearing for high-frequency signals in noise. The results are not meant to imply that a wide dynamic range of hearing does not exist at a frequency of 1 kHz in the cat, but rather that the mechanism underlying the wide dynamic range does not involve the medial olivo-cochlear efferent system. As pointed out by May and McQuone (1995), the density of efferent innervation in cat cochlea is greater in the basal regions than in the apical regions.

The above discussion has largely focused on intensity acuity; that is, the just noticeable differences in changes of stimulus intensity. However, there is more to the understanding of hearing than simply the objective measurement of thresholds, and it should be emphasized that animals, including human listeners, function in an environment in which sounds generally exist at supra-threshold levels. In human listeners the perceptual attribute of sound level is loudness; and as the level of a sound increases above threshold, there is a compressive growth in loudness that follows a power law (Stevens, 1956) as measured using magnitude estimation. Subjective perceptions are more difficult to address in animals, but behavioral techniques based on response-latency have been developed to measure loudness functions in animals.

The response-latency technique was pioneered by Stebbins (1966) and is based on measuring the reaction time to sounds that vary over a range of sound pressure levels. Latency-intensity functions generally display an inverse-exponential relationship: reaction times are short in response to high-intensity sounds, whereas reaction times become longer as the intensity of the sound decreases. The latency-intensity functions obtained for tones of various frequencies, for example, are interpreted to reflect the perception of loudness; that is, equal latencies are interpreted to indicate equal loudness. From these latency-intensity functions, equal latency contours can be generated. Pfingst *et al.* (1975) have demonstrated in human listeners that equal-latency contours are well matched to equal-loudness contours. These latency-intensity functions have been generated for tones in monkeys (Stebbins, 1966; Pfingst *et al.*, 1975), rabbits (Martin *et al.*, 1980), house finches (Dooling *et al.*, 1978), and cats (May *et al.*, 2009).

As mentioned above, the growth of loudness with increasing intensity follows a power law in human listeners, in which the exponent is around 0.3 (Stevens, 1956). That is, the loudness-intensity function is compressive. Dooling *et al.* (1987) applied a multidimensional scaling analysis to response latencies in order to derive a loudness scaling function in budgerigars; and, similar to humans, the loudness function in budgerigars can also be described by the power law with an exponent of 0.28. Compressive loudness functions have also been described for rats and chinchillas (Pierrel-Sorrentino and Raslear, 1980; Raslear *et al.*, 1983) and for cats (May *et al.*, 2009). Thus, while animals are generally less sensitive to changes in intensity than are human listeners, the perceptual dimensions of intensity (i.e. loudness) appear to be similar between humans and other animals. The similarity in the growth of loudness between humans and animals presumably reflects similarities in cochlear compression, whereas the higher acuity of humans for intensity discrimination may reflect more optimal processing of firing rate changes in the auditory nerve by the human central auditory system.

Related to intensity discrimination, in which the overall level of a sound changes, is spectral profile analysis. In profile analysis, overall level changes cannot be used as a cue; rather, comparisons across frequency channels must be made in order to determine whether or not an increment (or decrement) in a frequency component exists. Thus, in profile analysis, the subject cannot detect the presence of a signal by the use of absolute intensity changes, but must rely on relative intensity changes across frequencies. Profile analysis has not been widely studied across animal species. One profile analysis study has been carried out in birds. In this study, zebra finches and budgerigars had to detect a decrease in the amplitude of one component of a multi-component, harmonic complex tone; the thresholds obtained for birds were not significantly different from those obtained in human listeners for the same stimuli (Lohr and Dooling, 1998). In a similar experiment (Amagai *et al.*, 1999), budgerigars had to discriminate between a tone complex comprising 201 equal-amplitude components from a tone complex made of the same frequency components, but which varied in amplitude by a logarithmically spaced spectral ripple. Thresholds were measured for the depth of the spectral ripple. Because overall level was varied, the birds had to analyze the profile of the spectral ripple across frequency channels. Ripple detection thresholds for the birds were equal to or lower than those obtained from human listeners in the same behavioral procedure (Amagai *et al.*, 1999).

7.5 Speech discrimination and perception

While many birds and mammals produce vocalizations for communication, the production of speech is uniquely human. One of the long-running debates in the literature is whether the human nervous system possesses specialized neural mechanisms that have specifically evolved for processing speech sounds. Whereas it seems probable that the human nervous system has specializations for processing language, the question of whether or not it possesses neural mechanisms specialized for speech processing at the phonetic level has been much debated (e.g. Trout, 2001). Behavioral studies of speech discrimination in non-human animals have provided important insights into the processing of speech by human listeners.

Given that humans are a species in the biological order Primates, comparison of speech discrimination abilities between humans and other primates is a logical comparison. The discrimination of steady-state vowels in quiet has been obtained from several species of primates, including baboons (Hienz and Brady, 1988) and Old World monkeys (Sinnott, 1989).

Both groups of primates showed a performance greater than 90% correct for discriminating between pairs of vowels. In addition to primates, cats (Hienz et al., 1996a), gerbils (Sinnott and Mosteller, 2001), and blackbirds and pigeons (Hienz et al., 1981) can accurately discriminate between pairs of steady-state vowels. Higher discrimination performance is usually related to larger spectral differences between vowel formant frequencies. However, it is interesting to note that, for a given vowel pair, discrimination is better when the vowels are presented in such a way that there is an increase in formant frequencies compared to presenting the same vowels so that the formants decrease in frequency (Hienz et al., 1981, 1996a). In general, increasing the overall level of the vowels had no effect on vowel discrimination performance (Sinnott, 1989; Hienz et al., 1996a). Vowel discrimination in quiet is not affected by surgical sectioning of the olivoco-chlear efferent system (Dewson, 1968). Normal cats are able to discriminate vowels in the presence of broadband noise (Dewson, 1968; Hienz et al., 1996a), but discrimination performance for vowel discrimination in noise is poorer in cats following surgical sectioning of the olivocochlear efferent system (Dewson, 1968). This latter finding again suggests the importance of the medial olivocochlear efferent system in processing sounds in noise.

Formant frequency discrimination differs from vowel discrimination, in that only the frequency of a single formant is changed in the former, rather than the frequencies of all formants. Formant discrimination has been carried out in monkeys (Sommers et al., 1992), baboons (Hienz et al., 2004) and cats (Hienz et al., 1996b). The results from these studies indicate a difference between animal and human listeners for formant discrimination compared to pure-tone frequency discrimination. Sommers et al. (1992) trained monkeys to discriminate frequency changes of the first- or second-formant; the first formant of the vowel sound was 500 Hz and the second formant was 1400 Hz. Monkeys also discriminated the frequencies of pure tones having the same frequencies as the formants. Figure 7.4 compares DLs for formant discrimination with pure-tone frequency discrimination for monkeys. Note that for monkeys, the thresholds for formant discrimination (open bars in Fig. 7.4) are *lower* than those for pure-tone frequency discrimination (filled bars in Fig. 7.4). Similar results have been obtained in cats (Hienz et al., 1996b) and monkeys (Sinnott and Kreiter, 1991). For comparison, human thresholds for single-formant discrimination (Kewley-Port and Watson, 1994) and pure-tone frequency discrimination (Wier et al., 1977) at similar frequencies to the monkey data are also illustrated in Fig. 7.4. Note that for human listeners, the thresholds for formant discrimination (open bars) are *higher* than those for pure-tone frequency discrimination (filled bars). Thus, humans are more sensitive to frequency changes of pure tones than to vowels, but animals are more sensitive to frequency changes of vowels than to pure tones. It is also interesting to note in Fig. 7.4 that comparison of single-formant frequency discrimination thresholds for monkeys and humans are more similar than are pure-tone frequency discrimination thresholds between the two groups. The findings suggest that humans and non-human mammals use similar mechanisms for discriminating complex spectral shapes, such as vowels, but the mechanisms underlying pure-tone frequency discrimination may differ between the two groups. It is interesting to note here that the exquisite ability to discriminate pure tones by human listeners does not translate into a vastly improved ability over that of other non-human mammals to discriminate formant frequencies.

Discrimination of the frequency of the second formant for vowels in the presence of background noise has been studied in cats (Hienz et al., 1998). Thresholds increase as the background noise level increases. More interestingly, when lesions at the level of the floor of the 4th ventricle were made, there was little or no effect on second formant discrimination in quiet and at low noise levels. However, there was a significant increase in thresholds at high levels of background noise. These results argue that the medial olivocochlear efferent system plays an important role in speech processing in high levels of background noise.

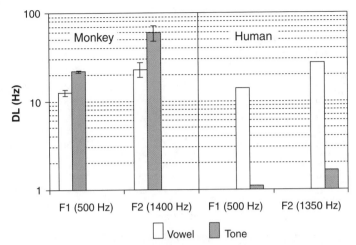

Fig. 7.4 Bar graphs showing frequency discrimination thresholds for pure tones and for single vowel formants obtained from monkeys and humans. Pure-tone thresholds are shown by the gray-filled bars; formant frequency thresholds are shown by the open bars. For monkeys, the standard frequencies of the pure tones and formants were 500 Hz and 1400 Hz; the sound levels of the tones and vowels were 76 dB SPL and 86 dB SPL, respectively. For humans, the standard frequencies were 500 Hz and 1350 Hz; the sound levels of the tones and vowels were 80 dB SPL and 77 dB SPL, respectively. Monkey data are from Sommers *et al.*, (1992); human tone data are from Wier *et al.*, (1977); human vowel data are from Kewley-Port and Watson (1994).

One of the distinct characteristics of speech perception by human listeners is that phonetic units can be perceived categorically. For example, the time between a consonant and a vowel is known as the 'voice-onset time' (VOT). If the VOT is made to exist along a continuum and systematically increases from 0 ms to 80 ms, for example, the corresponding perception of the sounds does not change systematically. Instead, as the VOT increases, the percept of the sound remains constant, and then abruptly changes to another percept as the VOT crosses a phonemic boundary. Further increases in VOT do not result in a change in the percept. For example, suppose a VOT of 0 ms is perceived as /da/ and a VOT of 80 ms is perceived as /ta/. As the VOT of the consonant–vowel increases from 0 to 80 ms, the listener's perception would be categorical, first hearing a series of /da/s followed by a series of /ta/s.

One of the first studies to address categorical perception of speech sounds in animals was carried out by Kuhl and Miller (1975). Chinchillas were trained to discriminate /da/ (having a VOT of 0 ms) from /ta/ (having a VOT of 80 ms). Animals were then tested in a stimulus generalization paradigm with VOTs ranging from 10 to 70 ms. Generalization gradients obtained were S-shaped with steep slopes, indicating a clear phonetic boundary (Fig. 7.5). Interestingly, generalization gradients and the location of the phonetic boundaries were similar between chinchillas and human listeners. The existence of phonetic boundaries has been described for quail (Kluender *et al.*, 1987; Kluender, 1991), budgerigars (Dent *et al.*, 1997*a*), chinchillas (Kuhl and Miller, 1978; Ohlemiller *et al.*, 1999), and monkeys (Sinnott *et al.*, 1976; Sinnott and Adams, 1987; Sinnott and Brown, 1997). Figure 7.6 summarizes the phonetic boundaries obtained from several studies in which both animals and humans were tested along a VOT continuum. Comparison of phonetic boundaries shows a close similarity between animals and humans, although there is a tendency for animal boundaries to be less than human boundaries, i.e. data points in Fig. 7.6 tend to fall below the diagonal line.

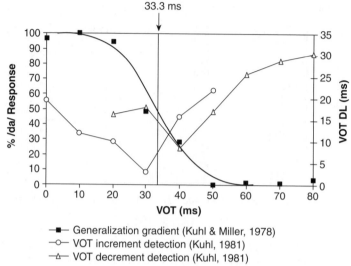

Fig. 7.5 Generalization gradients and psychometric functions for VOT demonstrating categorical perception obtained from chinchillas. Filled squares show the percent of responses labeled as /da/. Percent /da/ responses were converted to Z-scores and a linear regression was applied; the heavy solid line shows the gradient obtained from this analysis. The phonetic boundary of 33.3 ms is indicated by the vertical line and arrow. Also shown by the thin lines and open symbols are the VOT-DLs (see text for details).

The presence of a clear phonemic boundary is, by itself, insufficient to demonstrate categorical perception. If sounds are perceived categorically, then discrimination acuity across the phonetic boundary (i.e. across categories) should be easy, whereas discrimination within categories should be difficult. Kuhl (1981) measured VOT discrimination thresholds (i.e. VOT DLs) for chinchillas for different VOT-standards. Figure 7.5 compares thresholds for VOT increments and decrements. For VOT increments, the comparison or test stimulus had an increase in VOT relative to the standard; for VOT decrements, the test stimulus had a decrease in VOT relative to the standard.

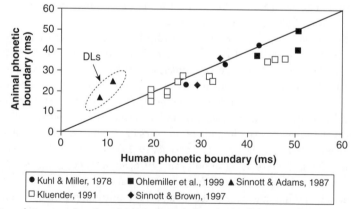

Fig. 7.6 Scatter plot comparing the phonetic boundaries obtained from birds (open symbols) and mammals (filled symbols) to human phonetic boundaries obtained from VOT continua. The diagonal line indicates equivalent boundaries between animals and humans.

The open circles in Fig. 7.5 show that when the standard VOT was 30 ms, and the test stimulus was an increase in VOT, then the VOT DL was 3 ms (i.e. VOT of 33 ms for the test). Note that a VOT of 33 ms is near the phonetic boundary of 33.3 ms that defines the two categories (i.e. /da/ vs. /ta/). As the standard VOT moves further from the phonetic boundary, VOT DLs increase. The open triangles in Fig. 7.5 show VOT discrimination thresholds for VOT decrements. These two functions show that discrimination is relatively easy for standard stimuli near the phonetic boundary, but discrimination becomes more difficult as the standard stimuli move further away from the boundary. This difference in discrimination abilities along the generalization gradient demonstrates the existence of categorical perception in the chinchilla. Thus, categorical perception of VOT cannot be explained by mechanisms that are unique or special to humans. Better discrimination near phonetic boundaries has also been reported for second-formant transitions, rather than VOT, along the /bae-dae-gae/ continuum in monkeys (Kuhl and Padden, 1993).

7.6 Binaural hearing

The central auditory system receives information about sound sources from two ears. Interaural time and interaural intensity cues provide important information about the location of sound sources along the horizontal plane, whereas the spectral cues produced by pinnae filtering provide information about localization along the vertical plane (see Chapter 6). Many of the psychophysical studies in non-human animals related to binaural hearing have addressed questions concerning sound localization in the free field (see Popper and Fay (2005) for recent reviews of sound localization in vertebrates). Sound localization studies in non-human animals generally fall into two categories: (1) acuity studies in which animals typically make left/right discriminations, and (2) accuracy studies in which animals make eye or head orientations to indicate the perceived location of a sound source.

One of the advantages of the comparative approach is that deficits in behavioral performance can be studied systematically following ablations along the central auditory pathway, and this approach has been used to study the functional role of auditory nuclei in sound localization. Jenkins and Masterton (1982) examined the effects of unilateral lesions along the auditory pathway on the ability of cats to localize sounds in the free field. Deficits in behavioral performance were produced no matter where the lesion was made. However, unilateral lesions above the superior olivary complex resulted in deficits in the sound field *contralateral* to the lesion, whereas lesions at the superior olivary complex resulted in bilateral deficits. Interestingly, when the lesion was limited to the trapezoid body (i.e. ventral acoustic stria), the deficit in sound localization occurred in the *ipsilateral* sound field. It is well known that the trapezoid body contains the axons of bushy cells in the anteroventral cochlear nucleus which project to the superior olivary complex. Thus, this study demonstrates behaviorally that the anteroventral cochlear nucleus plays an essential role in sound localization along the horizontal plane. In contrast, lesions of the intermediate and dorsal acoustic striae in cats have been shown to cause deficits in sound localization performance along the vertical plane (May, 2000). It is known that the dorsal acoustic stria is made of axons of neurons from the dorsal cochlear nucleus. Although the neurophysiological evidence has suggested the anteroventral cochlear nucleus is important for horizontal sound localization and the dorsal cochlear nucleus is likely to play a role in vertical sound localization, it is the results from these types of behavioral studies (Jenkins and Masterton, 1982; May 2000) which demonstrate that indeed the anteroventral and dorsal cochlear nuclei are involved functionally in horizontal and vertical sound localization, respectively.

The ability of mammals to localize sound along the vertical plane is thought to be due to the spectral filtering of the pinnae which results in the so-called head-related transfer functions.

Because the spectral notches in the head-related transfer functions vary with vertical position of the sound source, the pinnae provide the necessary cues for vertical localization. Heffner *et al.*, (1996) demonstrated that the pinnae are necessary for vertical sound localization. Sound localization performance was measured behaviorally in chinchillas before and after removal of the pinnae. The removal of the pinnae had no effect on sound localization performance in the horizontal plane (i.e. left/right discriminations), but produced large deficits in performance for front/back discriminations and localization along the vertical plane. The results of Heffner *et al.*, (1996) demonstrate that the pinnae are necessary for vertical sound localization, but that they do not play any substantial role in generating interaural cues used for horizontal localization.

Finally, the role of head movements in sound localization accuracy has been studied in monkeys (Populin, 2006) and cats (Tollin *et al.*, 2005). These studies compared sound localization performance in orienting tasks in which the head was fixed (i.e. restrained) or unrestrained. Localization accuracy was measured as the error between where the sound source was actually located and where the animal indicated behaviorally that the source was located. Both of these studies indicate that mammals were more accurate in sound orienting tasks when the head was unrestrained. That is, head movements play an important role in accurate sound localization in non-human animals.

Although interaural time and intensity cues are necessary for sound localization along the horizontal plane, there is more to binaural hearing than solely the free-field localization of sounds in space. Indeed, a large number of studies in human listeners that address questions regarding binaural processing present stimuli over headphones in order to independently control stimuli between the two ears. It is not surprising that a major reason that most of the research on binaural hearing in animals has focused on free-field sound localization over other aspects of binaural hearing is due to the difficulty in getting animals to wear headphones.

One important binaural phenomenon that has been well studied in humans listening through headphones is the binaural masking level difference (BMLD). The BMLD demonstrates that the detection threshold for a signal masked by a noise can be lower when the signal is presented dichotically and the noise is presented diotically (i.e. $S_\pi N_0$) compared to the signal and noise both being presented diotically (i.e. $S_0 N_0$). In this paradigm, if the phase of the background noise is the same at the two ears, but the phase of the signal at the two ears differs, then the detection thresholds will be lower than if the signal is presented in phase at the two ears. The improvement in signal detection occurs because the phase difference evokes a perception that the signal and noise are coming from different locations. Thresholds also are lower when the signal is presented monaurally and the noise is presented diotically (i.e. $S_m N_0$) compared to the condition when the signal and noise are both presented monaurally (i.e. $S_m N_m$).

The BMLD appears to be related to the 'cocktail party effect' originally described by Cherry (1953). Hulse *et al.* (1997) have shown that songbirds can identify conspecific songs in a background of heterospecific songs, i.e. an 'avian cocktail party'. However, the importance of detecting a signal in a background of noise for animals is not limited to vocal communication. Fay (1994) has argued that the primitive function of the auditory system is not for vocal communication, but 'to obtain information on the identities and locations of the objects in the immediate world that produce or scatter sound'. All animals have a need to determine the presence of signals from background noise, and the binaural auditory system helps facilitate this process.

In the mid-1970s, several studies in cats, adapted to wear leather helmets containing earphones, addressed questions directly related to the BMLD (Hoppe and Langford, 1974; Wakeford and Robinson, 1974; Cranford, 1975; Geesa and Langford, 1976). Thus, stimuli could be controlled independently to the ears. The results of these studies indicated that the phenomenon of BMLDs occurred in cats, but the release from masking was less in cats than in humans. That is, the

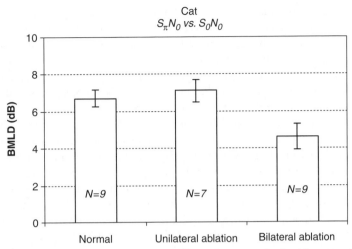

Fig. 7.7 Bar graphs showing the binaural masking level differences obtained from cats before (normal) and after cortical ablations. Data are from Cranford *et al.* (1978).

BMLDs in cats were smaller than those obtained from humans. More recently, BMLD has also been examined in the rabbit (Early *et al.*, 2001). The BMLDs for tonal signals measured in cats and rabbits are typically < 10 dB, whereas the BMLDs in humans are typically > 10 dB. In human listeners, as the signal frequency increases, there is a decrease in the BMLD; however, over the same frequency range of 500–1500 Hz, the BMLDs in cats remain relatively constant (Wakeford and Robinson, 1974). Unilateral lesions of the auditory cortex in cats did not produce a significant effect on BMLDs (for $S_{\pi}N_0$ vs. S_0N_0), but bilateral lesions of the auditory cortex significantly reduced the amount of BMLD (see Fig. 7.7). The reduction, but not elimination, of the BMLDS following bilateral cortical ablation, suggests that the release from masking is not entirely a cortical process, but that subcortical processes are also involved (Cranford *et al.*, 1978).

The BMLD is a lateralization phenomenon that occurs when stimuli are presented over headphones. A phenomenon related to the release from masking of the BMLD is spatial unmasking or free-field binaural unmasking. In spatial unmasking, there is a decrease in the detection threshold of a signal as the spatial positions between the signal and the noise masker increase. Monaural conditions can be produced by the use of earplugs or surgical ablation of one cochlea. For example, consider two loudspeakers both playing a coherent noise, but only speaker 1 plays a tonal signal in addition to the noise. Comparison of tonal detection thresholds when speaker 1 is located 90° to the right of the subject and speaker 2 is located 90° to the left with detection thresholds when both speakers are located 90° to the right show a release of masking of approximately 10 dB for the ferret (Hine *et al.*, 1994). Using this technique, Dent *et al.* (1997) have shown that budgerigars show spatial unmasking. This finding suggests that birds use similar binaural mechanisms as mammals, even though their interaural distances are generally smaller than most mammals.

Finally, in reverberant environments, sound propagates to the ears through multiple paths. That is, there is a direct path from the sound source to the ear, and multiple indirect paths that occur from sound reflections. Sound reflections have the potential of providing additional interaural cues that could interfere with a listener's ability to accurately localize a sound source. Depending on the delay between the direct and indirect sounds, the reflections are often not perceived as echoes. If the delay is small, then the direct and indirect sounds are fused together perceptually and heard as a single sound source; the location in space of this fused source is largely determined by the interaural cues of the direct sound source. This phenomenon is known as 'the law of the first wavefront' or the precedence effect, and several behavioral studies have examined the precedence effect in non-human animals.

Tollin and Yin (2003) studied the localization accuracy of cats using a scleral-search coil to measure saccadic eye movements toward the target. Using this technique, cats made saccadic eye movements to the location of a sound source that was played from an array of 15 loudspeakers. Cats displayed accurate sound localization abilities to 10-ms noise bursts in the horizontal and vertical planes when a single-noise source was presented. When this single-noise source was paired with a second noise burst which was delayed and presented through a different loud-speaker (i.e. a reflected noise source), sound localization ability was still accurate. Moreover, when the delay of the second, lag-noise source was between 0.4 and 10 ms, the saccades of the cat were directed consistently and rapidly toward the speaker location of the lead-noise source. That is, cats showed localization dominance in which the perceived location was largely determined by the speaker location of the lead-noise source (Tollin and Yin, 2003). This response is consistent with the precedence effect. When the delay of the lag-noise source was greater than 10 ms, the saccades became more variable, indicating that cats could perceive the location of the delayed noise source; that is, the echo threshold had been reached and the lag-noise source could be perceived as an echo (Tollin and Yin, 2003). Similar findings indicating the existence of the precedence effect have also been described for budgerigars (Dent and Dooling 2003a,b) and barn owls (Spitzer et al., 2003; Spitzer and Takahashi 2006).

Related to the precedence effect is another illusion that occurs in reverberant conditions, known as the 'Franssen effect'. In the Franssen effect, a transient tone with an instantaneous onset and a ramped offset is presented at one spatial location (e.g. from the left speaker) and a sustained tone of the same frequency with a ramped onset is presented from a different spatial location (e.g. from the right speaker). The sustained tone can be played for several seconds. Even after a transient tone has ended, listeners still localize the sound as being played from the location of the transient tone. Dent et al. (2004) studied the ability of cats to localize Franssen stimuli. Similar to human listeners, cats localized consistently to the location of the transient tone, but unlike humans the frequencies that evoked the illusion were ≥ 2.5 kHz (Dent et al., 2004).

7.7 Periodicity discrimination and pitch perception of complex sounds

Discussions regarding pitch often begin with pure-tone frequency discrimination and perception. It is well known that pure-tone frequency DLs for humans are lower than those of non-human animals (e.g. Sinnott et al., 1985; Hienz et al., 1993). In human listeners, a single pure tone evokes the perception of 'spectral pitch', and the perception of tonal frequency (i.e. spectral pitch) has been studied in several species of non-human animals. A perceptual dimension corresponding to tone frequency has been shown to exist for rats (Blackwell and Schlosberg, 1943), pigeons (Jenkins and Harrison, 1960), starlings (Cynx, 1993), and budgerigars (Dooling et al., 1987). Behavioral data obtained using simple pure tones for spectral pitch can be directly related to the topographic map of frequency-to-place along the basilar membrane.

Temporal periodicities are found in the waveforms of many different complex sounds, including speech and music, and a periodic acoustic waveform can evoke the perception of pitch. That is, pitch is related to the repetition rate of a complex sound. Moreover, a variety of different complex sounds can evoke a similar pitch; sounds that have spectral differences, but similarities in their periodicities, will evoke similar pitches. Thus, although the topographic map of frequency along the basilar membrane corresponds to a pitch map for pure tones, it does not correspond to a pitch map for complex sounds. Understanding pitch perception is fundamental to our understanding of how the auditory nervous system functions.

One type of complex sound that has been used widely to study pitch is the harmonic-tone complex (see Chapter 4). When human listeners are simultaneously presented with a series of tones that are harmonically related to a fundamental frequency (F0), the perception that is evoked is one of a single sound source having a pitch equal to the F0. When the frequency components of the tone complex are resolved by the auditory system, then the pitch is referred to as 'periodicity pitch'; if the components are unresolved, the pitch is known as 'residue pitch'. F0 discrimination has been studied in chinchillas for a harmonic-tone complex containing a 250-Hz F0 component (Shofner, 2000). Similar to results for human listeners, the DLs obtained from chinchillas for F0 discrimination were lower than DLs for the 250-Hz pure tone, suggesting similar neural mechanisms of F0 discrimination between humans and chinchillas. Tomlinson and Schwartz (1988) applied a generalization procedure in rhesus monkeys and showed that a gradient in behavioral responses occurred as the F0 of the comparison tone complex changed. This finding is consistent with the existence of a perceptual dimension in the monkey related to F0.

In human listeners, when the F0 component of a tone complex is removed, the perceived pitch of the complex remains matched to the F0; this is known as the 'pitch of the missing fundamental'. Interestingly, when the F0 component of the tone complex was removed from the comparison tone, monkeys continued to respond as if the F0 was present (Tomlinson and Schwartz, 1988). That is, monkeys appeared to have a pitch perception corresponding to the missing fundamental. Similar findings have been reported for songbirds (Cynx and Shapiro, 1986) and cats (Heffner and Whitfield, 1976; Whitfield, 1980). In cats having bilateral ablations of the auditory cortex, tone complexes were no longer discriminated based on the missing F0, but could be discriminated based on frequency discrimination of the spectral components (Whitfield, 1980). This finding suggests that the auditory cortex plays an important role in the perception of the missing fundamental, but is not necessary for frequency discrimination. It should be noted, however, that no study in non-human animals has used masking noise centered at the missing F0. The persistence of the pitch of the missing fundamental in human listeners in the presence of masking noise around the F0 is an essential demonstration that the perception is the result of neural processing mechanisms rather than the result of mechanical distortion products in the cochlea.

Another type of complex sound that has been widely used to investigate human pitch perception is rippled noise. Rippled noises are generated when broadband noise is delayed, attenuated, and added to (or subtracted from) the original, undelayed version of the noise. Each successive operation of delay–attenuate–add is called 'an iteration'. The spectra of rippled noises are continuous with peaks occurring at frequencies related to the delay. Rippled noises are pseudo-periodic sounds in that there exists temporal regularities in the waveform, but these regularities are not repeated in a periodic manner. In human listeners, the pitches evoked by rippled noises are referred to as 'repetition pitches'; the pitch is related to the delay, and the saliency or pitch strength is related to the number of iterations or the amount of attenuation used during stimulus generation.

Discrimination of rippled noise from flat-spectrum, wideband noise has been studied in chinchillas (Shofner and Yost, 1995) and budgerigars (Amagai et al., 1999). In these experiments, the delay is fixed and the attenuation of the delayed version of the noise is varied. More attenuation results in smaller spectral ripple depths and less periodicity strength in the stimulus. Budgerigar attenuation thresholds were similar to human thresholds and were lower than chinchilla thresholds.

When rippled noises are bandpass-filtered, behavioral performance in chinchillas is best when the center frequencies of the bandpass filter correspond to the 3rd–5th harmonic of the delay; that is, there appears to be a dominance region similar to that in human listeners (Shofner and Yost, 1997). In human listeners, as the attenuation is increased, there is a decrease in the strength of the pitch percept, and stimulus generalization gradients obtained from chinchillas indicate that a perceptual dimension related to periodicity strength also exists in non-human animals (Shofner et al., 2005), although chinchillas must learn to listen to information in low-frequency (i.e. resolved) auditory filters (Shofner and Whitmer, 2006). However, when chinchillas discriminate a cosine-phase, harmonic-tone complex from wideband noise, they appear to rely primarily on information in high-frequency (i.e. unresolved) auditory filters (Shofner and Whitmer, 2006).

Do rippled noises evoke a perception dimension in animals similar to that of pitch in human listeners? The existence of a perceptual dimension corresponding to rippled-noise delay has been investigated in goldfish (Fay, 2005) and chinchillas (Shofner et al., 2007) using stimulus generalization paradigms. Although goldfish can discriminate between rippled noises of different delays with thresholds similar to those of human listeners (Fay et al., 1983), no generalization gradient was obtained when animals were trained to detect a rippled noise of one delay and tested with rippled noises of different delays (Fay, 2005). Fay (2005) concluded that in goldfish the lack of a generalization gradient related to rippled-noise delay indicated that the pitch percept evoked by rippled noise was weaker than the noise percept evoked by rippled noise.

In contrast, stimulus generalization gradients related to delay have been obtained in chinchillas (Shofner et al., 2007) when positive and negative iterated rippled noises were employed. Positive rippled noises are generated when the iterations are in a delay–attenuate–*add* operation, whereas negative rippled noises are generated when the iterations are in a delay–attenuate–*subtract* operation. When chinchillas were trained to discriminate between positive rippled noises and tested with other positive rippled noises, gradients in behavioral responses were obtained. When chinchillas were trained to discriminate between negative rippled noises and tested with other negative rippled noises, gradients in behavioral responses were also obtained. The existence of generalization gradients related to delay indicates the existence of a perceptual dimension related to delay. However, when chinchillas were trained to discriminate between *positive* rippled noises and tested with other *negative* rippled noises, generalization gradients were not obtained, suggesting that other perceptual cues such as timbre may dominate the pitch cues when negative rippled noises are presented in the context of positive rippled noises. It should also be noted that the repetition pitch scale for chinchillas is linear on a semilog plot of performance as a function of frequency, which is similar in shape to the pure-tone pitch scale obtained for human listeners and budgerigars (Dooling et al., 1987) as well as starlings (Cynx, 1993).

Finally, another type of stochastic stimulus that evokes a pitch perception in human listeners is sinusoidal amplitude-modulated (SAM) noise. SAM noise is generated when wideband noise is amplitude-modulated by a single tone; in this sound, periodicity information exists in the stimulus envelope, but not in the fine structure. The long-term spectrum of SAM noise is flat and does not contain a spectral peak at the modulation frequency; hence the pitch evoked by SAM noise is called 'nonspectral pitch'. Discrimination of modulation frequencies of SAM noise has been studied in monkeys (Moody, 1994), chinchillas (Long and Clark, 1984), and budgerigars (Dooling and Searcy, 1981). Monkey and budgerigar thresholds are close to those obtained in human listeners over a range of similar modulation frequencies. The existence of a perceptual dimension corresponding to the modulation frequency has not been investigated using stimulus generalization procedures.

7.8 Concluding remarks

This chapter has provided an overview of research in animal psychophysical experiments in hearing. When discussing hearing in non-human animals, there is often a strong emphasis on the link between communication sounds and the auditory system. Indeed, one of the criticisms of comparative psychoacoustics research is that unlike natural calls and vocalizations, the stimuli presented are artificial and have no biological meaning to the animal. With the exception of speech, which has no inherent biological significance to non-human animals, no attempt was made by the authors to review the literature on acoustic communication in animals. However, there is more to vertebrate hearing than simply the processing of communication sounds. Like human listeners, animals use their auditory systems not only in acoustic communication, but in acquiring acoustic information about what objects are present in the environment. This has been described as the general, primitive function of vertebrate hearing (Fay, 1994). Although physiological experiments can be carried out in animals and are essential for our understanding of the neural mechanisms of hearing, hearing per se is perception and behavior. If an organism cannot detect, identify, and make the appropriate behavioral response to an environmental sound, then hearing, by definition, has not taken place. Psychoacoustic approaches provide important insights into auditory processing, not only for human listeners, but for all vertebrate animals. Unlike the ethological approach which often emphasizes the specializations that exist in the auditory systems of animals, the psychoacoustic approach places an emphasis on the generalizations that exist among the auditory systems of non-human animals.

References

Amagai, S., Dooling R. J., Shamma, S., Kidd, T. L., and Lohr, B. (1999). Detection of modulation in spectral envelopes and linear-rippled noises by budgerigars (*Melopsittacus undulatus*). *Journal of the Acoustical Society of America* **105**:2029–35.

Au, W. W. L. and Moore, P. W. B. (1990). Critical ratio and critical bandwidth for the Atlantic bottlenose dolphin. *Journal of the Acoustical Society of America* **88**:1635–8.

Blackwell, H. R. and Schlosberg, H. (1943). Octave generalization, pitch discrimination, and loudness thresholds in the white rat. *Journal of Experimental Psychology* **33**:407–19.

Cherry, E. C. (1953). Some experiments on the recognition of speech, with one and with two ears. *Journal of the Acoustical Society of America* **25**:975–9.

Clack, T. D. (1966). Effect of signal duration on the auditory sensitivity of humans and monkeys (Macaca mulatta). *Journal of the Acoustical Society of America* **40**:1140–6.

Clark, W. W. and Bohne, B. A. (1986). Cochlear damage: Audiometric correlates. In *Sensorineural Hearing Loss: Mechanisms, Diagnosis, and Treatment* (ed. M. J. Collins, T. J. Glattke, and L. A. Harker), pp. 59–82. Iowa City: University of Iowa Press.

Clopton, B. M. (1972). Detection of increments in noise intensity by monkeys. *Journal of Experimental Analysis of Behavior* **17**:473–81.

Costalupes, J. A. (1983). Broad band masking noise and behavioral pure tone thresholds in cats. *Journal of the Acoustical Society of America* **74**:758–64.

Cranford, J. L. (1975). Auditory masking-level differences in the cat. *Journal of Comparative and Physiological Psychology* **89**:219–23.

Cranford, J. L., Stramler, J., and Igarishi, M. (1978). Role of neocortex in binaural hearing in the cat. III. Binaural masking-level differences. *Brain Research* **151**:381–5.

Cynx, J. (1993). Auditory frequency generalization and a failure to find octave generalization in a songbird, the European starling (Sturnus vulgaris). *Journal of Comparative Psychology* **107**:140–6.

Cynx, J. and Shapiro, M. (1986). Perception of missing fundamental by a species of songbird (Sturnus vulgaris). *Journal of Comparative Psychology* 100:356–60.

Dent, M. L. and Dooling, R. J. (2003a). Investigations of the precedence effect in budgerigars: Effects of stimulus type, intensity, duration, and location. *Journal of the Acoustical Society of America* 113: 2146–58.

Dent, M. L. and Dooling, R. J. (2003b). Investigations of the precedence effect in budgerigars: The perceived location of auditory images. *Journal of the Acoustical Society of America* 113:2159–69.

Dent, M. L., Brittan-Powell, E. F., Dooling, R. J., and Pierce, A. (1997a). Perception of synthetic /ba/–/wa/ speech continuum by budgerigars (Melopsittacus undulatus). *Journal of the Acoustical Society of America* 102:1891–7.

Dent, M. L., Larsen, O. N., and Dooling, R. J. (1997b). Free-field binaural unmasking in budgerigars (Melopsittacus undulatus). *Journal of Comparative Psychology* 111:590–8.

Dent, M. L., Tollin, D. J., and Yin, T. C. T. (2004). Cats exhibit the Franssen illusion. *Journal of the Acoustical Society of America* 116:3070–4.

Dewson, J. H. III (1968). Efferent olivocochlear bundle: Some relationships to stimulus discrimination in noise. *Journal of Neurophysiology* 31:122–30.

Dooling, R. J. and Okanoya, K. (1995). The method of constant stimuli in testing auditory sensitivity in small birds. In *Methods in Comparative Psychoacoustics* (ed. G. M. Klump, R. J. Dooling, R. R. Fay, and W. C. Stebbins), pp. 161–9. Basel: Birkhauser Verlag.

Dooling, R. J. and Saunders, J. C. (1975). Hearing in the parakeet (Melopsittacus undulatus): Absolute thresholds, critical ratios, frequency difference limens, and vocalizations. *Journal of Comparative and Physiological Psychology* 88:1–20.

Dooling, R. J. and Saunders, J. C. (1975). Auditory intensity discrimination in the parakeet (Melopsittacus undulatus). *Journal of the Acoustical Society of America* 58:1308–10.

Dooling, R. J. and Searcy, M. H. (1981). Amplitude modulation thresholds for the parakeet (Melopsittacus undulatus). *Journal of Comparative Physiology* 143:383–8.

Dooling, R. J., Zoloth, S. R., and Baylis, J. R. (1978). Auditory sensitivity, equal loudness, temporal resolving power, and vocalizations in the house finch (Carpodacus mexicanus). *Journal of Comparative and Physiological Psychology* 92:867–76.

Dooling, R. J., Okanoya, K., Downing, J., and Hulse, S. (1986). Hearing in the starling (Sturnus vulgaris): Absolute thresholds and critical ratios. *Bulletin of the Psychonomic Society* 24:462–4.

Dooling, R. J., Brown, S. D., Park, T. J., Okanoya, K., and Soli, S. D. (1987). Perceptual organization of acoustic stimuli by budgerigars (Melopsittacus undulatus): I. Pure tones. *Journal of Comparative Psychology* 101:139–49.

Dyson, M. L., Klump, G. M., and Gauger, B. (1998). Absolute hearing thresholds and critical masking ratios in the European barn owl: a comparison with other owls. *Journal of Comparative Physiology A* 182:695–702.

Early, S. J., Mason, C. R., Zheng, L., Evilsizer, M., Idrobo, F., Harrison, J. M., and Carney, L. H. (2001). Studies of binaural detection in the rabbit (Oryctolagus cuniculus) with Pavlovian conditioning. *Behavioral Neuroscience* 115:650–60.

Egan, J. P. and Hake, H. W. (1950). On the masking pattern of a simple auditory stimulus. *Journal of the Acoustical Society of America* 22:622–30.

Ehret, G. (1976). Critical bands and filter characteristics of the ear of the housemouse (Mus musculus). *Biological Cybernetics* 24:35–42.

Evans, E. F., Pratt, S. R., Spenner, H., and Cooper, N. P. (1992). Comparisons of physiological and behavioral properties: Auditory frequency selectivity. In *Auditory Physiology and Perception* (ed. Y. Cazals, K. Horner, and L. Demany), pp. 159–69. New York: Pergamon Press.

Farabaugh, S. M., Dent, M. L., and Dooling, R. J. (1998). Hearing and vocalizations of wild-caught Australian budgerigars (Melopsittacus undulatus). *Journal of Comparative Psychology* 112:74–81.

Fay, R. R. (1988). *Hearing in Vertebrates: A Psychophysics Databook*. Winnetka, IL: Hill-Fay Associates.

Fay, R. R. (1994). Comparative auditory research. In *Comparative Hearing: Mammals* (ed. R. R. Fay and A. N. Popper), pp. 1–17. New York: Springer-Verlag.

Fay, R. R. (2005). Perception of pitch by goldfish. *Hearing Research* 205:7–20.

Fay, R. R., Yost, W. A., and Coombs, S. (1983). Psychophysics and neurophysiology of repetition noise processing in a vertebrate auditory system. *Hearing Research* 12:31–55.

Finneran, J. J., Schlundt, C. E., Carder, D. A., and Ridgway, S. H. (2002). Auditory filter shapes for the bottlenose dolphin (Tursiops truncatus) and the white whale (Delphinapterus leucas) derived with notched noise. *Journal of the Acoustical Society of America* 112:322–8.

Fletcher, H. (1940). Auditory patterns. *Reviews of Modern Physics* 12:47–65.

Geesa, B. H. and Langford, T. L. (1976). Binaural interaction in cat and man. II. Interaural noise correlation and signal detection. *Journal of the Acoustical Society of America* 59:1195–6.

Gourevitch, G. (1965). Auditory masking in the rat. *Journal of the Acoustical Society of America* 37:439–43.

Gourevitch, G. (1970). Detectability of tones in quiet and in noise by rats and monkeys. In *Animal Psychophysics: The Design and Conduct of Sensory Experiments* (ed. W. C. Stebbins), pp. 67–97. New York: Appleton-Century-Crofts.

Hall, J. W., Haggard, M. P., and Fernandez, M. A. (1984). Detection in noise by spectro-temporal pattern analysis. *Journal of the Acoustical Society of America* 76:50–6.

Halpern, D. L. and Dallos, P. (1986). Auditory filter shapes in the chinchilla. *Journal of the Acoustical Society of America* 80:765–75.

Hamilton, P. M. (1957). Noise masked thresholds as a function of tonal duration and masking noise band width. *Journal of the Acoustical Society of America* 29:506–11.

Hawkins, J. H. and Stevens, S. S. (1950). The masking of pure tones and of speech by white noise. *Journal of the Acoustical Society of America,* 22:6–13.

Heffner, H. E. and Heffner, R. S. (1995). Conditioned avoidance. In *Methods in Comparative Psychoacoustics* (ed. G. M. Klump, R. J. Dooling, R. R. Fay, and W. C. Stebbins), pp. 79–93. Basel: Birkhauser Verlag.

Heffner, H. and Whitfield, I. C. (1976). Perception of the missing fundamental by cats. *Journal of the Acoustical Society of America* 59:915–19.

Heffner, R. S., Koay, G., and Heffner, H. E. (1996). Sound localization in chinchillas III: Effect of pinna removal. *Hearing Research* 99:13–21.

Hienz, R. D. and Brady, J. V. (1988). The acquisition of vowel discrimination by nonhuman primates. *Journal of the Acoustical Society of America* 84:186–94.

Hienz, R. D. and Sachs, M. B. (1987). Effects of noise on pure tone thresholds in blackbirds (Agelaius phoeniceus and Molothrus ater) and pigeons (Columba livia). *Journal of Comparative Psychology* 101:16–24.

Hienz, R. D., Sinnott, J. M., and Sachs, M. B. (1980). Auditory intensity discrimination in blackbirds and pigeons. *Journal of Comparative and Physiological Psychology* 94:993–1002.

Hienz, R. D., Sachs, M. B., and Sinnott, J. M. (1981). Discrimination of steady-state vowels by blackbirds and pigeons. *Journal of the Acoustical Society of America* 70:699–706.

Hienz, R. D., Sachs, M. B., and Aleszczyk, C. M. (1993). Frequency discrimination in noise: Comparison of cat performances with auditory-nerve models. *Journal of the Acoustical Society of America* 93:462–9.

Hienz, R. D., Aleszczyk, C. M., and May, B. J. (1996a). Vowel discrimination in cats: Acquisition, effects of stimulus level, and performance in noise. *Journal of the Acoustical Society of America* 99:3656–68.

Hienz, R. D., Aleszczyk, C. M., and May, B. J. (1996b). Vowel discrimination in cats: Thresholds for the detection of second formant changes in the vowel /ɛ/. *Journal of the Acoustical Society of America* 100:1052–8.

Hienz, R. D., Stiles, P., and May, B. J. (1998). Effects of bilateral olivocochlear lesions on vowel formant discrimination in cats. *Hearing Research* 116:10–20.

Hienz, R. D., Jones, A. M., and Weerts, E. M. (2004). The discrimination of baboon grunt calls and human vowel sounds by baboons. *Journal of the Acoustical Society of America* 116:1692–7.

Hine, J. E., Martin, R. L., and Moore, D. R. (1994). Free-field binaural unmasking in ferrets. *Behavioral Neuroscience* 108:196–205.

Hoppe, S. A. and Langford, T. L. (1974). Binaural interaction in cat and man. I. Signal detection and noise cross correlation. *Journal of the Acoustical Society of America* 55:1263–5.

Houtgast, T. (1974). Lateral suppression in hearing: A psychophysical study on the ear's capability to preserve and enhance spectral contrasts. Ph.D. Thesis. Free University of Amsterdam: Academische Pers. BV.

Houtgast, T. (1977). Auditory-filter characteristics derived from direct-masking and pulsation-threshold data with a rippled-noise masker. *Journal of the Acoustical Society of America* 62:409–15.

Hulse, S. H., MacDougall-Shackleton, S. A., and Wisniewski, A. B. (1997). Auditory scene analysis by songbirds: Stream segregation of birdsong by European starlings (Sturnus vulgaris) *Journal of Comparative Psychology* 111:3–13.

Jenkins, H. M. and Harrison, R. H. (1960). Effect of discrimination training on auditory generalization. *Journal of Experimental Psychology* 59:246–53.

Jenkins, W. M. and Masterton, R. B. (1982). Sound localization: Effects of unilateral lesions in central auditory system. *Journal of Neurophysiology* 47:987–1016.

Jesteadt, W., Wier, C. C., and Green, D. M. (1977). Intensity discrimination as a function of frequency and sensation level. *Journal of the Acoustical Society of America* 61:169–77.

Johnson, C. S. (1968). Masked tonal thresholds in the bottle-nosed porpoise. *Journal of the Acoustical Society of America* 44:965–7.

Kewley-Port, D. and Watson, C. S. (1994). Formant-frequency discrimination for isolated English vowels. *Journal of the Acoustical Society of America* 95:485–96.

Kittel, M., Wagner, E., and Klump, G. M. (2000). Hearing in the gerbil (Meriones unguiculatus): Comodulation masking release. *Zoology* 103(Suppl. III):68.

Kittel, M., Wagner, E., and Klump, G. M. (2002) An estimate of the auditory filter bandwidth in the Mongolian gerbil. *Hearing Research* 164:69–76.

Kluender, K. R. (1991). Effects of first formant onset properties on voicing judgments result from processes not specific to humans. *Journal of the Acoustical Society of America* 90:83–96.

Kluender, K. R., Diehl, R. L., and Killeen, P. R. (1987). Japanese quail can learn phonetic categories. *Science* 237:1195–7.

Klump, G. M. (2001). Comodulation masking release in the Mongolian gerbil. *Association for Research in Otolaryngology Abstracts* 24:84.

Klump, G. M. and Langemann, U. (1995). Comodulation masking release in a songbird. *Hearing Research* 87:157–64.

Klump, G. M., Dooling, R. J., Fay, R. R., and Stebbins, W. C. (eds) (1995). *Methods in Comparative Psychoacoustics*. Basel: Birkhauser Verlag.

Kuhl, P. K. (1981). Discrimination of speech by nonhuman animals: Basic auditory sensitivities conducive to the perception of speech-sound categories. *Journal of the Acoustical Society of America* 70:340–9.

Kuhl, P. K. and Miller, J. D. (1975). Speech perception by the chinchilla: Voiced-voiceless distinction in alveolar plosive consonants. *Science* 190:69–72.

Kuhl, P. K. and Miller, J. D. (1978). Speech perception by the chinchilla: Identification functions for synthetic VOT stimuli. *Journal of the Acoustical Society of America* 63:905–17.

Kuhl, P. K. and Padden, D. M. (1983). Enhance discriminability at the phonetic boundaries for the place feature in macaques. *Journal of the Acoustical Society of America* 73:1003–10.

Kuhn, A. and Saunders, J. C. (1980). Psychophysical tuning curves in the parakeet: A comparison between simultaneous and forward masking procedures. *Journal of the Acoustical Society of America* 68:1892–4.

Langemann, U., Klump, G. M., and Dooling, R. J. (1995). Critical bands and critical-ratio bandwidth in the European starling. *Hearing Research* 84:167–76.

Langemann, U. and Klump, G. M. (2001). Signal detection in amplitude-modulated maskers. I. Behavioural auditory thresholds in a songbird. *European Journal of Neuroscience* 13:1025–32.

Lemonds, D. W., Au, W. W. L., Nachtigall, P. E., and Roitblat, H. L. (2000). High-frequency auditory filter shapes in an Atlantic bottlenose dolphin. *Journal of the Acoustical Society of America* 108:2614.

Levitt, H. (1971). Transformed up–down methods in psychoacoustics. *Journal of the Acoustical Society of America* 49:467–77.

Lin, J. Y., Dooling, R. J., and Dent, M. L. (1997). Auditory filter shapes in the budgerigar (Melopsittacus undulatus) derived from notched-noise maskers. *Journal of the Acoustical Society of America* 101:3124.

Lohr, B. and Dooling, R. J. (1998). Detection of changes in timbre and harmonicity in complex sounds by zebra finches (Taeniopygia guttata) and budgerigars (Melopsittacus undulatus). *Journal of Comparative Psychology* 112:36–47.

Long, G. R. (1977). Masked auditory thresholds from the bat, Rhinolophus ferrumequinum. *Journal of Comparative Psychology* 116:247–55.

Long, G. (1980). Some psychophysical measurements of frequency processing in the greater horseshoe bat. In *Psychophysical, Physiological, and Behavioral Studies in Hearing* (ed. G. van der Brink and F. H. Bilsen), pp. 132–5. Delft: Delft University Press.

Long, G. R. and Clark, W. W. (1984). Detection of frequency and rate modulation by the chinchilla. *Journal of the Acoustical Society of America* 75:1184–90.

McGee, T., Ryan, A., and Dallos, P. (1976). Psychophysical tuning curves of chinchillas. *Journal of the Acoustical Society of America* 60:1146–50.

Martin, G. K., Lonsbury-Martin, B. L., and Kimm, J. (1980). A rabbit preparation for neuron-behavioral auditory research. *Hearing Research* 2:65–78.

May, B. J. (2000). Role of the dorsal cochlear nucleus in the sound localization behavior of cats. *Hearing Research* 148:74–87.

May, B. J. and McQuone, S. J. (1995). Effects of bilateral olivocohlear lesions on pure-tone intensity discrimination in cats. *Auditory Neuroscience* 1:385–400.

May, B. J., Kimar, S., and Prosen, C. A. (2006). Auditory filter shapes of CBA/CaJ mice: Behavioral assessments. *Journal of the Acoustical Society of America* 120:321–30.

May, B. J., Little, N., and Saylor, S. (2009). Loudness perception in the domestic cat: Reaction time estimates of equal loudness contours and recruitment effects. *Journal of the Association for Research in Otolaryngology* 10:295–308.

Miller, J. D. (1964). Auditory sensitivity of the chinchilla in quiet and in noise. *Journal of the Acoustical Society of America* 36:2010.

Moody, D. B. (1994). Detection and discrimination of amplitude-modulated signals by macaque monkeys. *Journal of the Acoustical Society of America* 95:3499–510.

Moody, D. B., Beecher, M. D., and Stebbins, W. S. (1976). Behavioral methods in auditory research. In *Handbook of Auditory and Vestibular Research Methods* (ed. C. A. Smith and J. A. Vernon), pp. 439–97. Springfield, IL: Charles C. Thomas.

Moore, B. C. J. and Glasberg, B. R. (1983). Suggested formulae for calculating auditory-filter bandwidths and excitation patterns. *Journal of the Acoustical Society of America* 74:750–3.

Niemiec, A. J. (2001). The effects of increasing masker temporal regularity on co-modulation masking thresholds in chinchillas. *Association for Research in Otolaryngology Abstracts* 24:85.

Niemiec, A. J. and Moody, D. B. (1995). Constant stimulus and tracking procedures for measuring sensitivity. In *Methods in Comparative Psychoacoustics* (ed. G. M. Klump, R. J. Dooling, R. R. Fay, and W. C. Stebbins), pp. 65–77. Basel: Birkhauser Verlag.

Niemiec, A. J., Yost, W. A., and Shofner, W. P. (1992). Behavioral measures of frequency selectivity in the chinchilla. *Journal of the Acoustical Society of America* 92:2636–49.

Niemiec, A. J., Winter, A. Q., and Florin, Z. P. (1999). Chinchillas do not show masking release in co-modulated noise. *Association for Research in Otolaryngology Abstracts* 22:22.

Niemiec, A. J., Florin, Z. P., and Winter, A. Q. (2000). The use of spectral and temporal cues by chinchillas in co-modulation masking experiments. *Association for Research in Otolaryngology Abstracts* 23:27.

Ohlemiller, K. K., Jones, L. B., Heidbreder, A. F., Clark, W. W., and Miller, J. D. (1999). Voicing judgements by chinchillas trained with a reward paradigm. *Behavioral Brain Research* 100:185–95.

Okanoya, K. and Dooling, R. J. (1985). Colony differences in auditory thresholds in the canary. *Journal of the Acoustical Society of America* 78:1170–6.

Okanoya, K. and Dooling, R. J. (1987). Hearing in passerine and psittacine birds: A comparative study of absolute and masked auditory thresholds. *Journal of Comparative Psychology* 101:7–15.

Okanoya, K. and Dooling, R. J. (1988). Hearing in the swamp sparrow (Melospiza Georgiana) and the song sparrow (Melospiza melodia). *Animal Behavior* 36:726–32.

O'Loughlin, B. J. and Moore, B. C. J. (1981). Off-frequency listening: Effects on psychoacoustical tuning curves obtained in simultaneous and forward masking. *Journal of the Acoustical Society of America* 69:1119–25.

Patterson, R. D. (1976). Auditory filter shapes derived with noise stimuli. *Journal of the Acoustical Society of America* 59:640–54.

Patterson, R. D. and Nimmo-Smith, I. (1980). Off-frequency listening and auditory-filter asymmetry. *Journal of the Acoustical Society of America* 67:229–45.

Pfingst, B. E., Hienz, R., Kimm, J., and Miller, J. (1975). Reaction-time procedure for measurement of hearing. I. Suprathreshold functions. *Journal of the Acoustical Society of America* 57:421–30.

Pierrel-Sorrentino, R. and Raslear, T. G. (1980). Loudness scaling in rats and chinchillas. *Journal of Comparative and Physiological Psychology* 94:757–66.

Pickles, J. O. (1975). Normal critical bands in the cat. *Acta Otolaryngologica* 80:245–54.

Pickles, J. O. (1979). Psychophysical frequency resolution in the cat as determined by simultaneous masking and its relation to auditory nerve resolution. *Journal of the Acoustical Society of America* 66:1725–32.

Popper, A. N. and Fay, R. R. (2005). *Sound Source Localization.* New York: Springer.

Populin, L. C. (2006). Monkey sound localization: Head-restrained versus head-unrestrained orienting. *Journal of Neuroscience* 26:9820–32.

Raslear, T. G., Pierrel-Sorrentino, R., and Rudnick, F. (1983). Loudness scaling and masking in rats. *Behavioral Neuroscience* 97:392–8.

Reed, C. M. and Bilger, R. C. (1973). A comparative study of S/N_0 and E/N_0. *Journal of the Acoustical Society of America* 53:1039–44.

Ruggero, M. A. and Temchin, A. N. (2005). Unexceptional sharpness of frequency tuning in the human cochlea. *Proceedings of the National Academy of Sciences USA* 102:18614–19.

Ryan, A., Dallos, P., and McGee, T. (1979). Psychophysical tuning curves and auditory thresholds after hair cell damage in the chinchilla. *Journal of the Acoustical Society of America* 66:370–8.

Salvi, R. J., Ahroon, W. A., Perry, J. W., Gunnarson, A. D., and Henderson, D. (1982a). Comparison of psychophysical and evoked-potential tuning curves in the chinchilla. *American Journal of Otolaryngology* 3:408–16.

Salvi, R. J., Giraudi, D. M., Henderson, D., and Hamernik, R. P. (1982b). Detection of sinusoidally amplitude modulated noise by the chinchilla. *Journal of the Acoustical Society of America* 71:424–9.

Saunders, J. C., Else, P., and Bock, G. R. (1978). Frequency selectivity in the parakeet (Melopsittacus undulatus) studied with psychophysical tuning curves. *Journal of Comparative and Physiological Psychology* 92:406–15.

Saunders, J. C., Rintelmann, W. F., and Bock, G. R. (1979). Frequency selectivity in bird and man: A comparison among critical ratios, critical bands and psychophysical tuning curves. *Hearing Research* 1:303–23.

Saunders, S. S., Shivapuja, B. G., and Salvi, R. J. (1987). Auditory intensity discrimination in the chinchilla. *Journal of the Acoustical Society of America* 82:1604–7.

Schafer, T. H., Gales, R. S., Shewmaker, C. A., and Thompson, P. O. (1950). The frequency selectivity of the ear as determined by masking experiments. *Journal of the Acoustical Society of America* 22:490–6.

Scharf, B. (1970). Critical bands. In *Foundation of Modern Auditory Theory*, Vol. 1 (ed. J. V. Tobias), pp. 159–202. New York: Academic Press.

Seaton, W. H. and Trahiotis, C. (1975). Comparisons of critical ratios and critical bands in the monaural chinchilla. *Journal of the Acoustical Society of America* 57:193–9.

Serafin, S. V., Moody, D. B., and Stebbins, W. C. (1982). Frequency selectivity of the monkey's auditory system: Psychophysical tuning curves. *Journal of the Acoustical Society of America* 71:1513–18.

Shera, C. A., Guinan, J. J., and Oxenham, A. J. (2002). Revised estimates of human cochlear tuning from otoacoustic and behavioral measurements. *Proceedings of the National Academy of Sciences USA* 99:3318–23.

Shofner, W. P. (2000). Comparison of frequency discrimination thresholds for complex and single tones in chinchillas. *Hearing Research* 149:106–14.

Shofner, W. P. and Sheft, S. (1994). Detection of bandlimited noise masked by wideband noise in the chinchilla. *Hearing Research* 77:231–5.

Shofner, W. P. and Whitmer, W. M. (2006). Pitch cue learning in chinchillas: The role of spectral region in the training stimulus. *Journal of the Acoustical Society of America* 120:1706–12.

Shofner, W. P. and Yost, W. A. (1995). Discrimination of rippled-spectrum noise from flat-spectrum noise by chinchillas. *Auditory Neuroscience* 1:127–38.

Shofner, W. P. and Yost, W. A. (1997). Discrimination of rippled-spectrum noise from flat-spectrum noise by chinchillas: evidence for a spectral dominance region. *Hearing Research* 110:15–24.

Shofner, W. P., Yost, W. A., and Sheft, S. (1993). Increment detection of bandlimited noises in the chinchilla. *Hearing Research* 66:67–80.

Shofner, W. P., Whitmer, W. M., and Yost, W. A. (2005). Listening experience with iterated rippled noise alters the perception of 'pitch' strength of complex sounds in the chinchilla. *Journal of the Acoustical Society of America* 118:3187–97.

Shofner, W. P., Yost, W. A., and Whitmer, W. M. (2007). Pitch perception in chinchillas (Chinchilla laniger): Stimulus generalization using rippled noise. *Journal of Comparative Psychology* 121:428–39.

Sinnott, J. M. (1989). Detection and discrimination of synthetic English vowels by Old World monkeys (Cercopithecus, Macaca) and humans. *Journal of the Acoustical Society of America*, 86:557–65.

Sinnott, J. M. and Adams, F. S. (1987). Differences in human and monkey sensitivity to acoustic cues underlying voicing contrasts. *Journal of the Acoustical Society of America* 82:1539–47.

Sinnott, J. M. and Brown, C. H. (1997). Perception of the American English liquid /ra–la/ contrast by humans and monkeys. *Journal of the Acoustical Society of America* 102:588–602.

Sinnott, J. M. and Kreiter, N. A. (1991). Differential sensitivity to vowel continua in Old World monkeys (Macaca) and humans. *Journal of the Acoustical Society of America* 89:2421–9.

Sinnott, J. M. and Mosteller, K. W. (2001). A comparative assessment of speech sound discrimination in the Mongolian gerbil. *Journal of the Acoustical Society of America* 110:1729–32.

Sinnott, J. M., Beecher, M. D., Moody, D. B., and Stebbins, W. B. (1976). Speech sound discrimination by monkeys and humans. *Journal of the Acoustical Society of America* 60:687–95.

Sinnott, J. M., Petersen, M. R., and Hopp, S. L. (1985). Frequency and intensity discrimination in humans and monkeys. *Journal of the Acoustical Society of America* 78:1977–85.

Smith, D. W., Moody, D. B., and Stebbins, W. C. (1987). Effects of change in absolute signal level on psychophysical tuning curves in quiet and noise in patas monkeys. *Journal of the Acoustical Society of America* 82:63–8.

Smith, D. W., Moody, D. B., and Stebbins, W. C. (1990). Auditory frequency selectivity. In *Comparative Perception: Basic Mechanisms*, Vol. 1 (ed. M. A. Berkley and W. C. Stebbins), pp. 67–95. New York: Wiley Interscience.

Sommers, M. S., Moody, D. B., Prosen, C. A., and Stebbins, W. C. (1992). Formant frequency discrimination by Japanese macaques (Macaca fuscata). *Journal of the Acoustical Society of America* **91**:3499–510.

Southall, B. L., Schusterman, R. J., and Kastak, D. (2000). Masking in three pinnipeds: Underwater, low-frequency critical ratios. *Journal of the Acoustical Society of America* **108**:1322–6.

Southall, B. L., Schusterman, R. J., and Kastak, D. (2003). Auditory masking in three pinnipeds: Aerial critical ratios and direct critical bandwidth measurements. *Journal of the Acoustical Society of America* **114**:1660–6.

Spitzer, M. W. and Takahashi, T. T. (2006). Sound localization by barn owls in a simulated echoic environment. *Journal of Neurophysiology* **95**:3571–84.

Spitzer, M. W., Bala, A. D. S., and Takahashi, T. T. (2003). Auditory spatial discrimination by barn owls in simulated echoic conditions. *Journal of the Acoustical Society of America* **113**:1631–45.

Stebbins, W. C. (1966). Auditory reaction time and the derivation of equal loudness contours for the monkey. *Journal of Experimental Analysis of Behavior* **9**:135–42.

Stebbins, W. C. (1995). Uncertainty in the study of comparative perception: A methodological challenge. In *Methods in Comparative Psychoacoustics* (ed. G. M. Klump, R. J. Dooling, R. R. Fay, and W. C. Stebbins), pp. 331–41. Basel: Birkhauser Verlag.

Stevens, S. S. (1956). The direct estimation of sensory magnitudes—Loudness. *American Journal of Psychology* **69**:1–25.

Suthers, R. A. and Summers, C. A. (1980). Behavioral audiogram and masked thresholds of the megachiropteran echolocating bat, Rousettus. *Journal of Comparative Physiology* **136**:227–33.

Terhune, J. M. and Ronald, K. (1971). The harp seal, Pagophilus groenlandicus (Erxleben, 977). X. The air audiogram. *Canadian Journal of Zoology* **49**:385–90.

Terhune, J. M. and Ronald, K. (1975). Masked hearing thresholds of ringed seals. *Journal of the Acoustical Society of America* **58**:515–16.

Terry, M. and Moore, B. C. J. (1977). Suppression effects in forward masking. *Journal of the Acoustical Society of America* **62**:781–4.

Tollin, D. J. and Yin, T. C. T. (2003). Psychophysical investigation of an auditory spatial illusion in cats: The precedence effect. *Journal of Neurophysiology* **90**:2149–62.

Tollin, D. J., Populin, L. C., Moore, J. M., Ruhland, J. L., and Yin, T. C. T. (2005). Sound-localization performance in the cat: The effect of restraining the head. *Journal of Neurophysiology* **93**:1223–34.

Tomlinson, R. W. W. and Schwartz, D. W. F. (1988). Perception of the missing fundamental in nonhuman primates. *Journal of the Acoustical Society of America* **84**:560–5.

Trout, J. D. (2001). The biological basis of speech: What to infer from talking to the animals. *Psychological Review* **108**:523–49.

Uexküll, J. von (1921). *Umwelt und Innenwelt der Tiere*. Berlin: J. Springer.

Wagner, E. (2002). Across-channel processing in auditory perception: A study in gerbils (Meriones unguiculatus) and cochlear-implant subjects. Ph.D. Thesis. Munchen: Technischen Universitat.

Wakeford, O. S. and Robinson, D. E. (1974). Detection of binaurally masked tones by the cat. *Journal of the Acoustical Society of America* **56**:952–6.

Watson, C. S. (1963). Masking of tones by noise for the cat. *Journal of the Acoustical Society of America* **35**:167–72.

Whitfield, I. C. (1980). Auditory cortex and the pitch of complex tones. *Journal of the Acoustical Society of America* **67**:644–7.

Wier, C. C., Jesteadt, W., and Green, D. M. (1977). Frequency discrimination as a function of frequency and sensation level. *Journal of the Acoustical Society of America* **61**:178–84.

Zwicker, E., Flottorp, G., and Stevens, S. S. (1957). Critical bandwidth in loudness summation. *Journal of the Acoustical Society of America* **29**:548–57.

Chapter 8

Auditory organization

Benjamin J. Dyson

8.1 Introduction

The auditory system is essentially faced with two major problems in terms of perceptual organization. At the moment, I am receiving continuous and indiscriminate acoustic input at each ear, yet am able to hear out discrete sound sources such as the inevitable drilling taking place somewhere on campus, the music from my speakers in front of me, the seagulls circling high above in the courtyard outside my office, the tap of my fingers on the keyboard, and the occasional knock on my door. One way to think about perceptually organizing this auditory scene is in terms of two broad steps (Bregman, 1990). First, there is the task of segregating low-level aspects of the sound world in terms of common spatial, temporal, and spectral properties. Second, there is the job of integrating these individual auditory features to form specific acoustic objects or streams. In this way, I am able to perceive the low-frequency and distant rumble as the worker's drill, or the closer and higher frequency shriek as the seagull's call. In the last decade, there have been numerous review papers that cover acoustic separation, acoustic grouping, and the factors that influence them (Darwin, 1997; Moore and Gockel, 2002; Carlyon, 2004). Therefore, in addition to providing an overview of auditory segregation and integration, this chapter will also reach for cognitive and neuroimaging data as a way of providing further insight into the mechanisms involved in auditory perceptual organization. I will also stop to look at one particular case study of perceptual organization that is both contemporary and contentious: the relationship between auditory *what* and *where* information in the brain.

8.2 Perceptual organization within acoustic attributes

As established in the Introduction, one problem the auditory system faces is with respect to segregation: sounds arrive at the ear like the contents of an acoustic mixing bowl and we have the rather messy task of picking out (or segregating) the white bits from the yellow bits, the crumbly bits from the runny bits, with the aim of identifying the flour and eggs that made up the mixture. Thankfully, there are many acoustic properties we can use to help us go about this process of separation. To return to the initial example, the drill is further away than the seagull (i.e. differences in intensity), the seagull's squawk occurs at different times from the drill (i.e. differences in stimulus onset), and the bird's call is a radically different sound than the hammer of a pneumatic drill (i.e. differences in spectrotemporal structure). This is by no means an exhaustive list of acoustic cues that aid segregation, but it would be relatively exhausting to attempt to describe them all in depth (see Bregman, 1990). Therefore, this chapter focuses on the principles of perceptual organization related to frequency, and how we might go about organizing this kind of information in the presence of multiple frequencies at the same time point, multiple frequencies across time, and, finally, multiple frequencies across space. Chapter 9 provides additional discussion of the organization cues of harmonicity, onset time, and spatial location with respect to speech perception.

8.2.1 Organizing simultaneous sound

Although historically auditory experiments have dealt with an impressive array of different sounds, the acoustic stimuli heard within the soundproof booth of the psychophysicist (or cognitivist, for that matter) are often far less complex than even the first sounds a baby hears. Simply put, the pure tone observed in the laboratory is rarely produced naturally in the outside world (Gibson, 1966). Instead, natural sounds tend to be complex, in that a number of different frequencies emanate from the some source at the same time. However, there is a useful regularity within many naturally occurring sounds that the auditory system takes advantage of, in that individual frequency components that make up a single natural sound tend to be *harmonically related* to one another. In other words, higher frequencies produced by the sound source tend to be (roughly) integer multiples of lower frequencies produced by the same source (e.g. 800 Hz, 600 Hz, and 400 Hz are all multiple integers of 200 Hz). This leads us to the question of exactly how the auditory system might deal with the segregation of multiple frequencies presented at the same time.

One type of investigation that has proved particularly useful in studying the perceptual organization of multiple, concurrently presented frequencies is the mistuned harmonic paradigm. Here, participants are typically played complex auditory stimuli built up from a number of pure-tone components and asked to make certain kinds of psychoacoustic judgement relating to the sounds (such as pitch matching; e.g. Darwin *et al.*, 1995). A critical distinction is made between *tuned stimuli* in which all tonal components are integer multiples of the fundamental frequency (F0), and *mistuned stimuli* in which one or more partials are not integer multiples of the F0 (Fig. 8.1). Estimates of around 2–4% mistuning have been cited as sufficient for the detection of lower mistuned partials of a complex sound (Moore *et al.*, 1985, 1986). However, perhaps of greater interest in terms of perceptual organization is the phenomenological experience related to these sounds. The harmonicity of a complex is usually heard as a single 'buzz' for the tuned stimulus, and a 'buzz' with a separate pure-tone element for the mistuned stimulus (Moore *et al.*, 1986). In both the former and the latter cases, the buzz is the result of all harmonically related partials grouping together, while the pure-tone component heard after presentation of the mistuned stimulus represents the inharmonic partial that has been perceptually segregated from the harmonic partials. As a result of this perceptual phenomenon, the mistuned harmonic paradigm

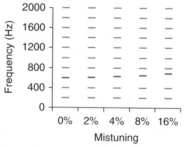

Fig. 8.1 Variations in concurrent sound segregation using five complex sounds composed of ten components each with a fundamental frequency (F0) of 200 Hz. The green marks indicate frequencies which are integer multiples of the F0 (i.e. tuned partials). The red marks indicate the third harmonic manipulated upwards by 0% (600 Hz), 2% (612 Hz), 4% (624 Hz), 8% (648 Hz), and 16% (695 Hz). Participants may be asked to categorize the sounds as either tuned or mistuned in order to provide a rough estimate of the degree of inharmonicity required for the detection of mistuning, and the number of objects within an acoustic scene.

has been used to distinguish between cases of singular and multiple concurrent objects within an auditory scene, with the tuned stimulus representing one object and the mistuned stimulus representing two (Alain *et al.*, 2002*a*; Dyson and Alain, 2004). In this way, we can begin to see how the mechanisms associated with *what* acoustic energy represents is closely related to *how many* independent sources of energy there are (Bregman and Steiger, 1980). To summarize, the perceptual organization of a complex sound on the basis of periodicity allows for the segregation between harmonically and inharmonically related frequencies, and the integration of harmonically related frequencies within a distinct percept (i.e. a buzz). With the basic effect established, concern now turns to the neural substrates underpinning concurrent sound segregation.

Object-related negativity (ORN)

Of particular interest in this regard is the auditory event-related potential (ERP) known as 'object-related negativity' (ORN; Alain *et al.*, 2001). While the presentation of both tuned and mistuned stimuli generate exogenous ERP components such as N1, mistuned stimuli tend to generate additional negativity around the same time. This means that when the average waveform generated by tuned stimuli is subtracted from that produced by mistuned stimuli, ORN is typically revealed (see Fig. 8.2). This component is characterized by negativity occurring approximately 180 ms after stimulus onset, and as shown in Fig. 8.2 has a scalp distribution both inferior and medial to the source of the N1, consistent with ORN generation in the medial planum

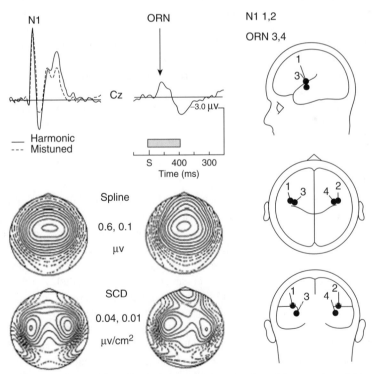

Fig. 8.2 In addition to exogenous auditory ERP components such as N1, complex mistuned stimuli generate additional negativity relative to complex tuned stimuli. This is known as 'object-related negativity' (ORN) and is characterized by negativity occurring approximately 180 ms after stimulus onset, with a scalp distribution both inferior and medial to the source of the N1, consistent with ORN generation in the medial planum temporale.

temporale (Alain *et al.*, 2001). ORN is thought to be intimately related to the perceptual mechanisms involved in concurrent sound segregation, since ORN both increases with the amount of mistuning within a complex sound and decreases when higher harmonics are used to carry the mistuned partial (Alain *et al.*, 2001), both of which are common psychophysical findings (Moore *et al.*, 1985; Hartmann *et al.*, 1990).

More recently, Johnson and colleagues (Hautus and Johnson, 2005; Johnson *et al.*, 2007) examined ORN using stimuli quite different from the complex sounds used in the mistuned harmonic paradigm. Here, participants were exposed to dichotic pitch stimuli composing broadband noise of 'interaurally identical amplitude spectra' (Hautus and Johnson, 2005, p. 275) between the two ears, in addition to a narrow frequency band that was shifted in location using an interaural time difference (ITD) between left and right ears (c.f., Cramer and Huggins, 1958). These *pitch stimuli* were compared to *control stimuli* in which no ITD was introduced for the narrow frequency band region. The resultant percept for the control stimuli was, therefore, a centralized noise, while for the pitch stimuli it was a centralized noise with a lateralized tone component. Therefore, despite differences in stimulus construction between this and the mistuned harmonic paradigm, the control stimuli (just like the tuned stimuli) represent one object, while the pitch stimuli (just like the mistuned stimuli) represent two objects. Despite slightly longer ORN latencies for cases of dichotic pitch relative to ORN elicited as a result of inharmonicity, Hautus and Johnson (2005) also found that ORN was larger for pitch stimuli relative to control stimuli. These recent studies support the idea that the observation of ORN is not limited to the comparison of tuned and mistuned stimuli, but rather may reflect more generic processes associated with the perceptual segregation of concurrently presented sounds. This is because in the case of the mistuned harmonic paradigm, discrimination between the two classes of stimuli (tuned and mistuned) is based on frequency relations; while in the case of the dichotic pitch paradigm, discrimination between the two classes of stimuli (pitch and control) is based on location. As Hautus and Johnson (2005) state, the ORN is likely to reflect 'fairly general mechanisms of auditory stream segregation that can broadly utilize a range of cues to parse simultaneous acoustic events' (p. 280). However, a note of caution is added by Carlyon (2004) who calls for further evidence to show that acoustic manipulations that do not generate differences in terms of single and multiple concurrently presented sounds also do not produce ORN.

Top-down effects

At this point, we can introduce an additional assumption regarding acoustic perceptual organization and the idea that at these primary stages of auditory scene analysis, low-level segregation mechanisms operate independently from attention (Bregman, 1990). Consequently, interest has turned to whether the production of ORN can be modulated by task demands (see Alain, 2007, for a full discussion of the role of top-down effects on concurrent sound segregation with respect to both attention and learning). In one set of cases (Alain *et al.*, 2001, 2002*a*), ORN amplitudes were calculated across both an active condition in which participants were required to categorize complex sounds as either one sound (tuned) or two (mistuned), and a passive condition in which participants were presented with the same sounds but now told to ignore them and allowed to read a book or watch a film as a distraction technique. Despite later auditory ERP components showing modulation as a consequence of task (e.g. larger P400 during active conditions), ORN amplitude was stable in both cases, supporting the idea that concurrent sound segregation is unaffected by the influence of attention. In a second set of papers (Alain and Izenberg, 2003; Dyson *et al.*, 2005*a*, Experiment 1), variations in ORN were examined across active tasks of varying difficulty. In Alain and Izenberg (2003), tuned and mistuned sounds were presented randomly to both ears and the tasks were auditory. Participants in the easy condition had to respond to the *detection* of shorter duration target sounds in one selected ear, while in the hard condition participants had to respond to the *identity* of shorter duration target sounds in one selected ear as either tuned or mistuned. In Dyson *et al.* (2005*a*), binaural tuned and mistuned sounds were presented randomly and the tasks were visual: in the easy condition, participants were presented with different coloured digits and asked to categorize each one as either above or below five; while in the hard condition, participants had to perform an *n-back* task in which they were required to respond to the previous numerical value of the number when the present digit was a certain colour. Once again, ORN amplitude did not significantly modulate on the basis of task difficulty (see also Hautus and Johnson, 2005). Johnson *et al.* (2007) have recently gone on to investigate task demands in the dichotic pitch paradigm, also showing no modulation of ORN according to task. It is important to note, however, that while ORN appears to be fairly resilient to global task demands, other auditory ERP components that occur around the same time (such as N1 and P2) are modulated by task demands, thereby reflecting something about the process-specific nature of ORN (Dyson *et al.*, 2005*a*). On the basis of this collection of studies then, it appears ORN is insensitive to global differences in attentional demands in terms of the presence or absence of the task, the level of difficulty of the task, and also whether the task makes demands on the auditory or visual system.

Although the ORN data suggest that the perceptual mechanisms involved in concurrent sound segregation cannot be modulated by top-down influences, quite different patterns of data have been demonstrated behaviourally in a variation of the mistuned harmonic paradigm. Darwin *et al.* (1995) invited participants to pitch-match complex sounds, with the target complex being preceded by a train of pure tones. When the train of pure tones was at the frequency of the mistuned harmonic contained within the target complex, the mistuned harmonic contributed less to the overall pitch of the target sound during pitch-matching relative to the absence of such a train (see also Darwin and Ciocca, 1992; Darwin *et al.*, 1994). These data indicate that the perceptual mechanisms involved in the concurrent grouping of frequency can be influenced by a previous context, thereby reducing the contribution of a mistuned partial to the overall pitch of the complex sound. In other words, prior exposure to the mistuned partial facilitated the segregation of concurrent acoustic energy, such that mistuned and tuned partials of the complex sound formed very distinct acoustic objects at the time of final concurrent segregation. This study is useful in highlighting a number of issues related to concurrent sound segregation. First, while these mechanisms related to simultaneous sound segregation can operate in the absence of attention, as the data from Darwin *et al.* (1995) show, this does not mean that they necessarily operate *independently* of attention. Second, it would be of additional interest to see whether neuroelectric measures of concurrent sound segregation such as ORN are modulated by preceding stimulus presentation. Third, it is not yet obvious to what extent the perceptual mechanisms involved in concurrent sound segregation simply relate to the specific demands placed on the participant. For example, pitch-matching (Darwin *et al.*, 1995) is an iterative process that makes rather heavy demands on auditory memory, relative to making a simple binary discrimination about the harmonic nature of the current stimulus (Alain *et al.*, 2001). Fourth, the Darwin *et al.* (1995) study is also useful as it introduces the notion of perceptual segregation occurring as a function of time, which now allows us to discuss the mechanisms involved in sequential sound segregation.

8.2.2 Organizing sequential sound

The classic paradigm for sequential sound presentation is shown schematically in Fig. 8.3. In its most basic form, four temporal intervals of equal spacing are used that may be filled with one of two frequencies (*A* or *B*), or silence (-). Typically, the A frequency is played in the first and third slots, the B frequency is played in the second slot, and silence fills the fourth slot, hence *ABA-*.

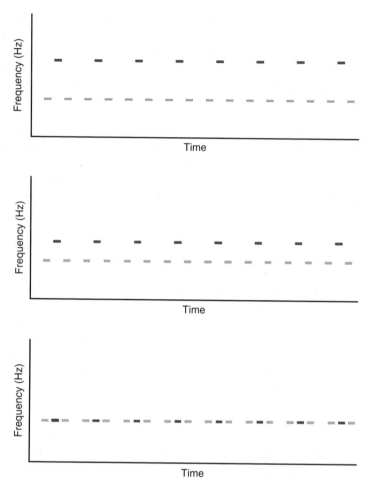

Fig. 8.3 An example of sequential sound segregation over four iterated temporal intervals, the first and third are filled with frequency A (in green), the second is filled with frequency B (in red), and the fourth is silence (blank). As the difference between A and B (Δf) increases (moving bottom to top on the figure), participants experience less of a galloping rhythm (horse percept; fusion) in which the two frequencies integrate to form a single stream of sound and more of a staccato rhythm (morse percept; fission) in which the two frequencies separate to form independent streams.

This sequence of sound is repeated over a number of iterations (i.e. *ABA-ABA-ABA-ABA-*) until one of two percepts are formed. One of the most critical factors in determining which percept is formed is the difference between the A and B frequencies or Δf (other factors include the rate of presentation, temporal envelope, and phase spectrum; see Moore and Gockel, 2002, for a thorough discussion of these additional influences). When the Δf is small, the percept participants typically have is of a galloping rhythm (informally referred to as the *horse* percept, formally known as 'fusion'), in which the two frequencies integrate to form a single stream of sound (i.e. both *A* and *B* frequencies combine to form 111-111-). This is in contrast to when the Δf is large and individuals hear a more staccato rhythm (informally referred to as the *morse* percept, formally known as 'fission'), in which the two frequencies separate to form independent streams (i.e. the A frequency is heard as 1-1-1-1- whereas the B frequency is heard as -2---2-). Typically, streaming requires a nominal amount of time to build up such that individuals hear fusion followed by fission if the Δf is large enough (see Snyder and Alain, 2007, for a review of sequential stream build-up). As Snyder *et al.* (2006) state, the mechanisms of sequential sound perception requires 'parsing sounds that originate from different physical objects and grouping together sounds that emanate from the same object' (p. 1). This is just in the same way that in the mistuned harmonic paradigm, harmonic partials group together while inharmonic partials separate to form independent acoustic percepts. However, in contrast to simultaneous organization, the grouping principles are now based on absolute frequency across time rather than periodic relations at the same time point.

Effects of attention

Once again, it is possible to ask again to what extent these low-level mechanisms of sequential auditory scene analysis operate independently of attention, and a recent series of behavioural studies by Cusack *et al.* (2004; see also Carlyon *et al.*, 2001) have tackled this question. Participants were played sequences of sounds for 20 seconds: in the left ear, tonal sequences were played in the manner described above in which the Δf was either 4, 6, 8, or 10 semitones. For the first 10 seconds of this sequence, noises were played in the same (left) or different (right) ear, which either increased or decreased in amplitude to give the perception of approaching or departing sounds, respectively. In *one-task* conditions, participants were required to ignore the noises throughout and simply attend to the tonal sequence, pressing a key at the start of the sequence whether it sounded more like one or two streams, and to make additional responses when the percept changed as streaming built up over time. In *two-task* conditions, participants were required to categorize the noises as either approaching or departing for the first 10 seconds and then switch to the tonal sequence and make streaming judgements for the last 10 seconds. Therefore, by comparing *one-task* and *two-task* conditions, Carlyon and colleagues were able to assess the effect of a 10-s build-up of streaming for the tonal sequence in the presence (*one-task*) or absence (*two-task*) of attention: if streaming was purely independent of attention, then the judgement of the tonal pattern as one or two streams at the 10-s mark should be identical for both *one-task* and *two-task* conditions. However, what Cusack *et al.* (2004) found was that despite the greater likelihood of responding two streams as a function of increasing Δf, the assumed 'automatic' build-up of evidence for either the tonal sequence as one or two streams was not apparent in the *two-task* condition. When attention was directed towards the tone sequence in the *one-task* condition, streaming built up over the first few seconds, so that listeners became increasing likely to judge the sequence as segregated (two streams) rather than fused (one stream). When attention was not directed towards the tone sequence in the *two-task* condition, segregation did not build up, so that when attention was switched to the sequence after 10 seconds the sequence was most likely heard as fused. In other words, when directed towards the noise, participants failed to accrue the same amount of evidence as to the 'horse' or 'morse' nature of the tones; in shifting attention to the tones at the 10-s mark, it was almost as though participants were hearing the tonal sequence for the first time. Similar results were obtained regardless of whether the tonal sequences and noise sequences were presented in the same or different ears, or whether they were contained within the same or different frequency channels, suggesting that these effects of attention were not contingent on the use of different peripheral channels.

Cusack *et al.* (2004) proposed a useful framework for thinking about the relationship between attention and sound segregation in their *hierarchical decomposition model* (see Fig. 8.4). They imagine an auditory scene in which three different sound sources are operational: a human speaker, a live band, and passing traffic. The suggestion is that attention essentially 'opens-up' an

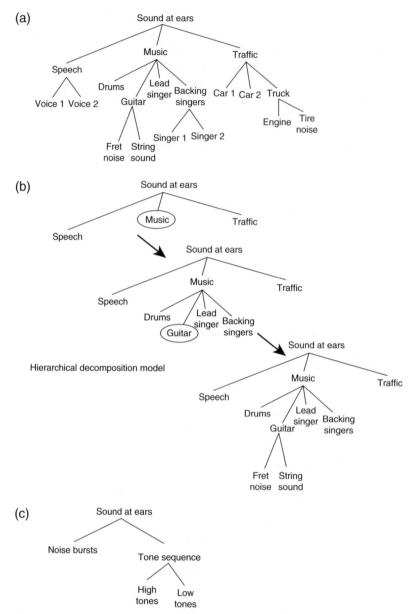

Fig. 8.4 The hierarchical decomposition model of Cusack *et al.* (2004) shows that the allocation of auditory attention allows for an increasingly fine-grained analysis of a selected sound source, while unattended sound sources remain at an undifferentiated level of analysis.

attended sound source to be decomposed into more and more detailed components. As shown in Fig. 8.4, the live band can be further broken down into various instruments, at which point attention can again be deployed (e.g. listen to the guitar as opposed to drums or singers), which can again lead to further decomposition and an even more precise attentional focus (e.g. attend to the string sound as opposed to fret noise). Meanwhile, in the absence of attention directed towards the other sound sources, there is no further elaboration or decomposition—we do not distinguish between the different kinds of traffic noise, nor do we analyse what the speaker might be saying. When attention is switched between sound sources, the previously decomposed sub-branches collapse back to a superordinate level, and decomposition on another source begins: we might distinguish between the truck and the car, and notice that one of the tyres on the car is sounding a little under-inflated. To return to the experimental stimuli (see Fig. 8.4c), when participants are engaged with noise categorization in the two-task condition, it becomes much more difficult to further decompose the unattended tones into their respective streams, thus perceptual evidence fails to build up over time to the same extent as it would if auditory attention had been directed to the tonal sequence from the outset. While clearly in its early stages of development, the hierarchical decomposition model is an interesting way of thinking about perceptual organization in complex acoustic scenes. The architecture of the model has obvious advantages in terms of processing capacity, in that the auditory system can only analyse one sound source in detail at any one time, leaving the other sources to blend together in an irrelevant mess; and also has important implications for theories of auditory attention since the notion of selection occurs at a very late stage of analysis, presumably incorporating semantic analysis.

Neuroimaging studies

Recent neuroimaging studies have also provided insights on how this build-up and re-setting of streaming as a function of auditory attention is represented at a neural level. Snyder *et al.* (2006) employed a paradigm similar to that shown in Fig 8.3, in which participants were presented with tri-tone sequences (*ABA-*) using a Δf of either 0, 4, 7, or 12 semitones over approximately 11 s, and recorded event-related potentials (ERPs) to the tones. Rather than manipulate attention on a trial-by-trial basis as in Cusack *et al.* (2004), Snyder *et al.* (2006) requested that participants complete both an active condition in which they responded to whether they heard one or two streams at the end of the sequences, and also a passive condition in which participants were exposed to the same stimuli but in the absence of task. The ERP data were generally in line with the hierarchial decomposition model of Carylon and colleagues, in that the perceptual organization of successive tones into independent streams was heavily contingent upon attention. First, a number of auditory ERP components including P1, N1, P2, and N1c were enhanced in situations that promoted morse-like percepts (i.e. increased Δf). Second, there was also an additional positivity observed across the acoustic ERP waveform, reflecting the supposed 'build-up' of streaming as the stimulus sequence played out. Importantly for the hierarchical decomposition model, this positivity was severely attenuated in the passive condition relative to the active condition, supporting the notion that perceptual integration requires at least some attention.

Elucidation of the neural mechanisms underlying sequential sound segregation have also benefited from an investigation of mismatch negativity (MMN; for a review see Picton *et al.*, 2000). MMN is a neural event generated when infrequently occurring *deviant sounds* are presented amongst frequently occurring *standard sounds*. In the simplest case, this might be a run of high-frequency tones (H) 'violated' by the presentation of a lower frequency tone (L) as in the stimulus chain: HHHHHL. Derived by subtracting the average ERP waveform of standard sounds from deviant sounds, *classic MMN* (in contrast to the relatively recent idea of *identity MMN*; for an example see Pulvermüller *et al.*, 2006) is typically characterized by negativity that occurs between 100 and 200 ms after deviant onset (Näätänen and Winkler, 1999), and is thought to index the automatic detection of mismatch between the incoming stimulus and what was expected based upon the previously presented stimuli (Ritter *et al.*, 1995).

However, in contrast to the somewhat simplistic statement made above regarding MMN elicitation, work by Sussman *et al.* (1999) showed that deviant change in frequency does not always bring about this neural correlate of change detection. As previously stated, the presentation of

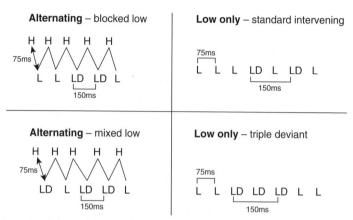

Fig. 8.5 A schematic of the various conditions used by Sussman (2005). In the alternating mixed–low condition (bottom left), double MMNs were elicited for the LD deviant, showing that stream segregation takes place prior to integration within streams.

HHHHHL should elicit an MMN for the L, with the idea being that the auditory system has detected a change relative to the acoustic stimulation that has gone before. However, Sussman *et al.* (1999) showed that MMN in this context can be abolished if the high and low tones form part of a more complex pattern, e.g. HHHHHLHHHHHL. In this case, it is the combination of low- and high-frequency tones that becomes the standard. Similar effects of context were studied in the comparison between *blocked* and *mixed* presentations (see Fig. 8.5). Here, particular interest was in whether double-deviants (i.e. LL) would elicit one or two MMNs. Blocked presentations in which double-deviants formed part of a more complex pattern with a standard run of high tones (i.e. HHHHLLHHHHLL) were shown to produce a single MMN. Conversely in mixed presentation, when double-deviants were mixed with single-deviants (i.e. HHHHLHHHHHLL), the double-deviant was shown to elicit two MMNs. Figure 8.5 provides a schematic of the primary experiment of Sussman (2005) in which these effects of context were compared in cases of single and multiple streams. The deviant was defined as a low-frequency tone (LD; 404 Hz) lower than both the standard low (L; 440 Hz) and standard high (H; 1508 Hz) -frequency tones. On the basis of previous work, in the 'low only' conditions, a double MMN should be observed for the standard intervening case, but only a single MMN should be observed for the triple-deviant. However, the 'alternating' condition provided a much more crucial manipulation in that the number of identifiable MMNs would help to reveal the order in which auditory segregation and integration takes place. In both alternating blocked low and alternating mixed low conditions, both of the dual LD stimuli violate the previous H stimuli, and therefore could be eligible for MMN. However, if streams were being integrated only after being segregated, then the second LD in the pair should only show MMN in the context of the alternating mixed low conditions. A single MMN was observed for double LD stimuli in blocked low cases, while double MMNs was observed for double LD stimuli in mixed low cases, consistent with the hypothesis of integration after segregation. It should also be noted that all these recordings took place under passive conditions, and, as such, strongly support the idea that segregation and integration operate at a pre-attentive stage of analysis. More recent research (Sussman *et al.*, 2007) has gone on to support this contention, with the additional proviso that the role of attention is essentially to initiate a more fine-grained analysis of the current stream of interest (cf. Cusack *et al.*, 2004). Couched in this way, we begin to see how both cognitive and neuroimaging research is starting to converge on a general model of auditory perceptual organization.

8.3 **Perceptual organization between acoustic attributes**

Whilst substantial progress has been made in understanding the mechanisms involved in concurrent and sequential sound segregation (although perhaps more so in the latter case; Carlyon, 2004), we have still only really shed light on the tiniest portion of the massively complex problem of auditory scene analysis. In the previous section, we have seen how frequency acts as a critical cue in the perceptual organization of sound, both at a single point in time as well as across time. We have also seen how the organizational principles of both segregation and integration apply equally to both concurrent and sequential sound segregation. In the case of concurrent sound segregation, frequencies may be simultaneously divided into harmonically related and inharmonically related partials, with the harmonically related partials grouping to form a unified percept. In the case of sequential sound segregation, frequencies may be divided across time according to Δf, with reoccurring frequencies becoming integrated to form independent streams of sound. However, there has been little discussion about how organization by frequency might interact with other acoustic attributes. Therefore, in the second half of the chapter, a different kind of segregation and integration will be discussed, namely, whether different types of acoustic information are processed separately and the extent to which effort is required to integrate these different properties together.

8.3.1 **Perceptual organization as a unitary phenomenon?**

One major assumption behind this section is that it possible to see perceptual organization in audition as essentially no different from perceptual organization in vision. Whilst this may be true to a certain degree, it is important to point out that critical differences between vision and audition have also been detailed that preclude the claim of exact isomorphism (Neuhoff, 2003). For instance, at a very basic level it would be hard to deny that the respective anatomical structures of the eye and the ear result in a number of radically different low-level mechanisms between vision and audition. As a result of this, Welch and Warren (1980) argued that vision seems suited to the perceptual organization of spatially based events, whilst audition appears to be specialized to the perceptual organization of temporally based events (see also Jones and Boltz, 1989; Large and Jones, 1999). Whilst the Welch and Warren (1980) distinction is one way to interpret the relative importance of space and time in vision and audition, other analogies have also been considered. If one considers both vision and audition to be intrinsically spatial *and* temporal in nature (see the dialogue between Handel, 1988*a*, *b* and Kubovy, 1988), then the idea of shared perceptual organizational mechanisms between the senses begins to make sense in terms of the need for an efficient processing system. Indeed, one unifying approach was put forward by Kubovy (1981), who provided a theory of perceptual processing abstracted from any particular modality. According to this model, both an optical array in vision and an acoustic field in audition can be thought of as variation along four dimensions: x and y spatial coordinates, time, and, wavelength (of light in the visual modality, or sound in the auditory modality). Here, both visual and auditory information processing are sensitive to similar kinds of variation and therefore have the opportunity to be dealt with by fundamentally similar mechanisms. Shamma (2001) has gone even further to argue that even if one accepts the view that space is intrinsically linked to the visual modality whilst time is intimately connected to the auditory modality *à la* Welch and Warren (1980), this does not necessary imply the use of fundamentally different neural systems. Specifically, it is possible that the basilar membrane transforms auditory temporal cues into spatial cues, so that both visual and auditory information may be processed by the same spatially based neural substrate.

To sum up then, at a relatively low level of analysis, rather obvious differences exist between the stimulus transducers employed for audition and vision. At a higher level of analysis however, the same underlying apparatus may well govern the processing of information from multiple senses (e.g. Cohen and Andersen, 2004). As Shamma (2001, p. 340) states: '. . . although anatomical differences are clearly significant early in these pathways (e.g. retina versus cochlear nucleus) . . . in more central neural structures, the theoretical views and anatomical studies support the notion of a unified proto-cortical plan for all primary sensory areas . . .' Therefore, while it is important to be sensitive to the differences between the sensory systems in terms of specific low-level perceptual mechanisms, it is equally important to be mindful of the notion that at a higher level of perceptual organization, audition may act in similar ways to vision.

8.3.2 Auditory events, objects, and streams

Continuing the theme of similar perceptual organizational principles across the different senses, Griffiths and Warren (2004) state that the notion of an object is important to all sensory systems, and may act as a unifying concept across the modalities. In other words, what we seem to have here is the proposal of one particular kind of representation that allows for integration across the senses. Auditory objects might be able to combine with visual objects (and objects from other domains) so that we may experience the rich, multisensory phenomenology that we often take for granted. However, as they warn 'attractive as such analogies might be in principle, it is not clear precisely what the analogous operations are, where they might be instantiated or how they might be achieved' (Griffiths and Warren, 2004, p. 890).

So what exactly is an object and what might an auditory one sound like? One specific definition of a perceptual object has been put forward by Kubovy and Van Valkenburg (2001, p. 102), who describe it as a representation 'which is susceptible to figure-ground segregation'. Thinking back to the previous sections on simultaneous and sequential sound analysis, we might begin to see how this figure-ground segregation can be applied to audition. In the case of simultaneous sounds, a mistuned partial creates a figure percept that is distinct from the homogenous periodic background from which it arises. Similarly, in the case of sequential sounds, sufficient Δf allows the B stream to perceptually segregate from the background A stream. Of course, in both cases attention can modulate the specific allocation of figure and ground to mistuned or tuned partials in the case of simultaneous analysis, and to A or B streams in the case of sequential analysis.

However, discussion of auditory objects is made problematic as a result of numerous similar sounding constructs within the literature, and by a lack of consistency between researchers. For example, according to Alain and Arnott (2000, p. 202) an auditory object is defined as a sound source over time, while an auditory event is defined as the perceptual dimensions of a sound at a particular point in time. In this respect, the former definition has a temporal aspect which the Kubovy and Van Valkenburg (2001) definition of an auditory object does not appear to have (although see Alain and Arnott, 2000, p. 203). Further confusion arises with further reading. In the case of Cusack et al. (2000), they find a unilateral neglect deficit in certain individuals for 'auditory objects separated only in time and not in space' (p. 1056). Once again, if auditory objects are separated in time, then this lacks the temporal aspect put forward by Alain and Arnott (2000). Similar conceptions of an auditory object as a perceptual snapshot of a particular sound at a particular time may be inferred in the description of 'temporally distributed auditory objects' provided by Ahveninen et al. (2007, p. 14609). Therefore, the current dilemma for researchers is whether an auditory object is understood in terms of a temporal dimension (making it more like an auditory stream) or whether an auditory object is understood independently of time (making it more like an auditory event). However, such statements can be immediately contradicted by previously published writing such as 'a stream is a perceptually bound collection of sounds that together constitute an event' (Griffiths and Warren, 2004, p. 889), and also by the additional idea that auditory perception should be concerned with sound events (e.g. hiss versus purr) rather than the objects that produce the sound events (e.g. cat).

From a cognitive perspective at least, these definitions of an auditory object fail to capture one critical aspect contained in the idea of a visual object, in that object-based representations tend to refer to the combination of a number of basic properties derived from a common origin. This is traditionally in contrast to feature-based representations, which tend to refer to the representation of basic properties unbound to any particular surface or source. Just to add another term to the mix then, other researchers have chosen to adopt the term 'conjunction' to distinguish between representations in which basic elements of the sensory system in question are combined, and 'feature' representations in which basic stimulus properties are assumedly left uncombined (Woods *et al.*, 1998; Dyson and Quinlan, 2003). However, as we shall see, problems in conceptualizing auditory conjunctions have also arisen, specifically with respect to the assumptions made about feature integration and the resultant percept.

8.3.3 Auditory features and conjunctions

Much of the empirical work on how various sound attributes might interact with one another may be thought of by evaluating the distinction between acoustic features and conjunctions. In this respect, the data owe much to certain principles of visual perceptual organizational, notably Treisman and Gelade's (1980) Feature Integration Theory (FIT; see Quinlan, 2004, for an extensive review). Under this scheme (see Fig. 8.6), visual object identification is determined by the combination of a number of feature maps. Upon the presentation of a visual scene, basic properties of individual objects (i.e. features) such as colour, orientation, and curvature are coded within individual spatially organized feature maps. When visual attention is directed towards a certain point in space, the contents of that particular space for each of the individual feature maps

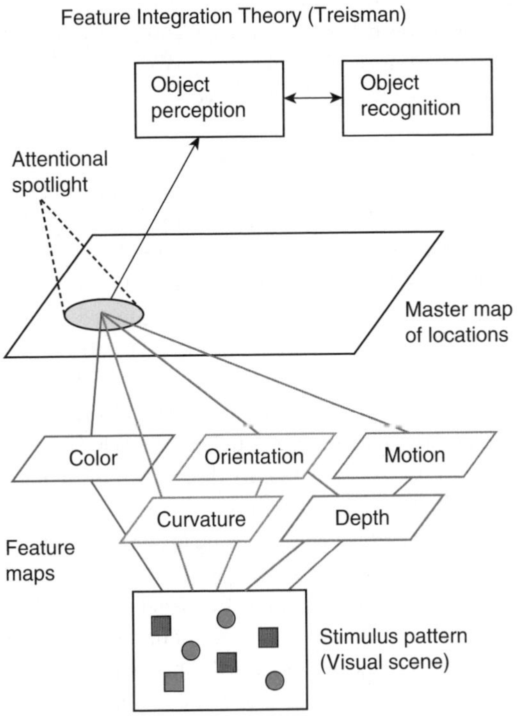

Fig. 8.6 Schematic of Treisman's Feature Integration Theory (FIT; Treisman and Gelade, 1980). While originally designed to account for visual processing, the framework has been applied with some success to the auditory domain albeit with modifications to suit the nature of acoustic stimuli.

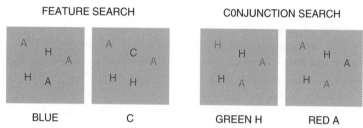

Fig. 8.7 Examples of visual feature search and conjunction search. (a) In feature cases, targets are discriminable from non-targets on the basis of a single feature (e.g. a colour; BLUE, or, a shape; C). (b) In the conjunction cases, targets are discriminable from non-targets only on the basis of combinations of features (e.g. a colour and a shape; GREEN H, or RED A).

integrate onto a master map of locations, thereby forming a conjunction. This integrated representation then leads the way to visual object perception and recognition.

Typically, support for the distinction between feature and conjunction processing has been derived from visual search paradigms. Here, participants are simultaneously presented with a number of spatially distributed items and asked to report the presence or absence of a predefined target (see Fig. 8.7). Under feature conditions, targets are discriminable from non-targets on the basis of a single feature (in Fig. 8.7(a), a specific colour (blue) or a specific shape (C)). Under conjunction conditions, targets are discriminable from non-targets only on the basis of a combination of features (in Fig. 8.7(b), a specific colour and shape (Green H or Red A)). Evidence is accrued for a two-stage model of visual perceptual processing, in which perceptual features are derived and then organized into integrated wholes, when responses to conjunction targets are longer than responses to feature targets (Treisman and Gelade, 1980). In considering the application of visual FIT to audition, a number of important issues are raised with respect to acoustic perceptual organization: What is the relation between feature and conjunction processing? Are observed processing differences between feature and conjunction processing really attributable to binding costs? and, Can acoustic features be incorrectly integrated?

The feature/conjunction relationship

Despite evidence that basic acoustic features such as location, frequency, and intensity appear to be picked up preattentively in a similar way to basic visual features (for a review see Wolfe, 1998), some of the earliest work on auditory feature integration by Woods and colleagues (Woods and Alain, 1993; Woods et al., 1994, 1998) suggests that this is where the analogy with visual perceptual organization ends. In Woods and Alain (1993), participants were required to detect the presence of a deviant target of pre-specified frequency and location defined by greater intensity than the standard tones. Therefore, for any target combination of frequency and location (e.g. left high), non-targets could either share no (e.g. right low), one (e.g. left low or right high), or both (e.g. left high) features with the target. Stimuli were presented at relatively fast rates and both behavioural and auditory ERP measures were recorded. In short, stimuli that shared either the frequency or the location value of the target tone produced neural activity within different cortical areas, lending weight to the idea of segregated processing for different acoustic features (see also Alain et al., 2002b). Neural responses to stimuli that shared both location and frequency with the target had a scalp distribution approximately halfway between those elicited for location or frequency. Since these conjunction ERPs developing some 30–40 ms later than feature ERPs, the time-course for feature and conjunction clearly overlapped. Therefore, the conclusion was that rather than there being discrete stages for auditory feature and conjunction processing, these mechanisms actually might run in parallel with one another. Further fuel to the fire was added by Woods *et al.* (1998). Using just behavioural measures, they were able to show that under certain conditions, responses to targets defined by conjunctions of frequency and location could actually be faster than responses to targets defined by location alone. Clearly the observation of a *conjunction benefit* as opposed to *conjunction cost* is problematic for any dual-process theory of auditory perceptual organization in which conjunctive (i.e. integrative) processes are contingent upon featural processes.

A second line of research also argues that auditory feature integration is substantially different from visual feature integration. Here, the argument runs that the development of a conjunction- or object-based representation in audition does not require attention, and may in fact be a result of mechanisms similar to those involved in the processing of auditory features (Näätänen and Winkler, 1999; Winkler *et al.*, 2005). As we have already seen, the ERP component known as MMN may serve as a useful indicator of what stimulus properties are available in the absence of any systematic attention directed towards the auditory system; and there is a substantial body of work documenting that MMNs arise as a consequence of *featural* differences between standard and deviant stimuli such as frequency, amplitude, duration, location, stimulus-onset asynchrony, and inter-stimulus-interval (Paavilainen *et al.*, 1991; Lëvanen *et al.*, 1996; Deouell and Bentin, 1998), which are exactly those properties that enable acoustic segregation. However, other studies have shown that MMN may also be elicited when a deviant differs from standard tones simply with respect to a unique *combination* of auditory features. For example, using the auditory dimensions of frequency and location, Sussman *et al.* (1998) presented participants with standard tones of 600 Hz Right, 700 Hz Middle, and 800 Hz Left, and a single deviant tone which was constructed from a recombination of standard frequency and location values—600 Hz Left. Despite the deviant differing from the standards only with respect to the specific pairing of frequency and location, MMN was produced under conditions of inattention. Gomes *et al.* (1997) also provide evidence of conjunction MMN using combinations of frequency and intensity under similar conditions.

While both ERP and behavioural data point to the idea that integration between acoustic features can occur on a preattentive basis and so may be viewed as distinct from dominant theories of visual object formation (although see Houck and Hoffman, 1986), one problem with interpreting this kind of data is that there is a rather large discrepancy between the way in which integration has been studied, namely the predominant use of a simultaneous paradigm in vision and the predominant use of a sequential paradigm in audition. Although the use of a sequential presentation paradigm is justifiable on the basis that peripheral masking at the cochlea will occur with simultaneous presentation (Woods *et al.*, 1998), as Hall *et al.* (2000) have warned '. . . although some form of feature integration appears to be needed for sequential events, the nature of the perceptual processes may be quite different from those typically described for vision and implied in FIT . . .' (p. 1245). For example, it is not yet clear whether the representation derived from these early binding mechanisms observed by Woods and colleagues is sufficient for stimulus identification (Dyson and Quinlan, 2003). However, a range of experiments have been offered up in an attempt to identify the conditions under which feature-binding costs might manifest themselves under sequential conditions, thereby resuscitating the FIT analogy with audition.

Alternative accounts of the conjunction effect

In Fig. 8.8, the top two tables represent feature and conjunction conditions in one experiment in which a conjunction benefit was demonstrated (Dyson and Quinlan, 2003—Experiment 1) and the bottom two tables represent feature and conjunction conditions in a second experiment in which a conjunction cost was shown (Dyson and Quinlan, 2003—Experiment 2). In the first

DYSON & QUINLAN (2003) EXPERIMENT 1

FEATURE CONDITION   CONJUNCTION CONDITION

Q&H		Green	Blue	Orange
	Ex. 1	Left	Centre	Right
A	E	NT1	T1	
C	D	T2		T3
H	B		T4	NT2

Q&H		Green	Blue	Orange
	Ex. 1	Left	Centre	Right
A	E	NT1		
C	D			
H	B	T1		NT2

DYSON & QUINLAN (2003) EXPERIMENT 2

FEATURE CONDITION   CONJUNCTION CONDITION

	Ex. 2	Left	Centre	Right
	E	T1	NT1	
	D			NT2
	B			T2

	Ex. 2	Left	Centre	Right
	E	T1		NT1
	D			
	B	NT2		T2

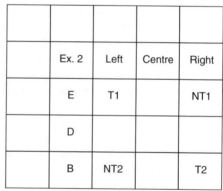

Fig. 8.8 Schematic representations of experimental designs that yield conjunction benefits (Dyson and Quinlan, 2003; Experiment 1, based on Quinlan and Humphreys (Q&H), 1987, Experiment 1) and conjunction costs (Dyson and Quinlan, 2003; Experiment 2) in audition. In both cases, acoustic stimuli varied in terms of location (left, centre, and right headphone presentation) and identity (vocal E, D, and B utterances). These manipulations show that transferring the same target/non-target relations from a visual simultaneous paradigm to an auditory sequential paradigm do not produce equivalent effects. NTx represent non-targets and Tx represent target stimuli.

example, the stimulus sets for feature and conjunction conditions were taken from a simultaneous visual paradigm reported in Quinlan and Humphreys, 1987—Experiment 1) and converted into a sequential auditory paradigm, replacing variation in colour (x-axis) and shape (y-axis) with location (x-axis) and vocal identity (y-axis), respectively. The conjunction benefit observed by Woods et al. (1998) was replicated, and focus turned to why auditory-feature binding might be acting in a different way to visual-feature binding. Comparing this study with the studies by Woods and colleagues, it was noted that differences in stimulus uncertainty (i.e. the number of stimuli) existed between feature and conjunction conditions. As Dyson and Quinlan (2003) stated: '. . . although this confound works against the standard experimental hypothesis of improved performance in the feature condition . . . it also provides a potential explanation of the data when the opposite result obtains . . .' (p. 258). Therefore, an alternative experiment was designed (depicted in the bottom half of Fig. 8.8) that equated for stimulus uncertainty and specifically the number of stimulus tokens per type. In having two targets and two non-targets, differences in stimulus uncertainty and stimulus exposure between feature and conjunction conditions could now be controlled for, and, under these conditions, a robust processing overhead associated with feature binding was observed. Two general conclusions then are that the perceptual integration mechanisms required for multiple stimulus features during sequential presentation are different from those required under conditions of simultaneous presentation (Hall et al., 2000), and that simple differences between the number of stimulus tokens presented across the various conditions in sequential auditory feature integration might go some way to account for the observation of either a conjunction benefit or conjunction cost. Dyson and Quinlan (2003) and Woods et al. (2001) discuss other potential methodological issues arising from the observation of conjunctive costs and benefits in audition.

Auditory illusory conjunctions

Further support for the idea that auditory perceptual organization is determined by a two-stage process, in which the independent pick-up of basic acoustic features is followed by their integration, is provided by the observation of illusory conjunctions (Treisman and Schmidt, 1982). Here, the assumption in audition is once again similar to that in vision, in that in contrast to featural processing, the processing of conjunctions operate under conditions of limited attentional capacity. Consequently, when the experimental situation demands more attentional capacity than is currently available, then there is an increased likelihood that features will become incorrectly bound to form an illusory conjunction. To return to the opening example, we might hear a drill flying overhead, or a seagull rumbling away in the distance.

One relatively famous form of auditory illusion that speaks to the notion of incorrect binding between acoustic features is the octave illusion (Deutsch, 1974). In its original form, participants were played for 20 seconds short (250 ms) pure tones that alternated in frequency as well as ear of delivery: when a high pitch (800 Hz) tone was played in the right ear a low pitch (400 Hz) was played in the left ear, and when a low pitch (400 Hz) tone was played in the right ear a high pitch (800 Hz) was played in the left ear. When asked to report what they heard, the majority of participants claimed that there had been a *single* tone changing with respect to both frequency and location, although not in the way of the original percept. Specifically at each presentation, the frequency of the single tone reported was determined by the dominant ear (typically the right ear for right handers), while the location of the tone reported was determined by the current location of the high tone (Deutsch and Roll, 1976). Therefore, a typical percept was a repeated high tone in the right ear followed by a low tone in the left ear (see Fig. 8.9). Although not originally discussed in terms of an auditory illusory conjunction, it is clear that these inaccurate perceptual combinations of location and frequency information support the idea that basic auditory attributes exist in some independent form such that they can be recombined into a percept that does not reflect actual acoustic stimulation (Deutsch and Roll, 1976). As discussion of this particular illusion 'characterized by large individual differences in perception' even by Deutsch (2004a, p. 355) rolls into a third decade, the interested reader is referred to the current dialogue between Chambers et al. (2004) and Deutsch (2004b), and the contrasting ideas that the octave illusion may be the result of either suppression (Deutsch, 2004a,b) or fusion (Chambers et al., 2004) between the two ears. What is particularly interesting, though, is that the octave illusion, like the studies

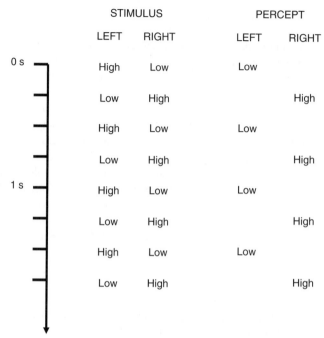

Fig. 8.9 A schematic of the original stimulus and the eventual percept resulting from the octave illusion. In the original stimulus, high-pitch and low-pitch tones alternate between left and right ears, although the eventual percept tends to be one of a single tone whose frequency is determined by the dominant ear and whose location is determined by the current location of the high tone (adapted from Deustch and Roll, 1976).

into auditory streaming, offer opportunities in which acoustic phenomenology can be matched to neurophysiological recordings on an individual-to-individual, trial-by-trial, and potentially even stimulus-by-stimulus basis.

Other recent work by Hall *et al.* (2000) and Thompson *et al.* (2001) have also demonstrated that such illusory combinations are possible using auditory features under more traditional paradigms. In Hall *et al.* (2000), participants were simultaneously presented with a number of spatially distributed auditory stimuli defined relative to pitch and instrument timbre. The design is particularly important here as the use of spatially distributed auditory stimuli closely resembles visual search, as opposed to sequential paradigms that have typically characterized the auditory feature integration literature. Responses were made to the presence of a pre-specified auditory target defined either by a single feature, or by the combination of features across the two dimensions. Whilst few errors were made in the feature case, the conjunction condition yielded substantial errors, especially when the auditory array contained recombinations of the pre-specified target stimulus. For example, participants may have been asked to listen out for a *262-Hz Trombone* sound, but when the auditory array contained a *262-Hz* violin sound and a *509-Hz Trombone* sound participants were more likely to (inaccurately) report the presence of that particular combination of features. In Thompson *et al.* (2001), tone sequences were employed and participants were presented with a primary sequence of two tones varying with respect to pitch and duration. This was followed by a probe tone, after which participants were required to indicate whether or not the probe tone had been present in the primary sequence. Again, error rates were generally low apart from the condition in which the probe tone was a recombination of features from the target sequence. For instance, the target sequence may have been a *G3 500-ms* note and a *C3 250-ms* note, whilst the probe tone was a *G3 250-ms* note.

Recently, however, some concern has been expressed as to the extent to which auditory illusory conjunctions are the product of differences in stimulus similarity between conditions, rather than errors in perceptual organization (Jamieson *et al.*, 2003). In this respect, alternative accounts related to stimulus similarity (e.g. Duncan and Humphreys, 1989) are being considered for auditory illusory conjunctions, in the same way similar accounts were put forward in accounting for the conjunction cost (see Dyson and Quinlan, 2003). Nevertheless, the work regarding auditory illusory conjunctions remain broadly consistent with a two-stage model of perceptual organization (although see Winkler *et al.*, 2005), in which features are processed in parallel and independently of one another, whilst feature-binding operates according to slower, capacity-limited operations (Treisman and Gelade, 1980; Bregman, 1990).

8.4 **Auditory *what* and *where* processing: A case study in perceptual organization**

We are now in a position to consolidate the previous discussions regarding perceptual segregation and integration by examining a popular distinction in the auditory literature between *what* and *where* processing. The basis for considering the processing of acoustic *what* and *where* information stems from similar distinctions in vision over 25 years ago (Ungerleider and Mishkin, 1982), stating that information regarding a visual object's identity (i.e. *what*) and location (i.e. *where*) are characterized by stronger activation in one of two processing streams within the brain, with *what* information predominately following a ventral pathway and *where* information predominately following a dorsal pathway. While the visual literature has since moved on to entertain a *how* (i.e. action-based) conceptualization of the dorsal stream (Milner and Goodale, 1995), work continues to investigate the putative separation of *what* and *where* systems as a general processing model which may be applied to the three major sensory systems (vision, audition, and touch; Kaas and Hackett, 1999).

8.4.1 **Neuroimaging data**

In addition to detailed theoretical arguments for the distinction between *what* and *where* pathways in audition (Kubovy and Van Valkenburg, 2001), there has also been an impressive array of neuroimaging work supporting this contention (e.g. Maeder *et al.*, 2001; Herrmann *et al.*, 2002). One early example is the work reported by Alain *et al.* (2001). Here, participants completed a same/different task under conditions of combined fMRI and ERP recording when stimulus classification was based upon either pitch (i.e. *what*) or location (i.e. *where*) information. Activation during pitch judgements was predominately found in the auditory cortex and the inferior frontal gyrus, whilst activation during location judgements was found in the posterior temporal cortex, parietal cortex, and superior frontal sulcus. As a result of these findings, Alain *et al.* (2001) concluded that there was good reason to support the basic conclusion that auditory *what* information predominately followed a ventral pathway, whilst auditory *where* information predominately followed a dorsal pathway.

Additional work continues to provide empirical evidence for the segregation of spatial and non-spatial acoustic information. For example, Ahveninen *et al.* (2006) recorded both haemodynamic and electromagnetic responses, while participants attended to the spatial or phonetic characteristics of Finnish vowels /æ/and /ø/ presented over headphones at 0° or 45° to the right. Pairs of stimuli were presented in which the second stimulus in the pair (probe) was different to the first stimulus in the pair (adaptor) according to spatial, phonetic, or neither attribute. In addition to responding to adaptor-probe pairings in these active conditions, participants were also exposed to the same stimuli under conditions of passive registration in order to assess the effect of task modulation on these putative pathways. Essentially, distinct pathways for spatial and phonetic activity were identified around 70–150 ms after stimulus onset, with spatial processing following a more posterior route and phonetic processing following a more anterior route. The selective nature of these pathways was also supported in that when adaptor and probe were not identical, neural adaptation was weaker in posterior regions during spatial change and weaker in anterior regions during phonetic change. Similar sentiments were conveyed by Altmann *et al.* (2007) in their analysis of haemodynamic and neuroelectric signals elicited by natural sound patterns (sheep and dog) presented 90° to the left or 90° to the right. The focus was once again on stimulus change and, particularly, the alteration of location, pattern, or location and pattern, after establishing runs of between 7 and 14 particular combinations of *what* and *where* information. Limiting their findings to the superior temporal lobe, Altmann *et al.* (2007) reported the activation of more anterior regions for pattern change and more posterior regions for location change.

De Santis *et al.* (2007) returned to the notion of pre-attentive segregation between spatial and non-spatial information, and examined ERP recordings purely in a passive condition. Participants were presented with sounds that varied again with respect to location (0° vs. 90°) and frequency (250 Hz vs. 500 Hz). Over a series of conditions, one attribute (e.g. location) was defined as 'relevant' in virtue of one value being presented over 80% of the trials (e.g. 0°) and the other over 20% of the trials (e.g. 90°), while the remaining attribute (e.g. frequency) was defined 'irrelevant' in virtue of both values (e.g. 250 Hz and 500 Hz) being presented with equal probability (50%). In this way, De Santis *et al.* (2007) were able to assess whether the auditory system was sensitive to acoustic context under conditions of passive registration (for a related demonstration of contextual sensitivity, see also Dyson *et al.*, 2005*b*). In an interesting comparison with Ahveninen *et al.* (2006), the authors found that between 100 and 160 ms after stimulus onset, *what* and *where* processing began to diverge, with selectivity for location information being found over the right temporoparietal cortices.

The likelihood of a dual-route model for auditory *what* and *where* information has been recently summarized by meta-analysis techniques (Arnott *et al.*, 2004). Figure 8.10 provides the image of interest, in which data from 36 studies (totalling 11 spatial and 27 non-spatial tasks) are evaluated with respect to five brain areas thought to be critical for the *what/where* distinction: inferior parietal lobe, anterior temporal lobe, posterior temporal lobe, inferior frontal lobe, and dorsal frontal lobe (after Rauschecker and Tian, 2000). Distinctions between spatial and

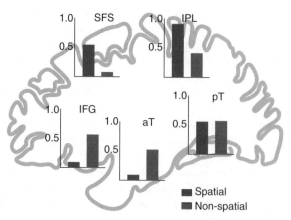

Fig. 8.10 Summary of a meta-analysis evaluating the dual-route hypothesis in audition (Arnott *et al.*, 2004). Distinctions between spatial and non-spatial processing begin after the posterior temporal lobe, in which *where* (i.e. spatial) processing follows a dorsal route to the superior frontal sulcus and *what* (i.e. non-spatial) processing follows a ventral route to the inferior frontal gyrus.

non-spatial processing begin after the posterior temporal lobe, with *where* (i.e. spatial) processing following a dorsal route to the superior frontal sulcus and *what* (i.e. non-spatial) processing following a ventral route to the inferior frontal gyrus. One remaining issue, however, is that the range of stimuli and tasks employed during non-spatial conditions are likely to be greater than the range of stimuli and tasks employed during non-spatial conditions, thereby leading to more diffuse activity along the ventral route for *what* processing relative to the dorsal route for *where* processing. Although Arnott *et al.* (2004) rule out the possibility of whether the predominance of linguistic stimuli in non-spatial tasks led to the differences between *what* and *where* pathways, it remains likely that the relatively limited remit of spatial processing relative to non-spatial processing led to a clearer dorsal pathway for *where* information. This comment is echoed by De Santis *et al.* (2007) who state that the acoustic attributes available for non-spatial segregation encompass a much wider range (e.g. frequency, intensity, duration) than those available during spatial segregation.

8.4.2 Alternative conceputalizations

However, it is also important to note that there is strong opposition to this view of auditory perceptual organization. In a development that strongly echoes the distinction between Ungerleider and Mishkin (1982) and Goodale and Milner (1992) in the visual literature, a debate has also opened up in the auditory literature as to the functionality of the dorsal stream (Romanski *et al.*, 2000). For example, Kaas and Hackett (1999) maintain that the dorsal stream is essentially concerned with the processing of localization akin to Ungerleider and Mishkin's (1982) *where* pathway. In contrast, Belin and Zatorre (2000) suggest that dorsal route processing is in fact concerned with *how* information. Although Belin and Zatorre (2000) in audition, and Goodale and Milner (1992) in vision, share the same label for the dorsal stream, substantially different conceptualizations of *how* information are employed in the two cases. In vision, *how* information represents details of motor control and action. In audition, *how* is interpreted as an analysis of spectral motion or the evolution of an auditory signal over time. Clearly, additional work is required to resolve the ambiguity associated with the functionality of the dorsal stream in auditory stimulus processing (Romanski *et al.*, 2000). Other researchers (Zattorre *et al.*, 2002; Hall, 2003) have seriously questioned the notion of dual-processing altogether. For example, Hall (2003) echoes previous comments regarding the ambiguity of the functionality of the dorsal route (i.e. *where* vs. *how*), but also goes on to point out that, in terms of anatomical independence, both the superior temporal sulcus and inferior temporal cortex offer opportunities for substantial interconnectivity between ventral and dorsal auditory streams. Zattorre *et al.* (2002) share a similar bleak view of this distinction and, whilst providing some support for dual-route processing in their own research, also state that these findings are equally compatible with a distributed account of processing in which the dorsal route may be able to process both *what* and *where* information (see also Table 8.1 in Clarke and Thiran, 2004, for a description of a *what* pathway that relies heavily on spatial processing).

8.4.3 Selective attention studies

So, what are we to make of all this? Does the processing of acoustic identity and location information require perceptual integration, or are the *what* and *where* of sound intimately linked at the earliest cortical level? Just like the neuroimaging literature, behavioural research examining the interaction between these acoustic dimensions has run into a similar impasse and two observations will suffice. In a series of studies reported by Dyson and Quinlan (2002; specifically see Experiment 3), evidence was provided for the separation of pitch and location information. Here, participants were required to distinguish between sequentially presented targets and non-targets under *within-dimensional* and *between-dimensional* conditions. In the within-dimensional conditions, all stimulus discriminations could be made on the basis of a single dimension (either pitch or location) across a block of trials, thereby enabling participants to essentially ignore the dimension that was irrelevant to the task. In the between-dimensional conditions, the locus of target/non-target discrimination varied randomly between dimensions across a block of trials, thereby prohibiting participants from ignoring either dimension in any systematic way. The idea was that if *what* and *where* were processed interdependently, then both pitch and location information should be recovered at each trial and there should be no cost in switching discriminative dimensions across trials in the between-dimensional conditions relative to the within-dimensional conditions. In contrast to this prediction, RTs in the within-dimensional conditions were found to be significantly faster than those in the between-dimensional conditions. This supported the idea that under certain experimental conditions, location information can be processed in the absence of pitch information and vice versa (see also Näätänen *et al.*, 1980, for further evidence regarding the independent processing of location and pitch). In a contrasting series of behavioural studies reported by Mondor *et al.* (1998), consistent evidence was provided for the interdependence between pitch and location information. In one experiment, participants were asked to categorize sounds according to either *what* or *where* information under two types of condition. In *control conditions*, participants only experienced variation along the task-relevant attribute while the task-irrelevant attribute was kept constant. In *selective attention conditions*, participants were exposed to stimuli that varied in both location and pitch (c.f. Garner, 1976). A general *filtering cost* was observed such that average responses were slower in the selective attention conditions relative to the control conditions. One additional and intriguing finding was that *what* and *where* information was equally disruptive when it irrelevantly varied in the selective attention conditions, despite overall differences in speed of processing for location and pitch such that *where* responses were completed faster than *what* responses (since replicated by Dyson and Quinlan, 2004). As a result, Mondor *et al.* (1998) argued that auditory *what* and *where* information is processed according to an attentional template (after Duncan and Humphreys, 1989), in which pitch and location information are always retrieved, even if some of this information is irrelevant to the task in hand. This close relationship between the retrieval of location and pitch information fits relatively uncomfortably with ideas of functionally separate dual-route processing. Taken at face value then, these two studies (Mondor *et al.*, 1998; Dyson and Quinlan, 2002) provide contradictory behavioural evidence for the perceptual organization of auditory *what* and *where* information, thereby reflecting similarly contrary findings in the neuroimaging literature.

In attempting to consolidate this literature, Dyson and Quinlan (2004) proposed a framework where the conditions under which the processing of acoustic location and identity information operate independently and interdependently were specified. This was achieved by a consideration of the trial-to-trial contingencies implicit within paradigms such as those used by Mondor *et al.* (1998). In Dyson and Quinlan (2004; Experiment 3), participants were played auditory stimuli that varied in both pitch (high, low) and headphone location (left, right), but once again participants were only required to categorize the stimuli on the basis of a single attribute. Two blocked conditions were completed in which responses were made either to pitch or location, and RT analysis was performed on the basis of trial pairs. Since both relevant and irrelevant dimensional values could change across consecutive trials, this yielded four inter-trial contingencies relative to the repetition (*Rep*) or change (*Chg*) of relevant (*Rel*) or irrelevant (*Irr*) dimensional values (see Fig. 8.11 for the matrix of possible outcomes). A theoretically important distinction was identified between pairs of trials in which the relevant dimensional value repeated across trials and cases where the relevant dimensional value changed (see also Huettel and Lockhead, 1999).

DYSON & QUINLAN (2004) EXPERIMENT 3

FREQUENCY CONDITION

TRIAL N+1

TRIAL N	Left High	Left Low	Right High	Right Low
Left High	RelRep-IrrRep	RelChg-IrrRep	RelRep-IrrChg	RelChg-IrrChg
Left Low	RelChg-IrrRep	RelRep-IrrRep	RelChg-IrrChg	RelRep-IrrChg
Right High	RelRep-IrrChg	RelChg-IrrChg	RelRep-IrrRep	RelChg-IrrRep
Right Low	RelChg-IrrChg	RelRep-IrrChg	RelChg-IrrRep	RelRep-IrrRep

LOCATION CONDITION

TRIAL N+1

TRIAL N	Left High	Left Low	Right High	Right Low
Left High	RelRep-IrrRep	RelRep-IrrChg	RelChg-IrrRep	RelChg-IrrChg
Left Low	RelRep-IrrChg	RelRep-IrrRep	RelChg-IrrChg	RelChg-IrrRep
Right High	RelChg-IrrRep	RelChg-IrrChg	RelRep-IrrRep	RelRep-IrrChg
Right Low	RelChg-IrrChg	RelChg-IrrRep	RelRep-IrrChg	RelRep-IrrRep

Fig. 8.11 Matrix to show all possible inter-trial contingencies in terms of task-relevant (*Rel*) and task-irrelevant (*Irr*) repetition (*Rep*) and change (*Chg*) in Dyson and Quinlan, 2004 (Experiment 3). All stimuli were combinations of *what* (frequency; high and low) and *where* (location; left and right lateralized headphone presentation) information. Failures of selective attention as represented by an RT difference between *IrrChg* minus *IrrRep* are only apparent when the task-relevant dimension is maintained, thereby demonstrating a constraint in observing the interdependence between *what* and *where* information in audition.

In this context, evidence for the interdependence between *what* and *where* information would be indexed by the failure of selective attention in terms of an RT difference between irrelevant dimensional value change (*IrrChg*) and irrelevant dimensional value repetition (*IrrRep*) trial pairs. However, an RT effect for irrelevant variation was contingent on the repetition of the task-relevant dimension, in that participants were significantly slower during *RelRep-IrrChg* trials relative to *RelRep-IrrRep* trials, but no such effect was found for relevant change trials due to the equivalence of RT between *RelChg-IrrRep* and *RelChg-IrrChg* responses.

These findings suggest that there can be no one way to talk about the relationship between *what* and *where* information in audition. The data from *RelRep* trials support the idea of Mondor *et al.* (1998) and interdependence between location and pitch in the auditory system. Conversely, the data from *RelChg* trials support the idea of Dyson and Quinlan (2002) and the independence of these acoustic properties. That is, both evidence for independence and interdependence between *what* and *where* information can be derived from the same experimental condition using exactly the same stimuli. In this way, the data provided by Dyson and Quinlan (2004) also supports the claim that any dual-route hypotheses (Arnott *et al.*, 2004) will eventually have to be consolidated with more distributed accounts of acoustic processing in which *what* and *where* information are closely related (Zattorre *et al.*, 2002). What will be critical for future research is the continued detailing of the temporal and configural relations under which these opposing states of interaction are more likely to manifest themselves.

8.5 Conclusions

The present chapter has reviewed some recent literature on auditory perceptual organization, examining the joint principles of segregation and integration and how these apply to organization both within acoustic attributes and between acoustic attributes. In the first case, segregation was shown to operate in both simultaneous and sequential sound presentation in the way tuned partials of a complex sound separate from mistuned partials in the former case, and in the way different frequencies separate from each other in the latter case. Integration was also in evidence for simultaneous sound presentation in the way multiple, harmonically related partials group together to form a unitary percept, and was also in evidence for sequential sound presentation in the way common frequencies group across time to form individual streams. Ideas of segregation and integration also applied to how different kinds of acoustic information were organized and whether additional processes were required to bind together assumedly disparate pieces of acoustic information. There was also some commentary on the extent to which ideas regarding perceptual organization in vision could apply to audition, specifically in relation to the distinction between feature and conjunction processing, and *what* and *where* processing pathways. This chapter will conclude by discussing one particular issue arising from neuroimaging research, in addition to providing some final thoughts about the structure of the auditory system itself.

8.5.1 Evaluating attention with ERPs

As is commonly stated, auditory ERPs confer an advantage over behavioural responses in terms of assessing the contribution of attention on auditory processing, since auditory ERPs can essentially be recorded in the absence of task and putatively outside the focus of attention. In such passive conditions, participants are invited to read a book or watch a muted, subtitled movie and told to simply ignore the sounds. However, there are a few problems with traditional passive conditions. First, there is no explicit assessment of the level of attention. In other words, we simply have no way of knowing to what extent participants 'sneak a little listen' (Carlyon, 2004, p. 468) to the ignored sounds. While this may seem innocuous enough, as Sussman *et al.* (2007) have warned, a brief moment of *covert attention* to the unattended channel may be all that one needs to start the stream segregation process. Therefore, while it is possible to manipulate relatively successfully the levels of attention during active tasks, it may be more difficult to draw clear distinctions between active and passive conditions. This may be somewhat less of a problem with experimental paradigms that employ the rapid presentation of large numbers of stimuli (e.g. Dyson and Alain, 2004; Dyson *et al.*, 2005b), where the systematic influence of attention is likely to be both marginalized and equally distributed across the conditions of interest. Second, there are the less-discussed issues of order effects. ERP correlates of attention are traditionally assessed by comparing various active (or task-based) conditions with a passive (or non-task-based) condition. In comparing these two types of condition, we can be led to relatively non-contentious conclusions, such as group-average ERP amplitudes to auditory stimuli recorded during the passive condition being significantly smaller than those during the active condition, but also to slightly more controversial statements, such as the automaticity of perceptual organization given the equivalence between passive and active ERP morphology. To control for order effects, it is necessary to counterbalance the order of these conditions, but this leads to the alternative problem of half the participants having the active task still 'ringing in their ears' while the passive condition is ongoing. A direct assessment of whether counterbalancing produces its own kind of problems can be remedied by entering task-order as an additional factor into future analyses comparing 'passive' versus 'active' auditory perceptual organization.

8.5.2 What guides the auditory system?

As was noted in the section on feature and conjunction processing, in visual FIT it is generally agreed that due to the spatiotopic organization of the visual system, feature and master maps are organized in terms of location, and it is attention directed at a particular position that gives rise to integrated features. With respect to auditory FIT, the application of spatially organized maps has been questioned since auditory spatial acuity is lower in resolution than visual spatial acuity (Woods and Alain, 2001). Consequently, researchers have argued for the use of guiding mechanisms other than location for auditory conjunction search (although see Hall *et al.*, 2000). For example, Woods *et al.* (2001) suggest that frequency serves as the acoustic property upon which attention must be focused before auditory features can be bound. That is, whilst visual features remain unbound in the absence of attention towards a point in space, auditory features remain unbound in the absence of attention directed on a specific frequency. Support for this frequency-based FIT (FB-FIT) is derived from the observation that the detection of a single frequency presented over multiple spatial positions is faster than the detection of multiple frequencies presented over a single spatial position (Woods *et al.*, 1998). What is not currently clear, however, is what happens when one of the attributes currently being integrated also happens to be the (putative) organizational factor in the feature integration model. This is, in part, due to a limited conceptualization of integration in which typically only two acoustic features are bound together (although see Woods and Alain, 2001), and further work will have to systematically address whether the binding mechanisms observed for basic features are equivalent to those when features that are critical to the organization of the perceptual system in question are invoked.

Further support for the unique nature of frequency information has also been hinted at in the behavioural studies of Mondor *et al.* (1998) and Dyson and Quinlan (2004). In both cases, a failure of selective attention was observed in processing location when variation in frequency was irrelevant to the task. However, the critical observation here was that in both experiments, pitch responses were overall significantly slower than location responses. Given standard horse-race accounts of processing (e.g. Mordkoff and Yantis, 1991), this simply should not be the case, and suggests a level of influence for frequency upon other acoustic attributes that transcends behavioural metrics of processing speed.

However, despite overwhelming evidence for tonotopic perceptual organization in audition, alternative conceptualizations have been put forward (e.g. Shamma, 2001). For example, Handel (1988*a*) argues that prioritizing the processing of location confers an evolutionary advantage that the processing of frequency does not. The idea that location may also act as a critical guiding factor in auditory perception is supported by additional evidence in which differences in ERP peak amplitude have been observed in the absence of behavioural differences. For example, Schröger and Wolff (1997) demonstrated that location MMN peaked sooner than frequency MMN, despite the differences in discriminability between spatial (300 μs) and non-spatial (60 Hz) values failing to reach statistical significance when participants were asked to detect location and pitch deviants. A similar finding was also observed by Altmann *et al.* (2007), who observed faster neuroelectric responses for location than for spectral pattern information. Again, the intriguing aspect of the data was that ERP effects were observed in the absence of significant behavioural differences in the detection of location change (556 ms) and spectral pattern change (547 ms). Ahveninen *et al.* (2007) also observed that *where* pathway activation occurred some 30 ms before *what* pathway activation, despite attempts to control for the relative discriminability between these attributes. This kind of data underscore that neuroimaging techniques are beginning to provide crucial insights into sensory system processes that have hitherto been unobservable with behavioural data. Nevertheless, future research needs to focus on assessing the validity of such an auditory 'anchoring' model in which the organization of auditory perceptual organization is laid bare, and more specifically, when and which kind of properties operate as effective guides for the rest of the auditory system (see Woods *et al.*, 2001).

Therefore, just by considering essentially two acoustic attributes (frequency and location) it has been possible to cover a range of materials and to detail some of the current complexities and ambiguities within the perceptual organization literature. Whilst *time* has been mentioned in passing, it is important to note that there are also additional models of acoustic perceptual organization that greatly emphasize the temporal aspects of auditory processing either in isolation (Large and Jones, 1999) or in combination with other properties (Griffiths and Warren, 2002). In short though, it will be the convergence of psychophysical, cognitive, and neuroimaging techniques that will allow us to fully appreciate the complexity of the auditory scene analysis problem in all its forms.

References

Ahveninen, J., Jääskelälnen, I. P, Raij, T., Bonmassar, G., Devore, S., Hämälälnen, M., Levanen, S., *et al.* (2006). Task-modulated 'what' and 'where' pathways in human auditory cortex. *Proceedings of the National Academy of Science USA* **103**:14608–13.

Alain, C. (2007). Breaking the wave: Effects of attention and learning on concurrent sound perception. *Hearing Research* **229**:225–36.

Alain, C. and Arnott, S. R. (2000). Selectively attending to auditory objects. *Frontiers in Bioscience* **5**:202–12.

Alain, C. and Izenberg, A. (2003). Effects of attentional load on auditory scene analysis. *Journal of Cognitive Neuroscience* **15**:1063–73.

Alain, C., Arnott, S. R., Hevenor, S., Graham, S., and Grady, C. L. (2001). 'What' and 'where' in the human auditory cortex. *Proceedings of the National Academy of Sciences USA* **98**:12301–6.

Alain, C., Schuler, B. M., and McDonald, K. L. (2002*a*). Neural activity associated with distinguishing concurrent auditory object. *Journal of the Acoustical Society of America* **111**:990–5.

Alain, C., Bernstein, L. J., Cortese, F., He, Y., and Zipursky, R. B. (2002*b*). Deficits in automatically detecting changes in conjunction of auditory feature in patients with schizophrenia. *Psychophysiology* **39**:599–606.

Altmann, C. F., Bledowski, C., Wibral, M., and Kaiser, J. (2007). Processing of location and pattern changes of natural sounds in the human auditory cortex. *NeuroImage* **35**:1192–200.

Arnott, S. R., Binns, M. A., Grady, C. L., and Alain, C. (2004). Assessing the auditory dual-pathway model in humans. *Neuroimage* **22**:401–8.

Belin, P. and Zatorre, R. J. (2000). 'What', 'where' and 'how' in auditory cortex. *Nature Neuroscience* **3**:965–6. [Letter to the editor.]

Bregman, A. S. (1990). *Auditory Scene Analysis.* Cambridge, MA: MIT Press.

Bregman, A. S. and Steiger, H. (1980). Auditory streaming and vertical localization: Interdependence of 'what' and 'where' decisions in audition. *Perception and Psychophysics* **28**:539–46.

Carlyon, R. P. (2004). How the brain separates sound. *Trends in Cognitive Sciences* **1**:465–71.

Carlyon, R. P., Cusack, R., Foxton, J. M., and Robertson, I. H. (2001). Effects of attention and unilateral neglect on auditory stream segregation. *Journal of Experimental Psychology: Human Perception and Performance* **27**:115–27.

Chambers, C. D., Mattingley, J. B., and Moss, S. A. (2004). Reconsidering evidence for the suppression model of the octave illusion. *Psychonomic Bulletin and Review* **11**:642–66.

Clarke, S. and Thiran, A. B. (2004). Auditory neglect: what and where in auditory space. *Cortex* **40**:291–300.

Cohen Y. E. and Andersen, R. A. (2004). Multimodal spatial representations in the primate parietal lobe. In *Crossmodal Space and Crossmodal Attention* (ed. C. Spence and J. Driver), pp. 154–76. Oxford: Oxford University Press.

Cramer, E. M. and Huggins, W. H. (1958). Creation of pitch through binaural interaction. *Journal of the Acoustical Society of America* **30**:412–17.

Cusack, R., Carlyon, R. P., and Robertson, I. H. (2000). Neglect between but not within auditory objects. *Journal of Cognitive Neuroscience* 12:1056–65.

Cusack, R., Deeks, J., Aikman, G., and Carlyon, R. P. (2004). Effects of location, frequency region, and time course of selective attention on auditory scene analysis. *Journal of Experimental Psychology: Human Perception and Performance* 30:643–56.

Darwin, C. J. (1997). Auditory grouping. *Trends in Cognitive Sciences* 1:327–33.

Darwin, C. J. and Ciocca, V. (1992). Grouping in pitch perception: effects of onset asynchrony and ear of presentation of a mistuned component. *Journal of the Acoustical Society of America* 91:3381–90.

Darwin, C. J., Ciocca, V., and Sandell, G. J. (1994). Effects of frequency and amplitude modulation on the pitch of a complex tone with a mistuned harmonic. *Journal of the Acoustical Society of America* 95:2631–6.

Darwin, C. J., Hukin, R. W., and Al-Khatib, B. Y. (1995). Grouping in pitch perception: Evidence for sequential constraints. *Journal of the Acoustical Society of America* 98:880–5.

De Santis, L., Clarke, S., and Murray, M. M. (2007). Automatic and intrinsic auditory 'what' and 'where' processing in humans revealed by electrical neuroimaging. *Cerebral Cortex* 17:9–17.

Deouell, L. Y. and Bentin, S. (1998). Variable cerebral responses to equally distinct deviance in four auditory dimensions: A mismatch negativity study. *Psychophysiology* 35:745–54.

Deutsch, D. (1974). An auditory illusion. *Nature* 251:307–9.

Deutsch, D. (2004a). The octave illusion revisited again. *Journal of Experimental Psychology: Human Perception and Performance* 30:355–64.

Deutsch, D. (2004b). Reply to 'Reconsidering evidence for the suppression model of the octave illusion', by C. D. Chambers, J. B. Mattingley, and S. A. Moss. *Psychonomic Bulletin and Review* 11:667–76.

Deutsch, D. and Roll, P. L. (1976). Separate 'what' and 'where' decision mechanisms in processing a dichotic tonal sequence. *Journal of Experimental Psychology: Human Perception and Performance* 2:23–9.

Duncan, J. and Humphreys, G. W. (1989). Visual search and stimulus similarity. *Psychological Review* 96:433–58.

Dyson, B. J. and Alain, C. (2004). Representation of concurrent auditory objects in human auditory cortex. *Journal of the Acoustical Society of America* 115:280–9.

Dyson, B. J. and Quinlan, P. T. (2002). Within- and between-dimensional processing in the auditory modality. *Journal of Experimental Psychology: Human Perception and Performance* 28:1483–98.

Dyson, B. J. and Quinlan, P. T. (2003). Feature and conjunction processing in the auditory modality. *Perception and Psychophysics* 65:254–72.

Dyson, B. J. and Quinlan, P. T. (2004). Stimulus processing constraints in audition. *Journal of Experimental Psychology: Human Perception and Performance* 30:1117–31.

Dyson, B. J., Alain, C., and He, Y. (2005a). Effect of visual attentional load on auditory scene analysis. *Cognitive, Affective and Behavioral Neuroscience* 5:319–38.

Dyson, B. J., Alain, C., and He, Y. (2005b). I've heard it all before: Perceptual invariance represented by early cortical auditory evoked responses. *Cognitive Brain Research* 23:457–60

Garner, W. R. (1976). Interaction of stimulus dimensions in concept and choice processes. *Cognitive Psychology* 8:98–123.

Gibson, J. J. (1966). *The Senses Considered as Perceptual Systems.* Boston: Houghton Mifflin.

Gomes, H., Bernstein, R., Ritter, W., Vaughan, H. G. Jr, and Miller, J. (1997). Storage of feature conjunctions in transient auditory memory. *Psychophysiology* 34:712–16.

Goodale, M. A. and Milner, A. D. (1992). Separate visual pathways for perception and action. *Trends in Neurosciences* 15:20–5.

Griffiths, T. D. and Warren, J. D. (2002). The planum temporale as a computational hub. *Trends in Neuroscience* 25:348–53.

Griffiths, T. D. and Warren, J. D. (2004). What is an auditory object? *Nature Reviews Neuroscience* 5:887–92.

Hall, D. A. (2003). Auditory pathways: are 'what' and 'where' appropriate? *Current Biology* 13:R406–8.

Hall, M. D., Pastore, R. E., Acker, B. E., and Huang, W. (2000). Evidence for auditory feature integration with spatially distributed items. *Perception and Psychophysics* 62:1243–57.

Handel, S. (1988a). Space is to time as vision is to audition: seductive but misleading. *Journal of Experimental Psychology: Human Perception and Performance* 14:315–17.

Handel, S. (1988b). No one analogy is sufficient: rejoinder to Kubovy. *Journal of Experimental Psychology: Human Perception and Performance* 14:321.

Hartmann, W. M., McAdams, S., and Smith, B. K. (1990). Hearing a mistuned harmonic in an otherwise periodic complex tone. *Journal of Acoustical Society of America* 88:1712–24.

Hautus, M. J. and Johnson, B. W. (2005). Object-related brain potentials associated with perceptual segregation of a dichotically-embedded pitch. *Journal of the Acoustical Society of America* 116:275–80.

Herrmann, C. S., Senkowski, D., Maess, B., and Friederici, A. D. (2002). Spatial versus object feature processing in human auditory cortex: a magnetoencephalographic study. *Neuroscience Letters* 334:37–40.

Houck, M. R. and Hoffman, J. E. (1986). Conjunction of color and form without attention: evidence from an orientation-contingent color aftereffect. *Journal of Experimental Psychology: Human Perception and Performance* 12:186–99.

Huettel, S. A. and Lockhead, G. R. (1999). Range effects of an irrelevant dimension on classification. *Perception and Psychophysics* 61:1624–45.

Jamieson, R. K., Thompson, W. F., Cuddy, L. L., and Mewhort, D. J. K. (2003). Do conjunction errors in auditory recognition imply feature migration? *Canadian Journal of Experimental Psychology* 57:125–30.

Johnson, B. W., Hautus, M. J., Duff, D. J., and Clapp, W. C. (2007). Sequential processing of interaural timing differences for sound source segregation and spatial localization: Evidence from event-related cortical potentials. *Psychophysiology* 44:541–51.

Jones, M. R. and Boltz, M. (1989). Dynamic attending and responses to time. *Psychological Review* 96:459–91.

Kaas, J. H. and Hackett, T. A. (1999). 'What' and 'where' processing in auditory cortex. *Nature Neuroscience* 2:1045–7.

Kubovy, M. (1981). Concurrent-pitch segregation and the theory of indispensable attributes. In *Perceptual Organization* (ed. M. Kubovy and J. R. Pomerantz), pp. 55–98. Hillsdale, NJ: Lawrence Erlbaum Associates.

Kubovy, M. (1988). Should we resist the seductiveness of the space:time::vision:audition analogy? *Journal of Experimental Psychology: Human Perception and Performance* 14:318–20.

Kubovy, M. and Van Valkenburg, D. (2001). Auditory and visual objects. *Cognition* 80:97–126.

Kubovy, M. and Van Valkenburg, D. (2003). In defence of the theory of indispensable attributes. *Cognition* 87:225–33.

Large, E. W. and Jones, M. R. (1999). The dynamics of attending: How people track time-varying events. *Psychological Review* 106:119–59.

Lëvanen, S., Ahonen, A., Hari, R., McEvoy, L., and Sams, M. (1996). Deviant auditory stimuli activate human left and right auditory cortex differently. *Cerebral Cortex* 6:288–96.

Maeder, P. P., Meult, R. A., Adriani, M., Bellman, A., Fornari, E., Thiran, J. P., *et al.* (2001). Distinct pathways involved in sound recognition and localization: A human fMRI study. *NeuroImage* 14:802–16.

Moore, B. C. J. and Gockel, H. (2002). Factors influencing sequential stream segregation. *Acta Acustica/Acustica* 88:320–33.

Moore, B. C. J., Peters, R. W., and Glasberg, B. R. (1985). Thresholds for the detection of inharmonicity in complex tones. *Journal of the Acoustical Society of America* 77:1861–7.

Moore, B. C. J., Glasberg, B. R., and Peters, R. W. (1986). Thresholds for hearing mistuned partials as separate tones inharmonic complexes. *Journal of Acoustical Society of America* **80**:479–83.

Mondor, T. A., Zatorre, R. J., and Terrio, N. A. (1998). Constraints on the selection of auditory information. *Journal of Experimental Psychology: Human Perception and Performance* **24**:66–79.

Mordkoff, J. T. and Yantis, S. (1991). An interactive race model of divided attention. *Journal of Experimental Psychology: Human Perception and Performance* **17**:520–38.

Milner, A. D. and Goodale, M. A. (1995). *The Visual Brain in Action*. Oxford: Oxford University Press.

Näätänen, R. and Winkler, I. (1999). The concept of auditory stimulus representation in cognitive neuroscience. *Psychological Review* **125**:826–59.

Näätänen, R., Porkka, R., Merisalo, A., and Ahtola, S. (1980). Location vs. frequency of pure tones as a basis of fast discrimination. *Acta Psychologica* **44**:31–40.

Neuhoff, J. (2003). Pitch variation is unnecessary (and sometimes insufficient) for the formation of auditory objects. *Cognition* **87**:219–24.

Paavilainen, P., Alho, K., Reinikainen, K., Sams, M., and Näätänen, R. (1991). Right hemisphere dominance of different mismatch negativities. *Electroencephalography and Clinical Neurophysiology* **78**:466–79.

Picton, T. W., Alain, C., Otten, L., Ritter, W., and Achim, A. (2000). Mismatch negativity: Different water in the same river. *Audiology and NeuroOtology* **5**:111–39.

Pulvermüller, F., Shtyrov, Y., Ilmoniemi, R. J., and Marslen-Wilson, W. D. (2006). Tracking speech comprehension in space and time. *NeuroImage* **31**:1297–305.

Quinlan, P. T. (2004). Visual feature integration theory: past, present, and future. *Psychological Bulletin* **129**:643–73.

Quinlan, P. T. and Humphreys, G. W. (1987). Visual search for targets defined by combinations of color, shape, and size: An examination of the task constraints of feature and conjunction searches. *Perception and Psychophysics* **41**:455–72.

Rauschecker, J. P. and Tian, B. (2000). Mechanisms and streams for processing of 'what' and 'where' in auditory cortex. *Proceedings of the National Academy of Sciences USA* **97**:11800–6.

Ritter, W., Deacon, D., Gomes, H., Javitt, D. C., and Vaughan, H. G. Jr, (1995). The mismatch negativity of event-related potentials as a probe of transient auditory memory: A review. *Ear and Hearing* **16**:52–67.

Romanski, L. M., Tian, B., Fritz, J. B., Mishkin, M., Goldman-Rakic, P. S., and Rauschecker, J. P. (2000). 'What', 'where' and 'how' in auditory cortex. *Nature Neuroscience* **3**:965–6. [Letter to the editor.]

Schröger, E. and Wolff, C. (1997). Fast preattentive processing of location: a functional basis for selective listening in humans. *Neuroscience Letters* **232**:5–8.

Shamma, S. (2001). On the role of space and time in auditory processing. *Trends in Cognitive Sciences* **5**:340–8.

Snyder, J. S. and Alain, C. (2007). Towards a neurophysiological theory of auditory stream segregation. *Psychological Bulletin* **133**:780–99.

Snyder, J. S., Alain, C., and Picton, T. W. (2006). Effects of attention on neuroelectric correlates of auditory stream segregation. *Journal of Cognitive Neuroscience* **18**:1–13.

Sussman, E. (2005). Integration and segregation in auditory scene analysis. *Journal of the Acoustical Society of America* **117**:1285–98.

Sussman, E., Gomes, H., Nousak, J. M. K., Ritter, W., and Vaughan, H. G., Jr, (1998). Feature conjunctions and auditory sensory memory. *Brain Research* **793**:95–102.

Sussman, E., Ritter, W. and Vaughan, H. G., Jr, (1999). An investigation of the auditory streaming effects using event-related potentials. *Psychophysiology* **36**:22–34.

Sussman, E. S., Horvath, J., Winkler, I., and Orr, M. (2007). The role of attention in the formation of auditory streams. *Perception and Psychophysics* **69**:136–52.

Thompson, W. F., Hall, M. D., and Pressing, J. (2001). Illusory conjunctions of pitch and duration in unfamiliar tone sequences. *Journal of Experimental Psychology: Human Perception and Performance* 27:128–40.

Treisman, A. and Gelade, G. (1980). A feature-integration theory of attention. *Cognitive Psychology* 12:97–136.

Treisman, A. and Schmidt, N. (1982). Illusory conjunctions in the perception of objects. *Cognitive Psychology* 14:107–41.

Ungerleider, L. G. and Mishkin, M. (1982). Two cortical visual systems. In *Analysis of Visual Behavior* (ed. D. J. Ingle, M. A. Goodale, and R. J. W. Mansfield), pp. 549–86. Cambridge, MA: MIT Press.

Welch, R. B. and Warren, D. H. (1980). Immediate perceptual response to intersensory discrepancy. *Psychological Bulletin* 88:638–67.

Winkler, I., Czigler, I., Sussman, E., Hórváth, J., and Balázs, L. (2005). Preattentive binding of auditory and visual stimulus features. *Journal of Cognitive Neuroscience* 17:320–9.

Wolfe, J. M. (1998). Visual search. In *Attention* (ed. H. Pashler), pp. 13–73. Hove: Psychology Press.

Woods, D. L. and Alain, C. (1993). Feature processing during high-rate auditory selective attention. *Perception and Psychophysics* 53:391–402.

Woods, D. L. and Alain, C. (2001). Conjoining three auditory features: An event-related brain potential study. *Journal of Cognitive Neuroscience* 13:492–509.

Woods, D. L., Alho, K., and Algazi, A. (1994). Stages of auditory feature conjunction: An event-related brain potential study. *Journal of Experimental Psychology: Human Perception and Performance* 20:81–94.

Woods, D. L., Alain, C., and Ogawa, K. H. (1998). Conjoining auditory and visual features during high-rate serial presentation: Processing and conjoining two features can be faster than processing one. *Perception and Psychophysics* 60:239–49.

Woods, D. L., Alain, C., Diaz, R., Rhodes, D., and Ogawa, K. H. (2001). Location and frequency cues in auditory selective attention. *Journal of Experimental Psychology: Human Perception and Performance* 27:65–74.

Zattorre, R. J., Bouffard, M., Ahad, P., and Belin, P. (2002). Where is 'where' in the human auditory cortex. *Nature Neuroscience* 5:905–9.

Chapter 9

Speech perception

Chris Darwin

Speech is conveniently located midway between thought and
action, where it often substitutes for both.
John Andrew Holmes (1927)

Speech serves us well. It requires little energy, it remains sufficiently intelligible in appalling listening conditions, it communicates our thoughts, emotional state, and social background, and is
learned well before we have to go to school. Its robustness, versatility, and flexibility are probably
a result of relatively recent species-specific adaptations building on substrates of sound production and perception that had evolved both separately and together over a much longer period.
This chapter will be predominantly concerned with the acoustic, auditory, and phonetic aspects
of speech perception. It will not attempt to cover the rich and rewarding areas concerned with
lexical access from speech (Gaskell and MarslenWilson, 1998; Stevens, 2002), and it will deal only
briefly with prosodic aspects of speech—the changes in pitch, rhythm, and stress that highlight
important information in speech and modulate the lexical (van Donselaar *et al.*, 2005), syntactic
(Cutler *et al.*, 1997), and pragmatic processing of an utterance as well as contributing to its emotional content. Previous reviews of the areas covered in this chapter are also available and will help
the reader to augment the necessarily cursory treatment given here to some areas (Diehl *et al.*,
2004; Galantucci *et al.*, 2006).

9.1 The sound of speech

The nature of the sound that reaches the ear of the listener from a talker is the result of very many
different influences, including both *intrinsic* factors, such as the way that the talker's vocal tract
moves, and *extrinsic* ones, such as the acoustics of the room or the incidental presence of other
talkers or sound sources (Fig. 9.1). Historically, early investigations during the 1940s and 1950s
focused on the intelligibility of speech in the face of extrinsic factors, such as noise (e.g. at cocktail
parties) and filtering. Later investigations catalogued the cues to phonetic categories and revealed
intrinsic factors, such as co-articulation. More recent work, motivated partly by the problem of
automatically recognizing speech in noise, moved back to problems caused by extrinsic factors,
such as how to separate speech from structured background sounds such as from another talker.

9.1.1 Intrinsic influences

The invention of the spectrograph in the 1940s showed the sound structure of speech to be quite
unlike our naïve, literate concept of it. Unlike music, where discretely written notes translate into
discrete sounds which become discrete perceptual entities, speech lacks discrete sounds. It is not
difficult to understand why.

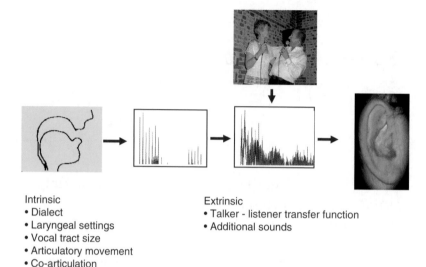

Fig. 9.1 When a talker speaks to a listener, the sound emerging from the talker's mouth is a result of intrinsic influences on the speech such as co-articulation, dialect, and vocal-tract length. But the sound arriving at the ear of the listener has been modified by the environmental transfer function from the talker to the listener, and has added to it whatever arbitrary extraneous sounds happen to be present.

We speak by exciting a variably shaped tube. We can excite this tube, the vocal tract, with brief, discrete sounds, as when we sing short *staccato* musical notes, but in normal speech the excitation is more continuous, as are the changes in shape of the tube, so the emerging sound is also continuous. The excitation either can be a buzzy sound that has a definite pitch or it can be noise. Both can be produced by the vocal cords in the larynx: they can either vibrate as the air flows between them to give a buzz, or remain static and cause the air to be noisily turbulent producing aspiration. Normal speech is a mixture of these voiced and voiceless sources; whisper has only the voiceless noise. In addition, for some consonants, such as those in 'sheaths', the vocal cords are silent and the noise is produced by constrictions elsewhere in the vocal tract. For others, such as the voiced fricatives ('There's veg …'), the vocal cords vibrate *and* there is a supralaryngeal constriction, giving a buzzy noise. Acoustically, the fricatives are rather complex (as are the nasal vowels and consonants where a second tube is added to the filter), but the simple laryngeal source followed by a single tube vocal-tract filter models most vowels and non-fricative consonants well.

Broadly speaking, there is continuous excitation during speech, with the larynx switching between periodic voiced buzz, and aspiration hiss, and fricatives coming and going. The only silence that normally happens in speech is during pauses (e.g. for breath) and during stop consonants, where the mouth is completely shut-off, stopping the flow of air that is necessary for sound production. Acoustically, the periodic buzz produced by the vibrating vocal cords consists of a series of harmonically related frequency components that are integer multiples of the rate at which the vocal cords are vibrating. If the vocal cords are vibrating at F0, then harmonic frequencies F0, 2 F0, 3 F0, etc. will be present in the sound coming from the vocal cords. If the vocal cords are producing a hiss, then the noise will consist of a random mixture of all frequencies and will not have harmonic structure.

The almost continuous source of sound from the vocal cords is filtered by the continually changing vocal tract. Movements of the tongue, jaw, and lips change the shape of the tract and consequently change its resonant frequencies (or formants), which amplify frequencies in the sound source that are near to them (Figs 9.2 and 9.3). Since the vocal tract is mainly made of compliant flesh, these formant resonances have a relatively broad bandwidth (c. 100 Hz), and since a (male adult) vocal tract is about 17.5-cm long, they occur on average about every 1000 Hz (odd half-wavelengths). If you say the neutral vowel /ʌ/ (as in southern English 'mud') your vocal tract has a roughly constant cross-sectional area along its length from the larynx to the lips, and the formants occur at roughly 500 Hz, 1500 Hz, 2500 Hz, etc. Moving your tongue, jaw, or lips changes the cross-sectional area profile and consequently the formants change their frequencies. Although the sound source changes abruptly from buzz to noise (and fricatives come and go), changes in formant frequencies are moderately continuous with occasional abrupt changes as stops, fricatives, or nasals start or stop. Consequently, a sentence such as 'We were away a year ago' has just a single episode of (near) silence during the stop /g/ of 'ago', otherwise it is a continuous voiced sound with smoothly changing formant frequencies.

The smooth change of the acoustic speech signal is in marked contrast to the discrete set of symbols that we are familiar with in alphabetic text. Speech is much more like semaphore than it is like alphabetic or phonetic text. In semaphore, each alphabetic letter is represented by a different angular arrangement of the two arms—like a particular time on a clock. The signaller moves his arms from one position to the next and this movement (or at least that of the flags he is holding) is visible to the observer. For a skilled signaller (and receiver) the arms will be in continuous motion. So it is with speech—the jaw, lips, and tongue move continuously and we hear the continuously changing acoustic consequence of that movement. The formant transitions generated by this movement carry a major burden in conveying the phonetic message (Strange et al., 1983; Strange 1987). Speech emphatically does not consist of a sequence of steady-state sounds. How we segment the continuous flow of speech into the discrete symbols of language is an unsolved problem.

The problem is made more difficult by the phenomenon of co-articulation. For most consonants (and sometimes for vowels too) their articulatory specification is incomplete. For example, in order to produce a bilabial stop (/b/ or /p/) you need to close your lips but your tongue can be just about anywhere, except between your lips. Consequently, the sound that emerges as your lips close and open (especially the formant transitions) will vary depending on where your tongue happens to be. In a simple vowel–consonant–vowel sequence such as 'abbey', the tongue will be moving from whatever vowel precedes the stop to whatever follows it (Öhman, 1966). So, the global configuration of the vocal tract at any instant reflects the co-articulation of more than one phonetic segment (Fig. 9.4). Such co-articulatory effects can extend for considerable distances: the sound of the /s/ in /stru/ can reflect lips rounded for /u/ while that in /stri/ the lips spreading in anticipation of /i/. Although the co-articulation of /b/ with some segment that specifies where the tongue should be is necessary, effects like the lip-rounding or spreading of /s/ may occur or not depending on language-specific or individual stylistic factors. For example, British English vowels may be optionally nasalized by co-articulation with neighbouring nasal consonants (such as /m/, /n/), but in French such nasalization could change the meaning of the word and so may be blocked. Co-articulation can extend in both directions (Mann and Soli, 1991). Lip-rounding of /s/ before /u/ is anticipatory, but, for example, the lip-rounding of /r/ can carry over to a following stop (Mann, 1980).

If co-articulation did not exist, the sound of speech could be thought of as an interpolation between distinct target states corresponding to the consonants and vowels of the language. But co-articulation undermines the idea of invariant acoustic targets. The articulatory manoeuvres

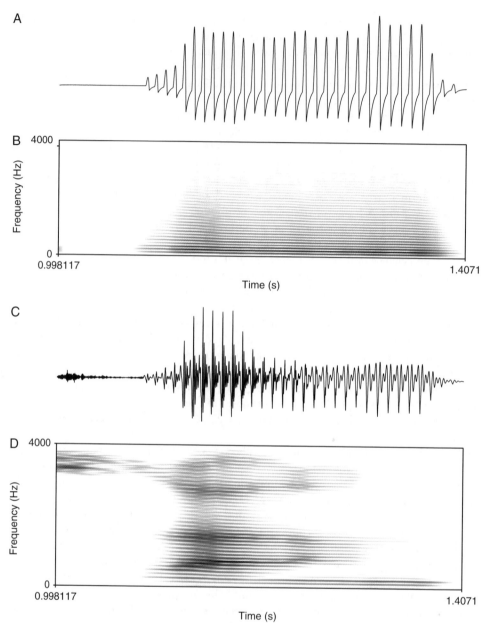

Fig. 9.2 Waveforms and their narrowband spectrograms produced by formant synthesis of the word 'sound'. A and B illustrate the sound emerging from the larynx, C and D from the lips. The periodic waveform emerging from the larynx (A) is roughly triangular with harmonic structure; the amplitude of the harmonics decreases smoothly with increasing frequency (B). The waveform emerging from the lips (C) has a more complex structure caused by the resonant frequencies of the vocal tract or 'formants' which appear as a darkening of the harmonics in D. Note that the noise for the 's' of 'sound' does not originate at the larynx and so is not present in A or B.

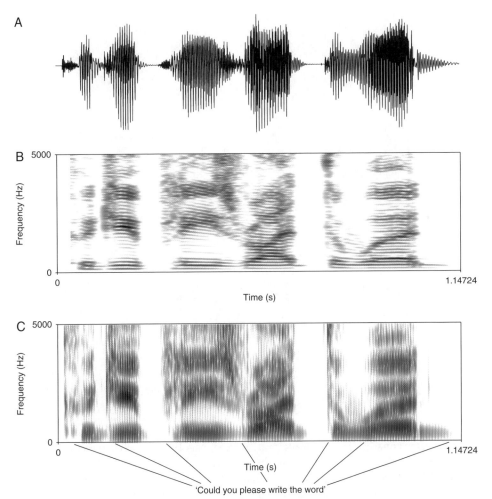

Fig. 9.3 The waveform at the lips (A) of the phrase 'Could you please write the word ...'. B shows a narrowband spectrogram (similar to Fig. 9.2D) where the harmonic structure is shown as the continuous horizontal lines, darkening when they are close to a formant frequency. C shows a wideband spectrogram, whose finer temporal resolution shows the amplitude modulation caused by individual laryngeal cycles as vertical striations (absent during the voiceless noise portion of the 'p' of 'please'), but at the expense of the harmonic structure. Formants appear as dark bands.

for nearby phonemes overlap, producing a sound stream in which the phonetic segments are, to use Liberman *et al.*'s (1967) term, 'encoded'. Perceptually, co-articulation brings costs and benefits. For example, the lip-rounding change to the spectrum of /s/, makes /s/ more spectrally variable, but gives the listener advance warning of the upcoming /u/ (for a computational approach to identifying co-articulatory phenomena see Coleman, 2003). The mechanisms that the brain uses to decode co-articulation have been the subject of a Manichaean opposition of speech-specific mechanisms to general auditory mechanisms which is discussed later (Fowler, 2006).

We adapt the clarity of our speech to suit the communicative context, reducing articulatory effort when it would be superfluous, or increasing it where necessary (Lindblom, 1990). Words spoken in a predictable context (such as 'nine' after 'a stitch in time saves ...') are less intelligible when excised and played in isolation than are words spoken in an unpredictable context

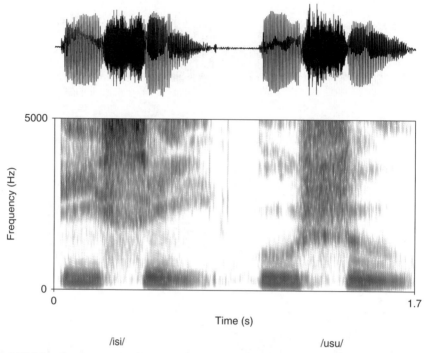

Fig. 9.4 Wideband spectrogram of /isi/ (vowel as in 'sea') and /usu/ (vowel as in 'Sue'). Notice that the spectral structure of the 's' differs substantially between the two due to co-articulation of the /s/ and the vowel.

('the train to Brighton will leave from platform ...') (Lieberman, 1963); vowels in speech addressed to infants are acoustically more distinct than are those in speech addressed to adults (Kuhl *et al.*, 1997).

So far we have described aspects of speech that lie within the speech of a single talker. But, of course, talkers differ. Men's vocal tracts are longer than women's by around 12–15% (Peterson and Barney, 1952) and their pharynxes relatively larger (Fant, 1964). Children's vocal tracts are smaller still. As a consequence there are global differences between the formant frequencies produced by men, women, and children, which are partly a multiplicative scaling due to overall size differences, and which partly depend on the vowel thanks to non-linear changes such as the relatively large male pharynx.

Talkers also differ in their dialect, which can differ dramatically in the vowel sounds that are used in particular words, and in their style of speech (Laver, 1980): for example, they may habitually talk with lips spread or protruded more than is usual, or with a harsher or breathier voice.

9.1.2 Extrinsic influences

Sounds, including speech, must also travel from their source to the listening ear. The acoustic transfer function produced by this journey can change both wide and narrow regions of the spectrum, and introduce echoes and reverberation. High frequencies are scattered more by water vapour and particles in the air, and bend round corners or propagate through walls less well than low frequencies, so distant sounds are muffled. In addition, the outer ear introduces narrow spectral notches whose frequencies vary with the angle at which the sound is arriving. Fortunately, thanks to the small size of our ears, these notches are in a frequency range (> c. 5 kHz) that is not important for speech. Reverberation smears out rapid changes in sound, so that abrupt offsets and onsets are made more gradual and the detailed frequency modulation of formants and of pitch blurred.

Like most other sounds, except perhaps our partner's snores, speech is usually heard against a background of other sounds. This background can be acoustically stable, such as the noise of a waterfall, or extremely complex, such as the speech of one or more other talkers. The sounds that are present at the same time as speech wreak havoc with the overall auditory input to the brain. Parts of the spectrum can be masked, and additional features introduced that could plausibly be part of the speech. The way that we detect and disentangle the auditory features of speech and track a particular talker over time are very active current areas of research, which pose not only a frustratingly complex intellectual challenge, but also have practical applications for speech recognition and for the design of hearing aids and cochlear implants.

9.2 Auditory coding of speech

9.2.1 Frequency analysis and formants

The auditory information that the brain receives about speech is crucially limited by the filtering action of the cochlea and the transmission limitations of the auditory nerve. To a first approximation, the cochlea acts like a filterbank with constant-Q of about 10 (Q = centre frequency/bandwidth), so that the energy around each frequency is averaged over a frequency window that is about one-tenth of that frequency wide; put another way, bandwidth is about one-tenth of centre frequency (see Chapter 2). Auditory coding thus resembles a traditional (fixed bandwidth) narrowband spectrogram in the lower frequencies (less than say 1 kHz for a male voice), but a broadband spectrogram in the higher frequencies. In the lower frequency region, the auditory spectral peaks correspond to the harmonics of the voice, whereas in the higher they correspond to the formants. Since a constant-Q filterbank with a Q of 10 will be able to resolve out the first 10 or so harmonics of any fundamental, auditory coding resolves out individual harmonics in roughly the first-formant region for a male voice (with a fundamental of about 100 Hz) but well into the second-formant region for a female voice (with a fundamental of about 200 Hz). Notice that both physically and perceptually the formant frequency corresponds more to the peak in the spectral *envelope* than to the frequency of the most intense harmonic (Carlson *et al.*, 1975; Darwin and Gardner 1985). Consequently there is no explicit coding of the first-formant frequency in voiced speech, and only explicit coding of high second formants in female voiced speech. Higher formants, however, *are* simply represented peripherally as an energy peak (see Fig. 9.3).

Although formants are habitually used as the control parameters for speech synthesis (Lawrence, 1953; Holmes *et al.*, 1964), and so are some of the explicitly manipulated parameters in studies of the cues underlying speech perception, their perceptual status is unclear. Arguing for listeners using formant frequencies as an abstract intermediate representation between the sound of speech and its linguistic representation in the brain is the phenomenon of sine-wave speech. An intelligible transformation of speech can be produced with two or three frequency- and amplitude-modulated sine waves that track the lower formant frequencies and their amplitudes (Bailey *et al.*, 1977a,b; Remez *et al.*, 1981). The percept of these sounds is initially of weird whistles, but, with a little exposure and encouragement, the percept flips to a moderately intelligible voice, albeit one with a bizarre whistling quality. However, attempts to demonstrate directly the perceptual reality of formant-frequency extraction have produced less support for the formant. When listeners are asked to adjust the formant frequency of a sound consisting of a single formant of a two-formant, vowel-like sound to match a similar target sound (Dissard and Darwin, 2000), interesting differences appear between formants containing resolved harmonics and those that contain unresolved ones. When the two sounds have the same F0, the variability of matches (within-subject standard deviation) for either the first or the second formant is around 1–3%, as previously found for formant-frequency discrimination thresholds (Kewley-Port, 1995). But when the two sounds are given different F0s, so that formant matches cannot be made on the basis of the sounds being identical, variability increases to around 8% for first-formant matches, but to only about 4% for second-formant matches. There seems to be a substantial perceptual cost in having to extract the spectral envelope from resolved harmonics in order to ascertain the first-formant frequency.

Algorithms used for speech recognition have made rather little use of the formant. Because formants are peaks in the transfer function of the vocal tract, their physical presence depends on energy near their frequency being present in the source excitation. Since such excitation is not always present, reliable automatic tracking of formants is notoriously difficult, and so more global parameters (such as cepstral coefficients) are often used instead in automatic speech recognition. However, changes to the spectrum of a sound produced by the transfer function between the talker and the listener can change such global measures and relative formant amplitudes, but have rather little effect on formant frequencies or on listeners' judgements of phonetic quality (Ainsworth and Miller, 1972; Klatt, 1979, 1985b; Darwin et al., 1989;). When labelling sounds as vowels, listeners generally behave as if they were extracting formant frequencies (Klatt, 1985a).

Simply for the perception of formant frequencies, the human auditory system would do better to have a broader bandwidth in the low-frequency region. Indeed, simple automatic speech recognition algorithms and patients, either with cochlear implants or with broadened auditory filters due to sensorineural hearing loss, can recognize speech quite well using remarkably broadband representations of speech (Shannon et al., 1995). Early attempts to enhance the performance of recognition algorithms by giving them an auditory front-end complete with narrow-band harmonic structure gave disappointingly little improvement. However, when additional sounds are present, such as another talker, the performance of recognition algorithms and implant users deteriorates substantially compared with that of algorithms and listeners with normal peripheral frequency analysis. For implant users, a larger number of channels is needed before performance asymptotes in noise than in quiet (Dorman et al., 1998). Speech recognition algorithms can also benefit from finer low-frequency analysis in order to segregate the required speech from other simultaneous sounds (Cooke and Brown, 1993).

Our finer frequency analysis brings not only improved detection of narrow-band features such as harmonics that have been masked by noise, but also with its resolution of low-numbered harmonics an improved percept of pitch (Houtsma and Smurzynski, 1990). The harmonic regularity of resolved harmonics provides a way to separate the voiced sounds of one talker from those of another. Because the range of the first formant is relatively narrow (roughly 200–800 Hz compared with the second formant of 800–2500 Hz), it is particularly difficult to identify the F1 frequencies of two simultaneous sounds when they are on the same F0. The substantial improvement in intelligibility gained by putting simultaneous talkers on a different fundamental frequency rather than the same one is largely due to having different harmonic series in the low-frequency, first-formant region. Only with large F0 differences is it also important that the high-frequency region of a talker has the same F0 as the low-frequency region (Culling and Darwin, 1993a; Bird and Darwin, 1998).

9.2.2 Auditory nerve

At the level of the auditory nerve, various non-linearities that affect speech are evident in the way that sound is coded (for a recent review see Young, 2008). The intensity compression produced by cochlear outer hair cells introduces complex suppression phenomena into the coding of complex sounds. One of the effects of this suppression is to enhance more intense sounds at the expense of less intense sounds, thereby emphasizing excitation near formant peaks (Sinex and Geisler, 1984).

A second non-linearity is temporal adaptation: the auditory nerve's rate of firing decreases sharply (in a few tens of ms) after the onset of a sound. Such adaptation allows the firing pattern to reflect not just the current value of a sound but its recent history; it serves to emphasize change rather than current values. The effects of such adaptation is evident in the way that the dynamic aspects of speech are represented in the auditory nerve (Delgutte and Kiang, 1984). There are various perceptual effects that may be at least partly (Palmer *et al.*, 1995) the consequence of such adaptation. One such (Summerfield *et al.*, 1984) neatly demonstrates that a flat-spectrum noise can be heard as having a vowel-like quality if it is immediately preceded by a noise with the complementary spectrum to the vowel (that is with spectral troughs where the vowel's formants provide spectral peaks). Auditory adaptation effects have also been invoked as a possible explanation of perceptual compensation for co-articulation (Lotto and Kluender, 1998). More generally, non-linearities in the auditory system provide a partial explanation of that most basic of phenomena in the perception of speech: categorical perception.

9.3 **Categorical perception**

For many simple perceptual dimensions such as loudness, or (for those who do not possess absolute pitch (Athos *et al.*, 2007)) pitch, our ability to discriminate similar sounds far exceeds our ability to label sounds in isolation. This seemingly general principle is spectacularly violated for the complex sounds that form a continuum between stop consonants differing in place of articulation (/ba/-/da/-/ga/) (Liberman *et al.*, 1957). Here our ability to discriminate sounds is predicted, at least in its general form, by whether the two sounds are heard as belonging to the same or to different phonemic categories. Discrimination is close to chance within a phoneme category, but very good between categories.

The phenomenon is a robust one; it applies to a variety of phonetic dimensions including both place of articulation and voicing, and it survives the application of fastidious psychophysical techniques (Macmillan 1987; Macmillan *et al.*, 1988). Categorical perception provided the ballistic impetus for intensive research into speech perception during the 1960s and 1970s, fuelled by the claim that such 'categorical perception' was unique to the human perception of speech (Liberman *et al.*, 1967).

Alternative views arose, that categorical perception was more general, being neither restricted to speech nor to its human perception. Non-speech analogues of sounds differing in voicing gave a similar relationship between discrimination and labelling in adult humans (Pisoni, 1977), a finding that was later extended to a variety of different complex auditory dimensions (Harnard, 1987; Burns and Campbell, 1994). In addition, both chinchillas and macaques were shown to have categorical perception-like behaviour (see Chapter 7). Chinchillas labelled a voiced–voiceless continuum of sounds in a very similar way to humans (Kuhl and Miller, 1978), while macaques showed discrimination peaks both at the stop consonant voicing boundary (Kuhl and Padden, 1982) and at place of articulation boundaries (Kuhl and Padden, 1983). Subsequently it became clear that, at least for the voicing dimension, there are significant non-linearities in the response of the chinchilla auditory nerve to the temporal features that distinguish voiced from voiceless stop consonants (Sinex *et al.*, 1991). This non-linear mapping, between the control parameters used to synthesize speech sounds and detectable changes in the response of the auditory nerve, defines regions where the auditory nerve output changes little as the sound's parameters are altered. Conversely, other regions may contain large auditory nerve changes. Such discontinuities

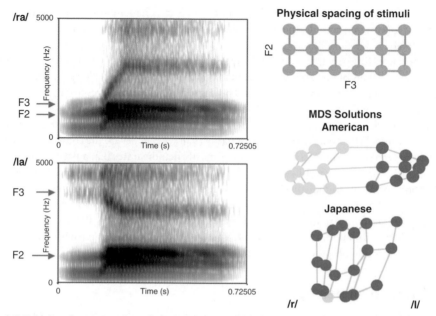

Fig. 9.5 Wideband spectrograms of synthetic /r/ and /l/ taken from a matrix of sounds that varied both F2 and F3 starting frequency. American and Japanese listeners were asked to identify individual items and to rate the similarity of pairs of items that physically were equally spaced (orange circles). The similarity ratings gave multidimensional scaling solutions that revealed very different perceptual spaces for American and Japanese listeners. The yellow and red circles represent sounds heard as /r/ or /l/, respectively. (Figures kindly provided by Paul Iverson.)

provide demarcation for natural categories (Rosch, 1973) and may well have been exploited in the evolution of language (Kuhl, 1988)[1].

Is categorical perception entirely due to such auditory discontinuities? Although such discontinuities help in the learning of phonemic categories by infants (Holt *et al.*, 2004), a variety of evidence indicates that it is not. Most strikingly, infants undergo a dramatic change in their perception of speech sounds during their first year of life (Werker and Tees, 1984; Werker, 1989) so that they can lose their neonatal ability to discriminate between sounds that lie within a phonemic category in their native language (Best *et al.*, 1988). The performance of adult listeners thus reflects both the global constraints imposed by the basic design of the auditory system and also culturally determined acquired similarity (and perhaps also differentiation (Kuhl *et al.*, 2006)). The inability of adult Japanese listeners to distinguish sounds differing in their F3 transitions, which native English-speaking listeners readily label differentially as /r/ and /l/, reflects a dramatic restructuring of phonetic space (Iverson *et al.*, 2003) that is unlikely to occur at a peripheral auditory level (Fig. 9.5). At what level of processing and where in the brain such changes occur are important questions.

---

[1] The evolution of phonemic boundaries may also have been influenced by similar non-linearities between changes in articulatory position and the resulting sound (Fant, G. (1970). *Acoustic Theory of Speech Production*. The Hague: Mouton; Stevens, K. N. (2000). *Acoustic Phonetics*. Cambridge, MA: The MIT Press). There are regions of articulatory space (for example, where the cavity-affiliation of formants changes) that give a more stable acoustic output in the face of articulatory variability and provide thereby a natural centre for both vowel and consonantal categories.

9.4 **Perception of co-articulation**

A recurring question in speech perception concerns the type of mechanisms responsible for the decoding of co-articulatory influences on the speech signal. On the one hand they have been attributed to mechanisms specific to speech, and on the other to adaptation-like mechanisms that serve to enhance auditory contrast. A particularly interesting and extensively investigated example derives from an experiment by Virginia Mann (1980). She explored the co-articulatory influence of a preceding /l/ or /r/ on the following stop /d/ or /g/ in syllables such /arda/. Since the tongue is generally further back in the mouth for /r/ than for /l/, the place in the mouth at which /d/ and /g/ are articulated differs depending on whether they are preceded by /l/ or /r/. In addition, the lips are rounded for /r/, but not for /l/, and can remain so into the following stop consonant. These differences are also evident in the sound, specifically in the formant transitions leading into the final vowel from the stop closure, which help to cue the /d/–/g/ distinction; a preceding /l/ makes the /g/ transitions more /d/-like. Mann showed that when a synthetic continuum of sounds from /da/ to /ga/ was preceded by /al/, listeners heard more sounds as /ga/ than when they were in isolation or preceded by /ar/. Such perceptual context effects could be explained, as Mann did, by mechanisms specific to the human processing of speech, which invoke our knowledge of the dynamic articulatory constraints on speech production (Fowler, 1986). A subsequent, ingenious experiment by Mann (1986) demonstrated that such articulatory knowledge must be more general than that associated with the listener's native language, since Japanese listeners, who do not distinguish English phonemes /r/ and /l/ in their production, and cannot hear the difference between them (Miyawaki et al., 1975), nevertheless also show similar perceptual effects of /r/ and /l/ on /d/ and /g/ to American listeners. The possibility that such compensation effects may derive from a language-universal rather than a language-specific body of implicit knowledge about vocal-tract constraints received support from the perception of speech by infants. Fowler and colleagues (Fowler et al., 1990) demonstrated a related shift in discrimination in infants too young (4 months old) to have developed the phoneme categories of their native language.

However, both the Mann (1980, 1986) and the Fowler results could have a yet more universal, namely auditory, explanation. The evidence comes from two types of experiment: those showing that non-human animals demonstrate similar effects, and those showing that a non-speech, but acoustically similar, precursor sound has similar effects on /d/–/g/ labelling to that produced by /al/ or /ar/. Lotto and colleagues (1997) trained four quail to distinguish isolated /da/ from /ga/ using synthetic sounds that differed in their third-formant (F3) transition. When the quail were then presented with ambiguous sounds preceded by /al/ or /ar/ (which are also distinguished by their F3 transitions), they showed shifts in their labelling of the now embedded /da/–/ga/ series that were similar to those shown by human listeners. The second type of experiment uses non-speech analogues of speech sounds. Specifically, Lotto and Kluender (1998) used two types of precursors: modulated and steady. The two different modulated precursors were single sine waves that were frequency-modulated to track the frequency of F3 in /al/ or /ar/. The two steady precursors were fixed at the final F3 frequency of /al/ or /ar/. Although such isolated sine waves sound like whistles rather than speech, both types of precursor gave shifts in the /d/–/g/ labelling in the same direction as those found with speech precursors. The authors attributed their results to a general auditory contrast mechanism rather than to speech-specific mechanisms concerned with implicit knowledge about the articulatory dynamics of vocal tracts. Although such contrast effects could be due to rapid adaptation in the auditory nerve, it is likely that they have a more central origin since /da/–/ga/ labelling shifts are still found when either a speech (Holt and Lotto, 2002) or non-speech (Lotto et al., 2003) precursor is put into the opposite ear. Nevertheless, some aspects of adaptation effects (Coady et al., 2003) echo the conclusion from auditory nerve experiments that adaptation at that level serves to enhance the characteristics of rapid changes (Delgutte and Kiang, 1984). Such dependence on auditory nerve characteristics is, of course, to be expected since the auditory nerve provides the input to higher centres.

Do these auditory adaptation effects explain the perception of co-articulation? A counter view is based on an ingenious experiment employing the robust and striking McGurk effect (McGurk and McDonald, 1976) in which the seen articulation of one syllable changes the percept of the heard syllable. For example, a sound that is heard as /ba/ with no visual input will change to /da/ while watching synchronized lips articulating /ga/. The effect provides a powerful tool for separating purely auditory from subsequent mechanisms. For example, Roberts and Summerfield (1981) used it to demonstrate that the adaptation that follows repeated presentation of a syllable is a purely auditory effect, and is not influenced by a McGurk-induced change in its perceived category. Fowler and colleagues (2000) compared the perception of a /da/–/ga/ continuum when preceded either by normal /al/ and /ar/ or by a syllable ambiguous between the two but disambiguated by a simultaneous visual presentation of a face hyperarticulating /al/ or /ar/. They found similar shifts in the labelling of the /da/–/ga/ continuum in both cases. Although, in principle, purely auditory mechanisms could not be responsible for the shift in the latter condition, an alternative explanation that does not require visual mediation of the phonetic context has been proposed by Holt and Lotto (Holt et al., 2005). They provide evidence that Fowler's result was due to concurrent visual information influencing the /d/–/g/ labelling directly rather than via the perception of /r/ vs. /l/. (Lotto and Holt, 2006). This claim has in turn been challenged (Fowler, 2006), and the challenge challenged (Lotto and Holt, 2006).

At issue lies the status of auditory mechanisms in the perception of speech. Fowler (2006) pits general auditory mechanisms against those specific to speech. But why are they viewed as alternatives? There has been a long tradition at Haskins Laboratories, which Fowler continues, to set the perception of speech apart from the perception of 'non-speech'. Such separation was understandably inspired by the early results of categorical perception, and was an important tool in Alvin Liberman's very effective nurturing of research into speech perception. But it risks leaving its contemporary proponents isolated from developments in auditory psychophysics and neuroscience. To quote Lotto and Holt 'it is necessary to move past gestural theories and examine speech communication within the framework of general perceptual and cognitive sciences' (Lotto and Holt, 2006, p. 182). Much of contemporary psychoacoustics has benefited from the application of models of the peripheral (Meddis et al., 1990; Meddis and O'Mard, 1997) and increasingly of more central parts of the auditory system (Roberts and Holmes, 2006). It is most unlikely that speech signals evade the various transformations that auditory signals undergo in the cochlea, brainstem, and mid-brain. Some of these transformations may well have evolved to help solve perceptual problems common to the perception of all sounds in a natural environment (Darwin, 1991; Roberts and Holmes, 2006). If we are to understand the perception of speech not only in the soundproof room but also in its more usual richly hostile environment, our theories of speech must build on our understanding of auditory neuroscience, not attempt to stand as an alternative.

9.5 Extrinsic influences

The sound arriving at the listener's ears is generally a mixture of the attended sound and those from the other sound sources that are incidentally present. Moreover, each of the sounds will have suffered filtering and produced additional echoes on its journey from its source. These extrinsic influences on the effective speech signal raise perceptual problems which are common to much of auditory perception.

A number of excellent recent reviews have addressed the problem of recognizing speech against a background of other sounds. Assmann and Summerfield (2004) have dealt with the problem of adverse conditions in general, whilst Bronkhorst (2000) has covered, in detail, the problem of recognizing speech against a background of other sounds.

There is a similar issue in automatic speech recognition, where a technology has arisen that is predicated on there being essentially only a single sound source present—the required talker. Barker (2006) provides a thorough overview of attempts to recognize speech in sound mixtures and of some of the relevant background psychological experimental work. Although recognition systems have developed a 'detailed knowledge of acoustics, grammar and discourse ... there is still no general solution to the problem of recognizing speech in the presence of competing sound sources. In this regard, speech recognition remains a brittle technology' (Barker, 2006, p. 297).

A remarkable characteristic of speech is its resistance to a variety of distortions. Summerfield and colleagues (2005, pp. 223–4) have listed six different types of static and dynamic filtering and additive noise (Miller, 1947; Warren et al., 1995) under which speech maintains 70–80% intelligibility for listeners with normal hearing. It can also remain partially intelligible under infinite peak-clipping (Licklider et al., 1948), reduction to amplitude-modulated noise in only three distinct, broad frequency bands (Shannon et al., 1995), or to two or three sine waves (Bailey et al., 1977a,b; Remez et al., 1981) and alternation with broadband noise (Miller and Licklider, 1950; Verschuure and Brocaar, 1983). You can even, as Melvyn Hunt demonstrated, recognize speech to some extent, if, through the resynthesis capabilities of linear predictive coding, a symphony orchestra is substituted for your larynx. It can also survive against a background of other structured sounds such as music and speech (Cherry, 1953; Cherry and Taylor, 1954; Cherry and Wiley, 1967).

It is possible that the driving force behind the evolution of this remarkable resistance of speech to bizarre and extreme distortions lies in its need to remain intelligible against arbitrarily complex and intense competing sounds, including echoes and reverberation. In addition, speech needs to remain intelligible in the face of changes to the transfer function between talker and listener, such as the relative attenuation of high frequencies produced by intervening objects and damp air. Combinations of background noises are arbitrary, so, in general, they will mask out arbitrary combinations of frequencies. Perhaps as an adaptation to this adulteration, we seem to be able to combine different frequencies independently. For stationary masking sounds, the intelligibility of speech is well predicted by the Speech Intelligibility Index (ANSI, 1997), which treats as independent (though with different fixed weights) the contribution made by each of several frequency bands. Listeners are also adept at perceiving speech which is being interrupted by noise (Miller and Licklider, 1950) even when the interruptions are asynchronous across different frequency channels, as in the case of 'checkerboard noise' (Howard-Jones and Rosen, 1993; Carlyon et al., 2002; Buss et al., 2004). Provided the speech is relatively predictable, intelligibility is improved by the presence of interrupting noise over interrupting silence when the noise is intense enough to have masked the missing speech (Miller and Licklider, 1950; Cherry and Wiley, 1967; Powers and Wilcox, 1977; Verschuure and Brocaar, 1983). The noise seems to allow the recognition system to permit the missing sensory data in a way that silence does not. In these situations, listeners find it difficult to identify what sounds were missing and what were not (Warren, 1970; Warren et al., 1972; Samuel, 1981; Warren, 1984).

Although the independence of frequency bands holds well when averaged over time, at any moment the important information about the speech signal will be very localized. Harmonics with high amplitude, by virtue of being close to formant peaks, will generally stand out more easily against the noise background, and may provide enough information for identification. Consequently, when two voices are mixed together at similar levels, the energy in any particular local frequency–time region (corresponding to a small region on a spectrogram) will be dominated

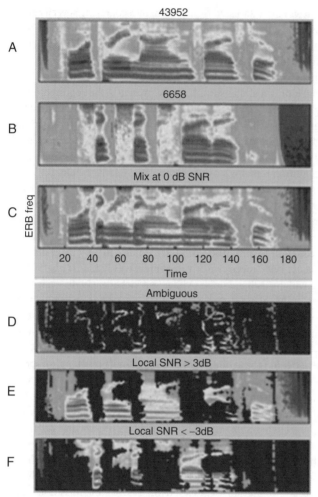

Fig. 9.6 The upper panels (A and B) show ERB-scale spectrograms (modelling the ear's frequency analysis) of two different spoken digit sequences '43952' and '6658'. Panel C shows a spectrogram of their mixture. The lower three panels show the result of subjecting the spectrogram of the mixture to a binary mask. For panel E the mask allows those local frequency-time regions where the energy level from the first digit sequence is >3 dB above that of second sequence. Panel F shows where it is >3 dB in favour of the second sequence, and D shows the ambiguous region where the levels from the two sequences are within 3 dB of each other. (Spectrograms kindly provided by Martin Cooke.)

by one of the signals. Although technically the mixture of the two voices is an additive mixture of the pressure waveforms, sparseness results in the mixture being closely approximated by the locally (in a frequency/time representation) most intense source. Such dominance is exaggerated by the roughly logarithmic intensity coding of sound by the brain, since if $a>>b$, then $\log(a+b) \sim \log(a)$. This view of speech masked by competing sounds corresponds to the idea of noisy speech being 'glimpsed', giving the listener occasional, relatively undistorted views of the signal scattered across the frequency–time plane (Miller and Licklider, 1950; Cooke, 2003, 2006; Assmann and Summerfield, 2004). The job of the listener then is to group together those glimpses which come from the same sound source.

Researchers addressing the difficult problem of recognizing speech mixed with other speech sounds have exploited this sparse representation of speech (Varga and Moore, 1991; Wang and Brown, 2006*b*) to recast the problem of speech separation. Wang (2005) has proposed that the creation of the ideal binary mask should be a defining goal in the separation of simultaneous sounds. Such a mask indicates which local frequency/time regions of a spectrogram are dominated by a particular sound source and is illustrated in Fig. 9.6. The value of this idea for understanding human perception is shown by the fact that, provided that the target speech is being masked by other speech rather than by noise (Brungart *et al.*, 2006*a*), speech resynthesized from just those patches identified by an ideal binary mask is remarkably intelligible and lacks audible interference from other sources. An interesting implication of this result is that, at least for listeners with normal auditory bandwidths, peripheral masking is not a limitation in perceiving one talker against another.

For the listener, as for the speech recognition algorithm, the ideal binary mask is not given; it is simply a convenient way of specifying the perceptual task of separating out those parts of the signal that are primarily due to the required sound source or talker. That such separation is necessary for recognition depends on the simple assumption that the brain stores information about speech in a source-specific way, so that only characteristics of the speech are saved, they are not mixed with characteristics of other sounds that were or might be present. How such separation can be achieved is the subject of extensive experimental work on human listeners into auditory scene analysis (ASA; Bregman, 1990), and into its computational equivalent (CASA; Wang and Brown, 2006*a*).

9.6 Auditory scene analysis for speech

Our ability to separate the speech of two talkers depends substantially on aspects of speech that are not essential for the intelligibility of the speech of a single talker. So, for example, although speech that has been reduced to three sinusoids that track the first three formants' frequencies and amplitudes is moderately intelligible, its intelligibility is relatively poorer than normal speech when it is part of a multi-talker mixture (Barker and Cooke, 1999; Brungart *et al.*, 2006*b*). Such 'sine-wave speech' lacks harmonic structure and the corresponding voice pitch. The same relative impairment also occurs for other transformations that remove the pitch of the voices (Brungart *et al.*, 2006*b*). In a similar vein, we habitually recognize speech whatever its absolute level or spatial location, but it is much easier to separate two talkers when they are talking at different overall levels—even when the quieter talker is the target (Egan *et al.*, 1954; Brungart, 2001) or from different locations (Plomp, 1976). There are then aspects of speech which are not essential for the intelligibility of a single talker, but which contribute substantially to its intelligibility when mixed with other sounds. These aspects can be used to help to increase the detection of speech features in background noise and to separate the frequency components of one talker from those of another.

The problems that arise in recognizing speech against a background of other sounds vary substantially with the type of background noise. For example, for a background of unstructured noise, the problem is mainly one of *detecting* the components of the source. Here, differences in source azimuthal location improve the signal-to-noise ratio by means of head shadow and of binaural interaction. High frequencies of noise are attenuated at the ear farther from the noise by head shadowing, and binaural interaction can improve the detectability of low-frequency components in noise (Plomp, 1976). Once a feature is detected there is no ambiguity about its provenance. But with a structured background, such as other talkers, the burden of the problem shifts from detection to allocation (Brungart *et al.*, 2006*a*). As we noted earlier, the sparseness of speech in the spectrotemporal plane preserves local features from a particular sound source in the presence of other sparse sources. But if the target and the masker consist of similar local features then decisions have to be made as to which features are from a common source. In addition, these sources must themselves be tracked over time, especially across silent gaps. A variety of different aspects of speech help in these tasks.

9.6.1 **Harmonicity**

Much of speech has a harmonic structure, thanks to the periodic vibration of the vocal cords at the F0. The F0 of speech varies continuously as we speak, so that two people talking at the same time will almost always have different F0s. Two simultaneous sounds are more difficult to hear separately when they are played on the same F0 than when they have different F0s, be they vowels (Scheffers, 1979, 1983; Assmann and Summerfield 1989, 1990) or the notes of musical instruments (Sandell and Darwin, 1996). The difficulty arises from the fact that their harmonics coincide and so physically add together in the ear, rather than being separated by frequency analysis.[2] A significant improvement in the identification of the individual sounds can be produced by a difference in F0 that is too small (half a semitone) for the harmonics to be resolved by the ear. The improvement here may be due to the brain intelligently interpreting the pattern of beats that these sounds generate (Culling and Darwin, 1994). For larger F0 differences, the separately resolved harmonics from the two F0 series can be perceptually segregated into groups which improve the estimation of the first-formant frequency for each of the talkers. For F0 differences larger than about four semitones, listeners can also use consistency of F0 between the first and higher formants to group together the formants from the same talker (Culling and Darwin, 1993a). Similar effects arise in continuous speech (Brokx and Nooteboom, 1982; Bird and Darwin, 1998) where additionally there is the problem of tracking a single talker over time. The continuity of the F0 contour can help in such tracking (Darwin, 1975; Darwin and Bethell-Fox, 1977; Darwin and Hukin, 2000). In natural situations the F0 contours of different talkers will cross, and in such situations a difference in timbre (such as vowel quality) between the sources helps to give the listener the correct, crossing percept (Culling and Darwin, 1993b).

9.6.2 **Onset time**

The auditory system is especially responsive to sound onsets—the auditory nerve response adapts rapidly in the first few hundredths of a second after a sound has started (Smith, 1979; Yates et al., 1985; Chimento and Schreiner, 1990). Partly as a consequence of such neural coding, sounds which start together are more difficult to hear separately than those that start at different times. The individual harmonics of a complex tone are readily heard if their consecutive onsets are staggered by, say, a tenth of a second. But the overall timbre of the sound is less clear than with simultaneous onsets. The effect that onset time has on vowel quality can be quantified by measuring first-formant phoneme boundaries for vowel pairs that differ mainly in their first formant. If one of the harmonics near the first-formant frequency starts a few hundredths of a second before the rest, the phoneme boundary between the two vowel categories shifts to a different (nominal) F1 value, implying that the leading harmonic is making less of a contribution to the vowel (Darwin, 1984). This reduction is not entirely due to frequency-specific adaptation at the frequency of the leading harmonic, since it partially reversed by making just the leading portion of that harmonic group with another sound that started with the leading sound but stopped when the remaining sounds started (Darwin and Sutherland, 1984). This grouping effect in turn, however, may be due to broadband inhibition operating centrally, perhaps at the level of the cochlear nucleus (Roberts and Holmes, 2006). It is an interesting question to what extent the low-level processing characteristics

---

[2] Similar problems arise at the octave (twice F0) or the twelfth (three times F0) as exploited by organs to create the blended sound of the Principal Chorus by adding together pipes with F0s at the fundamental, octave, and twelfth (octave quint).

of the auditory system make explicit those features of the (mixed) acoustic input that are in fact specific to individual sound sources.

9.6.3 Spatial differences

Although we hear a mixture of different simultaneous sounds remarkably veridically over a single loudspeaker, mixtures are generally easier to separate when there is a difference in spatial position—particularly in azimuth, the horizontal plane. Such differences are most apparent in helping us to track a particular sound source over time—following the attended talker. In experiments on simpler sounds, such as tones differing in frequency, a difference in perceived azimuth between alternate tones in a sequence will readily cause the creation of two separate auditory streams each with its own melodic contour (Bregman and Ahad, 1995, Demonstration 41; Hukin and Darwin, 2000; Sach and Bailey, 2004). Likewise, when two voices are mixed, attention to one of them can be easier when they come from different spatial directions. The tracking improvement due to spatial separation is greater when other cues that might help tracking are not present. Freyman (1999), for example, found that a perceived spatial difference gave a substantial improvement in tracking the target voice when he used two female voices who both spoke semantically anomalous sentences. Here, neither voice quality, nor semantic predictability could help the tracking problem. Spatial differences were less beneficial when another cue (a difference in level) was introduced between the two voices.

Under some circumstances, binaural cues can be less effective than harmonicity and onset-time in grouping sounds across frequency. Differences in level, especially the extreme case of dichotic presentation, are more effective than differences in the interaural time difference (ITD). The weakness of ITDs in separating simultaneous sounds is well demonstrated in an ingenious experiment by Culling and Summerfield (1995). They used four different noise bands that can be combined in different ways to give the first two formants of four different vowels. If two such bands are played to each ear, listeners have no difficulty in reporting the vowel that corresponds to the formants played to either ear. However, if the noise bands differ by ITDs rather than by which ear they are led to, listeners are unable to do the task. With extended practice, some listeners *can* learn to use ITDs in this way (Darwin, 2002; Drennan *et al.*, 2003), but for naïve listeners the contrast between dichotic presentation and the ITD condition is striking. This difference is all the more surprising when we consider that ITDs are the dominant cue for the localization of complex, wideband sounds such as speech in non-reverberant conditions (Wightman and Kistler, 1992).

The unreliability of ITDs in a particular frequency region in reverberant environments (Shinn-Cunningham *et al.*, 2005) may be a good reason for not relying on them as a primary cue for the simultaneous grouping of objects. An obvious, but significant, observation is that we almost never hear the different frequency regions of a sound coming from different directions. One way of helping sound sources to retain their spatial integrity is to localize sounds as a whole, rather than localizing their component parts independently (Woods and Colburn, 1992; Hill and Darwin, 1996; Best *et al.*, 2007). According to this scheme, different frequency regions are grouped together using grouping cues—such as harmonicity, onset time, or schema-based knowledge—and an estimate is then made of the object's location based on the values of the individual cues, such as interaural time and level differences in the frequency regions that make up that sound source.

Although, as we have seen, the natural spatial separation of attended and unattended sources improves detection and tracking of the attended source, a spatially separated distractor sound *can* cause a remarkable amount of disruption to selective attention. Brungart and Simpson (2002) asked listeners to respond to a target speech signal spoken by one of two competing talkers in one ear while ignoring a simultaneous masking sound in the other ear. When the masking sound in the unattended ear was noise, listeners were able to segregate the competing talkers in the target ear nearly as well as they could with no sound in the unattended ear. But when the masking sound in the unattended ear was speech, speech segregation in the target ear was very substantially worse than with no sound in the unattended ear. The presence of speech-like (Brungart et al., 2005) sounds in the unattended ear makes the separation of sounds in the attended ear much harder.

9.6.4 Schemata

Our accumulated knowledge guides our perception: predictable speech is more intelligible than unpredictable. Such knowledge probably also influences our ability to segregate speech from background sounds—Bregman (1990) recognizes the role that internal schemata can play in seg-regating sounds from mixtures. But we do not yet have a good understanding of how such specific knowledge interacts with the low-level heuristics outlined in the above sections.

This problem is currently occupying computer scientists seeking to interface CASA with tradi-tional methods of speech recognition that use Hidden Markov Models of speech patterns (Barker, 2006). The problem was originally tackled (Weintraub, 1987) by isolating the recognition stage, which has detailed knowledge of specific speech patterns, from the scene analysis stage, which uses general heuristics (Weintraub, 1987). An alternative approach (speech fragment decoding; Barker, 2006) uses stored specific speech knowledge to help to track, for example, an individual talker across intersecting pitch tracks. The questions raised in this area are potentially very rich ones for the interaction of computer science, psychophysics, and auditory neuroscience.

9.7 Summary

Speech perception raises difficult questions not only because of its intrinsic nature, but also because of extrinsic factors which are a result of us listening to it in a world of other sounds. The transfor-mations of the acoustic signal that are produced by early stages in auditory processing appear to help in the segregating of sound sources, and may also contribute to some of the intrinsic problems of speech itself. There are fundamental questions that remain unanswered. For example, the way that the sounds of speech are represented in the auditory system, which can only be answered by addressing—through a combination of computational science, psychophysics, and auditory neu-roscience—the problem of perceiving speech in a realistic acoustic environment.

References

Ainsworth, W. A. and Miller, J. B. (1972). The effect of relative formant amplitude on the identity of synthetic vowels. *Language and Speech* 15:328–41.

ANSI (1997). *ANSI S3.5–1997, Methods for calculation of the Speech Intelligibility Index.* New York: American National Standards Institute.

Assmann, P. F. and Summerfield, A. Q. (1989). Modeling the perception of concurrent vowels: Vowels with the same fundamental frequency. *Journal of the Acoustical Society of America* 85:327–38.

Assmann, P. F. and Summerfield, A. Q. (1990). Modeling the perception of concurrent vowels: Vowels with different fundamental frequencies. *Journal of the Acoustical Society of America* 88:680–97.

Assmann, P. F. and Summerfield, Q. (2004). The perception of speech under adverse conditions. In *Speech Processing in the Auditory System* (ed. S. Greenberg, W. A. Ainsworth, A. N. Popper and R. R. Fay), pp. 231–308. New York: Springer-Verlag.

Athos, E. A., Levinson, B., Kistler, A., Zemansky, J., Bostrom, A., Freimer, N., and Gitschier, J. (2007). Dichotomy and perceptual distortions in absolute pitch ability. *Proceedings of the National Academy of Sciences USA* 104:14795–800.

Bailey, P. J., Dorman, M. F., and Summerfield, A. Q. (1977a). Identification of sine-wave analogues of CV syllables in speech and nonspeech modes. *Journal of the Acoustical Society of America* 61:S66.

Bailey, P. J., Summerfield, Q., and Dorman, M. (1977b). On the identification of sine-wave analogues of certain speech sounds. *Haskins Laboratories Status Report* SR-51/52:1–25.

Barker, J. (2006). Robust automatic speech recognition. In *Computational Auditory Scene Analysis* (ed. D. L. Wang and G. J. Brown), pp. 297–350. Hoboken, NJ: Wiley.

Barker, J. and Cooke, M. (1999). Is the sine-wave speech cocktail party worth attending? *Speech Communication* 27:159–74.

Best, C. T., McRoberts, G. W., and Sithole, N. M. (1988). Examination of perceptual reorganization for nonnative speech contrasts—zulu click discrimination by English-speaking adults and infants. *Journal of Experimental Psychology: Human Perception and Performance* 14:345–60.

Best, V., Gallun, F. J., Carlile, S., and Shinn-Cunningham, B. G. (2007). Binaural interference and auditory grouping. *Journal of the Acoustical Society of America* 121:1070–6.

Bird, J. and Darwin, C. J. (1998). Effects of a difference in fundamental frequency in separating two sentences. In *Psychophysical and Physiological Advances in Hearing* (ed. A. R. Palmer, A. Rees, A. Q. Summerfield, and R. Meddis), pp. 263–9. London: Whurr.

Bregman, A. S. (1990). *Auditory Scene Analysis: the Perceptual Organization of Sound*. Cambridge, Mass: Bradford Books, MIT Press.

Bregman, A. S. and Ahad, P. A. (1995). *Compact Disc: Demonstrations of Auditory Scene Analysis*. Montreal: Department of Psychology, McGill University.

Brokx, J. P. L. and Nooteboom, S. G. (1982). Intonation and the perceptual separation of simultaneous voices. *Journal of Phonetics* 10:23–36.

Bronkhorst, A. W. (2000). The cocktail party phenomenon: a review of speech intelligibility in multiple-talker conditions. *Acustica* 86:117–28.

Brungart, D. S. (2001). Informational and energetic masking effects in the perception of two simultaneous talkers. *Journal of the Acoustical Society of America* 109:1101–9.

Brungart, D. S. and Simpson, B. D. (2002). Within-ear and across-ear interference in a cocktail-party listening task. *Journal of the Acoustical Society of America* 112:2985–95.

Brungart, D. S., Simpson, B. D., Darwin, C. J., Arbogast, T. L., and Kidd, G. (2005). Across-ear interference from parametrically-degraded synthetic speech signals in a dichotic cocktail-party listening task. *Journal of the Acoustical Society of America* 117:292–304.

Brungart, D. S., Chang, P. S., Simpson, B. D., and Wang, D. L. (2006a). Isolating the energetic component of speech-on-speech masking with an ideal time–frequency segregation. *Journal of the Acoustical Society of America* 120:4007–18.

Brungart, D. S., Lyer, N., and Simpson, B. D. (2006b). Monaural speech segregation using synthetic speech signals. *Journal of the Acoustical Society of America* 119:2327–33.

Burns, E. M. and Campbell, S. L. (1994). Frequency and frequency ratio resolution by possessors of realtive and absolute pitch: Examples of categorical perception? *Journal of the Acoustical Society of America* 96:2704–19.

Buss, E., Hall, J. W. 3rd, and Grose, J. H. (2004). Spectral integration of synchronous and asynchronous cues to consonant identification. *Journal of the Acoustical Society of America* 115(5, Pt 1):2278–85.

Carlson, R., Fant, G., and Granstrom, B. (1975). Two-formant models, pitch and vowel perception. In *Auditory Analysis and Perception of Speech* (ed. G. Fant and M. A. A. Tatham), pp. 55–82. London: Academic.

Carlyon, R. P., Deeks, J., Norris, D., and Butterfield. S. (2002). The continuity illusion and vowel identification. *Acta Acustica United with Acustica* 88:408–15.

Cherry, C. and Wiley, R. H. (1967). Speech communication in very noisy environments. *Nature* 214:1164.

Cherry, E. C. (1953). Some experiments on the recognition of speech, with one and with two ears. *Journal of the Acoustical Society of America* 25:975–9.

Cherry, E. C. and Taylor, W. K. (1954). Some further experiments upon the recognition of speech, with one and with two ears. *Journal of the Acoustical Society of America* **26**:554–9.

Chimento, T. C. and Schreiner, C. E. (1990). Time course of adaptation and recovery from adaptation in the cat auditory-nerve neurophonic. *Journal of the Acoustical Society of America* **88**:857–64.

Coady, J. A., Kluender, K. R., and Rhode, W. S. (2003). Effects of contrast between onsets of speech and other complex spectra. *Journal of the Acoustical Society of America* **114**(4, Pt 1):2225–35.

Coleman, J. (2003). Discovering the acoustic correlates of phonological contrasts. *Journal of Phonetics* **31**:351–72.

Cooke, M. (2003). Glimpsing speech. *Journal of Phonetics* **31**:579–84.

Cooke, M. (2006). A glimpsing model of speech perception in noise. *Journal of the Acoustical Society of America* **119**:1562–73.

Cooke, M. P. and Brown, G. J. (1993). Computational auditory scene analysis: Exploiting principles of perceived continuity. *Speech Communication* **13**:391–9.

Culling, J. F. and Darwin, C. J. (1993*a*). Perceptual separation of simultaneous vowels: within and across-formant grouping by F0. *Journal of the Acoustical Society of America* **93**:3454–67.

Culling, J. F. and Darwin, C. J. (1993*b*). The role of timbre in the segregation of simultaneous voices with intersecting Fo contours. *Perception and Psychophysics* **34**:303–9.

Culling, J. F. and Darwin, C. J. (1994). Perceptual and computational separation of simultaneous vowels: cues arising from low frequency beating. *Journal of the Acoustical Society of America* **95**:1559–69.

Culling, J. F. and Summerfield, Q. (1995). Perceptual separation of concurrent speech sounds: absence of across-frequency grouping by common interaural delay. *Journal of the Acoustical Society of America* **98**:785–97.

Cutler, A., Dahan, D., and vanDonselaar, W. (1997). Prosody in the comprehension of spoken language: A literature review. *Language and Speech* **40**(Pt 2):141–201.

Darwin, C. J. (1975). On the dynamic use of prosody in speech perception. In *Structure and Process in Speech Perception* (ed. A. Cohen and S. G. Nooteboom), pp. 178–94. Berlin: Springer-Verlag.

Darwin, C. J. (1984). Perceiving vowels in the presence of another sound: constraints on formant perception. *Journal of the Acoustical Society of America* **76**:1636–47.

Darwin, C. J. (1991). The relationship between speech perception and the perception of other sounds. In *Modularity and the Motor Theory of Speech Perception* (ed. I. G. Mattingly and M. G. Studdert-Kennedy), pp. 239–59. Hillsvale, NJ: Erlbaum.

Darwin, C. J. (2002). Auditory streaming in language processing. In *Genetics and the Function of the Auditory System (19th Danavox Symposium)* (ed. L. Tranebjaerg, T. Andersen, J. Christensen-Dalsgaard, and T. Poulsen), pp. 375–92. Denmark: Holmens Trykkeri.

Darwin, C. J. and Bethell-Fox, C. E. (1977). Pitch continuity and speech source attribution. *Journal of Experimental Psychology: Human Perception and Performance* **3**:665–72.

Darwin, C. J. and Gardner, R. B. (1985). Which harmonics contribute to the estimation of the first formant? *Speech Communication* **4**:231–5.

Darwin, C. J. and Hukin, R. W. (2000). Effectiveness of spatial cues, prosody and talker characteristics in selective attention. *Journal of the Acoustical Society of America* **107**:970–7.

Darwin, C. J., McKeown, J. D., and Kirby, D. (1989). Compensation for transmission channel and speaker effects on vowel quality. *Speech Communication* **8**:221–34.

Darwin, C. J. and Sutherland, N. S. (1984). Grouping frequency components of vowels: when is a harmonic not a harmonic? *Quarterly Journal of Experimental Psychology* **36A**:193–208.

Delgutte, B. and Kiang, N. Y. (1984). Speech coding in the auditory nerve: IV. Sounds with consonant-like dynamic characteristics. *Journal of the Acoustical Society of America* **75**:897–907.

Diehl, R. L., Lotto, A. J. and Holt, L. L. (2004). Speech perception. *Annual Review of Psychology* **55**:149–79.

Dissard, P. and Darwin, C. J. (2000). Extracting spectral envelopes: Formant frequency matching between sounds on different and modulated fundamental frequencies. *Journal of the Acoustical Society of America* **107**:960–9.

Dorman, M. F., Loizou, P. C., Fitzke, J., and Tu, Z. (1998). The recognition of sentences in noise by normal-hearing listeners using simulations of cochlear-implant signal processors with 6–20 channels. *Journal of the Acoustical Society of America* 104:3583–5.

Drennan, W. R., Gatehouse, S., and Lever, C. (2003). Perceptual segregation of competing speech sounds: the role of spatial location. *Journal of the Acoustical Society of America* 114(4, Pt 1):2178–89.

Egan, J. P., Carterette, E. C., and Thwing, E. J. (1954). Some factors affecting multi-channel listening. *Journal of the Acoustical Society of America* 26:774–82.

Fant, G. (1964). A note on vocal tract size factors and nonuniform F-pattern scalings. *Speech Transmission Laboratory, Stockholm STL–QPSR* 4:22–30.

Fant, G. (1970). *Acoustic Theory of Speech Production*. The Hague: Mouton.

Fowler, C. A. (1986). An event approach to the study of speech perception from the direct realism perspective. *Journal of Phonetics* 14:3–28.

Fowler, C. A. (2006). Compensation for coarticulation reflects gesture perception, not spectral contrast. *Perception and Psychophysics* 68:161–77.

Fowler, C. A., Best, C. T., and McRoberts, G. W. (1990). Young infants perception of liquid coarticulatory influences on following stop consonants. *Perception and Psychophysics* 48:559–70.

Fowler, C. A., Brown, J. M., and Mann, V. A. (2000). Contrast effects do not underlie effects of preceding liquids on stop-consonant identification by humans. *Journal of Experimental Psychology: Human Perception and Performance* 26:877–88.

Freyman, R. L., Helfer, K. S., McCall, D. D., and Clifton, R. K. (1999). The role of perceived spatial separation in the unmasking of speech. *Journal of the Acoustical Society of America* 106:3578–88.

Galantucci, B., Fowler, C. A., and Turvey, M. T. (2006). The motor theory of speech perception reviewed. *Psychological Bulletin and Review* 13:361–77.

Gaskell, M. G. and MarslenWilson, W. D. (1998). Mechanisms of phonological inference in speech perception. *Journal of Experimental Psychology–Human Perception and Performance* 24:380–96.

Harnard, S. A. (1987). *Categorical Perception: the Groundwork of Cognition*. New York: Cambridge University Press.

Hill, N. I. and Darwin, C. J. (1996). Lateralisation of a perturbed harmonic: effects of onset asynchrony and mistuning. *Journal of the Acoustical Society of America* 100:2352–64.

Holmes, J. N., Mattingly, I. G., and Shearme, J. N. (1964). Speech synthesis by rule. *Language and Speech* 7:127–43.

Holt, L. L. and Lotto, A. J. (2002). Behavioral examinations of the level of auditory processing of speech context effects. *Hearing Research* 167:156–69.

Holt, L. L., Lotto, A. J., and Diehl, R. L. (2004). Auditory discontinuities interact with categorization: implications for speech perception. *Journal of the Acoustical Society of America* 116:1763–73.

Holt, L. L., Stephens, J. D., and Lotto, A. J. (2005). A critical evaluation of visually moderated phonetic context effects. *Perception and Psychophysics* 67:1102–12.

Houtsma, A. J. M. and Smurzynski, J. (1990). Pitch identification and discrimination for complex tones with many harmonics. *Journal of the Acoustical Society of America* 87(1):304–10.

Howard-Jones, P. A. and Rosen, S. (1993). Uncomodulated glimpsing in checkerboard noise. *Journal of the Acoustical Society of America* 93:2915–22.

Hukin, R. W. and Darwin, C. J. (2000). Spatial cues to grouping in the Wessel illusion. *British Journal of Audiology* 34:109.

Iverson, P., Kuhl, P. K., Akahane-Yamada, R., Diesch, E., Tohkura, Y., Kettermann, A., and Siebert, C. (2003). A perceptual interference account of acquisition difficulties for non-native phonemes. *Cognition* 87:B47–57.

Kewley-Port, D. (1995). Vowel formant discrimination. *Journal of the Acoustical Society of America* 98:2948–9 (A).

Klatt, D. H. (1979). Perceptual comparisons among a set of vowels similar to /ae/: some differences between psychophysical distance and phonetic distance. *Journal of the Acoustical Society of America* 66:S86.

Klatt, D. H. (1985a). The perceptual reality of a formant frequency. *Journal of the Acoustical Society of America* 78:S81–82.

Klatt, D. H. (1985b). A shift in formant frequencies is not the same as a shift in the center of gravity of a multi-formant energy concentration. *Journal of the Acoustical Society of America* 77:S7.

Kuhl, P. K. (1988). Auditory perception and the evolution of speech. *Human Evolution* 3:19–43.

Kuhl, P. K. and Miller, J. D. (1978). Speech perception by the chinchilla: identification functions for synthetic VOT stimuli. *Journal of the Acoustical Society of America* 63:905–17.

Kuhl, P. K. and Padden, D. M. (1982). Enhanced discriminability at the phonetic boundaries for the voicing feature in macaques. *Perception and Psychophysics* 32:542–50.

Kuhl, P. K. and Padden, D.M. (1983). Enhanced discriminability at the phonetic boundaries for the place feature in macaques. *Journal of the Acoustical Society of America* 73:1003–10.

Kuhl, P. K., Andruski, J. E., Chistovich, I. A., Chistovich, L. A., Kozhevnikova, E. V., Ryskina, V. L., Stolyarova, E. I., Sundberg, U., and Lacerda, F. (1997). Cross-language analysis of phonetic units in language addressed to infants. *Science* 277:684–6.

Kuhl, P. K., Stevens, E., Hayashi, A., Deguchi, T., Kiritani, S., and Iverson, P. (2006). Infants show a facilitation effect for native language phonetic perception between 6 and 12 months. *Developmental Science* 9:F13–F21.

Laver, J. (1980). *The Phonetic Description of Voice Quality*. Cambridge: Cambridge University Press.

Lawrence, W. (1953). The synthesis of speech from signals which have a low information rate. In *Communication Theory* (ed. W. Jackson), pp. 460–9. London: Butterworths Scientific Publications.

Liberman, A. M., Harris, K. S., Hoffman, H. S., and Griffith, B. C. (1957). The discrimination of speech sounds within and across phoneme boundaries. *Journal of Experimental Psychology* 54:358–68.

Liberman, A. M., Cooper, F. S., Shankweiler, D. S., and Studdert-Kennedy, M. (1967). Perception of the speech code. *Psychological Review* 74:431–61.

Licklider, J. C. R., Bindra, D., and Pollack, I. (1948). The intelligibility of rectangular speech-waves. *American Journal of Psychology* 61:1–20.

Lieberman, P. (1963). Some effects of semantic and grammatical context on the production and perception of speech. *Language and Speech* 6:172–87.

Lindblom, B. E. F. (1990). Explaining phonetic variation: a sketch of the H&H Theory. In *Speech Production and Speech Modeling* (ed. H. J. Hardcastle and A. Marchal), pp. 403–39. Dordrecht: Kluwer.

Lotto, A. J. and Holt, L. L. (2006). Putting phonetic context effects into context: a commentary on Fowler (2006). *Perception and Psychophysics* 68:178–83.

Lotto, A. J. and Kluender, K. R. (1998). General contrast effects in speech perception: Effect of preceding liquid on stop consonant identification. *Perception and Psychophysics* 60:602–19.

Lotto, A. J., Kluender, K. R., and Holt, L. L. (1997). Perceptual compensation for coarticulation by Japanese quail (*Coturnix coturnix japonica*). *Journal of the Acoustical Society of America* 102:1134–40.

Lotto, A. J., Sullivan, S. C. and Holt, L. L. (2003). Central locus for nonspeech context effects on phonetic identification. *Journal of the Acoustical Society of America* 113:53–6.

McGurk, H. and McDonald, J. (1976). Hearing lips and seeing voices. *Nature* 264:746–8.

Macmillan, N. A. (1987). Beyond the categorical/continuous distinction: A psychophysical approach to processing modes. In *Categorical Perception* (ed. S. Harnad), pp. 53–87. New York: Cambridge.

Macmillan, N. A., Goldberg, R. F., and Braida, L. D. (1988). Resolution for speech sounds: Basic sensitivity and context memory on vowel and consonant continua. *Journal of the Acoustical Society of America* 84:1262–80.

Mann, V. A. (1980). Influence of preceding liquid on stop-consonant perception. *Perception and Psychophysics* 28:407–12.

Mann, V. A. (1986). Distinguishing universal and language-dependent levels of speech perception: evidence from Japanese listeners perception of English 'l' and 'r'. *Cognition* 24:169–96.

Mann, V. and Soli, S. D. (1991). Perceptual order and the effect of vocalic context on fricative perception. *Perception and Psychophysics* 49:399–411.

Meddis, R. and O'Mard, L. (1997). A unitary model of pitch perception. *Journal of the Acoustical Society of America* **102**:1811–20.

Meddis, R., Hewitt, M. J., and Shackleton, T. M. (1990). Implementation details of a computational model of the inner hair-cell/auditory nerve synapse. *Journal of the Acoustical Society of America* **87**:1813–16.

Miller, G. A. (1947). The masking of speech. *Psychological Bulletin* **44**:105–29.

Miller, G. A. and Licklider, J. C. R. (1950). The intelligibility of interrupted speech. *Journal of the Acoustical Society of America* **22**:167–73.

Miyawaki, K., Strange, W., Verbrugge, R., Liberman, A. M., Jenkins, J. J., and Fujimura, O. (1975). An effect of linguistic experience: the discrimination of /r/ and /l/ by native speakers of Japanese and English. *Perception and Psychophysics* **18**:331–40.

Öhman, S. E. G. (1966). Coarticulation in VCV utterances. *Journal of the Acoustical Society of America* **39**:151–68.

Palmer, A. R., Summerfield, Q., and Fantini, D. A. (1995). Responses of auditory-nerve fibers to stimuli producing psychophysical enhancement. *Journal of the Acoustical Society of America* **97**:1786–99.

Peterson, G. H. and Barney, H. L. (1952). Control methods used in a study of the vowels. *Journal of the Acoustical Society of America* **24**:175–84.

Pisoni, D. B. (1977). Identification and discrimination of the relative onset time of two component tones: implications for voicing perception in stops. *Journal of the Acoustical Society of America* **61**:1352–61.

Plomp, R. (1976). Binaural and monaural speech intelligibility of connected discourse in reverberation as a function of a single competing sound source (speech or noise). *Acustica* **34**:200–11.

Powers, G. L. and Wilcox, J. C. (1977). Intelligibility of temporally-interrupted speech with and without intervening noise. *Journal of the Acoustical Society of America* **61**:195–9.

Remez, R. E., Rubin, P. E., Pisoni, D. B., and Carrell, T. D. (1981). Speech perception without traditional speech cues. *Science* **212**:947–50.

Roberts, B. and Holmes, S. D. (2006). Asynchrony and the grouping of vowel components: captor tones revisited. *Journal of the Acoustical Society of America* **119**(5, Pt 1):2905–18.

Roberts, M. and Summerfield, Q. (1981). Audiovisual presentation demonstrates that selective adaptation in speech perception is purely auditory. *Perception and Psychophysics* **30**:309–14.

Rosch, E. H. (1973). Natural categories. *Cognitive Psychology* **4**:328–50.

Sach, A. J. and Bailey, P. J. (2004). Some characteristics of auditory spatial attention revealed using rhythmic masking release. *Perception and Psychophysics* **66**:1379–87.

Samuel, A. G. (1981). The role of bottom-up confirmation in the phonemic restoration illusion. *Journal of Experimental Psychology: Human Perception and Performance* **7**:1124–31.

Sandell, G. J. and Darwin, C. J. (1996). Recognition of concurrently-sounding instruments with different fundamental frequencies. *Journal of the Acoustical Society of America* **100**(4, Pt 2):2683.

Scheffers, M. T. (1979). *The Role of Pitch in Perceptual Separation of Simultaneous Vowels*. Annual Progress Report, Vol. 14, pp. 51–4. Eindhoven, The Netherlands: Institute for Perception Research.

Scheffers, M. T. (1983). *Sifting Vowels: Auditory Pitch Analysis and Sound Segregation*. The Netherlands: Groningen University.

Shannon, R. V., Zeng, F.-G., Kamath, V., Wygonski, J., and Ekelid, M. (1995). Speech recognition with primarily temporal cues. *Science* **270**:303–4.

Shinn-Cunningham, B. G., Kopco, N., and Martin, T. J. (2005). Localizing nearby sound sources in a classroom: binaural room impulse responses. *Journal of the Acoustical Society of America* **117**:3100–15.

Sinex, D. G. and Geisler, C. D. (1984). Comparison of the responses of auditory nerve fibers to consonant-vowel syllables with predictions from linear models. *Journal of the Acoustical Society of America* **76**:116–21.

Sinex, D. G., McDonald, L. P. and Mott, J. B. (1991). Neural correlates of nonmonotonic temporal acuity for voice onset time. *Journal of the Acoustical Society of America* **90**:2441–9.

Smith, R. L. (1979). Adaptation, saturation, and physiological masking in single auditory nerve fibers. *Journal of the Acoustical Society of America* **65**:166–78.

Stevens, K. N. (2000). *Acoustic Phonetics*. Cambridge, MA:The MIT Press.

Stevens, K. N. (2002). Toward a model for lexical access based on acoustic landmarks and distinctive features. *Joutnal of the Acoustical Society of America* 111:1872–91.

Strange, W. (1987). Information for vowels in formant transitions. *Journal of Memory and Language* 26:550–7.

Strange, W., Jenkins, J. J., and Johnson, T. L. (1983). Dynamic specification of coarticulated vowels. *Journal of the Acoustical Society of America* 74:695–705.

Summerfield, A. Q., Haggard, M. P., Foster, J., and Gray, S. (1984). Perceiving vowels from uniform spectra: phonetic exploration of an auditory after-effect. *Perception and Psychophysics* 35:203–13.

Summerfield, A. Q., Culling, J. F., and Assmann, P. F. (2005). The perception of speech under adverse conditions: Contributions of spectro-temporal peaks, periodicity, and inter-aural timing to perceptual robustness. In *Listening to Speech* (ed. S. Greenberg and W. A. Ainsworth), pp. 223–35. Oxford: Oxford University Press.

van Donselaar, W., Koster, M., and Cutler, A. (2005). Exploring the role of lexical stress in lexical recognition. *Quarterly Journal of Experimental Psychology A,* 58:251–73.

Varga, A. P. and Moore, R. K. (1991). Simultaneous recognition of concurrent speech signals using hidden Markov model decomposition. In *EUROSPEECH—1991*, September, Genova Italy.

Verschuure, J. and Brocaar, M. P. (1983). Intelligibility of interrupted meaningful and nonsense speech with and without intervening noise. *Perception and Psychophysics* 33:232–40.

Wang, D. L. (2005). An ideal binary mask as the computational goal of auditory scene analysis. In *Speech Separation by Humans and Machines* (ed. P. L. Divenyi), pp. 181–97. New York: Kluwer Academic Publishers.

Wang, D. L. and Brown, G. J. (2006a). *Computational Auditory Scene Analysis*. Hoboken, NJ: Wiley.

Wang, D. L. and Brown, G. J. (2006b). Fundamentals of computational auditory scene analysis. In *Computational Auditory Scene Analysis* (ed. D. L. Wang and G. J. Brown), pp. 1–44. Hoboken, NJ: Wiley.

Warren, R. M. (1970). Perceptual restoration of missing phonemes. *Science* 167:392–3.

Warren, R. M. (1984). Perceptual restoration of obliterated sounds. *Psychological Bulletin* 96:371–83.

Warren, R. M., Obusek, C. J., and Ackroff, J. M. (1972). Auditory induction: perceptual synthesis of absent sounds. *Science* 176:1149–51.

Warren, R. M., Riener, K. R., Bashford, J. A. Jr, and Brubaker, B. S. (1995). Spectral redundancy: intelligibility of sentences heard through narrow spectral slits. *Perception and Psychophysics* 57:175–82.

Weintraub, M. (1987). Sound separation and auditory perceptual organisation. In *The Psychophysics of Speech Perception* (ed. M. E. H. Schouten), p. 125–34. Dordrecht: Martinus Nijhoff.

Werker, J. F. (1989). Becoming a native listener. *American Scientist* 77:54–9.

Werker, J. F. and Tees, R. C. (1984). Cross-language speech perception: evidence for perceptual reorganization during the first year of life. *Infant Behaviour and Development* 7:49–63.

Wightman, F. L. and Kistler, D. J. (1992). The dominant role of low-frequency interaural time differences in sound localization. *Journal of the Acoustical Society of America* 91:1648–61.

Woods, W. A. and Colburn, S. (1992). Test of a model of auditory object formation using intensity and interaural time difference discriminations. *Journal of the Acoustical Society of America* 91:2894–902.

Yates, G. K., Robertson, D., and Johnstone, B. M. (1985). Very rapid adaptation in the guinea-pig auditory nerve. *Hearing Research* 17:1–12.

Young, E. D. (2008). Neural representation of spectral and temporal information in speech. *Philosophical Transactions of the Royal Society of London. Series B, Biological Sciences* 363:923–45.

Chapter 10

Music perception

W. Jay Dowling

10.1 Introduction

When we listen to music, as well as to other patterns of sound, many of the same principles of perception apply as in other domains like vision. We immediately encounter figure-ground relationships between the focal aspect of the pattern we are attending to, and the rest of the sounds that reach our ears. As an example, suppose we hear the piece shown in Fig. 10.1, the slow movement from Beethoven's 'Spring' sonata for violin and piano (*Sonata in F Major, op. 24*). When the piano begins to play, it stands out as a figure in contrast to other sounds in the room. You follow the undulating accompaniment pattern in the left-hand piano part, but this recedes into the background, like wallpaper, when the melody starts in the upper voice. The dynamic shape of the melody dominates the auditory scene, and though you may notice the quiet entry of the violin in the second measure, your attention reverts quickly to the melodic shape.

These are very simple observations, but already we encounter a distinct difference between audition and vision. At first our attention is drawn to the piano as a *sound source*, in contrast to all the other sound sources in the environment. But then the sound of the piano splits into two *sound objects*—the melody and the accompaniment—both coming from the same source. The piano as a sound source is located in physical space, along with the violin, the rattling of page turns, coughs in the audience, etc. The melody as a sound object is, in contrast, located in a kind of 'virtual space' of pitch and time, as is the background accompaniment. Melody and accompaniment have the same location in physical space, but different locations in pitch and time. Kubovy and Van Valkenburg (2001) provide a stimulating discussion of this contrast, pointing out that the closest auditory analog of shape perception in vision is the perception of melodic contours traced in pitch across time.

When the melody shifts to the violin in measure 10, melody and accompaniment come from different locations in physical space as well as occupying different pitch ranges (and contrasting in timbre—their instrumental tone color). These contrasts help clarify the musical structure; being present at a concert changes what we hear and understand of the music. As Vines *et al.* (2006) have documented, the gestures of the musicians while playing communicate aspects of the musical message, as well as reinforce the differentiation of sound sources. (This could be especially important in listening to a string quartet, where all the instruments have similar timbres, to help differentiate what each instrument is doing, or a rock band in which the instruments tend to mask one another's sound. The visual message helps us focus attention on a particular instrumental line as figure.)

The contour of the melodic line has what Mari Jones has called 'dynamic shape' in emphasizing its motion in time through the pitch space (Jones, Summerell, and Marshburn, 1987). The dynamic motion of the melody conveys feelings of tension and relaxation. The first phrase is felt as very relaxed. Then very quietly the tension increases, reaching a peak in the third two-bar phrase. Then it recedes as the eight-measure melody comes to an end on the very stable tonic

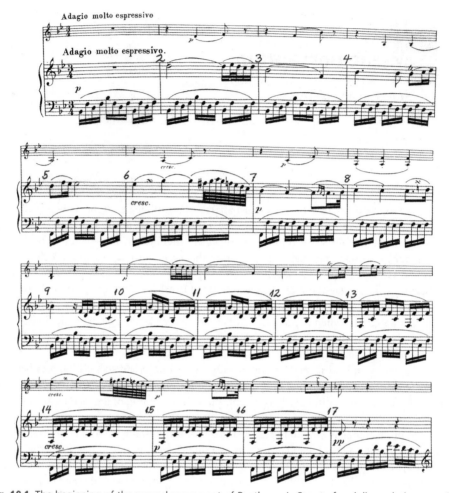

Fig. 10.1 The beginning of the second movement of Beethoven's *Sonata for violin and piano op. 24.*

pitch (Bb). Much of this increase and decrease in tension arises from the relative stability and instability of pitches in a tonal context. In tonal music (which includes the pitch-organizing systems of virtually all the world's folk and art music before the explorations of twentieth-century Europe), the pitches are arranged in a hierarchy, with the tonic (the first degree of the scale) as the central and most stable pitch. The less stable pitches are attracted in greater or lesser degree toward the more stable pitches. You encounter this kind of instability very strongly if you sing a nursery song like 'Twinkle, Twinkle' and stop before you reach the last note: 'How I wonder what you ...'. Stopping on the very unstable second degree of the scale makes you feel how strongly it needs to resolve to the stable tonic. We shall explore this further in looking at the work of Krumhansl (1990) who found that listeners are quite consistent in their judgments of the stability of pitches in a tonal context, and are even able to track their position in a virtual space of tonal pitch while listening to a piece that shifts from key to key (that is, from one tonal scale to another). The virtual space of pitch is well represented in the human brain (as Janata *et al.*, 2002, have shown).

Pitch and time as dimensions of the virtual space of audition have a feature that sets them apart from the physical space of vision: these dimensions are calibrated in terms of cognitive frameworks that help listeners keep track of the positions of the musical notes in the space. As Helmholtz

(1877/1954, p. 252) pointed out, 'Melody has to express a motion, in such a manner that the hearer may easily, clearly, and certainly appreciate the character of that motion ... This is only possible when the steps of this motion, their rapidity and their amount, are ... exactly *measurable* by immediate sensible perception.' As we shall see, pitch is heard in terms of motion along the musical scale framework that underlies the melody, and time and rhythm (the 'rapidity' of the motion) are heard in terms of a framework of beats. We feel the tension and stability of a melody in terms of its departures from and returns to the stable tonic region of the scale, and the temporal solidity of being on the beat.

Before we look in detail at how music is perceived, there is one more general feature of perception to consider. Perception is intimately bound up with memory, and is very difficult to conceive of as a separate process. In order for us to experience it, information from the outside world must be held in a memory buffer, and that information is registered in such a buffer as soon as it enters our nervous system. We do not experience raw, uninterpreted sensory data. The stimuli we experience have already been encoded in terms of our customary categories of perception ('assimilated', in Piaget's terms (see Inhelder and Piaget, 1958)). When we hear speech in our familiar language, we hear meaningful words, not uninterpreted speech sounds or babbling, and when we listen to tonal music we hear pitches in terms of their places in the tonal framework, and we hear them occurring in relation to a metrical framework of beats. The notes of a melody have already been encoded into our memory buffers by the time we experience them. Furthermore, what we acknowledge having heard depends on how long after the fact our memory system is queried; seconds make a difference in the answer.

There is another way in which memory has an immediate impact on our perception. We experience a piece of music as extended in time, and not present all at once in our auditory field (the way a picture is in the visual field). This means that as we continue listening we are continually evaluating (usually implicitly) the familiarity of what we are hearing, and understanding how it fits what preceded it. For each new phrase, we are implicitly asking, echoing William James (1890), 'Is that thingumabob again'? We are tracking the degree to which the present phrase is like what went before, and how it fits its context. Too much new and different material and the music becomes incomprehensible; too much similarity, and it becomes boring. There is good reason to believe that this tracking relies on our sense of familiarity with the new material, and not on explicit recollection of the previous phrases. (See Yonelinas, 2002, for the distinction between familiarity and recollection.)

It is clear from this discussion that music perception is multidimensional. Perceiving music leads the brain to combine patterns of features varying on several sensory dimensions at once. In this chapter we will look at those dimensions one at a time, and see how they fit together into a meaningful overall pattern. It is also clear that we hear music embedded in a particular culture. Our perceptual habits have been shaped by the regularities of the music we are used to hearing. Those habits lead us to expect certain continuations of what we are hearing, and so the things that surprise us are determined by what is usually done. The cognitive frameworks for pitch and time, so useful as aids in our understanding of the music we hear, are largely culture-specific. It takes considerable perceptual learning with the music of a new culture before we automatically encode the relevant features and contrasts that are built into it, just as it does with language.

10.2 Perceptual frameworks

When we listen to music from our own cultural tradition, what we experience is not a stream of undifferentiated sound, but sounds that are encoded in terms of the cultural system of categories. This is similar to what happens when we listen to speech in a language we know: the sounds enter

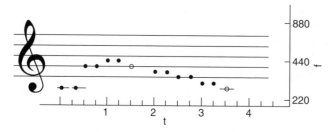

Fig. 10.2 The tune 'Twinkle, Twinkle, Little Star' presented at 4 beats/s (MM = 240 beats/min) displayed on a grid showing pitch and frequency in Hz (*f*) vs. time in s (*t*), with the musical staff notation superimposed on the y-axis.

our conscious experience already encoded as syllables, words, and sentences. To convince yourself that we hear musical pitches in terms of scale categories, sing 'Twinkle, Twinkle, Little Star' and stop on the next-to-last note: '… How I wonder what you.' The pattern sounds incomplete when it ends on *re* in the *do, re, mi* scale; it needs to get back to *do*, the tonic, to end in a stable place and sound finished. Traditional Chinese music is based on pentatonic scales, and Lao-Tse (1972) warns us that 'the five tones deafen the ear'—that we should try to hear things as they really are, and not in terms of conventional categories. In the twentieth century composers tried a variety of ways of breaking through our automatic encoding of pitches: by giving all 12 pitches in the octave equal weight so there was no longer a stable tonic to return to (Schönberg, 1967), by constructing scales with unfamiliar patterns of dividing the octave (Partch, 1974), or by constructing musical patterns out of sound objects found in nature and their transformations (*musique concrète*, Schaeffer, 1952). But the overwhelming preponderance of music we hear is constructed in our familiar tonal system, and our ears are well practiced in encoding it in terms of its categories.

The category systems of pitch and time divide our auditory space into a two-dimensional grid such as that shown in Fig. 10.2. The y-axis, pitch, represents a logarithmic scale of frequency along which the frequency doubles with every octave (going from an A at 220 Hz to an A an octave higher at 440 Hz, to an A another octave higher at 880 Hz). The x-axis, time, is divided into beats and their subdivisions. Time perception organized in terms of beats is much more precise, with a much smaller just-noticeable difference between similar time intervals, than time perception not so organized (Bharucha and Pryor, 1986). In our Western European tradition we are so used to beats occurring at absolutely regular intervals (such as in 'Twinkle, Twinkle' where beats are grouped by twos) that we don't often consider the possibility of unevenly timed divisions of the measure into groupings of 3 + 2, for example, that are characteristic of some Eastern European songs. Grouped in this way, 'Twinkle, Twinkle' would have a hitch in its rhythm: 'Twi-uncle, twinkle, lih-uh-tle star; howow I wonder wha-hat you are.' Hannon and Trehub (2005) showed that whereas American adults had difficulty noticing structural violations in the more complex 3 + 2 patterns, Bulgarian adults coped equally well with their familiar 3 + 2 patterns and the simpler 2 + 2 patterns (such as in Fig. 10.2). Six-month-olds, not yet acculturated to one or another pattern, also coped equally well. Just as the pitch categories on the y-axis of Fig. 10.2 are the result of acculturation (for example, in traditional Indonesia the pitch categories of the five- and seven-tone scale systems can even vary from village to village), so are the time categories on the x-axis.

10.2.1 Pitch

The pitches of tonal music, in whatever culture, are specified in terms of a hierarchical series of constraints, illustrated for European music in Fig. 10.3 (Dowling, 1978; Dowling and Harwood, 1986). We start with the non-musical *psychophysical scale*, which assigns perceived pitches to physical frequencies (the frequencies of sine waves, or the fundamental frequencies of harmonic

Psycho-
physical
function

Tonal
material

Tuning
system

Modal
scale

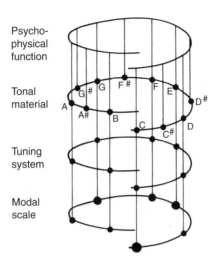

Fig. 10.3 Levels of analysis of the pitch material of music, illustrating the selection of culturally defined pitch categories in Shepard's helical psychophysical scale for pitch. Tone height in octaves is represented on the y-axis, and tone chroma (tonal scale value) is represented around the helix. (From Dowling and Harwood, 1986.)

complex tones—see Chapter 4). As a first approximation the psychophysical scale could be represented as a logarithmic scale relating pitch in octaves to frequency—doubling the frequency increases pitch by 1 octave. However, especially where music is concerned, pitches an octave apart are perceptually similar to each other, and serve the same functions in the tonal structure. When men and women sing together, they sing the same song but with the pitches an octave apart, and cultures that name their pitch categories give the same (or similar) names to pitches an octave apart. As Shepard (1982) pointed out, this octave equivalence means that the helix shown in Fig. 10.3 is a natural way to represent the relation of pitch and frequency. Pitches an octave apart are close to one another, and for every octave that the pitch ascends, it goes through a cycle of the helix, returning an octave higher to a point on the helix just above the point representing that pitch class in the lower octave. This allows us to classify each pitch in terms of its *pitch height* or octave level, the y-axis of the graph, and its specific functional pitch quality or *chroma*, which changes as we go around the curve of the helix.

The helix also captures another important fact about pitch perception, that what defines a melody is the pattern of relations among the pitches, and not the absolute pitch levels themselves. You can start 'Twinkle, Twinkle' on any pitch, and as long as you follow the same pattern of pitch intervals from note to note, it will still be 'Twinkle, Twinkle'. Those pitch intervals can be represented as movements back and forth around the helix. Shifting the tune to a new starting point, a new 'key', means translating that pattern of intervals in a screw-like motion along the helix. The helix has the very useful property that a tune (its interval pattern) can be shifted anywhere along it in this way without altering its shape.

Out of the infinity of pitches represented on the helix, the psychophysical scale, each culture selects a set of pitches for use in its music, which I have called the *tonal material*. In European music the tonal material consists of the chromatic scale that divides the 2/1 frequency ratio of the octave into twelve logarithmically equal steps, called *semitones* or half steps. Ascending 1 semitone along the chromatic scale involves multiplying the frequency by $2^{1/12} = 1.058463\ldots$; note that doing this twelve times lands us exactly 1 octave higher: $(2^{1/12})^{12} = 2$. This method of generating the tonal material in European music is called *equal temperament* because of the uniformly equal semitones that constitute the building blocks of all its tonal structures. Equal temperament was borrowed from China around 1720, and makes possible a shift in pitch of the tonal center (*tonic*) to any of the twelve pitches in the tonal material. Such a shift of the tonal center along with all of the tonal scale pitches related to it is called *modulation*.

Note that in defining the tonal material and the subsequent levels of analysis shown in Fig. 10.3, what is important is the *relative*, and not the absolute, pitches involved. This is easy for us to forget in the European tradition, where we think of the pitch A in the middle of the keyboard as having a fundamental frequency of 440 Hz. But this standardization of pitch levels is only about 100 years old (see Ellis's appendices to Helmholtz, 1877/1954). Unless one is among the small minority of the population with absolute pitch (the ability to name pitches out of context), small variations in the anchor points of the tonal material amid the infinity of possibilities in the psychophysical scale will not be noticeable.

Out of the tonal material, cultures often (but not universally) select a more restricted set of pitches, called a *tuning system*, as the basis for the formation of modal scales to be used in music. For example, in European music we could select the seven white keys on the piano (C, D, E, F, G, A, B) as a tuning system, one that could provide the basis for the keys of C major and A minor. In some cultures the tuning system is simply identical with the tonal material. For example, many Native American cultures use a tuning system (and tonal material) essentially the same as the pentatonic tuning systems of China and Europe (European white notes C, D, E, G, A, or black notes F#, G#, A#, C#, D#) from which modal scales and melodies can be formed.

The final step in this process, of moving from the abstract to the concrete in the selection of pitches with which to make a melody, is to form a *modal scale* from the tuning system. This involves establishing a tonal hierarchy (Krumhansl, 1990) on the pitches of the tuning system. For example, selecting C as a tonic in the set of white notes establishes the modal scale of C major, with a tonal hierarchy in which the most stable pitches are C, E, and G, and pitches D, F, A, and B are less stable (that is, have strong tendencies that 'pull' them toward the more stable pitches. To take the example of 'Twinkle, Twinkle' again, if the tune is in C major and begins on C, then the next-to-last note D has a strong tendency pulling it toward the C, that we feel when we stop short without resolving that tendency. Similarly, if we sing a *do-re-mi* scale beginning on C, and stop on the seventh pitch: *do, re, mi, fa, sol, la, ti* ... (C, D, E, F, G, A, B ...), we feel a very strong tendency pulling the B toward the upper C. These tonal tendencies have implications for how we perceive the pitches in the music we hear. Francès (1988, Experiment 2), for example, showed that if the pitches of a piece of music are altered in the direction of their tendencies in the tonal context, they are much less noticeable as 'out-of-tune' notes than pitches altered in the opposite direction.

The expectations we have of what pitches are coming next as we listen to music are engendered by our experience at the level of modal scales and the tonal hierarchy. The violation and resolution of these expectancies have strong emotional effects (Sloboda, 1998; Bharucha, 1999). Meyer (1956) called attention to this rise and fall of tension as an important source of our emotional response to music. If we return to the Beethoven sonata movement in Fig. 10.1, we can see examples of tonal tendencies and their resolution in the melody that starts in measure 2. The melody begins on D in the tonic chord Bb-D-F. The chord is stable, but the D is a little less stable than the tonic Bb, and this instability is resolved in the next measure to the Bb. The piece continues with pitches in the stable tonic chord until measure 5, where the harmony shifts to the dominant seventh chord F-A-C-Eb, in which the least stable pitch, Eb, is found in the melody. A very standard practice would be to resolve the dominant seventh to the tonic chord, with the Eb following its strong tendency downward to the D. However, at this point Beethoven defies gravity and takes the melody line to G in measure 6—an even less stable pitch in the context of the underlying F-A-C dominant chord, and one that generates acoustic dissonance with the neighboring scale notes F and A. The melody outlines the subdominant chord Eb-G-Bb against the dominant chord in the accompaniment, landing on the Bb in measure 7. This Bb, though the tonic, is now very unstable in the context of the continuing dominant chord (F-A-C), and needs to resolve downward to the A, which it does. We are now back to an unambiguous dominant harmony in both melody and accompaniment, which resolves peacefully to the tonic chord in measure 9. Thus in the course of eight measures Beethoven traces an excursion into very unstable tonal regions, and then back again to the stable tonic. This excursion gives the melody emotional energy that is immediately felt by the listener. These considerations of the tonal hierarchy show in detail how this is done, and there is clear evidence that musicians track the relationship of the pitches they hear in a piece to the tonal center (Toiviainen and Krumhansl, 2003) and that non-musicians as well as musicians track the rise and fall of tension in chord sequences (Bigand et al., 1996). Of course Beethoven has at his disposal techniques for even greater excursions; this is just a brief example in an eight-measure melody. In a movement lasting several minutes complications can be added by modulating to other keys (moving the pitch level of the tonic) and then back again, and by introducing contrasting melodic and rhythmic material. Musically trained listeners track such modulations, and Janata et al. (2002) have shown how that tracking is represented in the brain. And non-musicians provide evidence of knowing implicitly what key they are in during the middle of a continuously modulating piece, in that they respond quickly and accurately to out-of-key pitches when they occur (Janata et al., 2003). Listeners have an implicit knowledge of musical structure, and that knowledge, applied through the fulfillment and violation of expectancies, leads them to experience the ebb and flow of tension in the music, as Meyer (1956) theorized.

10.2.2 Time

Our perceptual and memory systems impose constraints on the temporal framework in terms of which we hear music. The sequence of sounds must not go too fast—somewhere between 10 and 20 notes/s it becomes a blur in which we lose track of individual pitches—and it must not go too slow, either. As a practical matter, we have difficulty recognizing familiar melodies when they go much faster than 6 notes/s (167 ms/note) or slower than about 0.6 note/s (1670 ms/note; Warren et al., 1991; Dowling et al., 2008). The notes simply do not hang together in a meaningful pattern at slower tempos. Furthermore, much music, especially songs and folk music, is organized into phrases, and the phrases are generally no longer than about 5 s, which is about the duration of material that can be stored in our auditory sensory memory buffer (Dowling and Harwood, 1986; Winkler and Cowan, 2005).

The temporal framework (Fig. 10.2) is organized into beats. We have a strong tendency to hear a beat in the music we listen to. Even if we hear just a series of evenly spaced clicks, we tend to group them perceptually into patterns of twos or threes or fours, set off by strong and weak beats (Fraisse, 1982). We find it easy to tap along with the beat in a piece of music, but only if there are sufficient cues in the music to where the beat is. Conversely, we can tap a complex rhythm along with a beat, but only if they are going at the same speed (that is, if they coincide periodically at the same spot in the pattern; Povel and Essens, 1985). Povel and Essens also showed that complicating the relationship between the rhythmic pattern and the beat makes the pattern more difficult to follow. They had listeners tap along with the upper line in Fig. 10.4; this was much easier for the simpler pattern (a) than for the more complex pattern (b).

A problem arises concerning how our internal beat is represented in the nervous system. The internal representation must be precise enough so that we can succeed in tapping along with the music, but it cannot be so rigid that it will fail to follow variations in tempo. Music is full of slight and large alterations in tempo from moment to moment, often introduced in the interest of emotional expression, aesthetic impact, and naturalness (see Gabrielsson and Lindström, 2001). A piece in

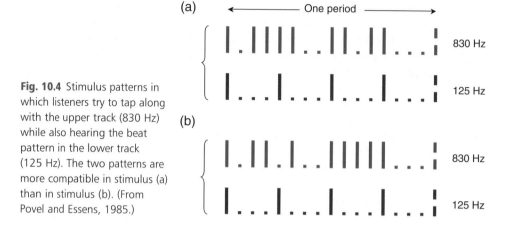

Fig. 10.4 Stimulus patterns in which listeners try to tap along with the upper track (830 Hz) while also hearing the beat pattern in the lower track (125 Hz). The two patterns are more compatible in stimulus (a) than in stimulus (b). (From Povel and Essens, 1985.)

which the beats and notes occur with rigid temporal regularity sounds dull and mechanical. Hence the grid illustrated in Fig. 10.2 is an oversimplification of what occurs in practice. How do we track the sequence of beats, and remain synchronized with the continually varying music? Large and Jones (1999) have proposed a solution in their theory of internal oscillators. They propose that we tune internal oscillators to temporal regularities in the environment. However, unlike a rigid beat structure, the oscillators continually update their relationship to the rhythmic events. They generate expectancies, that are then checked against reality and the oscillators are reset to continue tracking the events. An oscillator produces a periodic signal controlled by two parameters which can be reset: its tempo and its phase. If the oscillator is set to correct tempo to match the event sequence, but is out of sync with the events, its phase can be reset to achieve synchronization. This resetting is typically automatic, but can also be done intentionally to anticipate a hitch in the rhythm (Repp, 2002). The system copes with expressive timing changes such as a *ritardando* at the end of a phrase by gradually resetting the tempo.

10.3 Attention

The frameworks of pitch and time assist the direction of attention to important aspects of the musical pattern. When we are familiar with a style of music, our attention is directed automatically to regions in pitch and time where important events are likely to occur. This is similar to what happens when we learn a language: through practice we learn to direct our attention to important details in the stream of speech, so that what had formerly been an undifferentiated stream of sound becomes a comprehensible stream of words and phrases. We can see the effects of such learning with musical patterns in the examples of Fig. 10.5. In Fig. 10.5(a) we see two familiar melodies interleaved in time: 'Frère Jacques' (odd notes) and 'Twinkle, Twinkle' (even notes) played in two different octaves. It is easy to direct our attention to one or the other and perceive it clearly (Bregman, 1990); see also Chapter 8. In Fig. 10.5(b) the two melodies are interleaved in the same pitch range. Now it is very difficult to hear either one. However, with less than an hour's practice most people, musicians and non-musicians alike, can come to hear one or the other target melody when they are interleaved as in Fig. 10.5(b), provided they know what melody to listen for (Dowling, 1973). Knowing the target melody makes it possible to aim our attention at points in pitch and time where notes of that melody are likely to occur, and verify whether they did. As we would expect from Large and Jones's (1999) oscillator theory, it is easier to discern an

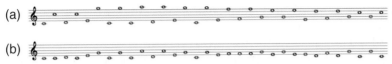

Fig. 10.5 (a) The tunes 'Frère Jacques' (red notes) and 'Twinkle, Twinkle' (blue notes) interleaved in time in separate octaves, presented at 8 notes/s. (b) The same two tunes interleaved in the same pitch range.

interleaved target when its notes occur on the beat (odd notes) than when they are off the beat (even notes; Dowling *et al.*, 1986). Our attentional system is apparently able to aim at a series of little windows in the pitch and time grid, and select the information that occurs there. This is illustrated by another experiment of Dowling *et al.* (1987). On each trial the pattern shown in Fig. 10.6 was presented at about 6 notes/s. The target note was the E in the middle of the pattern. When the pattern was repeated, it was interleaved with distractor notes, and the E moved to another pitch. Finally a probe tone was presented, and the listener judged whether the probe was higher or lower or the same in pitch as the pitch of the target. When the target moved within two semitones up or down, responses were relatively accurate; but on the few occasions when the target moved outside the limits of the pattern (to a higher or lower A), the listeners completely lost track of the target and performance fell to chance. Within the focus of attention, pitch judgment was affected by expectancies based on the system shown in Fig. 10.3. As long as the target landed on a pitch in the tonal material (D, D#, F, F#), judgment of the probe was relatively accurate. If the target landed on a quarter step (0.5 semitone) between those pitches, however, the pitch judgments were assimilated to neighboring tonal scale steps. That is, if the target was a pitch midway between D and D#, the probe D was judged equal to it. This indicates that when pitch encoding is hurried (because of the immediately following distractor note), the pitch encoding system takes the nearest scale note as a default value. This suggests that in listening to music, our auditory system will 'clean up' slight intonation errors in rapid passages.

There is considerable evidence that the perception of expected musical events is faster and more accurate than for unexpected events, due to the preparation for processing that expectancy sets in motion. For example, Bigand *et al.* (1999) presented chord sequences followed by target chords

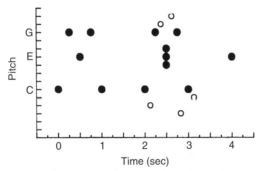

Fig. 10.6 Stimulus pattern in which the target pattern is first played alone at 4 tones/s (filled symbols), and then with interleaved distractor notes (open symbols). The center tone of the target is presented at a new pitch, higher or lower (multiple filled circles). Finally, a probe tone is presented, and the listener judges the pitch of the probe relative to that of the target tone. (From Dowling, 1992).

that were in-tune or out-of-tune (with the fifth of the chord raised by a semitone—a relatively obvious mistuning). Both musicians and non-musicians were better at detecting the mistunings in expected chords than in unexpected chords, with correct responses around 10 percentage points greater and 100 ms faster. Our experience with a particular musical style develops our attentional habits, which facilitate the processing of musical patterns within that style.

10.4 **What we perceive**

We have the subjective impression of perceiving things in the world just as they are, but as Treisman (2006, p. 317) points out, we are able to maintain this impression because we are seldom tested at those awkward moments when our finished perceptions—the world as we will remember it—are still under construction. Brunswik (1956, 2001) developed a 'lens' model of perception (Fig. 10.7), characterizing the coherent representation of the world we experience as achieved across a seemingly chaotic complex of sensory processing. Not only does our mental representation of events in music depend on what we select for attention, but it depends on the continued processing of a phrase even after subsequent phrases have entered the auditory sensory buffer. We can see this in the results of Dowling *et al.* (2001) who presented listeners with the beginnings of classical minuets. One of the initial phrases would be a target phrase to be tested later. The music continued, and a high-pitched signal indicated the occurrence of a test phrase, which was either a replica of the target phrase, a similar lure with the same melodic contour and rhythmic pattern as the target but at a different pitch level, or a different phrase. Figure 10.8 shows examples of these types of test in Beethoven's Minuet in G. Listeners had to say whether the test phrase was exactly the same as the target they had heard. In general, they found it easy to say that target test phrases were the same and different test phrases were different, no matter how long the delay between target and test (up to 30 s). However, the responses to the similar lures varied with delay. When interrupted after a 5-s delay, listeners confused the similar lures with the targets, shown in a high proportion of 'same' responses (false alarms). But when posed the same

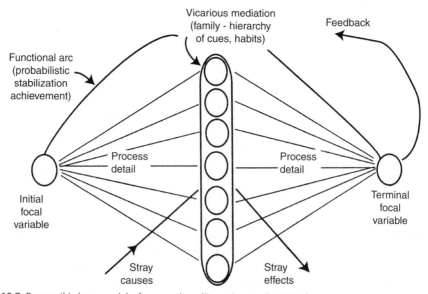

Fig. 10.7 Brunswik's lens model of perception. (From Brunswik, 2001.)

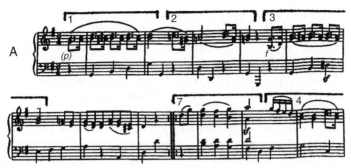

Fig. 10.8 The start of Beethoven's *Minuet in G* illustrating the structure of stimuli from Dowling *et al.* (2001), with a possible target phrase (bracket 1), a possible test item testing the target with a similar lure (bracket 3), and a possible different lure (bracket 7). (From Dowling *et al.*, 2001.)

question after 15 s their confusion had disappeared, and listeners no longer thought they had recently heard the similar lure. In the 10 s that had elapsed since the initial question was posed, it seems likely that the memory representation of the target phrase had gained in coherence and detail. For example, if we take the initial phrase (bracket 1) in Fig. 10.8 as a target, it could be tested after a 5-s delay with the phrase in bracket 3 as a similar lure. The melody in the lure has the same contour and rhythm as in the target, the accompaniment patterns are very similar, and both are in the same key. The main difference is that the melody in bracket 3 is attached to the tonal scale in a different place from the melody in bracket 1; the former centers on the third degree of the scale (B), whereas the latter centers on the fifth degree of the scale (G). Otherwise these two phrases match in key, melodic contour, and rhythm. It appears that the response given after 5 s is based on those feature matches, and that the response after 15 s takes account of the relationship of the contour to the scale. I think the development during the additional delay of a richer and more detailed representation of the phrase is responsible for the change in responses. This is an example of the answer to the question 'What did you perceive?' depending on when the listener is asked.

Once a coherent, meaningful representation of a phrase is formed, it can be stored in a relatively permanent form, to be called up into working memory when needed for comparison with other phrases, manipulated, or used in thinking about the piece and its structure (Winkler and Cowan, 2005; Treisman, 2006). Proust, an avid student of the psychology in the 1890s, has provided an excellent introspective account of the initial stages of cognitive processing of a melodic phrase. He begins by describing the initial experience of vague fleeting shapes that 'have vanished before these sensations are well-enough formed in us to avoid being submerged by following ... notes.' He continues: 'It was as if memory, like a worker striving to erect a solid foundation in the midst of a flood, while making facsimiles of these fleeting phrases, would not allow us to compare them to those that follow, and to differentiate them.' But shortly afterward, the listener's 'memory gave him a provisional and summary transcript of it, even while he continued listening. He took a good enough look at the transcript while the piece continued, so that when the same impression suddenly returned, it was no longer impossible to grasp' (Proust, 1999, p. 173, as cited in Dowling *et al.*, 2001, pp. 272–3).

10.4.1 The perceptual/memory representation

The content of our experience is a memory representation at some stage of encoding. Hence the question arises concerning the content of that representation: what features are encoded and brought to mind? Some 20 years ago our answer would have been that the representation of a melody is fairly abstract. Clearly what allows us to identify 'Twinkle, Twinkle' is a pattern of pitches that can be transposed to start on any note; when we sing 'Happy Birthday' it is rarely in the same key as the time before. We thought that what we remember consists of a melodic and rhythmic contour attached to a tonal scale in the appropriate mode (major or minor; Dowling, 1978). However, we have now learned that when the tune is one that we have always heard in the same key, our memory is quite literal, and the tune is represented much as we have always perceived it. Levitin (1994) discovered this in an experiment in which he brought students into a lab with a display of currently popular CDs on the wall. He had them pick out their favorite album, and then think of their favorite song on that album, and then sing it. Levitin found that they sang the song within a semitone or two of the key of the original. Moreover, they sang it at more or less the original tempo (Levitin and Cook, 1996). It seems likely that in the early stages of encoding the pop songs, the contour and tonal scale were encoded as separate features, and then combined, as in the Dowling et al. (2001) experiment described above. Levitin's result suggests that the scale in question is not just the general pattern of the major scale, for example, but fixed at least to some degree in its pitch level. It may take many repetitions for the scale to be absolutely fixed, however, since Dowling and Tillmann (in preparation), in a replication of Dowling et al. (2001), varied the key of the test item up or down 1 semitone without a noticeable effect on recognition performance. We do know that varying the pitch of the test item by much more than a semitone is disruptive of performance in recognizing novel melodies (Dowling and Fujitani, 1971).

It is tempting to suppose that the pitch pattern of a melody is initially encoded in terms of its contour plus the exact sizes of intervals from note to note. This view is widely expressed in the music cognition literature. In this view the results of Dowling et al. (2001) described above would mean that when tested after a 5-s delay listeners base their responses on contour alone, but at 15 s respond in terms of both contour and interval sizes. However, when the features of interval pattern and tonal framework are separately controlled at brief delays, the tonal framework has strong effects, which would not be the case if the initial encoding were simply in terms of contour, or of contour plus interval sizes, without regard to the scale framework (Bartlett and Dowling, 1980). Furthermore, there is converging evidence that melody recognition occurs in situations where interval sizes have been eliminated as cues, as in the interleaved melodies of Fig. 10.5(b) (Dowling, 1973), and in a similar experiment in which the pitches of a familiar melody are randomly assigned to different octaves (that is, 'Twinkle, Twinkle' would still consist of C-C-G-G-A-A-G as in Fig. 10.2, but the Cs and Gs, etc., would all be in different octaves; Dowling and Hollombe, 1977). There is also evidence that intervals are very difficult to identify out of context, and are remembered in terms of familiar tunes that feature them, rather than the tunes being remembered in terms of the intervals (Smith et al., 1994). And the tonal hierarchy, including the dynamic tendencies of pitches in the scale noted above, operates in terms of pitch classes, and not intervals. That is, in Fig. 10.2, when we stop on the next-to-last note of 'Twinkle, Twinkle' the pull we feel toward the tonic is due to the fact that the next-to-last note is the second degree of the scale, and not to the fact that it is 2 semitones above the tonic and 2 semitones below the third degree. The seventh degree of the scale pulls upward to the tonic, but not because it is 1 semitone lower; the third degree is 1 semitone below the fourth, and doesn't pull upward in the same way. The expectancies we have of where a melody is going are based on the tonal values of the pitches, and not on the interval pattern. I believe the evidence shows that we remember melodies in terms of a contour attached to a scale framework, and the contour and scale are among the principal perceptual features that we use in our early encoding of the melody into the representation we experience.

10.5 **Consonance and dissonance**

The issue of consonance and dissonance is closely related to the rise and fall of musical tension discussed above. We usually distinguish two types of consonance and dissonance in music: tonal or acoustic, and aesthetic. Acoustic dissonance is produced by the interaction of two or more simultaneous tones when they enter the auditory system, and creates a state of tension that can be resolved by moving to a more acoustically consonant combination of tones. Acoustic dissonance can characterize a single simultaneous tone cluster presented out of context. Aesthetic dissonance depends on musical context, and involves the very sources of instability and tension discussed above in relation to the tonal hierarchy. A single tone (like the next-to-last note of 'Twinkle, Twinkle') can be aesthetically dissonant if it is unstable and requires resolution to another tone, but it cannot be acoustically dissonant. In practice, European composers use acoustic dissonance and aesthetic dissonance in tandem, so that the least stable points in a progression of chords are also usually the most acoustically dissonant. For example, in measure 6 of the Beethoven sonata movement (Fig. 10.1), the harmony contains the pitches F-A-C-Eb-G—including four adjacent pitches in the scale (Eb-F-G-A)—which is a very acoustically *and* aesthetically dissonant combination. This occurs at the peak of tension in his melody, which gradually subsides into the cadence reaching the tonic in measure 9.

The acoustic dissonance of a pair of tones is not directly related to the musical interval between them. If it were, the function relating the size of the most dissonant interval to the frequency level of the tones would be a straight line with a positive slope representing the proportional frequency change of the interval, like the dotted line in Fig. 10.9. (Note that all equal musical intervals in equal temperament represent equal frequency ratios—1.05946 for the semitone, 2.0 for the octave, etc.) A second hypothesis, suggested by Helmholtz (1877/1954), is that dissonance is caused by beats between adjacent tones with a frequency difference around 40 Hz, which produces a very rough sensation. In that case, the most dissonant intervals would be represented by a constant difference between frequencies, shown in the horizontal dashed line in Fig. 10.9. (Note that all these considerations apply to dissonance between pairs of sine waves—pure tones. We will consider complex tones below.) Plomp and Levelt (1965) found that neither of these hypotheses is correct. The curve they found (the solid line in Fig. 10.9) follows the constant musical interval rule in the upper register, but flattens out in the lower register. It follows the curve for one-quarter of the critical bandwidth, a parameter of the auditory system summarizing a large amount of converging evidence concerning the interaction and mutual interference of adjacent tones (see Chapter 2). One consequence of the shape of the curve is that in the middle and upper registers of music it makes sense to think of some intervals (like perfect fourths and fifths) as being quite consonant across a wide range of frequencies, and of other intervals (like those of 1 and 2 semitones) as being fairly dissonant, but that this rule will not hold in the lower register. As we go lower, the proportionate size of the most dissonant frequency interval becomes greater, so that even thirds and fourths become quite dissonant. (You can imagine that if we transpose Bach chorales for a tuba quartet to play in their register, the result will be horrendous, even with excellent tuba players, because of the normally consonant thirds and fourths that abound in those pieces.) In practice, this leads composers to write with generally larger intervals between simultaneous bass notes than between the upper notes, as Plomp and Levelt documented in their report (and which is evident in Fig. 10.1).

Musical sounds are generally not pure tones, but rather harmonic complex tones, with a fundamental sine-wave frequency (which corresponds to the pitch) and a series of sine-wave harmonics (or 'overtones') at frequencies that are integer multiples of the fundamental. When two complex tones sound together, the dissonance produced is the sum of the dissonance produced

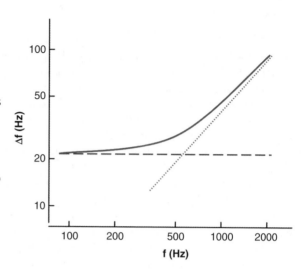

Fig. 10.9 The relationship of the most dissonant frequency interval (Δf) between two tones and the mean frequency (f) of the tones (solid line), which is approximately one-fourth of the critical bandwidth. The dotted line shows the results to be expected on the basis of a constant musical interval, and the dashed line shows a constant frequency difference (beat frequency).

by all the adjacent pairs of harmonics in the combination. There are two consequences of this that we should consider. First, combinations of complex tones will be less dissonant if their fundamental frequencies are small integer multiples of some common divisor, than if their relationships are more complicated. For example, consider two complexes in a 3/2 ratio: an E with components at 330, 660, 990, 1320, and 1650 Hz, and an A with components at 220, 440, 660, 880, 1100, and 1320 Hz. Either the adjacent components are sufficiently far apart not to interfere with each other (220, 330 and 440, etc.), or they coincide (at 660 and 1320). Not much dissonance is generated, and the combination, a perfect fifth, is consonant. But if we substitute an A# at 233, 466, 699, 932, and 1165 Hz, we get numerous clashes at 660–699, 1100–1165, etc., and the combination is quite dissonant. This is why *a capella* choirs and string quartets in slow passages tune their chords with simple whole number ratios rather than in equal temperament (where the perfect fifth has a ratio of 1.498 rather than the 1.5 of our example). The coincidence of the harmonics gives the chords a clarity and brilliance that they do not have in equal tempered tuning.

The second consequence of the interaction of adjacent harmonics concerns the dissonances in measures 9 and 10 of Fig. 10.1. Those dissonances (with pitches F-A-C-Eb-G-Bb, six of the seven pitches in the scale, simultaneously present or implied) do not stand out for the listener in the same way that they would if they all occurred clustered together in one octave, where they would have generated very strong acoustic dissonances. Because of the voicing of the chords (the distribution of pitches across several octaves), the harmonic components of the clashing notes are spread out, and not as much acoustic dissonance is generated as might have been. The aesthetic dissonance is subtle by comparison, and the eight-measure melody goes through changes in tension, but the effect is not at all jarring.

10.6 Timbre

Timbre involves qualities of sound apart from pitch and consonance. It is often called 'tone color' (*Klangfarbe* in German), and can be used to distinguish musical instruments and speech sounds. We can identify our favorite recordings within a tenth of a second on the basis of their timbre and texture (which instruments are playing in which registers, and how fast; Schellenberg *et al.*, 1999).

The psychophysics of timbre is multidimensional; that is, sound qualities cannot be arranged on a single dimension going from less to more. The cues involved in timbre perception consist of steady-state cues such as those that distinguish vowel sounds in speech, and transient cues, mostly in the first 50 ms after the onset of a sound, that distinguish initial consonants in speech (Dowling and Harwood, 1986). The steady-state cues depend largely on frequency regions in which the harmonics are strong due to resonances in the vocal tract or musical instrument, and are themselves multidimensional (Ladefoged and Broadbent, 1957; Slawson, 1968). Instruments are easily confused, however, if all the listener has are the steady-state cues. Saldanha and Corso (1964) demonstrated this by eliminating the onset transients from recordings of musical instruments, and found that discrimination among instruments as different as violins and trombones became very difficult when they were all playing the same pitch. Iverson and Krumhansl (1993) refined this result, finding that for the most part the same kinds of transient and steady-state cues are present in the onset of a tone and in the continuation of a tone as are present in the complete stimulus from beginning to end.

A major puzzle in the study of timbre perception has been the phenomenon of timbre constancy. The clarinet, for example, has different resonances and hence different steady-state cues in its upper and lower register, and yet it still sounds like a clarinet. But it seems likely that this is mainly true for musicians who have had years of experience hearing (or playing) clarinets in bands or orchestras. Steele and Williams (2006) had listeners distinguish a bassoon and a French horn, two instruments that Iverson and Krumhansl (1993) had found were easily confusable when they were playing in different octaves as well as playing the same pitch. Non-musicians had difficulty with this task, and their performance fell to chance when the pitch separation approached 2 octaves, whereas musicians' performance remained above 80% correct at 2.5 octaves separation. Timbre constancy clearly improves with perceptual learning.

10.7 Other topics

Several topics in the area of music perception have not been explored here for reasons of space. For issues concerned with loudness and sound localization the reader is referred to Dowling and Harwood (1986) and chapters in Deutsch (1999), as well as Bregman's (1990) book on auditory scene analysis that puts those issues into broader context. For music and the emotions, chapters in Juslin and Sloboda's (2001) volume provide broad, detailed coverage.

10.8 Summary

Music presents us with patterns of sound in a virtual space of pitch and time. Salient points on those dimensions—the tonal scale in pitch and the beat in time—give us a framework to track the organization of what we hear. We sense the degree of tension or relaxation in the music in relation to the stability of the pitches in the tonal and temporal frameworks. That instability can be enhanced by the addition of acoustic dissonance. Our familiarity with a genre of music provides expectancies by which we guide our attention to important aspects of the musical pattern. The distinctive timbres of the various voices and instruments also provide cues to musical organization; we can follow a particular melodic line more easily if its timbre contrasts with those in the background. The complexity of music and the extensive perceptual learning and acculturation involved in listening to and understanding it make music a fertile domain in which to study human cognition.

References

Bartlett, J. C. and Dowling, W. J. (1980). Recognition of transposed melodies: A key-distance effect in developmental perspective. *Journal of Experimental Psychology: Human Perception and Performance* 6:501–15.

Bharucha, J. J. (1999). Neural nets, temporal composites, and tonality. In *The Psychology of Music* (ed. D. Deutsch), pp. 413–40. San Diego: Academic Press.

Bharucha, J. J. and Pryor, J. H. (1986). Disrupting the isochrony underlying rhythm: An asymmetry in discrimination. *Perception ad Psychophysics* **40**:137–41.

Bigand, E., Parncutt, R., and Lerdahl, F. (1996). Perception of musical tension in short chord sequences: The influence of harmonic function, sensory dissonance, horizontal motion, and musical training. *Perception and Psychophysics* **58**:125–41.

Bigand, E., Madurell, F., Tillmann, B., and Pineau, M. (1999). Effect of global structure and temporal organization on chord processing. *Journal of Experimental Psychology: Human Perception and Performance* **25**:184–97.

Bregman, A. S. (1990). *Auditory Scene Analysis*. Cambridge, MA: MIT Press.

Brunswik, E. (1956). *Perception and the Representative Design of Psychological Experiments*. Berkeley: University of California Press.

Brunswik, E. (2001). *The Essential Brunswik* (ed. K. R. Hammond and T. R. Stewart). Oxford: Oxford University Press.

Deutsch, D. (ed.) (1999). *The Psychology of Music*. San Diego: Academic Press.

Dowling, W. J. (1973). The perception of interleaved melodies. *Cognitive Psychology* **5**:322–37.

Dowling, W. J. (1978). Scale and contour: Two components of a theory of memory for melodies. *Psychological Review* **85**:341–54.

Dowling, W. J. (1992). Perceptual grouping, attention and expectancy in listening to music. In *Gluing Tones: Grouping in Music Composition, Performance and Listening* (ed. J. Sundberg), pp. 77–98. Stockholm: Royal Swedish Academy of Music,

Dowling, W. J. and Fujitani, D. S. (1971). Contour, interval, and pitch recognition in memory for melodies. *Journal of the Acoustical Society of America* **49**:524–31.

Dowling, W. J. and Harwood, D. L. (1986). *Music Cognition*. Orlando, FL: Academic Press.

Dowling, W. J. and Hollombe, A. W. (1977). The perception of melodies distorted by splitting into several octaves: Effects of increasing proximity and melodic contour. *Perception and Psychophysics* **21**:60–4.

Dowling, W. J. and Tillmann, B. Memory improvement while hearing music: Effects of structural continuity on feature binding. (In preparation.)

Dowling, W. J., Lung, K. M.-T., and Herrbold, S. (1987). Aiming attention in pitch and time in the perception of interleaved melodies. *Perception and Psychophysics* **41**:642–56.

Dowling, W. J., Tillmann, B., and Ayers, D. (2001). Memory and the experience of hearing music. *Music Perception* **19**:249–76.

Dowling, W. J., Bartlett, J. C., Halpern, A. R., and Andrews, M. W. (2008). Melody recognition at fast and slow tempos: Effects of age, experience, and familiarity. *Perception and Psychophysics* **70**:496–502.

Fraisse, P. (1982). Rhythm and tempo. In *The Psychology of Music* (ed. D. Deutsch), pp. 149–80. New York: Academic Press.

Francès, R. (1988). *The Perception of Music* (transl. W. J. Dowling). Hillsdale, NJ: Erlbaum. [Original work published in 1958.]

Gabrielsson, A. and Lindström, E. (2001). The influence of musical structure on emotional expression. In *Music and Emotion: Theory and Research* (ed. P. N. Juslin and J. A. Sloboda), pp. 223–48. Oxford: Oxford University Press.

Hannon, E. E. and Trehub, S. E. (2005). Metrical categories in infancy and adulthood. *Psychological Science* **16**:48–55.

Helmholtz, H. L. F. von. (1877/1954). *On the Sensations of Tone* (transl. A. J. Ellis). New York: Dover.

Inhelder, B. and Piaget, J. (1958). *The Growth of Logical Thinking: From Childhood to Adolescence* (transl. A. Parsons and S. Milgram). New York: Basic Books.

Iverson, P. and Krumhansl, C. L. (1993). Isolating the dynamic attributes of musical timbre. *Journal of the Acoustical Society of America* **94**:2595–603.

James, W. (1890). *Principles of Psychology*. Boston: Henry Holt.

Janata, P., Birk, J. L., Van Horn, J. D., Leman, M., Tillmann, B., and Bharucha, J. J. (2002). The cortical topography of tonal structures underlying Western music. *Science* **298**:2167–70.

Janata, P., Birk, J. L., Tillmann, B., and Bharucha, J. J. (2003). Online detection of tonal pop-out in modulating contexts. *Music Perception* **20**:283–305.

Jones, M. R., Sommerell, L., and Marshburn, E. (1987). Recognizing melodies: A dynamic interpretation. *Quarterly Journal of Experimental Psychology* **39A**:89–121.

Juslin, P. N. and Sloboda, J. A. (eds) (2001). *Music and Emotion: Theory and Research*. Oxford: Oxford University Press.

Krumhansl, C. (1990). *Cognitive Foundations of Musical Pitch*. New York: Oxford University Press.

Kubovy, M. and Van Valkenburg, D. (2001). Auditory and visual objects. *Cognition* **80**:97–126.

Ladefoged, P. and Broadbent, D. E. (1957). Information conveyed by vowels. *Journal of the Acoustical Society of America* **29**:98–104.

Lao-Tse (1972). *Tao Te Ching* (trans. G.-F. Feng and J. English). New York: Vintage.

Large, E. W. and Jones, M. R. (1999). The dynamics of attending: How we track time-varying events. *Psychological Review* **106**:119–59.

Levitin, D. J. (1994). Absolute memory for musical pitch: Evidence from the production of learned melodies. *Perception and Psychophysics* **56**:414–23.

Levitin, D. J. and Cook, P. R. (1996). Memory for musical tempo: Additional evidence that auditory memory is absolute. *Perception and Psychophysics* **58**:927–35.

Meyer, L. B. (1956). *Emotion and Meaning in Music*. Chicago: University of Chicago Press.

Partch, H. (1974). *Genesis of a Music*. New York: Da Capo.

Plomp, R. and Levelt, W. J. M. (1965). Tonal consonance and critical bandwidth. *Journal of the Acoustical Society of America* **38**:548–60.

Povel, D. J. and Essens, P. (1985). Perception of temporal patterns. *Music Perception* **8**:411–40.

Proust, M. (1999). *À la Recherche du Temps Perdu* (edn in 1 vol.). Paris: Gallimard. [Original ref.: Proust, M. (1913). *Du côté de chez Swann*. Paris: Grasset.]

Repp, B. (2002). Automaticity and voluntary control of phase correction following event onset shifts in sensorimotor synchronization. *Journal of Experimental Psychology: Human Perception and Performance* **28**:410–30.

Saldanha, E. L. and Corso, J. F. (1964). Timbre cues and the identification of musical instruments. *Journal of the Acoustical Society of America* **36**:2021–6.

Schaeffer, P. (1952). *À la Recherche d'une Musique Concrète*. Paris: Éditions du Seuil.

Schellenberg, E. G., Iverson, P., and McKinnon, M. C. (1999). Name that tune: Identifying popular recordings from brief excerpts. *Psychonomic Bulletin and Review* **6**:641–6.

Schönberg, A. (1967). *Fundamentals of Music Composition*. New York: St Martins Press.

Shepard, R. N. (1982). Musical pitch. In *The Psychology of Music* (1st edn; ed. D. Deutsch), pp. 343–90. San Diego: Academic Press.

Slawson, W. (1968). Vowel quality and musical timbre as functions of spectrum envelope and fundamental frequency. *Journal of the Acoustical Society of America* **43**:87–101.

Sloboda, J. (1998). Does music mean anything? *Musicae Scientiae* **2**:21–31.

Smith, J. D., Nelson, D. G. K., Grohskopf, L. A., and Appleton, T. (1994). What child is this? What interval was that? Familiar tunes and music perception in novice listeners. *Cognition* **52**:23–54.

Steele, K. M. and Williams, A. K. (2006). Is the bandwidth for timbre invariance only one octave? *Music Perception* **23**:215–20.

Toiviainen, P. and Krumhansl, C. L. (2003). Measuring and modeling real-time responses to music: The dynamics of tonality induction. *Perception* **32**:741–66.

Treisman, A. (2006). Object tokens, binding, and visual memory. In *Handbook of Binding and Memory: Perspectives from Cognitive Neuroscience* (ed. H. D. Zimmer, A. Mecklinger, and U. Lindenberger), pp. 315–39. Oxford: Oxford University Press.

Vines, B. W., Krumhansl, C. L., Wanderley, M. M., and Levitin D. J. (2006). Cross-modal interactions in the perception of musical performance. *Cognition* **101**:80–113.

Warren, R. M., Gardner, D. A., Brubaker, B. S., and Bashford, J. A., Jr (1991). Melodic and nonmelodic sequences of tones: Effects of duration on perception. *Music Perception* **8**:277–90.

Winkler, I. and Cowan, N. (2005). From sensory to long-term memory: Evidence from auditory memory reactivation studies. *Experimental Psychology* **52**:3–20.

Yonelinas, A. P. (2002). The nature of recollection and familiarity: A review of 30 years of research. *Journal of Memory and Language* **46**:441–517.

Chapter 11

Auditory attention

Charles Spence and Valerio Santangelo

11.1 Introduction

One of the most fundamental questions in the fields of cognitive psychology and cognitive neuroscience concerns how it is that human beings can selectively attend to certain aspects of their environment, while at the same time ignoring, or inhibiting, the processing of other, currently less-relevant, stimuli (Kauramäki et al., 2007). Researchers first started to investigate the topic of auditory selective attention after the Second World War, in an attempt to try to understand why it was that fighter pilots sometimes failed to perceive perfectly audible messages presented to them over headphones. Cognitive psychologists such as Donald Broadbent, based at the Applied Psychology Unit in Cambridge, introduced a variety of selective listening tasks in order to simulate the kind of multi-message environments that were typically faced by pilots. While the majority of the research in the intervening years has tended to focus on understanding the mechanisms of selective attention that operate unimodally within the visual modality, there has been a resurgence of interest in the mechanisms of auditory attention over the last decade or so. What is more, many researchers now believe that many of the same principles (and perhaps even neural mechanisms) can be used to describe and/or explain selective attention in both sensory modalities (e.g. Mayer et al., 2006; Wu et al., 2007; Dalton and Spence, 2008; Shinn-Cunningham, 2008). In this chapter, we briefly review the key empirical findings to have emerged from studies of auditory selective attention over the last 50 years or so. Additionally, we highlight recent evidence demonstrating the connection between selective attention and working memory. We also review a number of the models and theories (both cognitive and neuroscientific) that have been put forward in order to try to explain how selective attention operates in audition.

11.2 The speech shadowing task

Colin Cherry (a cognitive scientist from Imperial College, London) first introduced the now-ubiquitous dichotic listening task to the field of cognitive psychology more than half a century ago (see Cherry, 1953, 1954). The participants in a typical study were instructed to repeat aloud, or 'shadow', the auditory message presented to one ear over headphones, while at the same time trying to ignore the distractor message presented simultaneously to their other ear. Cherry found that people could successfully shadow the target message when it was defined by its unique location (i.e. when instructed to 'shadow the voice presented to their right ear'), or by some other distinctive physical feature (i.e. 'shadow the woman's voice and ignore the man's voice'). However, the surprising result to emerge from Cherry's research was just how little participants were able to remember when, after having shadowed the relevant auditory stream, they were probed about their knowledge of the content of the 'unattended' message. They could only verbally report on the physical features of the irrelevant stream, such as the gender of the speaker, or that they had noticed that the speech had been replaced by a tone, or that the voice of a male speaker had been replaced by that of a female. By contrast, the majority of Cherry's participants failed to notice when the speaker in the unattended stream was replaced by another speaker of the same gender (see also Wood and Cowan, 1995a), or when the language of the distracting message happened to switch from English to German midway through shadowing. Only about one-third of people noticed if the speech stream playing in the unattended ear was reversed while they were shadowing (see Wood and Cowan, 1995a).

The results of early shadowing studies thus revealed that little, if any, of the semantic content of the unattended message could be reported explicitly by participants. Indeed, Neville Moray (1959) even demonstrated that participants failed to recognize a word that had been presented 35 times in the unattended ear. Results such as these led Broadbent (1958) to put forward his highly influential early selection model of attention. According to Broadbent, environmental information is filtered out of awareness if it is identified as being irrelevant to a person's current goals. Filtering appeared to be based on the superficial physical features of the unattended stream, such as its location, pitch, and intensity (though note that there is nothing particularly simple, or 'early', about the neural coding of auditory location; Allport, 1992). Selective attention was, then, viewed by Broadbent and others as a filter that prevented irrelevant information from being processed beyond its basic physical characteristics. Such filtering was deemed necessary in order to protect the limited capacity central processing resources from becoming overloaded by too much incoming sensory information.

The notion that auditory selective attention was based solely on the physical features of the auditory stimulus was, however, soon questioned by other researchers. For example, in his now classic paper, Moray (1959) demonstrated that one-third of participants noticed their own first name when it was surreptitiously inserted into the irrelevant (and putatively unattended) auditory stream. This phenomenon, known as the 'cocktail party effect',[1] has now been replicated by other researchers (Wood and Cowan, 1995b; Conway et al., 2001). Many other ingenious shadowing studies also provided converging evidence for the semantic processing of the stimuli presented in the 'unattended' stream (e.g. Corteen and Wood, 1972; MacKay, 1973; Corteen and Dunn, 1974; and see Driver, 2001, for a review). Results such as these led Deutsch and Deutsch (1963) to argue that selection actually occurs much later in information processing than had previously been thought. According to their 'neurophysiologically inspired' model, all sensory stimuli are, in fact, processed for their semantic meaning, and selection (i.e. filtering) occurs just prior to participants becoming aware of that information.

One reason for the enduring nature of the controversy over whether attentional selection occurs early or late in human information processing has been the fact that different researchers have used different measures of a participant's awareness, and these have given rise to differing answers. These measures have varied from the subjective report originally introduced by Cherry (1953) to semantic priming (Mackay, 1973), and from forced choice recognition (Moray, 1959) to physiological measures, such as the phasic changes in the galvanic skin response (GSR) induced by the presentation of words that had previously been associated (paired) with an electric shock (see Corteen and Wood, 1972; Corteen and Dunn, 1974).

In one particularly elegant study, Corteen and Dunn (1974) demonstrated both 'early' and 'late' selection within the same shadowing study by simultaneously assessing two different measures

---

[1] There is a degree of confusion in the literature as to exactly what the term 'cocktail party effect' actually refers. While the majority of researchers currently use the term to refer to one's name popping-out of an unattended speech stream, Cherry (1953) himself actually used the term when referring to the question of how humans can recognize what one person is saying when others are speaking at the same time.

of awareness. The participants in their study were initially conditioned with an electric shock every time they heard a city name. Next, they were presented with two messages, one to either ear over headphones (this is known as 'dichotic presentation'). The participants had to shadow one of these speech streams, while simultaneously trying to monitor both streams for the occurrence of a city name (though, unbeknownst to the participants, city names were only ever presented to the unshadowed ear). The participants virtually never indicated explicitly that they had heard a city name (in fact, only 1 out of the 114 city names was responded to across all participants). However, on 40% of occasions, the presentation of the city name gave rise to a measurable phasic GSR. What is more, this physiological response was shown to generalize to city names that had not previously been associated with shock, hence arguing that the words had been processed to a semantic level (i.e. rather than the response having been triggered simply by the acoustic signature of specific city names). Corteen and Dunn's results therefore demonstrate that part of the answer as to why selection sometimes appears to occur early but at other times appears to occur much later in human information processing may depend, at least in part, on just how a participant's 'awareness' of a particular stimulus happens to be assessed.

That said, researchers have put forward a number of intermediate theories and cognitive models to account for the growing body of compelling evidence for both early and late selection (e.g. Treisman, 1969; Johnston and Heinz, 1978). Treisman, for example, proposed that attentional filtering simply attenuated the processing of stimuli in the unattended ear, rather than blocking them out completely. She also introduced the notion of dictionary recognition units (DRUs) with varying thresholds in order to account for the fact that certain stimuli (e.g. one's own name, as well as various threat-related words) 'break through' from the unattended channel more easily than other words. Treisman was, however, criticized for providing insufficient evidence regarding the neural substrates for the various components of her model (e.g. she was unclear on exactly how DRUs were actually instantiated in the brain).

By contrast, Johnston and Heinz (1978) put forward the argument that the depth of processing of non-target information was not fixed, but instead varied as a function of the ease with which participants were able to discriminate the target from amongst the non-target stimuli (see also Johnston and Heinz, 1979). According to their theory, selection could occur anywhere along the continuum of auditory information processing from early to late. More recently, Nilli Lavie has put forward a similar suggestion regarding the flexibility of attentional selection, although the mechanism that she has proposed is quite different.

According to the perceptual load theory of selective attention (e.g. Lavie and Tsal, 1994; see Lavie, 2005, for a recent review), a person's attentional resources will always be fully deployed in the processing of any incoming sensory information. Hence, under conditions where a participant's primary task is not overly demanding, there may well be spare attentional resources available for the processing of other stimuli (such as the irrelevant distractor stream in a dichotic listening study). Lavie argued that under such 'low-load' conditions late selection may be observed. However, if the load of the primary task increases (e.g. if the complexity or presentation rate of the to-be-shadowed message increases), then participants will have to devote more resources to processing it, and hence less residual attentional resources will be available for the processing of other auditory stimuli. Under such 'high-load' conditions, Lavie argued, selection will occur relatively early in information processing instead.

Perceptual load theory certainly provides an intuitively plausible account for why selection might sometimes occur early and at other times (and/or in other studies) it occurs much later in human information processing. What is more, in the 15 years since Lavie and Tsal (1994) first proposed the theory, an impressively large number of studies, both behavioural and neuroimaging, have been published providing support for the theory (see Lavie, 2005, for a review; though see Eltiti *et al.*, 2004, for contradictory evidence). That said, the majority of studies of perceptual load have restricted themselves to the study of unimodal visual selective attention. Consequently, the claim that early selection will be observed in dichotic listening studies where the to-be-shadowed stream is perceptually/cognitively demanding has yet to be tested empirically.[2] Nevertheless, several recent studies have now provided empirical evidence regarding the utility of the theory of perceptual load in accounting for the effects of varying primary task load on the processing of irrelevant auditory stimuli (see Alain and Izenberg, 2003; Chan and Spence, 2009).

The participants in Chan and Spence's (2009) experiment had to listen to a rapidly presented series of 1–3 syllable words spoken in either a loud or quiet voice from a loudspeaker placed in front of them. In the low-load condition, the participants had to discriminate the intensity of each word as rapidly as possible. By contrast, in the high-load condition, the participants had to discriminate whether or not each word had two syllables. While the participants performed one of these two auditory discrimination tasks, an additional sound was presented that appeared to sweep repeatedly from one ear to the other over the headphones worn by participants (the apparent motion of this auditory stimulus was created by varying the interaural phase difference between the signals presented to the participant's ears). After the end of shadowing, the moving sound was replaced by a stationary sound localized to the centre of the participant's head. This sound briefly appeared to move in the direction opposite to that of the inducing auditory movement, and participants simply had to discriminate whether it appeared to move to the left or right. The strength of this auditory motion after-effect (MAE) provided an indicator of the extent to which participants processed the background auditory information.

Chan and Spence (2009) found that participants were significantly more likely to report the sound to have moved in the direction opposite to that experienced in the exposure period in the low-load condition than in the high-load condition (see Fig. 11.1). The fact that a more pronounced auditory MAE was observed in the low-load condition (indicating the enhanced processing of the background auditory stream) is entirely consistent with the predictions of perceptual load theory (cf. Rees *et al.*, 1997, for an analogous visual experiment). When taken together with the results of Alain and Izenberg's (2003) event-related potential (ERP) study, showing the dramatic effects of manipulating perceptual load on auditory scene analysis, it would therefore appear that perceptual load theory may well turn out to provide just as good an account of selective attention in the auditory modality as it has already done in the visual modality.

11.3 **Working memory and selective attention**

One question that has been the subject of growing research interest over the last few years concerns why it is that only a subset of participants actually hear their own name when it is presented in the unshadowed stream. Perhaps the most important research to be published on this question was reported by Conway *et al.* (2001). They tested 40 participants, 20 from the upper quartile and another 20 from the lower quartile of a much larger group of participants on the basis of their performance on an operation span task—a standard test used to measure working memory

---

[2] One caveat is that no objective measure of 'load' has as yet been provided. Instead, Lavie and her colleagues typically seem to use an operational definition, i.e. you know it when you see it. Of course, this raises the problem of circularity, because if a putative manipulation of perceptual load does not have the desired effect on the degree of processing of background stimuli, it is hard to know whether the load manipulation itself was simply not dramatic enough to give rise to a significant change in the processing of the background (or irrelevant) stimuli, or whether instead, perceptual load manipulations do not always modulate whether selection occurs early or late in human information processing.

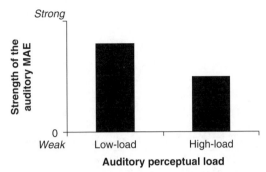

Fig. 11.1 (A) Schematic graph showing the pattern of results reported by Chan and Spence (2009) in their recent study investigating the effects of varying auditory perceptual load on the processing of background auditory stimuli. A significantly stronger auditory motion after-effect (MAE) was observed after participants had performed the low-load task (discriminating whether each word in a speech stream had been spoken in a quiet or loud voice) than after they had performed a more demanding (i.e. high-load) task (discriminating whether or not each word in the speech stream had two syllables or not). These results are consistent with the predictions of Lavie's (2005) theory of perceptual load.

(WM; the name given to a theoretical construct, a cognitive system containing storage buffers and a central executive that actively maintains goal-relevant information in the service of complex cognition; see Baddeley, 1986). Importantly, individual differences in WM capacity were found to correlate with measurable differences in a person's ability to selectively focus their auditory attention on a particular auditory stream. The participants in Conway *et al.*'s study had to shadow one of two auditory streams consisting of a series of monosyllabic words presented synchronously, one to either ear over headphones, at a rate of 60 words/second. The participant's first name (and that of one of the other participants in the study) were presented (to the unattended ear) after participants had shadowed the relevant ear for a few minutes. The low-span participants committed twice as many shadowing errors as the high-span participants, thus showing that they found the shadowing task to be more difficult. On being questioned about the contents of the irrelevant message after having completed the shadowing task, only 20% of the high WM-span participants reported having heard their own name in the irrelevant message, as compared to 65% of the low span participants.[3] By contrast, none of the participants reported hearing the yoked control participant's name.

Subsequent analysis of Conway *et al.*'s (2001) data revealed that the increased intrusion by the participant's own name in the low-span participants was not simply the result of their attention having wandered over to the irrelevant auditory stream in the moments prior to their name appearing there, since the low-span participants were no more likely to make an intrusion error for either of the two words immediately preceding the presentation of their own name than were the high-span participants (see Fig. 11.2). By contrast, those participants who reported hearing their own name in the unattended stream committed significantly more shadowing errors immediately after the presentation of their name than those who did not (see also Wood and Cowan, 1995*b*).

---

[3] This finding is surprising given that most people's intuition is that the higher WM group would have a greater capacity and therefore find it easier to process two streams of information at once; in fact, the opposite result was observed.

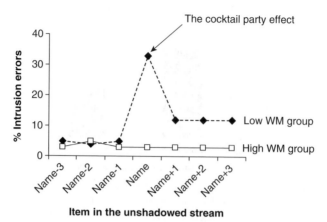

Item in the unshadowed stream

Fig. 11.2 Results from Conway *et al.*'s (2001) study of auditory selective attention and working memory. The figure schematically shows how often participants made an intrusion error for the speech items presented around the time that their name was presented in the unshadowed speech stream. Importantly, the results show that the low WM-span participants only made more intrusion errors than the high-span participants for items that followed the presentation of their own name and not for those items that preceded it.

These results would therefore appear to suggest that the attention of the relatively low-span participants was simply much more likely to be captured (exogenously; Spence and Driver, 1994) by the presentation of their own name when it was presented in the irrelevant auditory stream. Conway *et al.*'s results provided some of the first empirical evidence regarding the close link between working memory and attentional capture in audition. In particular, they suggest that low-span participants simply find it harder to filter out irrelevant information than those with a higher working memory span.

The link between attentional capture by irrelevant auditory stimuli and WM load/capacity first documented by Conway *et al.* (2001) has now been supported by a number of other studies (e.g. Berti and Schröger, 2003; Beaman, 2004; Muller-Gass and Schröger, 2007; Dalton *et al.*, 2009). For example, Dalton and her colleagues had their participants make speeded elevation discrimination responses to brief auditory targets presented unpredictably from either the left or right of fixation whilst simultaneously trying to ignore distractor sounds (Dalton *et al.*, 2009). The auditory distractors were always presented from the opposite side to the target and equiprobably from either the same or opposite elevation (see Fig. 11.3(A)). The participants were also given a list of digits to remember: In the low WM-load condition, the digits always consisted of the ascending numerical string '123456', whereas in the high-load condition, the order in which the digits (from 1 to 9) were presented was randomized from trial to trial. After having memorized a given digit list, the participants had to discriminate the elevation of 2–4 auditory targets before being presented with another pair of digits and deciding whether or not they had been presented in the same order in the preceding digit list. The results showed that the auditory distractors interfered significantly more (i.e. a larger congruency effect was observed) with participants' target elevation discrimination responses in the high WM-load condition than in the low-load condition (see Fig. 11.3(B)).

Although recent findings therefore converge on the conclusion that there is a close link between WM and (auditory) selective attention, the question of why exactly auditory selective attention should be impaired when WM resources are (for whatever reason) limited has not as yet been

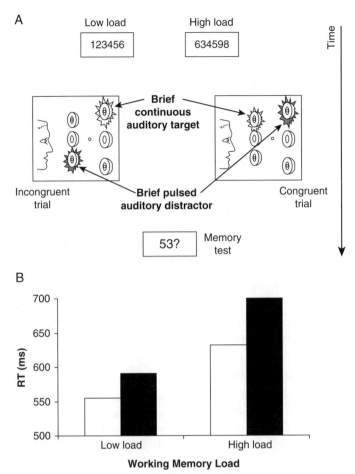

Fig. 11.3 (A) Schematic figure of the experimental design in Dalton *et al.*'s (2009) recent study of the effects of working memory load on auditory distractor interference. Participants were initially presented with either a predictable (low load) or unpredictable (high load) series of six digits to remember. Next, they had to make speeded elevation discrimination responses to a number of brief continuous auditory targets whilst simultaneously trying to ignore the elevation of the pulsed auditory distractors that were presented at the same time. Finally, another pair of digits was presented on the screen and participants had to decide whether they appeared in the same order as in the list of digits that were presented earlier. (B) Graph highlighting the results of Dalton *et al.*'s (2009) study. Mean RTs for congruent trials (where the target and distractor were presented from the same elevation) are presented in white, while mean RTs for the incongruent trials (where the target and distractor were presented from different elevations) are presented in black. The results show that distractor congruency effects (measured as the difference in performance between incongruent and congruent trials) were more pronounced under conditions of high working-memory load.

unequivocally resolved. According to de Fockert *et al.* (2001), loading WM deleteriously affects performance because it impairs a participant's ability to remember what his/her current task priorities are (i.e. to remember what constitutes the target and what the distractor; see also Lavie and de Fockert, 2005).[4] In other words, taxing WM is thought to result in participants being more likely to forget what their current task is, and, as a result, they will tend to get distracted more often. By contrast, those individuals with a higher WM capacity are thought to be capable of focusing/restricting their attention more efficiently on the stream/object that currently happens to be relevant, and hence are far less likely to suffer from breakthrough by information presented in the unattended stream.[5]

Interestingly, neuroimaging studies have now started to shed some light on the neural substrates of this interaction between WM and selective attention: For example, Todd *et al.* (2005) have demonstrated that loading WM (once again, by giving participants a digit string to remember) results in the suppression of neural activity in the right temporoparietal junction (TPJ), a region of the brain that is known to constitute a core structure in the ventrofrontoparietal attentional network (e.g. Corbetta and Shulman, 2002). The TPJ is thought to play a crucial role in the reorienting of our attention toward environmental events, no matter whether they happen to be relevant currently or not (see Berti and Schröger, 2003). Moreover, Johnson and Zatorre (2006) recently highlighted the key role played by the dorsolateral prefrontal cortex (a crucial area subserving executive functions, and in particular working memory; Curtis and D'Esposito, 2004) in dividing attentional resources between more than one to-be-attended stimulus, likely helping participants to maintain target-related information in working memory (see Petrides, 2000).

11.4 Auditory change deafness

Another dramatic example of the severe limitations on auditory information processing comes from studies of auditory change deafness (analogous to the phenomenon of 'change blindness' in vision; see Simons and Ambinder, 2005, for a review). Auditory change deafness has now been studied explicitly by a number of researchers using both simple and complex auditory displays (see Vitevitch, 2003; Eramudugolla *et al.*, 2005; Gregg and Samuel, 2008; Pavani and Turatto, 2008). For example, Vitevitch reported that 57% of the participants in one experiment failed to notice the change in the identity of a single speaker whom they happened to be shadowing. A subsequent control study demonstrated that this poor level of performance could not be attributed to problems with physically distinguishing between the voices of the two speakers (as participants performed at over 90% correct when explicitly judging whether they were the same or not). It is, however, still possible that Vitevitch's participants may actually have noticed the change in the speaker's voice, but simply have forgotten about this fact (which would presumably have seemed irrelevant to them at the time) in the interval between the occurrence of the voice switch and the experimenter subsequently quizzing them about what they had just heard (during

---

[4] Note that which stimulus constitutes the target, and which the distractor, often reverses from block to block in these studies, hence making the task of remembering what currently constitutes that target all the more difficult for participants.

[5] It should, however, be noted that this account does not readily explain Cowan *et al.*'s (2001) finding that those participants who noticed their own name (i.e. who showed a cocktail party effect) were no more likely to have switched their attention to the unattended stream for the words immediately preceding the presentation of their own name (see Fig. 11.2). What is more, this argument could also be turned around by suggesting that the poor performance on the WM task reflects a lack of attention to the WM task rather than a lack of capacity; i.e. that WM task performance is dependent on attention, not memory *per se.*

which time the participants had to shadow 50 words; cf. Norman, 1969; Corteen and Wood, 1972; Wood and Cowan, 1995a). Or, to put it another way, it is unclear whether Vitevitch's partici- pants' poor awareness of the physical attributes of the speech stimuli reflects 'attentional blind- ness' and/or 'attentional amnesia' (see Wolfe, 1999).

Fortunately, subsequent studies have done a much better job of isolating the genuinely percep- tual component of auditory change deafness and, what is more, they have achieved this under conditions in which the participants' *primary* task was to identify whether or not something had changed in the auditory displays that they were listening to. So, for example, the participants in a study by Eramudugolla *et al.* (2005) were presented with an auditory scene consisting of four, six, or eight distinct auditory objects (including the sounds of a trumpet, piano, female voice, clucking hen, etc., each seemingly presented from a different position) for five seconds (see Fig. 11.4(A)). Next, white noise was presented for 500 ms, followed by the presentation of a second auditory scene for a further five seconds. The two auditory displays were identical, except for the fact that on half of the trials one of the auditory objects was removed from the second display (sometimes it was replaced by another auditory object). On each trial, the participants simply had to decide whether or not one of the auditory objects was missing from the second display.

Eramudugolla *et al.*'s (2005) results showed that the accuracy (and sensitivity) of participants' auditory change detection responses dropped dramatically as the number of objects in the scene increased (see Fig. 11.4(B)). By contrast, participants' performance was unaffected by changes in set size under conditions where their spatial attention had been directed to the location where the potential change might occur in advance (by a visual cue, e.g. the word 'cello' when that was the

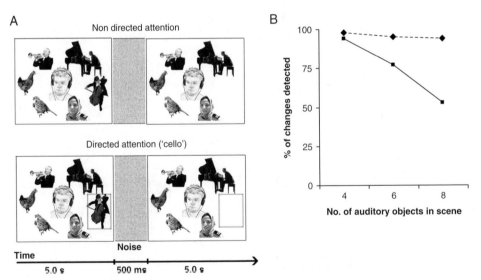

Fig. 11.4 (A) Shows the experimental set-up used in Eramudugolla *et al.*'s (2005) study of auditory change deafness. Note that the auditory stimuli were presented in virtual auditory space over headphones. Each trial consisted of the presentation of an auditory scene made up of four, six (shown here), or eight objects. (B) Graph highlighting the pattern of results obtained when the participants were not told which item in the display might change (non-directed attention condition; solid line), their performance deteriorated dramatically as the display size increased. By contrast, when the participants were informed in advance which item in the display might change (directed attention condition; dotted line), their performance was near-perfect no matter what the set size. Panel A reprinted from Eramudugolla *et al.*, 2005, Figure 1, with permission.

relevant item in the display). The excellent performance seen under the latter conditions confirmed that the decrement in performance observed in the former (uncued) condition was attentional in nature, rather than reflecting some form of energetic masking between the various simultaneously presented auditory stimuli (see Chan *et al.*, 2005; Shinn-Cunningham, 2008).

Eramudugolla *et al.* (2005) went on to argue that the presentation of the white noise burst between the two auditory displays likely masked the transients that might otherwise have cued the participants' attention to the change taking place in the display. However, subsequent research by Pavani and Turatto (2008) has shown that change deafness occurs regardless of whether or not white noise is introduced between two sequentially presented auditory displays, and (perhaps more surprisingly) that it even occurs when there is no temporal gap between them (see Fig. 11.5). Gregg and Samuel (2008) have reported that familiarity with the auditory objects presented in a scene does not facilitate people's change detection performance. Moreover, while Eramudugolla *et al.* reported enhanced change detection performance when the stimuli were presented from different (rather than the same) virtual spatial locations, a subsequent study by Gregg and Samuel (2008) actually reported the opposite result (i.e. change detection performance was better when all the sounds were presented from the same location). This discrepancy may, though, perhaps be attributable to differences in the duration of stimulus presentation in the two studies: For while Eramudugolla *et al.* presented their auditory displays for 5 seconds each, Gregg and Samuel presented theirs for only 1 second, and this may simply not have left their participants enough time

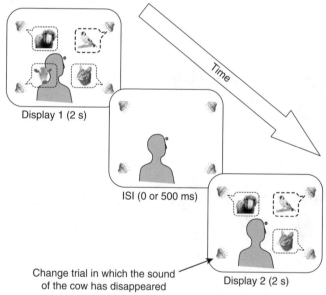

Display 1 (2 s)

ISI (0 or 500 ms)

Change trial in which the sound of the cow has disappeared

Display 2 (2 s)

Fig. 11.5 Schematic figure of the experimental design of Pavani and Turatto's (2008) study of auditory change deafness. On each trial, participants were presented with either three or four different animal sounds using real auditory scenes consisting of different sounds (taken from a set of 12 different animal calls), presented for 2 s from up to four different free-field loudspeakers arranged at the corners of a virtual square. Note that across experiments the interstimulus interval (ISI) was either filled with 500 ms of white noise or silence, or else was reduced to 0 ms (i.e. the second auditory display was presented immediately after the first). Once again, participants failed to notice a large proportion of the changes introduced between the two displays. Adapted from Pavani and Turatto, 2008, Figure 1.

to shift their attention between the various different items in the scene before each display was terminated (see Rhodes, 1987; Mondor and Zatorre, 1995).

Taken together, the results of these recent auditory change-detection studies therefore suggest that people may actually be unaware of the majority of the auditory information present in complex auditory scenes. These results are entirely consistent with the much older literature on speech shadowing (see above) showing that people are only aware of (or rather, only have conscious access to) the auditory information (i.e. to the auditory object or stream) that they happen to be attending to (Shinn-Cunningham, 2008), or which happens to capture their attention exogenously (i.e. in a stimulus-driven manner; Spence and Driver, 1994). Indeed, other recent research has shown that increasing the spatial separation between two speech streams enhances a person's ability to selectively listen to one of the speakers and ignore the other, while at the same time making it harder for them to divide their attention simultaneously between both streams (see Best et al., 2006; see also Ebata et al., 1968; Chan et al., 2005).

11.5 Auditory spatial attention

The research reported thus far clearly shows that people can voluntarily direct their auditory attention to a particular auditory stream (or object; see also Chapter 8; Shinn-Cunningham, 2008). However, it is important to note that people can also endogenously (or voluntarily) focus their auditory attention on a particular location (or side of space) in the absence (or, rather, prior to the presentation) of any auditory stimuli at that location (one can think of this distinction in terms of the debate between object- and space-based attention in vision). Voisin et al. (2006) have demonstrated that this form of spatial attentional orienting (or expectancy) can, nevertheless, lead to the selective activation of both the primary and secondary auditory cortical areas even in the absence of sound (presumably this pattern of activation reflects the brain's readiness to process an expected upcoming sound). Indeed, many studies have now shown that the processing of auditory stimuli is enhanced when they are presented at attended as opposed to unattended locations (e.g. Rhodes, 1987; Spence and Driver, 1994, 1996; Mondor and Zatorre, 1995; Quinlan and Bailey, 1995; Schröger and Eimer, 1997). For example, Spence and Driver (1994, 1996) used a variant of the Posnerian spatial cueing paradigm (see Posner, 1978) in order to investigate the consequences for perception of focusing spatial attention on either the left or right side of space (borrowing the analogy from vision, researchers often talk in terms of focusing the spotlight of auditory attention; see Spence and Driver, 1994; Best et al., 2006; Fritz et al., 2007). Participants were shown to discriminate the spatial location (either elevation or front vs. back) and the frequency of auditory targets that were presented on the attended (or expected) location more rapidly (and accurately) than when their attention had (invalidly) been directed to the other side (see Figs. 11.6(A), (B)).

Mayer et al. (2006) recently used functional magnetic resonance imaging (fMRI) to show that this form of auditory attentional reorienting (following the presentation of a spatially informative auditory cue to one or other ear; note that neuroimaging studies typically show greater brain activation following invalid, rather than valid, spatial cueing, because the reorienting of attention from one ear, or side, to the other is only required in the former case) is controlled by a bilateral parietal–prefrontal and right precuneous brain network (see Fig. 11.7(A)) similar to that identified previously by researchers studying the reorienting of visual attention (Corbetta and Shulman, 2002; Wu et al., 2007). It should, however, be noted that the cueing dimension in Mayer et al.'s study (i.e. left vs. right) was the same as the dimension along which participants had to make their target discrimination responses (again, left vs. right). Unfortunately, a response priming account of Mayer et al.'s results therefore cannot be ruled out (see Spence and Driver, 1994)—that is, the

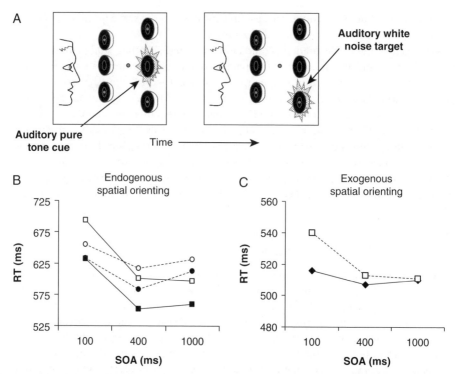

Fig. 11.6 (A) Schematic illustration of the orthogonal spatial-cueing paradigm used in Spence and Driver's (1994, 1997) studies of auditory spatial attention. Participants sat in front of an array of six target loudspeaker cones, three located in a column on either side of central fixation. On each trial, an auditory pure-tone cue (2000 Hz) was presented from the middle loudspeaker on either the left or right, shortly before a pulsed auditory white-noise target from one of the four corner loudspeakers which required a speeded manual elevation (up/down) discrimination response regardless of its side of presentation. (B) When the cue correctly predicted the target side in 75% of trials, the results show the facilitation of spatial discrimination (solid lines) and frequency discrimination responses (dashed lines) when the auditory target was presented on the validly (filled symbols), as opposed to invalidly, cued side (open symbols; Spence and Driver, 1994, Experiments 4 and 6, respectively). (C) Results from Spence and Driver's (1997; Experiment 3) exogenous auditory spatial cueing study in which the cue was now made non-predictive with regard to the likely target location (i.e. the target was equally likely to come from the same or opposite side as the cue). Results showed a short-lasting exogenous spatial cueing effect for auditory targets (validly cued trials, solid line; invalidly cued trials, dashed line).

auditory cue may simply have primed the appropriate behavioural response (since on the majority, 75%, of trials, the participants had to make the response signalled by the cue). It is only by using an experimental design in which the identity (or location) of the cue provides no information with regard to the likely target response, such as the discrimination of target elevation following the presentation of a lateralized cue in Spence and Driver's *orthogonal* cueing studies, that such a non-attentional explanation of any observed cueing effects can be unequivocally ruled out.

Spatial attention can also be captured exogenously (i.e. in a stimulus-driven manner) by salient environmental stimuli (e.g. Spence and Driver, 1994, 1997; McDonald and Ward, 1999). For example, Spence and Driver (1997) showed that participants could discriminate the elevation of auditory targets more rapidly and accurately when a spatially non-predictive auditory cue had

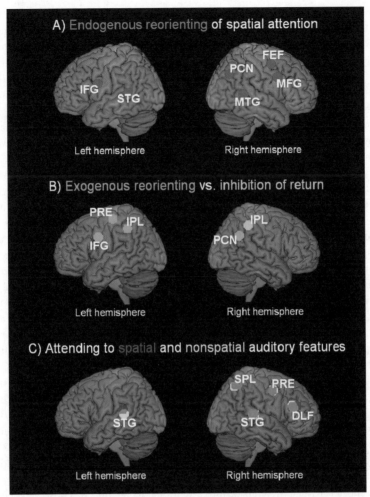

Fig. 11.7 Neural networks underlying spatial and non-spatial selective attention. (A) Cerebral areas activated by the endogenous reorienting (invalid minus valid trials) of spatial attention, including on the left hemisphere the inferior frontal gyrus (IFG) and superior temporal gyrus (STG), and on the right hemisphere the frontal eye-fields (FEF), precuneus (PCN), middle frontal and temporal gyri (MFG and MTG, respectively); Mayer *et al.* (2006). (B) Cerebral regions recruited either by the exogenous reorienting (attentional capture) of spatial attention, including on the left hemisphere the premotor area (PRE), inferior parietal lobule (IPL), inferior frontal gyrus (IFG), and the right precuneus (PCN), or by the inhibition of return effect (right inferior parietal lobule (IPL); Mayer *et al.* (2007). (C) Cerebral regions selectively activated by attending both spatial (location) and non-spatial (frequency) auditory features, including the bilateral superior temporal gyrus (STG), and on the right hemisphere the superior parietal lobule (SPL), premotor area (PRE), and dorsolateral frontal cortex (DLF); Zatorre *et al.* (1999).

been presented on the same, rather than opposite, side shortly before the target (see Fig. 11.6(C)). In contrast to the endogenous cueing effects reported above, exogenous cueing effects tend to be relatively short-lasting, typically dissipating within 2–300 ms of the presentation of the cue, and are observed even when participants are explicitly instructed to ignore the auditory cue as much as possible. Perhaps surprisingly, these auditory cues still appear to capture a participant's attention (albeit very briefly) when their location is made counterpredictive with respect to the likely location of the target sound (i.e. when the target is more likely to occur on the side opposite to the cue than on the same side). Spence and Driver showed that auditory attention was nevertheless directed exogenously to the cue side for a short while before endogenously being reoriented to the opposite (and more likely) side. Mayer et al. (2007; see also Mayer et al. 2006) have now shown that the exogenous reorienting of auditory spatial attention is associated with increased activation of a ventral frontoparietal brain network (more prominent in the left hemisphere; see Fig. 11.7(B)).

Interestingly, a number of studies have highlighted that exogenous spatial attentional orienting tends to have a more pronounced effect on performance when space is somehow relevant (either explicitly or implicitly) to a participant's task (see Rhodes, 1987; Spence and Driver, 1994; McDonald and Ward, 1999). Indeed, it is worth noting that spatial cueing effects are not always observed under those conditions in which a participant's task involves either the speeded detection or speeded non-spatial discrimination of the auditory target stimuli. One reason for this is that, unlike in vision, the earliest representations of auditory stimuli in the brain are tonotopic. As a consequence, participants may be able to respond on the basis of the neural activity in an early non-spatial auditory representation, and hence spatial cueing effects will not necessarily be observed. It is only when space is made relevant to the task, either explicitly (Spence and Driver, 1994) or implicitly (McDonald and Ward, 1999) that spatial cueing effects are reliably observed (see also Roberts et al., in press).

As the interval (or stimulus onset asynchronies, SOA) between the cue and target increases, exogenous attentional facilitation dissipates and sometimes, especially in simple speeded detection tasks, participants actually start to respond more slowly to targets on the cued than on the uncued side (see Fig. 11.8). This phenomenon, known as 'inhibition of return' (IOR), which tends to kick in at SOAs exceeding 300 ms, has now been documented in a number of auditory studies (e.g. Mondor et al., 1998a; Spence and Driver, 1998; McDonald and Ward, 1999; Mondor and Breau, 1999). While both auditory exogenous attentional orienting and auditory IOR appear to be linked with the activation of a brain network that includes the fronto-oculomotor areas, right premotor area, and the left postcentral sulcus (Mayer et al., 2007; Wu et al., 2007), the neural networks controlling exogenous orienting and IOR are by no means identical. Mayer et al. (2007), for instance, recently reported that certain parietal and frontal activations were only observed at shorter SOAs (where exogenous attentional facilitation was observed behaviorally), while the right inferior parietal lobule was selectively activated at the longer SOAs (where auditory IOR was observed behaviorally; see Fig. 11.7(B)).

It is important to note, however, that endogenous orienting, exogenous orienting, and IOR are not restricted to the spatial domain. In fact, all these attentional effects have now been shown to occur in the frequency domain as well. So, for instance, researchers have demonstrated that people can endogenously direct their attention to a particular frequency (or frequency band) in order to facilitate their perception of auditory stimuli that are subsequently presented at that frequency (see Greenberg and Larkin, 1968; Scharf et al., 1987; Scharf, 1998). Of course, under certain circumstances, selection may be guided by a combination of both frequency- and location-based cues (e.g. Mondor et al., 1998b; Woods et al., 2001), although frequency appears to be a more salient dimension for rapidly presented streams of auditory stimuli. Indeed, neuroimaging evidence suggests that they are both controlled by a similar network of cortical regions, typically involving the auditory cortex bilaterally, right superior parietal, right dorsolateral frontal, and right premotor regions (Zatorre et al., 1998; see Fig. 11.7(C)).

Todd Mondor and his colleagues have also shown that auditory attention is oriented exogenously to the frequency of a non-predictive auditory cue (at short cue–target SOAs). And, once again, at longer intervals, this facilitatory effect is sometimes replaced by frequency-specific IOR

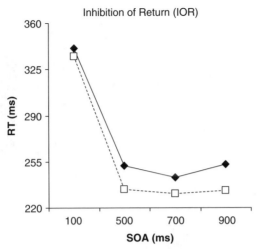

Fig. 11.8 Graph highlighting the results of Spence and Driver's (1998; Experiment 1A) study demonstrating auditory inhibition of return (IOR). Participants in this study had to make a speeded detection response to an auditory target appearing on either the left or right of fixation. A spatially non-predictive auditory cue was presented on either the same (50% of trials) or opposite side (50% of trials) in each trial. The results show that participants responded more slowly on the validly cued trials (solid line) than on the invalidly cued trials (dashed line). This difference reached significance ($p < 0.05$) at the three longer SOAs.

(see Mondor *et al.*, 1998a; Mondor and Breau, 1999). Although beyond the scope of the present chapter it should also be noted that auditory attention can be directed to many other stimulus features such as timbre (Ebata *et al.*, 1968; Mondor and Lacey, 2001), intensity, and duration as well (Mondor and Lacey, 2001; see also Fritz *et al.*, 2007).

11.6 Is exogenous spatial cueing really automatic?

While it has often been claimed that exogenous attentional orienting (or capture) effects such as those reported by Spence and Driver (1994) reflect the *automatic* capture of a participant's spatial attention following the presentation of a peripheral auditory cue, the latest research has shown that auditory cues do not always capture attention. For example, Santangelo *et al.* (2007) recently demonstrated that auditory spatial capture no longer occurs if a participant performs a concurrent attention-demanding auditory (or for that matter visual) perceptual task when the peripheral auditory cue happens to be presented. The participants in Santangelo *et al.*'s study made speeded auditory elevation discrimination responses following the presentation of a spatially non-predictive auditory cue, just as in Spence and Driver's (1994) earlier study (see above). However, in other blocks of trials, a rapid sequential auditory presentation (RSAP) stream of compressed speech sounds was also presented at fixation at a rate of 85 ms per item (see Fig. 11.9(A)). The participants had to monitor this stream of distractor letters for occasionally presented target digits. Importantly, on any given trial, the participants only had to make a single response—either to identify a target digit presented in the RSAP stream, or else to discriminate the elevation of a peripheral auditory target (that is, only one target was presented on each trial, though the type of target was unpredictable).

Santangelo *et al.*'s (2007) results showed a normal pattern of exogenous spatial attentional cueing effects in the single task—no-load—condition (thus replicating Spence and Driver, 1994).

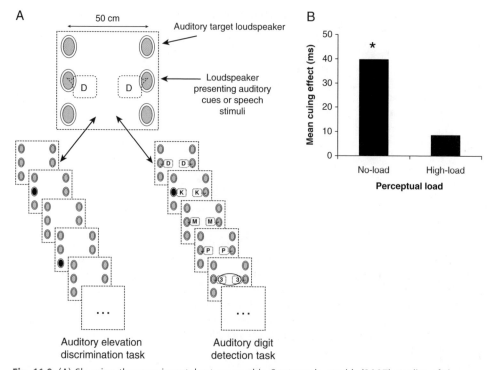

Fig. 11.9 (A) Showing the experimental set-up used in Santangelo et al.'s (2007) studies of the effects of varying perceptual load on exogenous auditory spatial attentional capture effects. In the no-load condition, participants performed an auditory elevation discrimination task (up vs. down). A spatially non-predictive auditory cue consisting of a pure tone (1100 Hz) was delivered for 50 ms from the middle loudspeaker equiprobably on either side. Spatial targets consisted of a burst of white noise delivered for 50 ms from one of the four corner loudspeakers. In the high-load condition, along with the elevation discrimination task, participants performed an auditory digit detection task. Compressed speech stimuli were presented simultaneously from the middle loudspeakers, thus giving the impression of being presented from the centre of the screen. (B) The results show a significant cueing effect in the no-load condition, which is eliminated in the high-load condition in which the participants also had to monitor the central RSAP stream for occasionally presented spoken target digits. Asterisks indicate a significant cueing effect ($p < 0.05$).

By contrast, no such spatial attentional capture was observed under those conditions in which participants simultaneously had to monitor the centrally presented auditory RSAP stream (i.e. high-load condition; see Fig. 11.9(B)). These results therefore demonstrate that spatial attentional capture in the auditory modality is not as 'automatic' as many researchers had previously claimed. It should, however, be remembered that an auditory cue was presented on each and every trial in Santangelo et al.'s study (just as in most typical exogenous spatial cueing studies). It therefore remains an interesting question for future research to determine whether or not non-predictive auditory cues would be any more likely to break through and capture a participant's spatial (or for that matter non-spatial) attention when they happen to be performing another attention-demanding task at the same time (see Ho and Spence, 2008, on this point) if they were presented very infrequently (and hence were far less predictable).

Santangelo et al.'s (2007) results are consistent with Lavie's perceptual load theory, if it is assumed that the presentation (and monitoring) of the RSAP task required all of a participant's

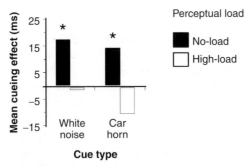

Fig. 11.10 Graph summarizing the results of Ho *et al.*'s (2009) study of exogenous spatial cueing and perceptual load, showing that a semantically meaningful car horn does not give rise to any larger cueing effect than does a semantically meaningless white-noise burst. The results also show that neither cue was capable of capturing the spatial attention of participants in the high-load condition (when they were monitoring a central steam of letters for the occasionally presented target digit). Asterisks indicate a significant cueing effect ($p < 0.05$).

attentional resources, thus leaving no spare resources for the processing of any task-irrelevant auditory stimuli, hence eliminating spatial cueing. Their results are, however, also consistent with claims that attentional capture may be contingent on an observer's attentional control settings (Quinlan and Bailey, 1995; Dalton and Lavie, 2004, 2007). The contingent capture of attention (at least when attention is captured by a feature singleton in a rapidly presented auditory stimulus stream) is associated with the activation of a dorsal frontoparietal brain network (see Watkins *et al.*, 2007). By contrast, a ventral network (comprising the superior temporal and inferior frontal cortices) appears to respond to acoustic variability regardless of its attentional significance. Meanwhile, in terms of spatial attentional capture by irrelevant background auditory signals, changes in the activation of the medial part of the planum temporale appears to be particularly important (Deouell *et al.*, 2007).

From an applied perspective (i.e. when thinking about the design of auditory warning signals to capture the attention of distracted drivers more effectively; see Ho and Spence, 2005, 2008), it is surprising to see just how many of the studies of exogenous attention reported to date have investigated the consequences of presenting auditory cues that are essentially semantically meaningless (e.g. such as pure-tone cues or white-noise bursts). *A priori*, one might have anticipated that the presentation of more meaningful auditory cues, or icons (see Gaver, 1986), such as, for example, the sound of a car horn (see Ho and Spence, 2005), or someone calling your name (Moray, 1959) would be more likely to break through and capture *spatial* attention. However, somewhat surprisingly, Ho *et al.* (2009) recently found that car horn sounds do not capture exogenous spatial attention any more effectively than (semantically meaningless) white-noise bursts (see Fig. 11.10).[6] What is more, auditory capture by the car horn sound was also shown to be eliminated under those conditions in which participants had to perform another attention-demanding perceptual task at the same time.

---

6 It would also be interesting in future research to investigate whether a person's own name would exogenously capture a person's auditory spatial attention in a Posnerian-cueing paradigm if they were performing a highly attention-demanding primary task at the same time (cf. Moray, 1959; Santangelo *et al.*, 2007; Ho *et al.*, 2009).

11.7 **Summary**

In summary, more than half a century of empirical research has highlighted the critical role that selective attention plays in modulating people's awareness of auditory stimuli. Many studies now show that people are only aware of (i.e. can only effectively attend to) one auditory object at a time (see Shinn-Cunningham, 2008). While people's auditory perception may look very impressive in simple laboratory settings, it should be borne in mind that the majority of laboratory studies typically involve the presentation of no more than one or two auditory stimuli in an otherwise silent environment. What is more, stimulation is rarely presented in any other modality (see Chapter 12). The research reviewed here suggests that our awareness of the various stimuli in more complex auditory environments is far sparser than our everyday intuitions would lead us to believe. Indeed, the latest research on the phenomenon of auditory change deafness unequivocally shows that in the absence of attention, people simply have no conscious awareness of the majority of the auditory stimuli around them. Given the limited capacity of attentional resources, it seems that people simply need to focus their attention on a subset of the available sensory information (normally just a single object or stream) in order to make sense of the world around them.

One of the central debates running through the last 50 years of research concerns the question of whether selection takes place early or late in auditory information processing. Currently, the theory of perceptual load (Lavie and Tsal, 1994; Lavie 2005) would appear to offer the most plausible account for the various divergent findings suggesting that selection can occur both early and late in human information processing. The available auditory research is currently consistent with the view that any manipulation that increases the perceptual load of a participant's primary task will result in the reduced processing of other stimuli in the environment. By contrast, increasing a person's 'cognitive load' (e.g. by giving them a series of digits to remember) has, somewhat paradoxically, been shown to increase distractor processing instead (Lavie, 2005; see also Muller-Gass and Schröger, 2007). Other research has shown that an increase in one's perceptual load dramatically reduces the probability that exogenous cues will capture spatial attention (Santangelo et al., 2007; Ho et al., 2009; Santangelo and Spence, 2008). In fact, one of the most interesting areas of research currently involves trying to gain a better understanding how top-down and bottom-up biases interact in the moment-by-moment control of our auditory attention (e.g. Fritz et al., 2007; Shinn-Cunningham, 2008).

Researchers have made impressive progress in recent years in terms of furthering our understanding of the neural systems underlying auditory selective attention and auditory attentional capture (see Fig. 11.7). The complex interplay between attentive and preattentive auditory information processing is a particularly important area of study for neuroscientists at the moment. We are now starting to get a better sense of the neural substrates of auditory attention (see Fritz et al., 2007, for a review of the literature on this rapidly expanding topic). Electrophysiological and neuroimaging studies have shown that attending to both spatial and non-spatial acoustic features appears to result in the activation of similar neural substrates (e.g. Zatorre et al., 1998; Watkins et al., 2006; Mayer et al., 2007; see Fig. 11.7(C)), thus supporting a model whereby auditory attention would appear to operate at a level at which separate features have already been integrated into unitary representations (see also Shinn-Cunningham, 2008). However, the results of other studies have demonstrated that directing auditory attention to individual acoustic features (such as frequency or duration) can modulate neural responses as early as the primary auditory cortex (Zatorre et al., 2002; Deouell et al., 2007; Kauramäki et al., 2007; see also Woldorff et al., 1993). Such results suggest that attention can also operate (if required by task-demands) at earlier stages of processing, affecting neurons in primary auditory cortex. For instance, Kauramäki et al. (2007) have shown that auditory attention operates, at least in part, by increasing both the neural gain (i.e. by increasing neuronal activity) and by changing the frequency selectively of neurons in auditory cortex. Future neuroimaging studies of auditory attention combining those imaging techniques that can offer both good spatial and temporal resolution (such as by combining MEG with fMRI) will hopefully soon resolve which level(s) auditory attention can actually operate at (i.e. before or after the integration of single acoustic features in a unitary representation), and what exact role task-demands (and perceptual/cognitive load, see Lavie, 2005) play in mediating selection within the auditory modality.

References

Alain, C. and Izenberg, A. (2003). Effects of attentional load on auditory scene analysis. *Journal of Cognitive Neuroscience* 15:1063–73.

Allport, D. A. (1992). Selection and control: A critical review of 25 years. In *Attention and Performance: Synergies in Experimental Psychology, Artificial Intelligence, and Cognitive Neuroscience*, Vol. 14 (ed. D. E. Meyer and S. Kornblum), pp. 183–218. Hillsdale, NJ: Erlbaum.

Baddeley, A. (1986). *Working Memory*. Oxford: Oxford University Press.

Beaman, C. P. (2004). The irrelevant sound phenomenon revisited: What role for working memory capacity? *Journal of Experimental Psychology: Learning, Memory and Cognition* 30:1106–18.

Berti, S. and Schröger, E. (2003). Working memory controls involuntary attention switching: Evidence from an auditory distraction paradigm. *European Journal of Neuroscience* 17:1119–22.

Best, V., Gallun, F. J., Ihlefeld, A., and Shinn-Cunningham, B. G. (2006). The influence of spatial separation on divided listening. *Journal of the Acoustical Society of America* 120:1506–16.

Broadbent, D. E. (1958). *Perception and Communication*. Elmsford, NJ: Pergamon.

Chan, J. S. and Spence, C. (2009). Auditory perceptual load. *Journal of Experimental Brain Research* [Submitted].

Chan, J. S., Merrifield, K., and Spence, C. (2005). Auditory spatial attention assessed in a flanker interference task. *Acta Acustica United with Acustica* 91:554–63.

Cherry, E. C. (1953). Some experiments upon the recognition of speech with one and two ears. *Journal of the Acoustical Society of America* 25:975–9.

Cherry, E. C. (1954). Some further experiments upon the recognition of speech, with one and with two ears. *Journal of the Acoustical Society of America*, 26:554–9.

Conway, A. R. A., Cowan, N., and Bunting, M. F. (2001). The cocktail party phenomenon revisited: The importance of working memory capacity. *Psychonomic Bulletin and Review* 8:331–5.

Corbetta, M. and Shulman, G. L. (2002). Control of goal-directed and stimulus-driven attention in the brain. *Nature Reviews Neuroscience* 3:201–15.

Corteen, R. S. and Dunn, D. (1974). Shock-associated words in a nonattended message: A test for momentary awareness. *Journal of Experimental Psychology* 102:1143–4.

Corteen, R. S. and Wood, B. (1972). Autonomic responses to shock-associated words in an unattended channel. *Journal of Experimental Psychology* 94:308–13.

Curtis, C. E. and D'Esposito, M. (2004). The effects of prefrontal lesions on working memory performance and theory. *Cognitive, Affective and Behavioral Neuroscience* 4:528–39.

Dalton, P. and Lavie, N. (2004). Auditory attentional capture: Effects of singleton distractor sounds. *Journal of Experimental Psychology: Human Perception and Performance* 30:180–93.

Dalton, P. and Lavie, N. (2007). Overriding auditory attentional capture. *Perception and Psychophysics* 69:167–71.

Dalton, P. and Spence, C. (2008). Selective attention in vision, audition, and touch. In *Learning and Memory: A Comprehensive Reference* (series ed. J. Byrne); Vol. 1: *Learning Theory and Behavior* (ed. J. Byrne), pp. 243–57. Oxford: Elsevier.

Dalton, P., Santangelo, V., and Spence, C. (2009). The role of working memory in auditory selective attention. *Quarterly Journal of Experimental Psychology*. 62:2126–32.

de Fockert, J. W., Rees, G., Frith, C. D., and Lavie, N. (2001). The role of working memory in visual selective attention. *Science* **291**:1803–6.

Deouell, L. Y., Heller, A. S., Malach, R., D'Esposito, M., and Knight, R. T. (2007). Cerebral responses to change in spatial location of unattended sounds. *Neuron* **55**:958–96.

Deutsch, J. A. and Deutsch, D. (1963). Attention: Some theoretical considerations. *Psychological Review* **70**:80–90.

Driver, J. (2001). A selective review of selective attention research from the past century. *British Journal of Psychology* **92**:53–78.

Ebata, M., Sone, T., and Nimura, T. (1968). Improvement of hearing ability by directional information. *Journal of the Acoustical Society of America* **43**:289–97.

Eltiti, S., Wallace, D., and Fox, E. (2004). Selective target processing: Perceptual load or distractor salience? *Perception and Psychophysics* **67**:876–85.

Eramudugolla, R., Irvine, D. R. F., McAnally, K. I., Martin, R. L., and Mattingley, J. B. (2005). Directed attention eliminates 'change deafness' in complex auditory scenes. *Current Biology* **15**:1108–13.

Fritz, J. B., Elhilali, M., David, S. V., and Shamma, S. A. (2007). Auditory attention – focusing the searchlight on sound. *Current Opinion in Neurobiology*, **17**:437–55.

Gaver, W. W. (1986). Auditory icons: Using sound in computer interfaces. *Human–Computer Interaction* **2**:167–77.

Greenberg, G. Z. and Larkin, W. D. (1968). Frequency-response characteristic of auditory observers detecting signals of a single frequency in noise: The probe–signal method. *Journal of the Acoustical Society of America* **44**:1513–23.

Gregg, M. K. and Samuel, A. G. (2008). Change deafness and the organizational properties of sounds. *Journal of Experimental Psychology: Human Perception and Performance* **34**:974–91.

Ho, C. and Spence, C. (2005). Assessing the effectiveness of various auditory cues in capturing a driver's visual attention. *Journal of Experimental Psychology: Applied* **11**:157–74.

Ho, C. and Spence, C. (2008). *The Multisensory Driver: Implications for Ergonomic Car Interface Design*. Aldershot: Ashgate Publishing.

Ho, C., Santangelo, V., and Spence, C. (2009). Multisensory warning signals: When spatial correspondence matters. *Experimental Brain Research* **195**:261–72.

Johnson, J. A. and Zatorre, R. J. (2006). Neural substrates for dividing and focusing attention between simultaneous auditory and visual events. *Neuroimage* **31**:1673–81.

Johnston, W. A. and Heinz, S. P. (1978). Flexibility and capacity demands of attention. *Journal of Experimental Psychology: General* **107**:420–35.

Johnston, W. A. and Heinz, S. P. (1979). Depth of nontarget processing in an attentional task. *Journal of Experimental Psychology: Human Perception and Performance* **5**:168–75.

Kauramäki, J., Jääskeläinen, I. P., and Sams, M. (2007). Selective attention increases both gain and feature selectivity of the human auditory cortex. *PLoS ONE* **2**:1–10.

Lavie, N. (2005). Distracted and confused? Selective attention under load. *Trends in Cognitive Sciences* **9**: 75–82.

Lavie, N. and de Fockert, J. (2005). The role of working memory in attentional capture. *Psychonomic Bulletin and Review* **12**:669–74.

Lavie, N. and Tsal, Y. (1994). Perceptual load as a major determinant of the locus of selection in visual attention. *Perception and Psychophysics* **56**:183–97.

McDonald, J. J. and Ward, L. M. (1999). Spatial relevance determines facilitatory and inhibitory effects of auditory covert spatial orienting. *Journal of Experimental Psychology: Human Perception and Performance* **25**:1234–52.

Mackay, D. G. (1973). Aspects of the theory of comprehension, memory and attention. *Quarterly Journal of Experimental Psychology* **25**:22–40.

Mayer, A. R., Harrington, D., Adair, J. C., and Lee, R. (2006). The neural networks underlying endogenous auditory covert orienting and reorienting. *Neuroimage* **30**:938–49.

Mayer, A. R., Harrington, D. L., Stephen, J., Adair, J. C., and Lee, R. R. (2007). An event-related fMRI study of exogenous facilitation and inhibition of return in the auditory modality. *Journal of Cognitive Neuroscience* 19:455–67.

Mondor, T. A. and Breau, L. M. (1999). Facilitative and inhibitory effects of location and frequency cues: Evidence of a modulation in perceptual sensitivity. *Perception and Psychophysics* 61:438–44.

Mondor, T. A. and Lacey, T. E. (2001). Facilitative and inhibitory effects of cuing sound duration, intensity, and timbre. *Perception and Psychophysics* 63:726–36.

Mondor, T. A. and Zatorre, R. J. (1995). Shifting and focusing auditory spatial attention. *Journal of Experimental Psychology: Human Perception and Performance* 21:387–409.

Mondor, T. A., Breau, L. M., and Milliken, B. (1998a). Inhibitory processes in auditory selective attention: Evidence of location-based and frequency-based inhibition of return. *Perception and Psychophysics* 60:296–302.

Mondor, T. A., Zatorre, R. J., and Terrio, N. A. (1998b). Constraints on the selection of auditory information. *Journal of Experimental Psychology: Human Perception and Performance* 24:66–79.

Moray, N. (1959). Attention in dichotic listening: Affective cues and the influence of instructions. *Quarterly Journal of Experimental Psychology* 11:56–60.

Muller-Gass, A. and Schröger, E. (2007). Perceptual and cognitive task difficulty has differential effects on auditory distraction. *Brain Research* 1136:169–77.

Norman, D. A. (1969). Memory while shadowing. *Quarterly Journal of Experimental Psychology* 21:85–93.

Pavani, F. and Turatto, M. (2008). Change perception in complex auditory scenes. *Perception and Psychophysics* 70:619–29.

Petrides, M. (2000). The role of the mid-dorsolateral prefrontal cortex in working memory. *Experimental Brain Research* 133:44–54.

Posner, M. I. (1978). *Chronometric Explorations of Mind*. Hillsdale, NJ: Erlbaum.

Quinlan, P. T. and Bailey, P. J. (1995). An examination of attentional control in the auditory modality: Further evidence for auditory orienting. *Perception and Psychophysics* 57:614–28.

Rees, G., Frith, C. D., and Lavie, N. (1997). Modulating irrelevant motion perception by varying attentional load in an unrelated task. *Science* 278:1616–19.

Rhodes, G. (1987). Auditory attention and the representation of spatial information. *Perception and Psychophysics* 42:1–14.

Roberts, K. L., Summerfield, A. Q., and Hall, D. A. (2009). Covert auditory spatial orienting: An evaluation of the spatial relevance hypothesis. *Journal of Experimental Psychology: Human Perception and Performance* 35:1178–91.

Santangelo, V. and Spence, C. (2008). Is the exogenous orienting of spatial attention truly automatic? A multisensory perspective. *Consciousness and Cognition* 17:989–1015.

Santangelo, V., Olivetti Belardinelli, M., and Spence, C. (2007). The suppression of reflexive visual and auditory orienting when attention is otherwise engaged. *Journal of Experimental Psychology: Human Perception and Performance* 33:137–48.

Scharf, B. (1998). Auditory attention: The psychoacoustical approach. In *Attention* (ed. H. Pashler), pp. 75–117. London: Psychology Press.

Scharf, B., Quigley, S., Aoki, C., Peachey, N., and Reeves, A. (1987). Focused auditory attention and frequency selectivity. *Perception and Psychophysics* 42:215–23.

Schröger, E. and Eimer, M. (1997). Endogenous covert spatial orienting in audition: 'Cost–benefit' analyses of reaction times and event-related potentials. *Quarterly Journal of Experimental Psychology* 50A:457–74.

Shinn-Cunningham, B. G. (2008). Object-based auditory and visual attention. *Trends in Cognitive Sciences* 12:182–6.

Simons, D. J. and Ambinder, M. S. (2005). Change blindness: Theory and consequences. *Current Directions in Psychological Science* 14:44–8.

Spence, C. J. and Driver, J. (1994). Covert spatial orienting in audition: Exogenous and endogenous mechanisms facilitate sound localization. *Journal of Experimental Psychology: Human Perception and Performance* **20**:555–74.

Spence, C. and Driver, J. (1996). Audiovisual links in endogenous covert spatial attention. *Journal of Experimental Psychology: Human Perception and Performance* **22**:1005–30.

Spence, C. and Driver, J. (1997). Audiovisual links in exogenous covert spatial orienting. *Perception and Psychophysics* **59**:1–22.

Spence, C. and Driver, J. (1998). Auditory and audiovisual inhibition of return. *Perception and Psychophysics* **60**:125–39.

Todd, J. J., Fougnie, D., and Marois, R. (2005). Visual short-term memory load suppresses temporo-parietal junction activity and induces inattentional blindness. *Psychological Science* **16**:965–72.

Treisman, A. (1969). Strategies and models of selective attention. *Psychological Review* **76**:282–99.

Vitevitch, M. S. (2003). Change deafness: The inability to detect changes between two voices. *Journal of Experimental Psychology: Human Perception and Performance* **29**:333–42.

Voisin, J., Bidet-Caulet, A., Bertrand, O., and Fonlupt, P. (2006). Listening in silence activates auditory areas: A functional magnetic resonance imaging study. *Journal of Neuroscience* **26**:273–8.

Watkins, S., Dalton, P., Lavie, N., and Rees, G. (2007). Brain mechanisms mediating auditory attentional capture in humans. *Cerebral Cortex* **17**:1694–700.

Woldorff, M. G., Gallen, C. C., Hampson, S. A., et al. (1993). Modulation of early sensory processing in human auditory cortex during auditory selective attention. *Proceedings of the National Academy of Sciences USA* **90**:8722–6.

Wolfe, J. M. (1999). Inattentional amnesia. In *Fleeting Memories* (ed. V. Coltheart), pp. 71–94. Cambridge, MA: MIT Press.

Wood, N. L. and Cowan, N. (1995*a*). The cocktail party phenomenon revisited: Attention and memory in the classic selective listening procedure of Cherry (1953). *Journal of Experimental Psychology: General* **124**:243–62.

Wood, N. L. and Cowan, N. (1995*b*). The cocktail party phenomenon revisited: How frequent are attention shifts to one's name in an irrelevant auditory channel? *Journal of Experimental Psychology: Learning, Memory, and Cognition,* **21**:255–60.

Woods, D. L., Alain, C., Diaz, R., Rhodes, D., and Ogawa, K. H. (2001). Location and frequency cues in auditory selective attention. *Journal of Experimental Psychology: Human Perception and Performance* **27**:65–74.

Wu, C. T., Weissman, D. H., Roberts, K. C., and Woldorff, M. G. (2007). The neural circuitry underlying the executive control of auditory spatial attention. *Brain Research* **1134**:187–98.

Zatorre, R. J., Mondor, T. A., and Evans, A. C. (1998). Auditory attention to space and frequency activates similar cerebral systems. *Neuroimage* **10**:544–54.

Zatorre, R. J., Bouffard, M., Ahad, P., and Belin, P. (2002). Where is 'where' in the human auditory cortex? *Nature Neuroscience* **5**:905–9.

Chapter 12

Auditory perception: Interactions with vision

Charles Spence and Salvador Soto-Faraco

12.1 Introduction

The last few years have seen a dramatic growth of research addressing the question of how the processing of information in the auditory modality is affected by the simultaneous stimulation of one or more of the other senses, such as, for example, vision or touch (see Calvert *et al.*, 2004; Spence and Driver, 2004, for reviews). Cognitive neuroscientists have identified a number of important factors that increase the likelihood that various non-auditory stimuli will impact significantly upon a person's perception of auditory events. In fact, many researchers now believe that one cannot really hope to gain a full understanding of human perceptual experience (or its underlying neural substrates, see Ghazanfar and Schroeder, 2006; Kayser and Logothetis, 2007) simply by focusing on the perceptual/attentional processing taking place in each sensory modality in isolation. Instead, the view currently held by many researchers is that one needs to study how the brain processes the information impinging on each of an observer's senses, and critically, to develop an understanding of the rules governing multisensory interactions and sensory dominance in order to understand many of the constraints/limitations on real-world perception (e.g. Churchland *et al.*, 1994; Pascual-Leone and Hamilton, 2001).

Recent years have seen much progress in this regard, and researchers are now increasingly able to predict (or at least model) how dramatically the presentation of a variety of different non-auditory signals will modulate a person's auditory experience (see Battaglia *et al.*, 2003; Alais and Burr, 2004; Körding *et al.*, 2007). At the same time, the results of recent neuroimaging studies are starting to provide an increasingly detailed account of both how and where these multisensory interactions take place in the human brain (e.g. Kayser *et al.*, 2007; Driver and Noesselt, 2008). The disposition of an observer's attention to a particular sensory modality has also been shown to influence his/her ability to respond to, or discriminate, sensory inputs in that modality, as well as affecting the processing of inputs presented to the other sensory modalities (e.g. Spence and Driver, 1997; Spence *et al.*, 2001). What is more, the existence of crossmodal links in spatial attention means that people typically find it easier to direct their attentional focus in different sensory modalities to the same, rather than different, spatial locations (Spence and Read, 2003; see Spence and Driver, 2004, for a review). Researchers have also started to gain a better understanding of the neural underpinnings of these attentional effects in the human brain (e.g. Shomstein and Yantis, 2004; Spence and Driver, 2004; Johnson and Zatorre, 2005, 2006).

In this chapter, we highlight some of the key studies demonstrating how auditory processing in humans can be modified by the presentation of visual stimuli. We have chosen to focus on interactions between audition and vision both for reasons of space and also because, as it happens, the majority of the research published to date has tended to focus on crossmodal interactions in human information processing between these two senses. We will review several sources of

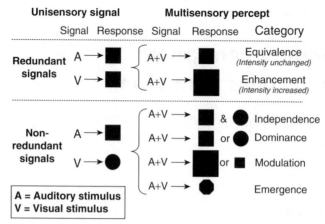

Fig. 12.1 Schematic figure illustrating some of the key ways in which the presentation of a visual stimulus can influence a person's auditory (multisensory) perception. Redundant signals are presented in the upper part of the figure, non-redundant signals in the lower part. The left part of the figure shows perceptual responses to the two signals (auditory and visual) when presented separately. The right part of the figure shows the multimodal perceptual response. In this figure, shape is used to signify the perceived identity of a stimulus, while size gives a schematic indication of the perceived intensity of the stimulus. Results showing equivalence or independence would suggest that there is little interaction between the senses. However, the majority of the studies reported in this chapter show one of the other forms of multisensory interaction. Enhancement has been shown in studies of audiovisual speech perception; dominance has been shown in studies of the Colavita effect; modulation has been shown in studies of spatial ventriloquism; while emergence has been demonstrated by studies of the McGurk effect. (Adapted and redrawn from Partan and Marler, 1999.)

evidence showing that the presentation of visual stimuli can have a variety of qualitatively different effects on a person's auditory (or perhaps more appropriately, multisensory) perception (see Fig. 12.1). So, for example, researchers have shown that the sight of appropriate visual information can result in the enhancement of auditory perception (as when the addition of lip movements enhances auditory speech perception in noise by an amount equivalent to amplifying the signal by as much as 15 dB; see Sumby and Pollack, 1954; Ross *et al.*, 2007). The addition of a visual stimulus can also enhance auditory detection (e.g. Lovelace *et al.*, 2003). Other research has, however, shown that adding visual events can also result in the inhibition, or even extinction, of auditory perception (e.g. Colavita, 1974; Koppen and Spence, 2007; Sinnett *et al.*, 2007, 2008). Meanwhile, in other situations, the addition of vision results in auditory illusions such as the ventriloquism effect (see Bertelson and de Gelder, 2004), or even in the emergence of an entirely new auditory percept (as in the McGurk effect; see McGurk and MacDonald, 1976; Jones and Jarick, 2006). Given the variety of potential outcomes when visual stimuli are combined with auditory stimuli, it is clearly important that we develop a solid understanding of the principles governing audiovisual interactions in human information processing.

12.2 **Sensory dominance**

In everyday life, multisensory cues regarding a particular environmental object or event usually provide *convergent* and partially redundant information (though see Welch *et al.*, 1986; Sugita and Suzuki, 2003, for naturally occurring exceptions). This typically strong correlation between the different sensory signals arising from a common multisensory event makes it difficult for researchers to assess the individual contribution of each participating sense to a person's final perception. As a consequence, many scientists have resorted to situations of artificially induced intersensory conflict, in which non-convergent, or discrepant, cues about a given object property are provided to each sensory modality. The goal here is to examine how the human perceptual system deals with these conflicting sensory inputs (for instance, integrating versus segregating them). One of the most popular questions concerns whether the sensory information presented to each sense is weighted equally during (multisensory) perception, or whether instead one sensory modality tends to dominate over the inputs provided to the other senses. The results of many studies have now shown that visual stimuli often (but not always) dominate (or strongly modulate) people's perception of multisensory objects and events.

12.3 The ventriloquism effect

One of the best known examples of the dominance of vision over audition occurs when a conflict is introduced between the spatial origin of auditory and visual stimuli. For example, in the cinema, we typically perceive the voices of the actors in the film as originating from their lips on the screen, even though the sounds are often physically presented from loudspeakers situated elsewhere in the auditorium. This illusion, known as the 'ventriloquism effect' (see Bertelson and de Gelder, 2004, for a review), shows that people (and for that matter, even frogs; Narins *et al.*, 2005) tend to mislocalize sounds toward their apparent visual source. On the other hand, spatially discrepant sounds normally have very little, if any, effect on an observer's visual localization responses, thus demonstrating that vision tends to dominate our perception whenever audiovisual spatial information conflicts.

Spatial ventriloquism effects are particularly strong in the case of audiovisual speech (presumably due to the highly correlated nature of the auditory and visual inputs resulting from the rich temporal structure inherent to speech stimuli), although similar intersensory biasing effects have now been reported for an extensive variety of spatially discrepant audiovisual stimuli, ranging from the sight and sound of whistling steaming kettles (Jackson, 1953), through to pure-tone beeps paired with spatially incongruent flashes of light (Radeau and Bertelson, 1987; Bertelson and Aschersleben, 1998; Recanzone, 1998; Slutsky and Recanzone, 2001). Unfortunately, however, the majority of spatial ventriloquism studies that have been published are open to a potential non-perceptual response bias explanation (see Choe *et al.*, 1975; Bertelson and Aschersleben, 1998; Bertelson and de Gelder, 2004, on this point). That is, the fact that people point more toward the location of the visual stimulus under conditions of intersensory conflict does not necessarily mean that they actually experience the sound as coming from that location. An alternative possibility is that observers may be well aware of the disparate origin of events but simply assume that what they see and hear should go together, and hence point toward the light simply because in everyday life vision typically provides a more reliable cue to location than sound (Bertelson and de Gelder, 2004).

Over about the last decade, however, a number of studies have successfully isolated the purely perceptual component of the audiovisual ventriloquism effect using a variety of different psychophysical techniques (e.g. see Bertelson and Aschersleben, 1998; Recanzone, 1998; Alais and Burr, 2004). So, for example, Bertelson and Aschersleben used a psychophysical staircase procedure in which the participants had to decide whether a sound had been presented from the left or right of fixation (see Fig. 12.2(A)). The sounds were initially presented from the far left or right and, after each correct response on a given staircase, the sound was moved one step toward the centre, whereas if participants made an erroneous response, the sound on that staircase was moved one step away from the centre. Thus, assuming good auditory localization, after a number

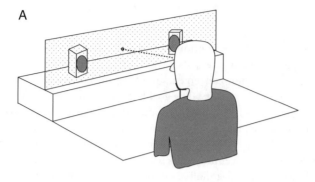

A

B

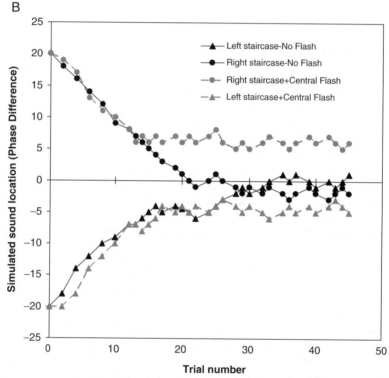

Fig. 12.2 (A) Schematic figure showing the experimental layout used in Bertelson and Aschersleben's (1998) study of the ventriloquism effect. On each trial, the participants had to decide whether a stereophonically presented sound had been presented from the left or right of central fixation. (B) Illustrative results from one idealized observer, adapted from the results' graphs presented in Bertelson and Aschersleben (1998). Multiple interleaved staircases were presented, some starting from the far left and others from the far right. After each correct response, the sound on a given staircase was moved one step down (toward fixation in the beginning of the sequence; thus making the auditory discrimination task a little harder), whereas the staircase moved one step in the opposite direction after each response reversal. Under such conditions, a participant's performance should hover around the point of uncertainty when s/he is no longer able to tell which side the sound came from (the zig-zag part of the graphs on the right). Bertelson and Aschersleben found that this point of uncertainty occurred further from fixation under those conditions in which an irrelevant visual event was presented at fixation concurrent with the target sound (due, they argued, to the spatial ventriloquism of the sound toward the centrally presented light). That is, performance was near-perfect (staircases ended up around zero) in the no-sound condition (black lines), but tailed off several degrees from fixation in the synchronous flash condition (grey lines).

of iterations the participant's responses would end up alternating between left and right as the sound approached the centre (thus defining the point of uncertainty). In Bertelson and Aschersleben's study, a visual stimulus was presented at fixation in synchrony with the sound on several of the different staircases that were randomly interleaved during the experiment.

Bertelson and Aschersleben's (1998) results (see Fig. 12.2(B)) showed that participants reached the point of uncertainty (i.e. they started to become uncertain of the side on which the sound had been presented) further away from the centre when the visual event was presented than when it was not, or else when it was desynchronized with the to-be-localized sound. These results are consistent with the claim that the simultaneous presentation of the visual stimulus resulted in the ventriloquism of the perceived position of the sound toward the centre, thus making it difficult to tell whether the sound had actually been presented from the right or left of fixation. Crucially, it is difficult to see how a response bias could systematically have influenced participants' performance under these conditions, given that the visual event (always presented from the centre) was neutral with respect to the response set (left or right), and the relevant measurement was made at the point of uncertainty regarding the location of the sound. It is therefore interesting to note that the visually induced shift of auditory location reported under such conditions (e.g. about 3° in Bertelson and Aschersleben's, 1998, study) is much smaller than the visual capture effects that have typically been reported in the literature, thus hinting at just how much response biases may have contributed to the results reported in earlier (and, unfortunately, also many present-day) studies of the ventriloquism effect.

An elegant psychophysical study by Alais and Burr (2004) has shown that the spatial ventriloquism effect actually reflects the near-optimal statistical integration of the component auditory and visual signals. While vision normally dominates audition in the spatial domain, Alais and Burr reported a shift from visual to auditory dominance (thus, demonstrating auditory capture) in their study by blurring the visual stimulus (see Fig. 12.3), hence making its localization less reliable as compared to that of the sound. That is, it appears as if the inputs from the different senses are combined by the human brain in order to minimize the variability associated with the final (multisensory) perceptual estimate (though see also Battaglia et al., 2003; Roach et al., 2006). The beauty of Alais and Burr's work is that it has finally provided a mathematical formalization of the classical idea of modality appropriateness which has been debated for decades (see Welch and Warren, 1980, 1986). The maximum likelihood estimation approach that Alais and Burr (amongst others) have espoused now allows researchers to predict how a particular pair of signals will interact with each other simply by estimating the variability associated with each of the individual signals (see Ernst and Bülthoff, 2004; Heron et al., 2004).

It should, of course, be borne in mind that the presentation of a single auditory and visual event in Alais and Burr's (2004) study (and in the majority of other studies of the spatial ventriloquism effect) profoundly simplifies the multisensory binding (or pairing) problem typically faced by the human brain in real-world settings. Note that under everyday conditions (i.e. outside the average psychophysicist's laboratory) our senses are bombarded by multiple sensory inputs at more or less the same time, and hence deciding which of the many visual stimuli should be bound with which of the many auditory stimuli that may be available simultaneously becomes a non-trivial problem. Computational modellers have recently started to address this question using both computational tools as well as psychophysics (cf. Körding et al., 2007).

Several studies have demonstrated that correlated (i.e. in terms of their temporal patterning) sensory inputs give rise to more pronounced multisensory integration than do signals that are uncorrelated (e.g. Thomas, 1941; Radeau and Bertelson, 1987). Radeau and Bertelson, for example, have shown that the correlation between the temporal profile of auditory and visual stimuli also influences the visual capture of audition seen in the spatial ventriloquism effect. The participants

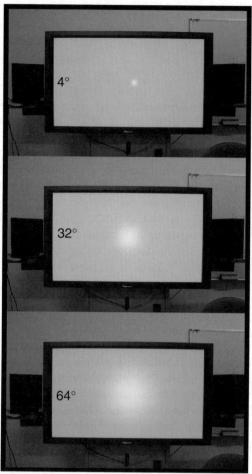

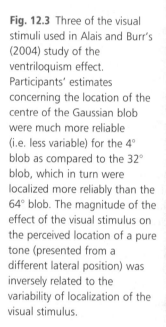

Fig. 12.3 Three of the visual stimuli used in Alais and Burr's (2004) study of the ventriloquism effect. Participants' estimates concerning the location of the centre of the Gaussian blob were much more reliable (i.e. less variable) for the 4° blob as compared to the 32° blob, which in turn were localized more reliably than the 64° blob. The magnitude of the effect of the visual stimulus on the perceived location of a pure tone (presented from a different lateral position) was inversely related to the variability of localization of the visual stimulus.

in Radeau and Bertelson's study were presented with pairs of spatially misaligned auditory and visual stimuli on each trial (see Fig. 12.4(A)). The temporal configuration (or pattern) of the stimulus presented in each sensory modality was varied from trial to trial. On each trial, the participants had to decide whether the sound had been presented to the left or right of the midline. The results showed that the visual biasing of the perceived location of the auditory stimulus was larger when the temporal configuration of the stimuli presented in the two sensory modalities matched than when it did not (see Fig. 12.4(B)).[1]

Cognitive neuroscientists have recently started to investigate the neural underpinnings of this spatial interaction between auditory and visual stimuli (e.g. Macaluso et al., 2004; Bonnath et al., 2007). For example, Bonath et al. conducted a combined event-related potential and event-related functional magnetic resonance imaging study of the ventriloquism effect, demonstrating,

---

[1] The high degree of correlation between auditory and visual information may also explain why the audio-visual integration of speech information (as, for example, measured by studies of the McGurk effect) seems to be so little affected by even very large spatial separation between auditory and visual inputs (see Jones and Jarick, 2006).

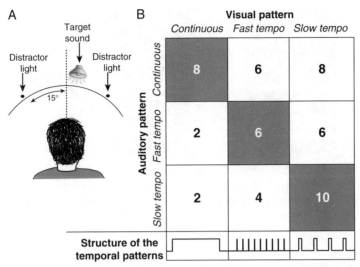

Fig. 12.4 (A) Schematic diagram illustrating the experimental set-up used in Radeau and Bertelson's (1987) study of the influence of temporal correlation (or patterning) of auditory and visual stimuli on the spatial ventriloquism effect. In the conditions of interest to us here, the auditory target was presented 1°, 3°, or 5° to one or the other side of the midline, together with a distractor light situated 15° to either the left or right of the midline. On each trial, the participants judged whether the sound had been presented to the left or right. The temporal pattern (continuous, fast tempo, or slow tempo) of the sounds and the lights was varied systematically. (B) The table highlights the nine possible combinations of three auditory and three visual temporal patterns presented to participants. The value in each cell provides a measure of the visual biasing of auditory localization, expressed as the difference between the number of 'right' judgements on those trials where the visual distractor was presented on the right versus on the left (thus, the bigger the value, the larger the visual biasing of auditory localization). Note that vision typically influences perceived sound location maximally when the temporal pattern presented in both sensory modalities coincided (the shaded cells in the table). (Adapted and redrawn from Spence, 2007, Figure 3.)

on a trial-by-trial basis, that a precisely timed biasing of the left–right balance of auditory cortex activity by spatially mismatching visual events (presented on either the left or right side) correlated with the ventriloquism illusion. Specifically, on those trials in which the visual stimulus elicited a ventriloquism effect (pulling the sound toward the side on which the light was presented; though note that the possible influence of response bias was not ruled out in this study), Bonnath et al. observed a relative reduction in the amplitude of the response (in both the BOLD and ERP signals) in the planum temporale (PT) of the hemisphere ipsilateral to the visual stimulus. This gave rise to a relative enhancement in the response at the PT contralateral to the side of the shifted auditory percept (note that a similar asymmetrical neural response was also observed in response to sounds that were actually presented on that side). Interestingly, this interaction in terms of the neural correlates of the ventriloquism effect was observed in a relatively narrow time window (230–270 ms) after the onset of the stimuli, thus leading Bonnath et al. to suggest that this particular illusion-related asymmetry (attributable to the visual influence on auditory spatial processing) was likely mediated by pathways from the visual cortex to multisensory association areas and from there back to the auditory cortex.

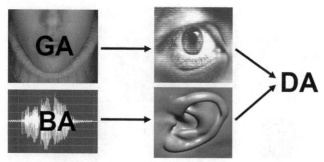

Fig. 12.5 The McGurk effect: When the lip movements corresponding to the syllable [GA] are cross-dubbed with the soundtrack of the syllable /BA/, people will often hear the syllable /DA/, i.e. a fusion between the two original unimodal sources of information (see McGurk and MacDonald, 1976; Jones and Jarick, 2006).

12.4 The McGurk effect

McGurk and MacDonald (1976) used the intersensory conflict methodology to study the relative contributions of audition and vision to speech perception. Participants in their study heard a voice uttering a particular syllable (e.g. 'ba'), while they simultaneously saw synchronized lip movements associated with another syllable (e.g. 'ga'). Surprisingly, most participants reported hearing a syllable (e.g. 'da') that was different from what had been presented in either modality (e.g. in this case, the multisensory integration of non-redundant auditory and visual information led to the 'emergence' of a new percept, see Fig. 12.1), thus demonstrating that the phoneme people *hear* can be modulated by the lip movements that they *see* (see Fig. 12.5). One of the most remarkable aspects of the McGurk effect is that it occurs even when people are perfectly aware that what they are hearing and seeing is incongruent, thus suggesting that the audiovisual integration leading to speech perception may occur rather automatically (though see Alsius *et al.*, 2005, 2007, on this point). In terms of the neural underpinnings of these audiovisual interactions in speech perception, a number of neuroimaging studies have now shown that the auditory cortex (even possibly A1; particularly on the left side) is not only activated by hearing speech sounds but also by watching lip movements and other facial articulatory gestures (e.g. Calvert *et al.*, 1997; Bernstein *et al.*, 2002; Pekkola *et al.*, 2005). Such findings suggest the existence of modulatory signals on sound processing originating either directly or indirectly from visual areas.

In the years since McGurk and MacDonald (1976) published their now-seminal study, similar effects have also been reported in a number of other non-speech domains. For example, Saldaña and Rosenblum (1993) observed a similar visual biasing effect of auditory perception when their participants (who were all trained musicians) observed plucking and bowing movements on a string instrument. Meanwhile, de Gelder and Vroomen (2000) reported that people's judgement of the emotional tone in which a sentence was spoken (i.e. happy vs. fearful) was modulated by the simultaneous sight of a face displaying either extreme happiness or fear. This result shows that judgments about *vocal* emotion can be modified by affective visual information.

12.5 The Colavita effect

One particularly striking demonstration of just how profoundly visual signals can affect (dominate) auditory perception comes from research on the Colavita visual dominance effect (see Colavita, 1974). In Colavita's original study, participants were presented with an unpredictable

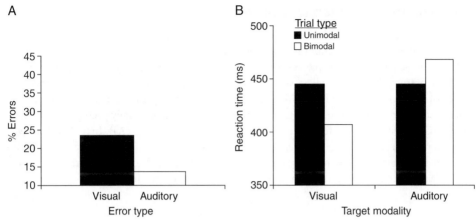

Fig. 12.6 (A) Accuracy data from one of Sinnett et al.'s (2007) experiments on the Colavita visual dominance effect. Note the imbalance between the proportion of erroneous responses to bimodal stimuli consisting of responding 'visual alone' (frequent error type) and 'auditory alone' (infrequent error type), instead of responding 'audiovisual'. (B) Results from Sinnett et al.'s (2008) study showing that, for the same stimuli that give rise to the Colavita visual dominance effect in terms of the accuracy data, RT measures on correct responses reveal that an accessory sound speeds up visual detection responses while an accessory visual stimulus actually slows down responses to auditory stimuli.

sequence of auditory (tone) and visual (flash) events, and were instructed to press one button as quickly as they could whenever they heard the tone, and another button whenever they saw the light. The majority of trials were unimodal (auditory or visual) but a small number (5 out of 35) of bimodal trials (consisting of the simultaneous presentation of the tone and flash) were interspersed throughout the experiment. The striking result reported by Colavita was that, despite the fact that participants experienced absolutely no problem in responding to the sounds when they were presented in isolation (and with a response latency that was, if anything, faster than the latency of their visual responses), they failed to respond to the sound on the majority of the bimodal trials (i.e. they failed to respond on 49 out of 50 trials across all 10 participants in the experiment). Instead, the participants only pressed the visual response button.

Although the methodological design and procedure in Colavita's (1974) original study were subject to a number of confounding factors (see Koppen and Spence, 2007; Sinnett et al., 2007), the basic Colavita visual dominance effect has survived many replications and methodological improvements over the intervening years (see Fig. 12.6(A); Koppen and Spence, 2007; Sinnett et al., 2007, 2008; Koppen et al., 2008).[2] It is almost as if the presentation of the visual stimulus somehow extinguishes (to borrow a term from the neuropsychology literature) participants' awareness of the sound on a certain proportion of the bimodal trials. The latest research has suggested that the Colavita visual dominance effect may be caused, at least in part, by the fact that while the presentation of a sound can speed up a participant's awareness of a visual stimulus (as indexed, for example, by simple detection latencies), the presentation of a visual stimulus actually slows their responses to a sound (see Fig. 12.6(B); Sinnett et al., 2008).

---

2 Although it should be noted that the magnitude of the effect reported in more recent studies has tended to be smaller than that described by Colavita (1974) in his original study.

12.6 **Crossmodal dynamic capture**

Researchers have demonstrated that the visual capture of audition is more pronounced for moving stimuli than for static stimuli (as most commonly used in traditional studies of the spatial ventriloquism effect). For example, Soto-Faraco *et al.* (2002) reported a series of experiments in which the presentation of a visual apparent motion stream consisting of the sequential presentation of two light flashes (one from either side of fixation) strongly influenced the direction in which an auditory apparent motion stream, consisting of two sequentially presented tones (one presented from either side of fixation) appeared to move (see Fig. 12.7(A)). In a typical study of what has now become known as 'the crossmodal dynamic capture effect', participants judge the direction of movement of the auditory apparent motion stream (left- or right-ward) while simultaneously trying to ignore an irrelevant visual apparent motion stream moving in either the same

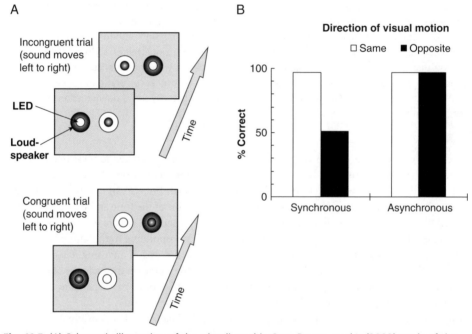

Fig. 12.7 (A) Schematic illustration of the stimuli used in Soto-Faraco *et al.*'s (2002) study of the audiovisual crossmodal dynamic capture effect. On each trial, a sound (100 ms duration) was presented sequentially from each of two loudspeakers (at an SOA of 150 ms), and each LED was also illuminated sequentially with the same timings. The order of presentation (i.e. left or right first) of the stimuli in either sensory modality was entirely unpredictable. The participants' task involved trying to discriminate whether the sound moved from left-to-right (as in the example illustrated in (A)), while trying to ignore the apparent movement of the visual distractors which could move in conflicting (or incongruent, top) or congruent direction (bottom). Grey rectangles represent the stimuli presented at a given moment in the trial, with the inner circles representing the LEDs (white represents off, shaded represents lit) and outer circles representing the loudspeakers (same coding). (B) The results of a typical crossmodal dynamic capture experiment. The graph represents the percentages of correct sound motion direction-discrimination responses for those trials in which visual apparent motion was presented in conflicting or congruent direction, either synchronous (example shown in (A)) or asynchronous (not shown) in time with the sounds.

(i.e. *congruent*) or opposite (i.e. *incongruent*) direction. The ability of participants to discriminate the direction of auditory apparent motion in Soto-Faraco *et al.*'s study was shown to be profoundly impaired when the visual apparent motion stream moved in the opposite, rather than the same, direction (see Fig. 12.7(B)), at least when the target and distractor streams were presented simultaneously.

Soto-Faraco and his colleagues have argued that this crossmodal dynamic capture effect (defined as the magnitude of the difference in performance between incongruent and congruent direction trials) reflects the mandatory integration of visual and auditory motion signals. Interestingly, however, while performance on congruent crossmodal trials typically tends to hover around ceiling (i.e. 100% correct) in the majority of the studies of the crossmodal dynamic capture effect (as it does on unimodal auditory direction of motion discrimination trials), performance on conflicting trials tends to fall in the range of 40–60% correct. It is important to note that the interference caused by the visual motion stream cannot simply be attributed to attentional distraction (i.e. to participants simply being unsure of the direction of the sound when visual stimuli are presented on directionally incongruent trials), since the crossmodal dynamic capture effect is just as strong on those trials in which the participants report being confident about their response (about which direction the sound moved in; see Soto-Faraco *et al.*, 2004). Taken together, these results suggest a partial, rather than a complete, capture of the direction of auditory apparent motion by the distracting visual apparent motion stream.

Crossmodal dynamic capture effects are somewhat larger when the stimuli in the different sensory modalities are presented from the same (rather than from a different) set of spatial locations (Soto-Faraco *et al.*, 2002; see also Meyer *et al.*, 2005), and when the auditory and visual streams are presented at approximately the same time, rather than asynchronously (e.g. Soto-Faraco *et al.*, 2002). What is more, the crossmodal dynamic capture effect is not restricted to the perception of apparent motion; it has been shown to influence the perception of the direction of continuous (i.e. real) motion stimuli as well (e.g. Soto-Faraco *et al.*, 2004). By contrast, however, little effect of auditory distractors has been reported on judgements of the direction of visual apparent motion, even when the strength (or quality) of apparent motion has been matched across the auditory and visual modalities (see Soto-Faraco *et al.*, 2004; though see also Freeman and Driver, 2008).

The results of the research reviewed in this section therefore show that the perception of auditory motion can be profoundly influenced by the dynamic stimuli that happen to be presented in the visual modality at around the same time. While the effects reported in certain of the early studies likely reflect some unknown combination of perceptual and decisional effects (such as response bias), researchers have now documented that this particular form of crossmodal interaction still occurs when the potential influence of response biases has been ruled out or at least strongly diminished (e.g. Mateeff *et al.*, 1985; Kitagawa and Ichihara, 2002; Soto-Faraco *et al.*, 2005; Sanabria *et al.*, 2007). Researchers are now starting to understand the neural correlates of crossmodal dynamic capture (e.g. Alink *et al.*, 2008). Interestingly, in accord with the conclusions from psychophysical research, Alink *et al.* have demonstrated that certain of the neural correlates of crossmodal dynamic capture can be seen in brain areas devoted to the perceptual analysis of motion in each of the two sensory modalities involved. In particular, trials where the crossmodal dynamic capture illusion is experienced by participants correlated with a BOLD increase in the visual motion areas together with the deactivation of auditory motion areas.

12.7 Crossmodal perceptual grouping

The fact that the binding of auditory and visual information appears to be stronger for dynamic stimuli (as in the crossmodal dynamic capture effect) than for static stimuli (as in traditional studies of the ventriloquism effect) may be explained in terms of the additional cues for crossmodal perceptual grouping that are available in the former, as compared to the latter, case (see Spence et al., 2007, for a review). O'Leary and Rhodes (1984) have looked more directly at the question of whether the grouping (or perceptual organization) of stimuli presented in one sensory modality influences how the stimuli presented in another modality are grouped or organized. The participants in their study heard a repeating sequence of six tones (see Fig. 12.8(A))

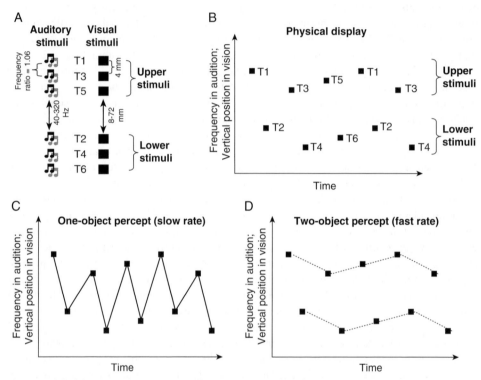

Fig. 12.8 (A), (B) Schematic illustration of the sequence of auditory and visual stimuli used in O'Leary and Rhodes' (1984) study of crossmodal influences on perceptual organization. T1–T6 indicate the temporal order (from 1, first, to 6, last) in which the six stimuli were presented in each sensory modality. Half the stimuli corresponded to the upper group (frequency in sound, spatial location in vision) and half to the lower group. The visual and auditory stimuli were presented in sequence alternating between events from the upper and lower groups, either presented individually (unimodal condition) or else together (in the bimodal stimulation condition). (C), (D) Perceptual correlates associated with different rates of stimulus presentation. In either sensory modality, at slow rates of stimulus presentation (C), a single stream (acoustic or visual) was perceived (as shown by the continuous line connecting the points). Faster rates of stimulus presentation (D), however, led to the perception of two separate concurrent streams, one in the upper (frequency or spatial, for sound or vision, respectively) range and the other in the lower range. In the bimodal condition, at intermediate rates of stimulus presentation subjective reports of whether participants perceived one or two streams in a given sensory modality were influenced by their perception of one or two streams in the other modality. These results were taken by O'Leary and Rhodes to argue that the nature of the perceptual organization in one sensory modality can influence how the perceptual scene may be organized (or segregated) in another modality (though see Spence et al., 2007). (Adapted and modified from Spence et al., 2007, Figures 1 and 2.)

where upper and lower frequency tones were presented in alternation (see Fig. 12.8(B)), just like in auditory streaming experiments (e.g. Bregman, 1990). At slow rates of stimulus presentation the participants heard a single variable-frequency auditory stream (see Fig. 12.8(C)), whereas faster rates gave rise to perceptual segregation between two auditory streams instead (see Fig. 12.8(D)): one higher frequency (alternating between the three higher frequency tones) and the other involving the grouping of the three lower frequency tones.

The participants in O'Leary and Rhodes' (1984) study were also presented with sequences of visual stimuli. In Analogy to the auditory displays, one group of three visual stimuli were presented from the upper part of the visual display while the rest were presented from the lower part of the display. At the slower rates of stimulus presentation, participants reported seeing a single object alternating in elevation between the upper and lower parts of the screen, while at faster presentation rates, participants reported seeing two segregated visual objects instead (one moving across the upper part of the screen while the other moved across the lower part of the screen).

Initially, the thresholds (in terms of the stimulus onset asynchrony, SOA) for perceiving one versus two streams were determined individually for each sensory modality by varying both the magnitude of the separation between the higher and lower stimuli (either in the frequency domain for auditory stimuli, or spatially for the visual stimuli), and the timing between successive stimuli in the sequence. Next these thresholds were assessed under conditions of bimodal stimulus presentation. Note that in the bimodal conditions, the highest frequency sound was presented in synchrony with the uppermost visual stimulus, the second highest tone with the second highest visual stimulus, and so on. O'Leary and Rhodes (1984) reported that the presentation of visual displays that were perceived by participants as consisting of two moving objects (i.e. visual streams where segregation had taken place) caused participants to report that the concurrent auditory displays were also perceived as two streams (i.e. as segregated) at presentation rates that yielded reports of a single perceptual stream when the accompanying visual sequence was perceived as a single stream, and vice versa. These results are consistent with the view that the perceptual organization taking place within the visual modality can have a significant effect on the perceptual organization of stimuli that happen to be presented in the auditory modality. Many subsequent studies have now confirmed that human multisensory perception reflects the consequences of a constant interplay between intramodal and crossmodal perceptual grouping (see Spence et al., 2007, for a review; though see also Huddleston et al., 2008).

12.8 The unity effect

It has long been argued that whenever two or more sensory inputs are perceived as being highly consistent (i.e. related in a way that implies that they are likely to have originated from the same environmental event), people will be more likely to bind them (e.g. Jackson, 1953; Welch and Warren, 1980). Until recently, however, all studies that have tried to investigate the 'unity assumption' or 'unity effect' (see Vatakis et al., 2008) were open to a response bias interpretation (see Bertelson and de Gelder, 2004), and/or failed to match the amount of information that was presented in the various different conditions. Take, for example, Jackson's (1953) early study in which he documented a larger spatial ventriloquism effect when participants had to localize a steaming whistling sound paired with the sight of a steaming kettle than when they had to localize the sound of a buzzer paired with a flash of light. It has been argued that Jackson's results provide convincing evidence in support of the unity assumption (since participants presumably had more reason to assume that the sight and sound of the kettle went together than they did to associate the sound of the bell with the flash of light). It should, however, be noted that these results are subject to both of the above-mentioned confounds. First, there was simply more information (e.g. temporal variation) in the sight and sound of a steaming kettle (cf. Radeau and Bertelson, 1987). Second, the results are open to the response bias interpretation outlined earlier—that is, participants may simply have pointed to the location of the steaming kettle because they assumed that is where the whistling sound ought to have come from, despite being aware of the spatial disparity.

Recently, however, more convincing evidence that the 'unity effect' can modulate certain kinds of multisensory integration has come from a series of experiments reported by Vatakis and her colleagues (Vatakis and Spence, 2007, 2008; Vatakis et al., 2008). The participants in these experiments were presented with an auditory and visual speech stimulus (the sight or sound of someone uttering a syllable or word) which had been desynchronized. On each trial, the participants had to make an unspeeded temporal order judgement (TOJ) concerning whether the auditory or visual speech stream had been presented first. In all trials, the content of the syllables coincided in vision and audition; but whereas on half of the trials the auditory and visual aspects were identity-matched (such that the sight and sound of a particular woman or man uttering a specific speech event were presented), on the remainder of the trials a man's voice was dubbed onto a woman's face or vice versa. Note here that, on average, exactly the same amount of information was presented on both congruent and incongruent trials. What is more, any bias to assume that the matched face and voice ought to go together could not lead to any systematic bias in terms of 'audition first' or 'vision first' responses. Thus, Vatakis and Spence were able to rule out the two main confounds that have pervaded previous studies in this area.

The participants' temporal resolution (measured in terms of the just noticeable difference, JND) was significantly poorer when judging the identity-matched audiovisual speech events than when judging the mismatching events. Vatakis and Spence (2007) argued that participants were simply more likely to bind the auditory and visual cues when they appeared to originate from the same speaker than when they did not, thus making it more difficult to resolve their actual temporal order of occurrence. In particular, Vatakis and Spence hypothesized that the increased likelihood of multisensory binding on the matching trials may have resulted in a more pronounced temporal attraction of the auditory and visual events (known as 'temporal ventriloquism'; Morein-Zamir et al., 2003), hence presumably making it harder for participants to correctly resolve their actual timing. These results therefore provide evidence that the unity effect can lead to enhanced multisensory integration for matching unisensory cues.

Interestingly, however, there are some important limitations to the unity effect. First, it seems to be specific to human speech signals (at least when tested on human observers), as no such effect has been reported in follow-up studies where participants judged the temporal order of videos showing a variety of different object actions (Vatakis and Spence, 2008)[3] or animal vocalizations (Vatakis et al., 2008). Second, even for human audiovisual speech events, there is no perfect correspondence between the temporal window for multisensory integration and the capacity of the observers to resolve the temporal order of auditory and visual events (Soto-Faraco and Alsius, 2007, 2008). This means that even under optimal conditions for assuming auditory–visual unity, there is still some residual access to the information in each separate modality.

Parise and Spence (2009) have recently demonstrated that synaesthetically congruent[4] auditory and visual stimuli also show enhanced multisensory binding as compared to synaesthetically

---

[3] Note that Vatakis and Spence's (2008) results suggest that Jackson's (1953) results with the steaming and whistling kettles did indeed reflect a response bias after all (i.e. as suggested by Bertelson and de Gelder, 2004; see also Vatakis and Spence, 2007).

[4] Synaesthetic congruency refers to the associations that are shared by most people between specific dimensions in different sensory modalities (see Walker and Smith, 1984; Marks, 2004). So, for example, people share a synaesthetic association between elevation in vision and pitch in audition (cf. O'Leary and Rhodes, 1984).

incongruent stimuli (see also Marks, 2004). The normal (i.e. non-synaesthetic) participants in Parise and Spence's study were presented with a pair of auditory and visual stimuli on each trial. The visual stimulus consisted of either a small or large circle (2.1 or 5.2° of visual angle, respectively), while the auditory stimulus consisted of either a low- or high-pitched sound (300 vs. 4500 Hz, respectively). The combination of stimuli presented on each trial varied, such that sometimes they were synaesthetically congruent (i.e. the small circle was paired with the high-pitched sound), while on other trials they were synaesthetically incongruent (i.e. the small circle was paired with the low-pitched sound; see Gallace and Spence, 2006). The SOA between the stimuli was varied on a trial-by-trial basis using the method of constant stimuli, and participants had to discriminate which stimulus had been presented second. The results showed impaired temporal sensitivity (i.e. larger JNDs indicating enhanced binding) when participants judged the temporal order of the synaesthetically congruent stimuli as compared to the synaesthetically incongruent stimulus pairs.

12.9 Modality-specific versus supramodal attentional resources

One of the fundamental questions in attention research concerns the extent to which people can selectively direct their attention toward a particular sensory modality—such as, for example, toward the auditory modality—at the expense of the processing of stimuli presented in one of the other modalities (Spence et al., 2001). Spence and his colleagues conducted a study in which they investigated whether attending to a particular sensory modality would facilitate behavioural performance for stimuli subsequently presented in that modality when compared to situations in which participants' attention was divided equally between several different modalities (audition, vision, and touch), or else had been misdirected to another sensory modality in advance of the target's presentation. The participants in this study were presented with a random sequence of auditory, visual, and tactile targets from one of two locations on either side of fixation. The participants had to make speeded left/right spatial discrimination responses to the target stimuli regardless of the modality in which the target on each trial had been presented (thus ensuring that the participants performed the *same* task in all three modalities). Targets in the three modalities were presented with equal probability in the 'divided attention' blocks. In the other blocks of trials, the probability of the stimuli in a given (target) modality (audition, touch, or vision) was increased, in order to encourage participants to focus their attention on that particular modality. The results showed that participants responded more rapidly (and somewhat more accurately) to the auditory targets in the 'attend audition' blocks than in the other blocks of trials where either visual or tactile targets were expected. Spence et al.'s results therefore show that voluntarily (i.e. endogenously) attending to the auditory modality can result in the facilitation of people's (speeded) responses to auditory stimuli when compared to situations in which their attention has been directed toward the visual or tactile modalities instead (see Spence and Driver, 1997).

More recently, however, Alais et al. (2006) have come to a somewhat different conclusion regarding the effects of attending to the auditory modality on performance. Participants in their study were either presented with auditory and visual stimuli at the same time (bimodal divided-attention condition) or else they were presented with separate blocks of trials in each sensory modality (unimodal focused-attention condition). The visual task consisted of 'low-level' contrast

---

This should not be confused with the experiences of synaesthetic individuals, for whom the presentation of a stimulus in one modality gives rise to an additional sensory experience (often in another sensory modality), as when the presentation of a particular speech sound or word gives rise to a very particular colour experience (see Robertson and Sagiv, 2005).

discrimination, while in the auditory modality the participants had to discriminate the pitch of auditory stimuli instead. The results showed that the auditory thresholds were slightly (but significantly) higher in the bimodal divided-attention condition than in the unimodal focused-attention condition (thus suggesting that there was a small, but nevertheless significant, cost associated with having to attend to stimuli presented in two sensory modalities simultaneously). By contrast, visual thresholds were unaffected by whether performance was assessed in the focused or bimodal divided-attention blocks (see Fig. 12.9). The relatively modest threshold increases observed in Alais et al.'s bimodal divided-attention condition contrasted with the far more dramatic threshold increases that were observed when the participants had to divide their attention unimodally, either between two different visual tasks, or else between two auditory tasks (unimodal divided-attention condition; see Fig. 12.9(C)).

The results of these two studies (Spence et al., 2001; Alais et al., 2006) are consistent with the view that focusing attention on a particular sensory modality only leads to relatively modest performance *benefits* when compared to dividing attention in order to monitor several modalities simultaneously. Interestingly, the majority of the attentional effects reported in Spence et al.'s study consisted of the performance costs on those trials in which the target happened to be presented in an unexpected modality. That is, the performance *costs* associated with directing attention to the wrong sensory modality were far greater than the performance *benefits* associated with correctly directing attention to the actual target modality on validly cued trials (measured relative to performance in the divided-attention baseline condition). Given that Alais et al. did not include an invalidly cued attention condition, they were unable to assess the attentional costs associated with misdirecting attention in their study.

Currently, the evidence supports the conclusion that focusing attention on a particular sensory modality may have a more pronounced effect on the performance of tasks that require speeded responding than on tasks requiring participants to make unspeeded perceptual judgements (see Alais et al., 2006, on this point). This idea links nicely to Prinzmetal et al.'s (2005) suggestion that selective attention may affect a participant's performance by influencing which sensory channel participants happen to attend to (and hence potentially respond to) first, rather than necessarily by enhancing the processing of signals in that modality.[5]

The results of a recent psychophysical study, in which participants had to make unspeeded synchrony judgements regarding auditory and visual stimuli, has provided evidence in support of the channel selection hypothesis (Zampini et al., 2005). Zampini et al. showed that endogenously attending to either the auditory or visual modality leads to a speeding-up of the relative time of arrival of stimuli presented in that sensory modality. On each trial in their study, a pair of stimuli was presented, one from either side of fixation (see Fig. 12.10(A)), at one of ten SOAs. The participants' attention was endogenously directed to either the visual or auditory modality on a block-by-block basis, by manipulating the relative proportion of visual or auditory stimuli in each block of trials. The participants made *unspeeded* discrimination responses concerning whether the two stimuli on each trial had been presented in synchrony or not. The results showed a small, but significant, prior entry effect (see Titchener, 1908; Shore and Spence, 2005) for the frequent (i.e. putatively attended) stimulus modality (see Fig. 12.10(B)). In other words, directing one's attention to the auditory modality resulted in visual stimuli having to be presented relatively earlier in time (by about 15 ms) in order for them to be judged as synchronous with a sound (see Fig. 12.10(C)) than when attention was directed to the visual modality.

---

[5] Prinzmetal et al. (2005) have introduced a distinction between 'channel selection' and 'channel enhancement'.

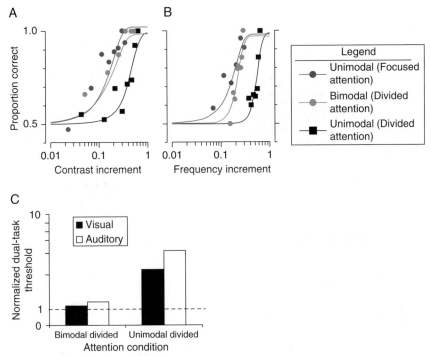

Fig. 12.9 Results of Alais *et al.*'s (2006) study showing that dividing attention between two tasks in the same modality (either audition or vision) leads to more pronounced performance costs (as shown by the increases in threshold) than dividing attention between two tasks in different sensory modalities. (A), (B) Sample psychometric functions from an observer for the visual task (contrast discrimination, (A), and the auditory task (pitch discrimination, (B)). In each panel, dark grey symbols/lines represent performance for the primary sensory modality when measured alone, while the two other curves show performance when the same task is measured together with a secondary task in the same (black symbols) or different modality (light grey symbols). The performance of a secondary task in the same modality shifted the psychometric functions markedly to the right, reflecting a marked increase in the contrast (or frequency) increment needed to perform the primary task. On the other hand, when the distractor task was presented in a different modality from the primary task, psychometric curves were quite similar to the results from the single-task condition. (C) Summarizes the mean primary thresholds in the dual-task conditions. The dual-task thresholds are shown as multiples of the thresholds measured in the single-task conditions (red curves in (A)), so that a value of 1.0 (dashed line) would indicate no change from single- to dual-task conditions. In all cases, secondary tasks in the same modality (Unimodal divided attention) raised primary thresholds considerably, while the crossmodal secondary tasks had little effect (Bimodal divided attention). (Adapted and redrawn with permission from Alais *et al.*, 2006, Fig. 1.)

In conclusion, there is now robust empirical evidence to demonstrate that people cannot always perform two tasks as effectively as they can perform each task in isolation when each of those tasks involves the processing of stimuli in different sensory modalities (here audition and vision). However, it is important to note that such dual-task costs across modalities are not always observed, and they are often weaker than within-modality dual-task costs (see Treisman and Davies, 1973; Martin, 1980; Alais *et al.*, 2006; Talsma *et al.*, 2006). Several factors influence how much of a dual-task deficit will be observed, including, for example, some degree of task specificity

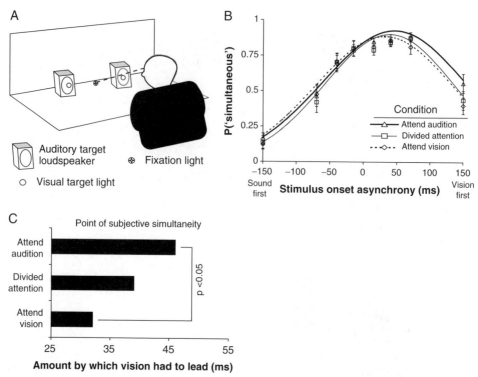

Fig. 12.10 (A) Experimental set-up used in Zampini *et al.*'s (2005) audiovisual prior entry study. Auditory and visual stimuli were presented randomly from either side of fixation. Participants reported whether the two stimuli on each trial had been presented simultaneously or not. (B) Psychometric functions fitted to the data from the attend audition, attend vision, and divided attention conditions plotted as a function of the SOA between the two stimuli. (C) The mean point of subjective simultaneity (PSS) values derived from the psychometric functions: The results show that participants perceived auditory stimuli 14 ms faster relative to visual stimuli when their attention had been directed to the auditory modality than when it had been directed to the visual modality instead. (Figure adapted from Zampini *et al.*, 2005.)

(see also Bonnel and Hafter, 1998). Generally speaking, tasks that require speeded responses to target stimuli seem to show more robust costs associated with the division of attention between different sensory modalities than do non-speeded tasks (Alais *et al.*, 2006; Johnston and Zatorre, 2006). Presenting the stimuli in different modalities from different locations has also been shown to increase dual-task costs under certain conditions (Spence and Driver, 1997; Spence and Read, 2003).

What then of the neural correlates of focusing attention on a particular sensory modality? Many researchers have now shown that when attention is drawn away from an auditory event by the presence of a visual stimulus, and particularly by attending to (performing) a visual task (when compared with a non-competitive baseline condition), the auditory cortex (particularly secondary auditory cortical areas) shows decreased activity in response to auditory stimuli (Woodruff *et al.*, 1996; Laurienti *et al.*, 2002; Shomstein and Yantis, 2004; Weissman *et al.*, 2004; Johnson and Zatorre, 2005). By analysing the functional connectivity between the visual and auditory cortical areas in visual and auditory tasks, Johnson and Zatorre (2005, 2006) were able to highlight a reciprocal inverse relationship, such that decreases in visual activation appear to be correlated with increases in auditory activation and vice versa. Meanwhile, it has recently been shown that even chinchillas show a decrease in cochlear sensitivity when performing a visual (but not when performing an auditory task), with the magnitude of this decrease correlating with the demands of the animal's visual task (see Delano *et al.*, 2007).

Johnson and Zatorre (2006) have also looked into the neural correlates of concurrently dividing one's attention between the auditory and visual modalities. In their study, they showed enhanced activation in dorsolateral prefrontal cortex (DLPFC) when participants had to divide their attention in order to monitor stimuli that were presented in two different modalities (a melody task was presented in the auditory modality, a shape task in the visual modality) at the same time, compared to when they had to focus their attention on the stimuli appearing in just a single sensory modality. The DLPFC only showed enhanced activity when the participants had to monitor both streams simultaneously and not when they only had to monitor one of the two streams (i.e. more DLPFC activity was observed under conditions of divided, but not focused, attention). Interestingly, while Johnston and Zatorre observed no performance decrement in the dual-task (i.e. divided attention) condition in their fMRI study, when compared to the single task condition (though note that an unspeeded recall task was used), the level of neural activity in DLPFC was shown to correlate inversely with the level of activation seen in sensory-specific cortices. This pattern of results would therefore appear to suggest that the recruitment of frontal areas might be necessary in order for participants to maintain the same level of behavioural performance under divided- (as compared to focused-) attention conditions.

Finally, researchers have also investigated which areas of the brain control the switching of a participant's attention from one sensory modality to another. So, for example, Shomstein and Yantis (2004) studied the patterns of brain activity associated with people *shifting* their attention between the visual and the auditory modality. They observed an increase of activity in the sensory cortex corresponding to the attended modality while at the same time noting a decrease of activity in the sensory cortex of the non-attended modality, when the participants shifted their attention from the visual to the auditory modality. What is more, superior prefrontal and posterior parietal cortices also exhibited a transient increase in activity that was time-locked to the onset of the voluntary (or endogenous) shift of attention between one modality and the other. These results led Shomstein and Yantis to suggest that the frontoparietal network that has been implicated previously in unimodal studies of visual and auditory attention (e.g. see Chapter 11) may also play a critical role in shifting attention between one sensory modality and another (see also Hunt and Kingstone, 2004; Brand-D'Abrescia and Lavie, 2008). A recent repetitive transcranial magnetic stimulation (rTMS) study has provided support for these conclusions (see Johnson *et al.*, 2007): Johnson *et al.* showed that participants' ability to divide their attention between unrelated auditory and visual inputs was indeed adversely affected after temporarily disrupting the DLPFC following 10 minutes of slow 1-Hz rTMS to this area, as would be expected if the DLPFC played a functional role in dividing attention between different sensory modalities. Following rTMS, the participants exhibited a pattern of behaviour consistent with their being able to attend to one or the other sensory modality, but not to both. Johnson *et al.* suggested that this brain area may support the increased load on working memory that is associated with divided, as compared to focused, attention.

12.10 **Crossmodal perceptual load**

As discussed in Chapter 11, Lavie's perceptual load theory (see Lavie, 2005, for a review) has provided a useful theoretical and empirical framework for explaining why selective attention sometimes appears to operate at relatively early stages of information processing, while at other times it appears to operate much later. To date, the majority of studies of perceptual load have focused on the selection taking place within a single sensory modality (primarily vision, but also to a lesser extent audition; see Chapter 11). A few studies have tackled the question of whether perceptual load affects human information processing in a modality-specific manner (see Wickens, 1980, 1992; Duncan et al., 1997), or instead consists of a common pool of processing resources that happen to be shared across the various senses (Spence and Driver, 1997; Spence et al., 2001; see also Brand-D'Abrescia and Lavie, 2008).

Unfortunately, however, the results of studies of crossmodal perceptual load that have been published to date have been rather mixed. For while some researchers have failed to observe reliable crossmodal effects of perceptual load (Rees et al., 2001; Tellinghuisen and Nowak, 2003), others have demonstrated a significant crossmodal load effect (Otten et al., 2000; Alsius et al., 2007; Santangelo et al., 2007; Sinnett et al., 2007). The variability in terms of the results may be related to the lack of any independent measure of the extent of the load imposed on the perceptual system by a particular task (see Sinnett et al., 2006, for a discussion on this point). It could, for example, be argued that any failure to demonstrate significant crossmodal perceptual load effects may be due to the particular studies in question simply using an insufficiently strong manipulation of perceptual load. Given these limitations, it would seem premature to draw any firm conclusions yet, especially given the general variability in the literature on the question of whether or not resources are shared between the different sensory modalities.

12.11 Summary

The evidence reviewed in this chapter demonstrates just how important it is to study perception in a multisensory (rather than just a unisensory) context. The majority of experiences in everyday life are multisensory and, as the results outlined here amply demonstrate, people simply cannot focus exclusively on what they hear and ignore any other sensory inputs that may be occurring at around the same time. Instead, if, as is often the case, the input arriving to the other senses conveys information that refers to the same external event then the brain appears to bind those sensory inputs, often adopting a statistically near-to-optimal strategy (e.g. see Alais and Burr, 2004; Roach et al., 2006; Körding et al., 2007; Wozny et al., 2008). This means that what we hear can often be dramatically influenced by what we see, as in the well-known spatial ventriloquism (e.g. Jackson, 1953; Bertelson and de Gelder, 2004) and McGurk illusions (e.g. McGurk and MacDonald, 1976; Jones and Jarick, 2006; see Fig. 12.1). At other times, even if the relevant information belongs to the attended auditory modality alone, other sensory inputs present in the environment need to be actively segregated in order to attain efficient perception and performance (Spence and Read, 2003; Spence and Driver, 2004).

Researchers have now highlighted a number of basic factors that appear to modulate the extent to which non-auditory (in this case visual) signals will alter/change a person's auditory perceptual experience. So, for example, visual signals are more likely to influence auditory perception if they happen to be presented from the same location at about the same time (see Spence, 2007, for a review). Visual signals are also more likely to influence auditory perception if they happen to have a similar temporal structure (Thomas, 1941; Radeau and Bertelson, 1987; Spence et al., 2007). The latest research has also shown that auditory and visual speech stimuli originating from the same speaker (and which may be subject to the unity effect; see Welch and Warren, 1980) show enhanced crossmodal binding (see Vatakis and Spence, 2007; Vatakis et al., 2008; see also Körding et al., 2007). Even the synaesthetic congruency between auditory and visual stimuli has been shown to modulate the degree of audiovisual temporal integration that is observed (e.g. Marks, 2004; Gallace and Spence, 2006; Parise and Spence, 2009). Finally, there is also some evidence that semantic congruency can influence the multisensory integration of auditory and visual signals under at least a subset of experimental conditions (e.g. Laurienti *et al.*, 2004; Koppen *et al.*, 2008; see Spence, 2007, for a recent review).

In terms of crossmodal attention, the consensus view that now seems to be emerging is that the limitations/constraints on dividing attention between two or more sources of information (or tasks) at the same time are more profound when those tasks are presented in the same modality than when they are presented to different sensory modalities (see Treisman and Davies, 1973; Wickens, 1980, 1992; Martin, 1980; Soto-Faraco and Spence, 2002; Alais *et al.*, 2006; Sinnett *et al.*, 2006; Talsma *et al.*, 2006). With regard to the concept of crossmodal perceptual load, the evidence is currently rather more mixed (see Lavie, 2005). However, the notion that there is a shared pool of resources for the processing of stimuli in different sensory modalities does have some explanatory validity (see Otten *et al.*, 2000; Arnell, 2006; Santangelo *et al.*, 2007; Sinnett *et al.*, 2006, 2007; Brand-D'Abrescia and Lavie, 2008). While it remains for future research to determine why null results have been reported in certain studies (e.g. Rees *et al.*, 2001; Tellinghuisen and Nowak, 2003), one plausible suggestion is simply that the extent of any crossmodal attentional limitations depends on the extent to which the tasks/stimuli presented to the different modalities require access to the same processing resources (or neural substrates). According to this suggestion, the more modality-specific[6] the task (such as the auditory pitch and visual contrast discrimination tasks used by Alais *et al.*, 2006), the more independent the resources in the different modalities will appear to be when participants have to combine the performance of tasks in different sensory modalities (see also Bonnel and Hafter, 1998). One other important conclusion to emerge from the literature reviewed here is that the more the tasks require speeded responding (e.g. Spence and Driver, 1997; Spence *et al.*, 2001; Levy *et al.*, 2006) the more likely it is that interference will be observed, whereas independence is more likely under conditions that allow for unspeeded responding (e.g. Duncan *et al.*, 1997; Soto-Faraco and Spence, 2002; Alais *et al.*, 2006; Johnson and Zatorre, 2006).

Recently, neuroimaging studies have started to reveal some of the neural substrates underlying the interaction between the senses that have been documented behaviourally. There is now extensive evidence that visual stimuli can modulate the activity seen in auditory cortex (Calvert *et al.*, 1997; Pekkola *et al.*, 2005; Kayser *et al.*, 2007). Indeed, some researchers have even started to question the appropriateness of distinguishing between modality-specific and multisensory cortex (Ghazanfar and Schroeder, 2006; Kayser and Logothetis, 2007). Furthermore, attending to the auditory (as compared to the visual) modality results in the enhancement of activity in modality-specific auditory cortical areas (e.g. Shomstein and Yantis, 2004; Johnson and Zatorre, 2005, 2006). While the division of attention between simultaneously presented auditory and visual sources may not always lead to an impairment of behavioural performance, neuroimaging research has revealed that this does not necessarily mean that the same neural substrates will be used under conditions of focused and divided auditory attention (see Johnson and Zatorre, 2006; Johnson *et al.*, 2007)

---

6 Note that to some degree the notion of the modality-specificity of a particular task equates with notions of low-level vs. high-level information processing (cf. Alais *et al.*, 2006). That is, the 'earlier' in information processing a task can be resolved, the more likely it is that it will require primarily modality-specific processing resources.

References

Alais, D. and Burr, D. (2004). The ventriloquist effect results from near-optimal bimodal integration. *Current Biology* 14:257–62.

Alais, D., Morrone, C., and Burr, D. (2006). Separate attentional resources for vision and audition. *Proceedings of the Royal Society B* 273:1339–45.

Alink, A., Singer, W., and Muckli, L. (2008). Capture of auditory motion by vision is represented by an activation shift from auditory to visual motion cortex. *Journal of Neuroscience* 28:2690–7.

Alsius, A., Navarra, J., Campbell, R., and Soto-Faraco, S. (2005). Audiovisual integration of speech falters under high attention demands. *Current Biology* 15:1–5.

Alsius, A., Navarra, J., and Soto-Faraco, S. (2007). Attention to touch weakens audiovisual speech integration. *Experimental Brain Research* 183:399–404.

Arnell, K. M. (2006). Visual, auditory, and cross-modality dual-task costs: Electrophysiological evidence for an amodal bottleneck on working memory consolidation. *Perception and Psychophysics* 68:447–57.

Battaglia, P. W., Jacobs, R. A., and Aslin, R. N. (2003). Bayesian integration of visual and auditory signals for spatial localization. *Journal of the Optical Society of America* 20:1391–7.

Bernstein, L. E., Auer, E. T. Jr, Moore, J. K., Ponton, C. W., Don, M., and Singh, M. (2002). Visual speech perception without primary auditory cortex activation. *Neuroreport* 13:311–15.

Bertelson, P. and Aschersleben, G. (1998). Automatic visual bias of perceived auditory location. *Psychonomic Bulletin and Review* 5:482–9.

Bertelson, P. and de Gelder, B. (2004). The psychology of multimodal perception. In *Crossmodal Space and Crossmodal Attention* (ed. C. Spence and J. Driver), pp. 141–77. Oxford: Oxford University Press.

Bonath, B., Noesselt, T., Martinez, A., Mishra, J., Schwiecker, K., Heinze, H.-J., and Hillyard, S. A. (2007). Neural basis of the ventriloquist illusion. *Current Biology* 17:1697–703.

Bonnel, A.-M. and Hafter, E. R. (1998). Divided attention between simultaneous auditory and visual signals. *Perception and Psychophysics* 60:179–90.

Brand-D'Abrescia, M. and Lavie, N (2008). Task coordination between and within sensory modalities: Effects on distraction. *Perception and Psychophysics* 70:508–15.

Bregman, A. S. (1990). *Auditory Scene Analysis: The Perceptual Organization of Sound*. Cambridge, MA: MIT Press.

Calvert, G. A., Bullmore, E. T., Brammer, M. J., Campbell, R., Williams, S. C., McGuire, P. K., Woodruff, P. W., Iversen, S. D., and David, A. S. (1997). Activation of auditory cortex during silent lipreading. *Science* 276:593–6.

Calvert, G. A., Spence, C., and Stein, B. E. (eds) (2004). *The Handbook of Multisensory Processes*. Cambridge, MA: MIT Press.

Choe, C. S., Welch, R. B., Gilford, R. M., and Juola, J. F. (1975). The 'ventriloquist effect': Visual dominance or response bias? *Perception and Psychophysics* 18:55–60.

Churchland, P. S., Ramachandran, V. S., and Sejnowski, T. J. (1994). A critique of pure vision. In *Large-scale Neuronal Theories of the Brain* (ed. C. Koch and J. L. Davis), pp. 23–60. Cambridge, MA: MIT Press.

Colavita, F. B. (1974). Human sensory dominance. *Perception and Psychophysics* 16:409–12.

de Gelder, B. and Vroomen, J. (2000). The perception of emotions by ear and eye. *Cognition and Emotion* 14:289–311.

Delano, P. H., Elgueda, D., Hamame, C. M., and Robles, L. (2007). Selective attention to visual stimuli reduces cochlear sensitivity in chinchillas. *Journal of Neuroscience* 27:4146–53.

Driver, J. and Noesselt, T. (2008). Multisensory interplay reveals crossmodal influences on 'sensory-specific' brain regions, neural responses, and judgments. *Neuron* 57:11–23.

Duncan, J., Martens, S., and Ward, R. (1997). Restricted attentional capacity within but not between sensory modalities. *Nature* 387:808–10.

Ernst, M. O. and Bülthoff, H. H. (2004). Merging the senses into a robust percept. *Trends in Cognitive Sciences* **8**:162–9.

Freeman, E. and Driver, J. (2008). Direction of visual apparent motion driven by timing of a static sound. *Current Biology* **18**:1262–6.

Gallace, A. and Spence, C. (2006). Multisensory synesthetic interactions in the speeded classification of visual size. *Perception and Psychophysics* **68**:1191–203.

Ghazanfar, A. A. and Schroeder, C. E. (2006). Is neocortex essentially multisensory? *Trends in Cognitive Sciences* **10**:278–85.

Heron, J., Whitaker, D., and McGraw, P. V. (2004). Sensory uncertainty governs the extent of audio-visual interaction. *Vision Research* **44**:2875–84.

Huddleston, W. E., Lewis, J. W., Phinney, R. E., and DeYoe, E. A. (2008). Auditory and visual attention-based apparent motion share functional parallels. *Perception and Psychophysics* **70**:1207–16.

Hunt, A. R. and Kingstone, A. (2004). Multisensory executive functioning. *Brain and Cognition* **55**:325–7.

Jackson, C. V. (1953). Visual factors in auditory localization. *Quarterly Journal of Experimental Psychology* **5**:52–65.

Johnson, J. A. and Zatorre, R. J. (2005). Attention to simultaneous unrelated auditory and visual events: Behavioral and neural correlates. *Cerebral Cortex* **15**:1609–20.

Johnson, J. A. and Zatorre, R. J. (2006). Neural substrates for dividing and focusing attention between simultaneous auditory and visual events. *Neuroimage* **31**:1673–81.

Johnson, J. A., Strafella, A. P., and Zatorre, R. J. (2007). The role of the dorsolateral prefrontal cortex in bimodal divided attention: Two transcranial magnetic stimulation studies. *Journal of Cognitive Neuroscience* **19**:907–20.

Jones, J. A. and Jarick, M. (2006). Multisensory integration of speech signals: The relationship between space and time. *Experimental Brain Research* **174**:588–94.

Kayser, C. and Logothetis, N. K. (2007). Do early sensory cortices integrate cross-modal information? *Brain Structure and Function* **212**:121–32.

Kayser, C., Petkov, C. I., Augath, M., and Logothetis, N. K. (2007). Functional imaging reveals visual modulation of specific fields in auditory cortex. *Journal of Neuroscience* **27**:1824–35.

Kitagawa, N. and Ichihara, S. (2002). Hearing visual motion in depth. *Nature* **416**:172–4.

Koppen, C. and Spence, C. (2007). Seeing the light: Exploring the Colavita visual dominance effect. *Experimental Brain Research* **180**:737–54.

Koppen, C., Alsius, A., and Spence, C. (2008). Semantic congruency and the Colavita visual dominance effect. *Experimental Brain Research* **184**:533–46.

Körding, K. P., Beierholm, U., Ma, W. J., Quartz, S., Tenenbaum, J. B., et al. (2007). Causal inference in multisensory perception. *PLoS ONE*, 2(9):e943.

Laurienti, P. J., Burdette, J. H., Wallace, M. T., Yen, Y.-F., Field, A. S., and Stein, B. E. (2002). Deactivation of sensory-specific cortex by cross-modal stimuli. *Journal of Cognitive Neuroscience* **14**:1–10.

Laurienti, P. J., Kraft, R. A., Maldjian, J. A., Burdette, J. H., and Wallace, M. T. (2004). Semantic congruence is a critical factor in multisensory behavioral performance. *Experimental Brain Research* **158**:405–14.

Lavie, N. (2005). Distracted and confused?: Selective attention under load. *Trends in Cognitive Sciences* **9**:75–82.

Levy, J., Pashler, H., and Boer, E. (2006). Central interference in driving: Is there any stopping the psychological refractory period? *Psychological Science* **17**:228–35.

Lovelace, C. T., Stein, B. E., and Wallace, M. T. (2003). An irrelevant light enhances auditory detection in humans: A psychophysical analysis of multisensory integration in stimulus detection. *Cognitive Brain Research* **17**:447–53.

Macaluso, E., George, N., Dolan, R., Spence, C., and Driver, J. (2004). Spatial and temporal factors during processing of audiovisual speech perception: A PET study. *Neuroimage* **21**:725–32.

McGurk, H. and MacDonald, J. (1976). Hearing lips and seeing voices. *Nature* **264**:746–8.

Marks, L. E. (2004). Cross-modal interactions in speeded classification. In *Handbook of Multisensory Processes* (ed. G. A. Calvert, C. Spence, and B. E. Stein), pp. 85–105. Cambridge, MA: MIT Press.

Martin, M. (1980). Attention to words in different modalities: Four-channel presentation with physical and semantic selection. *Acta Psychologica* **44**:99–115.

Mateeff, S., Hohnsbein, J., and Noack, T. (1985). Dynamic visual capture: Apparent auditory motion induced by a moving visual target. *Perception* **14**:721–7.

Meyer, G. F., Wuerger, S. M., Röhrbein, F., and Zetzsche, C. (2005). Low-level integration of auditory and visual motion signals requires spatial co-localisation. *Experimental Brain Research* **166**:538–47.

Morein-Zamir, S., Soto-Faraco, S., and Kingstone, A. (2003). Auditory capture of vision: Examining temporal ventriloquism. *Cognitive Brain Research* **17**:154–63.

Narins, P. M., Grabul, D. S., Soma, K. K., Gaucher, P., and Hödl, W. (2005). Cross-modal integration in a dart-poison frog. *Proceedings of the National Academy of Sciences USA* **102**:2425–9.

O'Leary, A. and Rhodes, G. (1984). Cross-modal effects on visual and auditory object perception. *Perception and Psychophysics* **35**:565–9.

Otten, L. J., Alain, C., and Picton, T. W. (2000). Effects of visual attentional load on auditory processing. *Neuroreport* **11**:875–80.

Parise, C. and Spence, C. (2009). 'When birds of a feather flock together': Synesthetic correspondences modulate audiovisual integration in non-synesthetes. *PLoS ONE* **4**(5):e5664. doi:10.1371/journal.pone.0005664.

Partan, S. and Marler, P. (1999). Communication goes multimodal. *Science* **283**:1272–3.

Pascual-Leone, A. and Hamilton, R. (2001). The metamodal organization of the brain. *Progress in Brain Research* **134**:427–45.

Pekkola, J., Ojanen, V., Autti, T., Jaaskelainen, I. P., Mottonen, R., Tarkianen, A., and Sams, M. (2005). Primary auditory cortex activation by visual speech: An fMRI study at 3T. *Neuroreport* **16**:125–8.

Prinzmetal, W., McCool, C., and Park, S. (2005). Attention: Reaction time and accuracy reveal different mechanisms. *Journal of Experimental Psychology: General* **134**:73–92.

Radeau, M. and Bertelson, P. (1987). Auditory-visual interaction and the timing of inputs. Thomas (1941) revisited. *Psychological Research* **49**:17–22.

Recanzone, G. H. (1998). Rapidly induced auditory plasticity: The ventriloquism aftereffect. *Proceedings of the National Academy of Science USA* **95**:869–75.

Rees, G., Frith, C., and Lavie, N. (2001). Processing of irrelevant visual motion during performance of an auditory attention task. *Neuropsychologia* **39**:937–49.

Roach, N. W., Heron, J., and McGraw, P. V. (2006). Resolving multisensory conflict: A strategy for balancing the costs and benefits of audio-visual integration. *Proceedings of the Royal Society B* **273**:2159–68.

Robertson, L. and Sagiv, N. (eds) (2005). *Synaesthesia: Perspectives from Cognitive Neuroscience*. Oxford: Oxford University Press.

Ross, L. A., Saint-Amour, D., Leavitt, V. M., Javitt, D. C., and Foxe, J. J. (2007). Do you see what I am saying? Exploring visual enhancement of speech comprehension in noisy environments. *Cerebral Cortex* **17**:1147–53.

Saldaña, H. M. and Rosenblum, L. D. (1993). Visual influences on auditory pluck and bow judgments. *Perception and Psychophysics* **54**:406–16.

Sanabria, D., Spence, C., and Soto-Faraco, S. (2007). Perceptual and decisional contributions to audiovisual interactions in the perception of apparent motion: A signal detection study *Cognition* **102**:299–310.

Santangelo, V., Belardinelli, M. O., and Spence, C. (2007). The suppression of reflexive visual and auditory orienting when attention is otherwise engaged. *Journal of Experimental Psychology: Human Perception and Performance* **33**:137–48.

Shomstein, S. and Yantis, S. (2004). Control of attention shifts between vision and audition in human cortex. *Journal of Neuroscience* **24**:10702–6.

Shore, D. I. and Spence, C. (2005). Prior entry. In *Neurobiology of Attention*. (ed. L. Itti, G. Rees, and J. Tsotsos), pp. 89–95. North Holland: Elsevier.

Sinnett, S., Costa, A., and Soto-Faraco, S. (2006). Manipulating inattentional blindness within and across sensory modalities. *Quarterly Journal of Experimental Psychology* 59:1425–42.

Sinnett, S., Spence, C., and Soto-Faraco, S. (2007). Visual dominance and attention: The Colavita effect revisited. *Perception and Psychophysics* 69:673–86.

Sinnett, S., Spence, C., and Soto-Faraco, S. (2008). The co-occurrence of multisensory competition and facilitation. *Acta Psychologica* 128:153–61.

Slutsky, D. A. and Recanzone, G. H. (2001). Temporal and spatial dependency of the ventriloquism effect. *Neuroreport* 12:7–10.

Soto-Faraco, S. and Alsius, A. (2007). Conscious access to the unisensory components of a cross-modal illusion. *Neuroreport* 18:347–50.

Soto-Faraco, S. and Alsius, A. (2008). Deconstructing the McGurk–Macdonald illusion. *Journal of Experimental Psychology: Human Perception and Performance* 35:580–7.

Soto-Faraco, S. and Spence, C. (2002). Modality-specific auditory and visual temporal processing deficits. *Quarterly Journal of Experimental Psychology A* 55:23–40.

Soto-Faraco, S., Lyons, J., Gazzaniga, M., Spence, C., and Kingstone, A. (2002). The ventriloquist in motion: Illusory capture of dynamic information across sensory modalities. *Cognitive Brain Research* 14:139–46.

Soto-Faraco, S., Spence, C., and Kingstone, A. (2004). Cross-modal dynamic capture: Congruency effects in the perception of motion across sensory modalities. *Journal of Experimental Psychology: Human Perception and Performance* 30:330–45.

Soto-Faraco, S., Spence, C., and Kingstone, A. (2005). Assessing automaticity in the audiovisual integration of motion. *Acta Psychologica* 118:71–92.

Spence, C. (2007). Audiovisual multisensory integration. *Acoustical Science and Technology* 28:61–70.

Spence, C. and Driver, J. (1997). On measuring selective attention to a specific sensory modality. *Perception and Psychophysics* 59:389–403.

Spence, C. and Driver, J. (eds) (2004). *Crossmodal Space and Crossmodal Attention*. Oxford: Oxford University Press.

Spence, C. and Read, L. (2003). Speech shadowing while driving: On the difficulty of splitting attention between eye and ear. *Psychological Science* 14:251–6.

Spence, C., Nicholls, M. E. R., and Driver, J. (2001). The cost of expecting events in the wrong sensory modality. *Perception and Psychophysics* 63:330–6.

Spence, C., Sanabria, D., and Soto-Faraco, S. (2007). Intersensory Gestalten and crossmodal scene perception. In *Psychology of Beauty and Kansei: New Horizons of Gestalt Perception* (ed. K. Noguchi), pp. 519–79. Tokyo: Fuzanbo International.

Sugita, Y. and Suzuki, Y. (2003). Implicit estimation of sound-arrival time. *Nature* 421:911.

Sumby, W. H. and Pollack, I. (1954). Visual contribution to speech intelligibility in noise. *Journal of the Acoustical Society of America* 26:212–15.

Talsma, D., Doty, T. J., Strowd, R., and Woldorff, M. G. (2006). Attentional capacity for processing concurrent stimuli is larger across modalities than within a modality. *Psychophysiology* 43:541–9.

Tellinghuisen, D. J. and Nowak, E. J. (2003). The inability to ignore auditory distractors as a function of visual task perceptual load. *Perception and Psychophysics* 65:817–28.

Thomas, G. J. (1941). Experimental study of the influence of vision on sound localization. *Journal of Experimental Psychology* 28:163–77.

Titchener, E. B. (1908). *Lectures on the Elementary Psychology of Feeling and Attention*. New York: Macmillan.

Treisman, A. M. and Davies, A. (1973). Divided attention to ear and eye. In *Attention and Performance*, Vol. 4 (ed. S. Kornblum), pp. 101–17. New York: Academic Press.

Vatakis, A. and Spence, C. (2007). Crossmodal binding: Evaluating the 'unity assumption' using audiovisual speech stimuli. *Perception and Psychophysics* **69**:744–56.

Vatakis, A. and Spence, C. (2008). Evaluating the influence of the 'unity assumption' on the temporal perception of realistic audiovisual stimuli. *Acta Psychologica* **127**:12–23.

Vatakis, A., Ghazanfar, A., and Spence, C. (2008). Facilitation of multisensory integration by the 'unity assumption': Is speech special? *Journal of Vision* **8**:1–11.

Walker, P. and Smith, S. (1984). Stroop interference based on the synaesthetic qualities of auditory pitch. *Perception* **13**:75–81.

Weissman, D. H., Warner, L. M., and Woldorff, M. G. (2004). The neural mechanisms for minimizing cross-modal distraction. *Journal of Neuroscience* **24**:10941–9.

Welch, R. B. and Warren, D. H. (1980). Immediate perceptual response to intersensory discrepancy. *Psychological Bulletin* **88**:638–67.

Welch, R. B. and Warren, D. H. (1986). Intersensory interactions. In *Handbook of Perception and Performance*, Vol. 1 (ed. K. R. Boff, L. Kaufman, and J. P. Thomas), pp. 25-1–25-36. New York: Wiley.

Welch, R. B., DuttonHurt, L. D., and Warren, D. H. (1986). Contributions of audition and vision to temporal rate perception. *Perception and Psychophysics* **39**:294–300.

Wickens, C. D. (1980). The structure of attentional resources. In *Attention and Performance*, Vol. 8 (ed. R. S. Nickerson), pp. 239–57. Hillsdale, NJ: Erlbaum.

Wickens, C. D. (1992). *Engineering Psychology and Human Performance* (2nd edn). NY: HarperCollins.

Woodruff, P. W., Benson, R. R., Bandettini, P. A., *et al.* (1996). Modulation of auditory and visual cortex by selective attention is modality-dependent. *Neuroreport* **7**:1909–13.

Wozny, D. R., Beierholm, U. R., and Shams, L. (2008). Human trimodal perception follows optimal statistical inference. *Journal of Vision* **8**(3):24, 1–11.

Zampini, M., Shore, D. I., and Spence, C. (2005). Audiovisual prior entry. *Neuroscience Letters* **381**:217–22.

Chapter 13

Auditory development and learning

Karen Mattock, Sygal Amitay, and David R. Moore

13.1 Introduction

Like all living systems, auditory system function is constantly changing in response to internal and external forces—genetic, disease, and experience. It has long been recognized, for example, that the fundamental measure of hearing, the pure-tone audiogram, is susceptible to both developmental and learning influences. Moreover, the deterioration of hearing sensitivity in later life is thought to be influenced by inheritance, acting synergistically with environmental (noise, toxins) and biological (ageing) processes.

Research into the long-term dynamics of hearing is, despite much increased effort and understanding over recent years, still in its infancy. The organization of this chapter mimics the history of research in the field. While we provide an overview of the most significant, older findings, the primary focus of our presentation is on the recent and, we think, exciting findings of the last decade. The bias of our work reflects our backgrounds, in experimental psychology and neuroscience. Those seeking alternative perspectives are directed to appropriate reviews in the overview that follows.

13.1.1 Stages of language acquisition

To infants, speech is incredibly salient, and cracking the speech code is seemingly effortless. Infants' success may be driven by biases that they bring to the task of language learning, built in part on prenatal experience with the low-frequency prosodic and rhythmic components of speech that are available *in utero* (Querleu *et al.*, 1988). Vouloumanos and Werker (2007) measured the rate of non-nutritive sucking to speech and non-speech stimuli and found that neonates have a speech bias. When given a choice of listening to speech, or equally complex sine-wave analogues, infants preferred speech, as indicated by consistent sucking rates to speech but not non-speech across the experiment.

Infants' initial sensitivities to phonetic contrasts are broad and unspecific—they routinely discriminate pairs of phones in the world's languages, regardless of their presence or absence in the ambient language. Adults, however, do not demonstrate such fluid abilities—their sensitivity is practised, fine-tuned, and optimized for perceiving only the acoustic differences between speech sounds that are significant for making distinctions between words in their native language. Thus, the first step to becoming a fluent perceiver and producer of language is to discover the subset of speech sounds (phones) that are functionally relevant to the language(s) you are learning. In Section 13.2 we discuss the perceptual shift in favour of the native language that occurs in the first year of life, the challenges faced by infants when applying their speech perception skills to the task of word learning, and the refinement of phonological representation in the second year of life and beyond (see Werker and Curtin, 2005). These baby steps to language, from birth to early school years, are presented in Fig. 13.1.

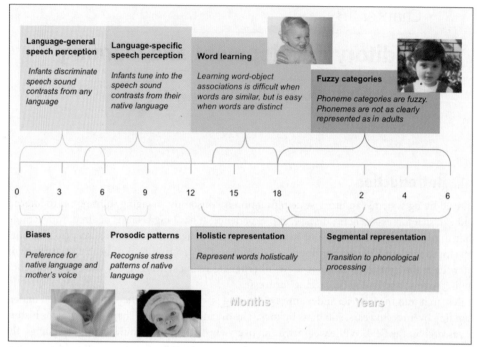

Fig. 13.1 Baby steps to language. Timeline of major achievements in speech perception during infancy (0–18 months) and early childhood (18 months–6 years).

13.1.2 **Development of hearing**

It is not entirely clear when human hearing begins, but behavioural indices, such as fetal movements in response to external sound, suggest that it is around the 25th week of gestation (Lecanuet *et al.*, 1995). However, this 'onset of hearing' marks but one significant event in a developmental sequence that begins at conception and continues, according to a recent cortical evoked-potential study (Poulsen *et al.*, 2007), to somewhere beyond 40 years of age. Despite this widely protracted period of development, it is clear that most major changes in auditory perception occur relatively early in a child's life. Newborn infants have tone-detection thresholds that are 30–70 dB higher than adults. Sensitivity then improves dramatically, so that, by 6 months, it is possible to observe thresholds for high-frequency sounds that are only 10 dB or so higher than those of young adults. But, while high-frequency sensitivity matures early (by around 2 years), low-frequency sensitivity continues to develop until about 10 years of age.

The presentation in this chapter reflects three general aspects of auditory development highlighted by the above data. The first is that the major period of development is the pre-school years. This includes fetal development and the all-important acquisition of language, also highlighted above. A crucial aspect of measuring hearing in these early years (see Section 13.2) is the typical inability to understand or follow instructions. The second aspect is older childhood (discussed in Section 13.3). When children reach school age, they are typically able to understand instructions, but attention and motivation can be variable, leading to uncertainties about the validity of data. Finally, linking all aspects of study of the development of hearing are the methodological challenges. These are introduced below (Section 13.1.3), but underpin much of the presentation throughout the chapter.

We have attempted to restrict ourselves, where possible, to the behavioural aspects of human auditory development. Inevitably, however, there are references to several closely related areas of developmental work: neurobiology (for a review, see Volume 2, Chapter 15; Rubel *et al.*, 1998), evoked potentials (see Burkhard *et al.*, 2006), and speech and language (Bishop, 1997; Jusczyk, 1997).

13.1.3 Methodological challenges

The very different time courses of various aspects of auditory development emphasize an equally important interpretive qualification. As discussed extensively by Wightman, Werner, and their colleagues (Wightman *et al.*, 1989; Werner and Rubel, 1992; Werner and Gray, 1998), behavioural responses to sounds are always a reflection of sensory and non-sensory factors, and the hearing abilities of children are particularly difficult to separate from their behavioural 'compliance'—the extent to which a response is indicative of having heard a sound. At this point it is useful to introduce the concept of 'listening'. We use this term to denote active hearing, by which we mean a cognitive engagement with an auditory stimulus. It is a matter of everyday experience that environmental sounds vary in audibility and salience, depending on their behavioural context. In the laboratory, the performance of highly motivated, trained, and intelligent young adult listeners tends to be relatively consistent and, for this reason, the performance of such listeners makes up at least 90% of the psychoacoustic literature. But even those listeners have occasional lapses of attention. For children, whether in the lab or in the community, variable attention and motivation place constraints on the interpretation of auditory test performance, while additional individual differences (age, other cognitive skills) need to be carefully monitored and, if possible, experimentally controlled.

It is arguable that researchers should place greater emphasis on the performance of all listeners under more typical conditions than the highly constrained measurements described above. In many instances, however, it is desirable to separate sensory from non-sensory aspects of listening. For example, if we are interested to know the extent to which maturation contributes to hearing, or whether learning-impaired children have a specific listening difficulty, it is desirable to measure and partial out the influence of variable attention as far as possible (see Fig. 13.2). Different investigators have used various methods to do this. These methods can be separated into what

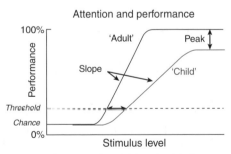

Fig. 13.2 Hypothetical psychometric functions for child and adult listeners. Both functions show a growth in performance with increasing stimulus 'level', where that means increases in detectability or discriminability rather than stimulus amplitude. Note that 'chance' performance is above zero, because we assume a multiple-choice task, and that 'threshold' differences between the listeners depend on stimulus level. The difference in slope of the rising phase of the functions and in peak performance has been used in the literature as indicators of the relative contribution of sensory and non-sensory factors to child and adult listening.

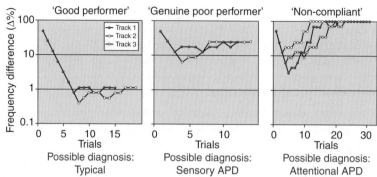

Fig. 13.3 Performance of children on a frequency discrimination task. An alternative perspective on children's listening abilities highlights individual variability as a key factor in understanding both normal development and listening problems. Each panel shows the performance of a different individual child (aged 6–8 years) on successive 'tracks' of 15–30 trials presented as an adaptive '3-down, 1-up' staircase. While the majority of children at all ages (6–11 years) show consistent, age-appropriate performance, some children show poorer performance, either without ('genuine poor performer') or with ('non-compliant') increased response variability. As might be expected, larger proportions of younger children express non-compliant performance. This schema is currently being investigated as a possible model for the diagnosis of two distinct types of 'auditory processing disorder' (APD). See text for further details (from Moore *et al.*, 2008).

may be called 'extrinsic' and 'intrinsic' measures of attention. Extrinsic methods are typically simple to administer (e.g. 'pencil and paper') and multifaceted, but are quite general tests of attention developed by cognitive psychologists (e.g. Test of Everyday Attention for Children—TEA-Ch; Manly *et al.*, 2001). Auditory scientists studying development have, however, generally preferred intrinsic methods (Fig. 13.3; see Moore *et al.*, 2008). These are estimates of attention based on performance variability on an auditory task, such as pure-tone frequency discrimination. Such intrinsic measures confirm quantitatively: (1) that children are poorer attenders than adults while performing lab-based listening tasks; (2) that, consequently or additionally, children's listening is less sensitive than that of adults; and (3) that these factors should be considered in measuring children's hearing, whether in the lab, the clinic, or the school.

Whatever the method of testing children's hearing, it is essential that their performance is compared against that of age-matched peers, that they are engaged in a task that is meaningful and motivating for them, that they are not asked to spend excessive time being tested, and that they are not too tired or otherwise distracted whilst performing the test.

13.1.4 Auditory learning

Auditory learning refers to change in perception of an acoustic stimulus with experience. By this simple and broad definition, we can immediately see that learning could occur on an ongoing and daily basis throughout the lifespan, and the evidence suggests that it does. Infants learn language (see Section 13.1.1), older children recover from middle ear infections (Hogan and Moore, 2003), and people of all ages learn to use hearing aids and cochlear implants (Sweetow, 2007). Note that in these three examples, specific training is unnecessary and, in fact, is rarely used. Laboratory studies of auditory learning, on the other hand, almost always manipulate auditory training, usually by varying the stimulus, as the independent variable of the experiment. However, we know from the above examples that many different environmental influences affect learning. A recent experiment (Amitay *et al.*, 2006*b*) showed, for example, that playing the visual spatial manipulation game Tetris led to improved pure-tone frequency discrimination. The assumption of experimental work is that specific training will further improve learning, but it is crucial to bear in mind the full range of influences that may be important, especially when designing clinical interventions.

In common with other studies in psychoacoustics (Plack, 2005) and perceptual learning (Fahle and Poggio, 2002), laboratory-based research in auditory learning tends to involve relatively short sessions of training using highly artificial stimuli (e.g. pure tones). These studies can tell us a great deal about the properties and mechanisms of auditory learning, but they provide only limited information about two critical aspects of the usefulness of learning: the transfer of training to the requirements of everyday listening, and the persistence of learning. The most challenging and one of the most common auditory tasks that most humans perform is listening to speech in a noisy environment, where the noise is itself composed of one or more speech signals. It is of great interest to know whether a given form of training influences this skill or one of its components (e.g. informational masking; Schneider *et al.*, 2007). The persistence of learning and its resistance to various forms of interference dictate the usefulness of a training programme—a certain amount of 'top up' training may be acceptable, but investment in training carries an expectation that the results will not be too short-lived. Unfortunately, these are areas where there is currently little information. An increase in translational research should place greater focus on both these practical problems which, of course, are also relevant to basic understanding.

Despite the focus of laboratory studies of perceptual learning on the trained stimulus, recent research suggests that training methods, rather than stimuli, may be of at least equal importance. Frequency discrimination improvement following Tetris training, cited above, is one example. Another, even more striking example from the same study (Amitay *et al.*, 2006*b*) is that training on identical stimuli can improve frequency discrimination to the same extent as adaptive training (see Section 13.4). A variety of results are consistent with the idea that training improves top-down processes, particularly attention, as much as bottom-up, specialist sensory processing. It is feasible, but not yet well established, that when we train we are mainly enhancing awareness. This could be general awareness, or wholly or partly limited to a specific modality, as major models of attention postulate (see Chapter 11).

13.1.5 Outline of chapter

The presentation that follows is organized into two sections (Sections 13.2 and 13.3) on the development of hearing and two (Sections 13.4 and 13.5) on auditory learning. There is inevitably some overlap in these presentations, for example in the acquisition and experience dependence of language (Section 13.2). However, there is also a surprising segregation, because most studies of auditory learning to date have examined adult listeners. There are various reasons for this, but probably the most influential, and noteworthy in this outline, is the different research cultures from which these fields have emerged. Studies of auditory development have mostly been conducted by developmental and cognitive psychologists and linguists. Auditory learning has, however, grown out of psychoacoustics, a branch of psychophysics. Psychophysics was conceived as a means for accurately measuring sensory ability and has evolved into an experimental approach of which the name speaks volumes, but the data rarely if ever achieve the implied level of precision. The synthesis presented here (Section 13.6) represents a growing recognition of the need to draw these research areas together. Like other chapters in this volume and series, it is intended to be comprehensive but, rather, to provide both a broad overview of the fields and a sense of current research issues and excitement.

13.2 **Fetal and infant hearing**

Acoustical recordings of the interuterine environment show that the maternal voice and external speech at 60 dB SPL can be differentiated, using measurement techniques, from uterine background noise (e.g. maternal respiratory and cardiovascular activity) above 100 Hz (Querleu *et al.*, 1988), and that the sound pressure level of the maternal voice is higher than that of the external voice (due to dual transmission—internal and airborne—of the maternal voice; Richards *et al.*, 1992). It is during late gestation that the human fetus is most influenced by the internal and external sound environment. Gerhardt and Abrams (1996) suggest that the fetus can detect components of speech and music that are below 500 Hz at 60 dB SPL or above. Generally, systematic observation of fetal responsiveness to sound is concerned with motor responses or heart rate changes in the fetus to startling stimulation, when vibroacoustic or airborne stimuli are presented at over 105 dB SPL, or to non-startling stimulation at 85–100 dB SPL.

13.2.1 **Fetal responsiveness to sound and postnatal auditory preferences**

During the third trimester, fetuses elicit motor and cardiac responses to brief presentations of high-pass filtered noise at 110 dB SPL, and respond differentially to differences between syllables 'babi' and 'biba' (Lecanuet *et al.*, 1997) and vowels 'ee' and 'ah' (Zimmer *et al.*, 1993). Furthermore, fetuses discriminate recordings of a rhyme spoken by their mother every day from week 33 to 37 of pregnancy when an unfamiliar female reads the familiar and an unfamiliar rhyme (DeCasper *et al.*, 1994). Kisilevsky *et al.* (2003) report differential fetal behaviour in response to the mother's voice and the voice of a stranger, indicating voice processing. Specifically, at 38 weeks, fetuses displayed heart rate acceleration to their mother's voice and heart rate deceleration to the voice of a stranger. Fetuses also show changes in cardiac reactions to non-speech auditory stimuli. For example, Lecanuet *et al.* (2000) showed that 36–39-week-old fetuses detect and respond with heart rate deceleration to the presentation of a low-pitched piano note, and a subsequent change to a second note.

Kisilevsky *et al.* (2000) found that fetuses at high risk of premature birth begin responding to sound at the same gestational age as low-risk fetuses; however, the nature of responsiveness is different for low- and high-risk fetuses. Fetuses born prematurely displayed increased heart rate variability and no cardiac acceleration in response to a startling 110 dB SPL sound at 33 weeks' gestation compared to fetuses at low risk of premature birth who showed cardiac acceleration.

There is some evidence that prenatal experience with sound affects postnatal speech preferences. Specifically, newborn infants seem to respond preferentially to speech that they were exposed to *in utero*. Using non-nutritive sucking paradigms it has been found that newborns have a preference for their mother's voice over the voice of a stranger (DeCasper and Fifer, 1980), their native language from a foreign language of a different rhythm class (Moon *et al.*, 1993), as well as stories read to them by their mother during the last weeks of pregnancy (DeCasper and Spence, 1986). The infants' experience with the prosodic and rhythmic components of the preferred speech is hypothesized to drive these preferences.

13.2.2 **Testing infants: Methods and acoustic considerations**

As discussed in Section 13.1, measuring auditory function in infants presents many challenges. Infants are limited by their inability to follow instructions, provide verbal responses, focus attention, and maintain a motivated state for the period of testing. Behavioural Observation Audiometry (BOA) and Visual Reinforcement Audiometry (VRA) are commonly used with infants and rely on measures of behavioural responses to determine the extremes of auditory function—whether the system is functional or not—rather than assessing specific responsiveness to particular sound levels, frequencies, or periodicities. BOA is best suited to infants aged 6–24 months. Typically, an auditory stimulus is played to the infant and several observers judge reflexive and orienting responses such as eye blink 'startle' responses. A downfall of the BOA methods is that infants habituate quickly to the auditory stimulus, meaning that the same response may not be achieved after repeated presentations.

By 5–6 months of age infants are able to localize sound, and make head turns reliably. VRA uses stimulus–response reinforcement to elicit recurring head-turns towards a visual reinforcer in response to sound. VRA has two phases: conditioning and testing. In the conditioning phase head-turns are shaped by making sound presentation and activation of the visual reinforcer contingent. Importantly, auditory stimuli must be above threshold, typically 30–70 dB SPL. Once the infant is reliably producing head-turns to a pre-established criterion, such as a number of correct consecutive head-turns, they progress to the test stage. In the test phase, signal intensity is decreased by 10 dB following correct head-turns and increased by 10 dB in the absence of head-turning. This adaptive, staircase procedure yields good test–retest reliability for the same child tested in multiple sessions and is suitable for 5-month-olds to 2.5-year-olds. VRA has been adapted for use in speech perception studies (e.g. Conditioned Head Turn procedure; Mattock and Burnham, 2006), where infants hear one category of speech sound played repeatedly and are trained to produce a head-turn when the speech sound changes to a different category.

It is a common finding that infants do not perform as well as adults during auditory processing tasks (see Aslin *et al.*, 1983). In fact, infants rarely achieve a 100% responding rate even in the face of large stimulus magnitude differences. Infant–adult differences may well be due to legitimate differences in auditory sensory capacity, or they may be due to non-sensory effects, such as infant–adult differences in motivation, attention, processing efficiency, memory, and response generation. Olsho *et al.* (1988) argue that infant capacities can only be compared to adults' when both groups are tested on similar tasks and under similar conditions. They found that adults trained to discriminate low frequencies performed significantly better than adults who were not trained. Analysis of infant performance in a frequency discrimination (adaptive staircase) task, where infants were trained to turn their heads to a mechanical toy when they heard a change in tone frequency, revealed that following training, differences between infants and adults in low-frequency discrimination performance were reduced only when the best performance of individual listeners was compared. Similarly, differences in the auditory performance of 3-year-olds and adults were reduced when each child's best performance was considered. Nozza (1995) used more rigorous psychophysical procedures to estimate the relative contributions of sensory and non-sensory factors to infant–adult differences. This included obtaining thresholds in quiet and in increasing masking noise, as well as determining the minimum masking level, for a 1-kHz tone. Infants were tested using an operant head-turn paradigm and adults were tested with an operant 'hand raising' paradigm. Tympanometry and other immittance measures were also taken to account for differences in ear canal sound pressure between infants and adults. In short, Nozza found that infant–adult differences in the behavioural threshold and minimum masking level are 12 dB and 8 dB, respectively: reasoning that 8 dB of the infant–adult difference in unmasked thresholds was due to sensory factors, and the remaining 4 dB attributable to non-sensory factors.

Overall, these findings highlight the importance of being mindful of the contributions of sensory and non-sensory factors when comparing auditory performance across infancy, and when evaluating studies where infant–adult differences are reported.

13.2.3 Hearing of non-speech sounds in infancy

Most infants are born into the world with a functional auditory system, but their hearing is not yet adult-like. Infants initially face problems with the higher frequencies and, although the inner ear is mature at birth, auditory signals are poorly transmitted through the brainstem contributing to a loss of information and poor frequency resolution. Specifically, brainstem evoked potentials are mature at low frequencies by 3 months, but maturity at higher frequencies is not evident until 6 months (Folsom and Wynne, 1987). With regard to frequency discrimination, 3-month-olds require a 120-Hz differential to detect a change in a 4000-Hz tone, whereas adults require a difference of only 40 Hz. At 1000 Hz, adults detect frequency changes of around 1%, however 6-month-olds need up to a 3% change (Aslin, 1989). These studies give the impression that infants' frequency discrimination is relatively mature by 6 months of age. However, as discussed later in Section 13.3, studies of older children that used cognitively challenging tasks, such as the three-alternative, forced-choice, fixed-tone procedures, show that children have higher sensory thresholds and a more variable performance due to poorer attention (see also Section 13.2.2 and Moore *et al.*, 2008; Halliday *et al.*, 2008).

Part of the problem with frequency discrimination has to do with frequency resolution. Frequency resolution is the ability to separate out sounds of different frequencies (see Chapter 2). Infants have higher thresholds for detecting a signal in broadband noise, but signal intensity relative to threshold is comparable to adult levels. Spetner and Olsho (1990) found that for 3-month-olds, 4000- and 8000-Hz tones were masked by a broader range of frequencies than for 6-month-olds and adults. In addition, 6-month-olds' frequency resolution was mature at all frequencies, whereas 3-month-olds showed mature frequency resolution only at 1000 Hz. However, obtained masked thresholds from 6.5-month-old infants, 2- and 5-year-old children, and adults for 800- and 4000-Hz signals presented in broad band and one-third octave maskers reveal a longer developmental trajectory. Critical band width was found to be 50% larger in infants than adults. Moreover, thresholds increased with masker bandwidth at both signal frequencies for children and adults, but only at 800 Hz for infants (Schneider *et al.*, 1990). The child–adult difference in masked thresholds was between 8 and 15 dB, of which only 1–2 dB were estimated to be due to variation in critical band width.

With regard to loudness (intensity) perception, neonates respond to intensity changes as small as 6 dB (Tarquinio *et al.*, 1990). Infants aged 7–9 months detect 6-dB intensity differences between 1000-Hz tones (Sinnott and Aslin, 1985), but need greater differences (9 dB) for broadband noise (Kopyar, 1997). In contrast, Werner and Boike (2001) showed that, on average, infants were relatively better at detecting changes in broadband noise than narrowband tones both under quiet and noise conditions. They suggested that infants have not yet developed the attention needed to detect narrowband sounds and that the multiple frequencies available in broadband noise were easier for them to detect.

Infants have difficulty with sound segregation, such as extracting a tone from broadband noise, and, unlike adults, this is even the case when the spectra of the noise and the tone do not overlap (Leibold and Werner, 2006). Infants can certainly separate out a relevant signal from irrelevant noise but they need a greater signal-to-noise ratio. There is some debate about whether difficulty in separating simultaneous sounds stems from problems with: (1) intensity coding, i.e. an inability to determine the addition of a tone to noise; (2) actually separating out the sound; or (3) attending selectively to one sound when two sounds are detected.

Sound localization is the ability to accurately identify where a sound is coming from. Locating a sound in the horizontal plane requires making a comparison of a sound wave that reaches one ear with the same wave (from the same source) to the other ear. Thus, if a sound is to the right of the subject, the sound wave will reach the right ear first, creating time and intensity differences between the two ears. Our brains then use this information to compute the location of the sound in the horizontal plane (see Chapter 6). Newborn infants readily make directional head-turns to sounds in the horizontal plane, but this initial ability is soon attenuated, re-emerging again at around 4 months of age (Muir and Field, 1979). The reason for this U-shape developmental pattern is unclear, but it is thought to be mediated by a shift from low-level reflexive responding by neonates to responding that is mediated by higher level processes at 4 months of age. Moreover, while infants become accurate at localizing the sound source, they also show rapid improvement at detecting the change in the position of the sound source. Infants detect changes around the midline of 5° by 18–24 months, and this improves to 1° by 5 years of age (Litovsky, 1997). However, infants have difficulty pinpointing where in a hemifield the sound is located (Morrongiello et al., 1994). This ability is not constrained by infants' insensitivity to interaural time differences (ITDs; Ashmead et al., 1991). Rather, the need to recalculate the direction of sound waves to both ears, taking into account head growth, is a possible reason for the U-shaped pattern of development. By the end of the first year, however, infants demonstrate substantial improvement in the localization of sound within a hemifield.

Several lines of research suggest that infants can process temporal cues. Temporal processing is needed for distinguishing between-category differences in speech sounds, and we know that infants can do this from very early in life (e.g. Eimas et al., 1971). Insight into temporal processing of non-speech sounds can be gleaned from findings that 5-month-old infants discriminate tone sequences with different temporal groupings, e.g. a 2–4 tone grouping with a 600-ms gap between the second and third tones from a 4–2 grouping where the gap lies between the fourth and fifth tones of a sequence (Chang and Trehub, 1977). There is evidence of more fine-grained temporal discrimination in infancy. Morrongiello and Trehub (1987) used the conditioned head-turn procedure to assess infants' duration discrimination. Six-month-old infants discriminated white-noise bursts and silence-duration differences of 20 ms following training. Older children require a 15-ms difference between noise bursts and adults a smaller difference of 10 ms. Difficulties in processing brief, rapid, spectrotemporal information have been linked to language disorders such as specific language impairment (SLI), and these have been found to occur early in life (although see Chapter 15, this volume for discussion).

Infants show advanced pitch perception abilities. Using the visually reinforced head-turn procedure, Clarkson and Clifton (1985) found that 7–8-month-old infants discriminated harmonic complexes from two pitch categories differing by 20%, and categorize spectrally diverse tonal complexes according to fundamental frequency (F0) information, thus demonstrating perceptual constancy for pitch. Similarly, in the music domain, Thorpe (1986) investigated whether infants could categorize variable two-tone sequences (tunes) on the basis of rising and falling pitch. Infants aged 7–10 months were tested for discrimination of two-tone rising sequences of various frequency intervals (6 and 2 semitones, 4 and 2 semitones, and 2 and 1 semitones) changing to two-tone sequences with falling frequency. Infants successfully detected directional changes in frequency for all intervals, and their performance was not influenced by the degree of frequency change. In another study, Trainor and Trehub (1992) played repeated transpositions of a 10-note melody to 8-month-old infants and adults for their detection of changes to the melody. Adults found a 4-semitone within-key change to the melody significantly more difficult to detect than a 1-semitone outside-key change, while infants discriminated both changes to the melody equally well. Trainor and Trehub proposed that adults' perception of melody is influenced by conventions associated with Western musical structure, whereas infants have not yet the musical experience to incorporate these constraints.

13.2.4 Speech perception

Sensitivity to spectrotemporal, duration, intensity, frequency, and periodicity information is paramount to speech perception. Perceiving vowels relies on the ability to detect and discriminate bands of energy in multiple, relatively invariant frequency regions (formants) and to process that information over time. Perceiving consonants relies on sensitivity to transient energy, and to the level of that energy. For example, voiceless 'h' and 'f' have less spectral energy than voiced 'b' and 'g', but the strident fricative 's' has a higher amplitude level than non-strident 'f'. Consonants can be broadband, such as fricatives, or they can be concentrated to a single frequency region, such as the low-frequency resonance of nasals with energy near the floor of the spectrogram (e.g. 'm' and 'n'). Stop consonants such as 'b' and 'p' have the additional acoustic cues of release burst (abrupt release of air) and transition from the burst to the formants.

Speech perception is complicated by the talker variability problem. For example, when 6-year-old Sally says 'cat' and 60-year-old Tom says 'cat', these enunciations are recognized as the same word, despite vast variation in acoustics due to differences in vocal tract size/shape, F0, and voice quality between speakers. Human listeners must compensate for these differences to be able to correctly perceive the linguistic message. But when does this ability develop?

Infants as young as 2 months demonstrate some capacity to handle talker variability. When infants were presented with 12 tokens each of the words /bug/ and /dug/ produced by six male speakers and six female speakers, they discriminated a change from /bug/ to /dug/ (and vice versa) words despite the talker variation. However, when a two-minute delay was introduced between the presentation of /bug/ tokens and the presentation of /dug/ tokens, infants could not discriminate the contrast. This highlights that infants show perceptual normalization for talker variation only when the processing resources for encoding and retrieving speech are not restricted (Jusczyk et al., 1992).

Categorical perception is fundamental to language processing because it assists the listener with categorizing or grouping invariance in the speech signal. Perceptual discrimination and identification along a speech continuum is heightened for subtle acoustic differences between speech sounds that straddle phonetic categories, such as the 10-ms difference in voice-onset time that changes /b/ to /p/, but not for the similar-sized acoustic differences that occur within phonetic categories (Liberman et al., 1957). Using the high-amplitude sucking procedure, Eimas et al. (1971) demonstrated that 1-month-olds categorically discriminate voicing differences between /ba/ and /pa/. Following the presentation of stop consonants from one phonetic category, infants increased their rate of sucking to a new stimulus from the contrasting phonetic category (between-category contrasts, /ba/ vs. /pa/) but not to a different stimulus token from the same phonetic category (within-category contrasts, /ba1/ vs. /ba2/).

Werker and Tees (1984) were the first to demonstrate how experience with the native language shapes the development of speech perception. They showed that English-learning infants easily discriminated non-native Hindi and Salish consonant contrasts at 6 months of age—in fact they discriminated as well as Hindi- and Salish-speaking adults—but between 6 and 12 months of age this ability progressively declined in the absence of experience hearing Hindi and Salish. Similar age-related attenuation in the ability to discriminate non-native speech sounds has been found between 6 and 12 months for other types of speech sounds. For example, Mattock and Burnham (2006) found a decline between 6 and 9 months of age for English infants' discrimination of non-native lexical tone contrasts, but no such age-related decline in Chinese infants' discrimination, as tone is used to distinguish words in tone languages such as Chinese. These findings highlight how infants' initial language-general speech perception abilities retreat to a language-specific pattern of listening as they learn to filter out the inappropriate sounds and attend to native speech sounds that are used functionally to distinguish words. Moreover, phonetic representation of native language phonetic contrasts is increasingly refined as a function of age, linguistic experience, and general cognitive development. For example, there is evidence for the influence of native language on the perception of vowels as early as 6 months of age (Kuhl et al., 1992) and for consonants, English infants show continued improvements in discrimination of the native 'd' versus 'th' contrast between 12 months and 4 years of age, and further improvement between 4 years and adulthood (Polka *et al.*, 2001).

While infants' speech perception is language-specific by around 1 year of age, infants are not yet making full use of their skills when beginning to learn words. English-learning 14-month-old infants fail to learn the association between novel words and novel objects when word labels are similar, 'bi' and 'di', but they succeed in learning the word–object pairing when the labels are dissimilar, 'lif' vs. 'neem' (Stager and Werker, 1997). Werker and Curtin (2005) assume that infants' sensitivity to native speech sound categories is maintained across development, but because word learning is cognitively demanding, infants' attention to fine phonetic detail suffers as a consequence of the cognitive load. Infants first process words holistically, which is why using dissimilar words makes word learning easier. As vocabulary expands, and phonetic space becomes more crowded, there is a need for clearer phonological representations and transition to phonological processing.

More than 30 years of infant speech perception research has shown us that young infants have a remarkable perception of speech sounds and syllables presented in isolation. Research during the last decade has focused on identifying at what age infants begin to locate and recognize isolated words in connected speech, and how they do this. Word recognition and word segmentation is easy for adults who have a store of lexical knowledge to support such segmentation, but for young infants, segmentation of the speech stream must be based on non-lexical cues. For example, in English about 90% of words have a strong–weak stress pattern and being able to recognize this pattern is helpful for segmenting multisyllabic sequences from continuous speech. Echols *et al.* (1997) familiarized 7- and 9-month-old English-learning infants to weak–strong–weak-stressed trisyllables and then tested them for their preference for variants of these trisyllables modified by the insertion of a pause before the stressed syllable yielding a strong–weak (English-like) pattern, or insertion of a pause after the stressed syllable thus yielding a weak–strong pattern. The 7-month-olds did not show a selective preference but the 9-month-old infants listened longer to the list containing strong–weak words, highlighting that segmentation abilities emerge around 9 months of age.

Hearing impairment impacts audibility of acoustic speech cues (see Chapters 14 and 15). Figure 13.4 plots the frequency of speech sounds at normal conversational level, and highlights how the perception of individual speech sounds is affected by the degree of hearing loss. For an infant with hearing impairment, these audibility problems are compounded by the fact that infants have not yet built up stable representations of phonetic, phonotactic, and prosodic patterns of their language. Conductive hearing loss due to otitis media with effusion (OME), an infection characterized by the presence of fluid in the middle ear space that compromises sound conduction, is very common in infancy with an estimated 75–85% of all infants experiencing at least one episode of OME by the age of 2 years (see Chapter 15, Fig. 15.5). Mild hearing loss of up to 15 dB can result, and this loss can be detrimental to the perception of voiceless consonants such as 'p', 'h,' and 'f' and fricative sounds such as 's' and 'z' as shown in Fig. 13.4. However, for infants, the presence of OME has even been found to affect the perception of voiced stop consonants, the speech sounds with the strongest energy. Polka and Rvachew (2005) found that infants experiencing OME on the day they participated in a speech perception study were worse at discriminating 'bu' from 'gu' than infants who were OME-free. Mild conductive hearing losses (such as those experienced during episodes of otitis media) muffle speech, making it unclear and difficult to attend to.

The presence of background noise is another factor that can impede access to speech patterns. Background noise reduces the audibility of specific speech elements and places additional cognitive load on selective attention. The outcome of numerous studies has highlighted that infants

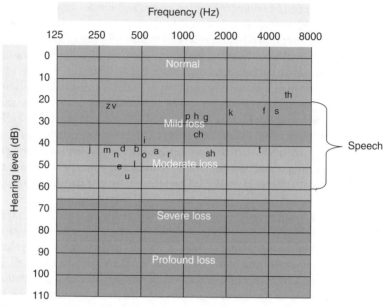

Fig. 13.4 Frequency of speech sounds plotted as a function of hearing loss. Coloured bands represent degree of hearing loss and speech sounds affected by such loss. Note that impaired perception of consonants is due mostly to high-frequency hearing loss and perception of vowels is due mostly to low-frequency hearing loss.

need substantially higher signal-to-noise ratios than adults to detect phonetic differences (e.g. Nozza *et al.*, 1991).

13.3 Hearing in older children

Speech and language development are closely linked to hearing and auditory processing. Children with hearing loss tend to perform more poorly on tasks assessing speech and language skills, and some children show disordered auditory processing despite normal hearing thresholds (see Chapter 15). In Section 13.2.4 it was shown that speech perception is associated with the identification of phonemes and words, as well as sensitivity to auditory features such as periodicity, duration, and intensity. This section highlights how auditory perception continues to be refined across childhood.

13.3.1 Frequency and temporal perception

In Section 13.1.2 we reported that high-frequency discrimination shows some improvement between birth and 6 months of age. However, the developmental course for low-frequency discrimination is also lengthy, and seems to develop as a product of increasing experience. Soderquist and Moore (1970) report that 5-year-olds' frequency discrimination of low-frequency pure tones is significantly poorer than that of 7- and 9-year-olds. However, following specific training, low-frequency discrimination improves, especially for the 5-year-olds, and by around 7 years of age low-frequency discrimination appears to be at adult levels. Converging evidence from 4- and 5-year-olds tested in an 'odd one out' procedure shows that, compared to adults, children's discrimination of a 440-Hz standard tone from comparison stimuli differing by 1–400 Hz is poorer and more variable. Frequency discrimination improves significantly by 6 years of age, but still falls short of adult levels (Jenson and Neff, 1993). Recent work with older children shows that pure-tone frequency discrimination thresholds in children aged 6–7 years, 8–9 years, and 10–11 years remain poorer than adults' at 1 kHz; and, despite improvements in discrimination following training, on average, even 10- to 11-year-olds do not have thresholds on a par with adults (Halliday *et al.*, 2008).

Frequency resolution approaches adult-like levels at a similar age to frequency discrimination. When 6- and 10-year-old children were tested for detection of a tone presented either in bandpass noise or spectrally notched noise, thresholds for both age groups were not significantly different from adult thresholds. However, 6-year-olds' performance on a backward masking task used to measure temporal resolution sensitivity revealed that 6-year-olds have thresholds that are 34 dB higher than adults. Thus, there is disparity in the development of adult-like frequency and temporal resolution—6 years and 10 years, respectively (Hartley *et al.*, 2000).

Duration discrimination of brief-duration tones may not reach maturity until 11 years of age. In a study using a two-alternative, two-interval forced choice procedure, thresholds were measured for 1000-Hz tones with pulse durations of 200, 50, and 20 ms for children aged 5, 7, 9, and 11 years, and adults. Overall, 5-year-olds found the task most difficult and many failed to complete the task. Of those 5-year-olds who completed the task, larger duration differences were needed for them to detect differences between stimuli. The 7-year-olds performed similarly to 5-year-olds, and showed poorer discrimination compared to older children and adults whose performance was similar (Thompson *et al.*, 1999). Further evidence for an age-related improvement in duration discrimination comes from Elfenbein *et al.* (1993) who measured difference limens in adults and in children aged 4, 6, 8, and 10 years of age. Listeners were presented with a broadband noise burst of 350 ms as the standard for comparison in a forced-choice procedure. Duration discrimination improved as a function of age, and adult-like discrimination was emergent between 8 and 10 years of age. Children's difficulty with temporal resolution has been proposed to underlie their higher backward masking thresholds than of adults. However, a systematic study by Hill *et al.* (2004) shows that, in 9–10-year-olds, threshold differences are explained by children's difficulty in processing 'efficiency' (the involvement of non-sensory factors), rather than difficulty in extricating rapidly presented sounds (see also Section 13.3.4).

Auditory fusion or 'gap detection', that is, whether consecutive sounds are perceived as one or two events, is another measure of temporal resolution that shows systematic improvement with age. A study by Davis and McCroskey (1980) revealed that interpulse intervals of 22–24 ms were needed for 3-year-olds to discern two auditory events. Intervals shorter than 22 ms were perceived as a single event. Interval differences of 11–15 ms were perceived by 6-year-olds as two events, compared to 6–8-ms differences for adults. A subsequent study by Irwin *et al.* (1985) reports that gap detection is adult-like by 11–12 years of age. Gap thresholds were 5.6 and 5.7 ms at 40 dB SPL for 11-year-old children and adults, respectively. Temporal acuity improved for both 11-year-old children and adults at 60 dB SPL, with gap thresholds decreasing to 3.6 ms for children and 3.4 ms for adults.

Overall, the studies discussed here highlight that temporal resolution, whether measured in tone-duration discrimination or gap-detection tasks, is adult-like by 11 years of age.

13.3.2 Spectral pattern discrimination

Attending to spectral cues is important for the discrimination of amplitude and frequency, and more broadly, for speech perception. Relative to adults, young children show poorer and more variable discrimination of both non-speech tones with sinusoidal-rippled amplitude spectra, and synthetic consonants and vowels presented in quiet or in noise (Allen and Wightman, 1992).

Young children also show poorer attentional selectivity to auditory targets. In a study by Stellmack *et al.* (1997), children were required to attend to a target tone in the presence of two distracters and identify in which distracter the target tone was higher pitched. Compared to adult listeners, preschool children found this task significantly more difficult when the 1000-Hz target was placed between distracters of 250 and 4000 Hz. However, children did not find the task more difficult than adults when distracters of 200 and 4000 Hz or 270 and 4320 Hz were used.

13.3.3 Perception in noise

In instances where the listening environment is challenging, young children's performance is compromised in comparison to adults. Children's compromised performance can be explained by many factors including lower motivation, inattention, and inefficient listening strategies. This finding is consistent across speech recognition and tasks requiring detection of a tone in quiet versus masking noise. For example, children's thresholds for detection of a 500-Hz pure tone in the presence of a 20-Hz wide Gaussian low-fluctuating narrowband noise centred at 500 Hz are higher than adult thresholds, and are not lowered when the fluctuations of noise are reduced (Buss *et al.*, 2006).

13.3.4 Speech perception in older children

As discussed in Section 13.2.4, young infants' lexical representations are underspecified and undifferentiated; in part, because with such a small vocabulary there is no need to represent words in such detail, and also because such detailed phonetic representation is beyond the attentional and memory capabilities of the infant. Metsala and Walley (1998) propose that young infants recognize words holistically and that word learning shifts attention from phonetic detail to semantics. Consequently, young infants' lexical representations are phonologically underspecified. As vocabulary expands and phonetic space becomes more crowded, the need for clearer phonological representations becomes imperative. This is known as lexical restructuring and is important for early development of phonological awareness.

Transition from holistic to segmental/phonological processing following lexical restructuring is not an easy one for children, and they continue to display less sensitivity to phonetic differences and more fuzzy phoneme categories than adults. For example, Zlatin and Koenigsknecht (1976) found that 2-year-old children require larger acoustic differences than 6-year-olds and adults to discriminate differences between 'goat' and 'coat', and Nittrouer and Studdert-Kennedy (1987) found that 3–5-year-olds have greater difficulty discriminating fricatives than 7-year-olds and adults. Walley and Metsala (1990) reported that 5-year-olds also struggle more than 8-year-olds at detecting mispronunciations of later acquired words.

Over childhood, word recognition abilities gradually move from holistic to segmental strategies. The gating paradigm—where steady increases in the amount of speech input are revealed from word onset and the listener has to respond with word identity after the gated trial–has been used to emphasize that young children need more speech input to correctly recognize spoken words than adults, even if the word being revealed is well known to them (Elliott *et al.*, 1987). Moreover, the amount of speech input needed to correctly recognize the words decreases progressively between 7, 9, and 11 years of age, although even 11-year-olds need more speech input than adults (Metsala, 1987).

Studies with 4-, 6- and 8-year-old children show that language-specific speech perception is positively correlated to age-related reading ability (Burnham, 1986, 2003). Learning to read requires mastery of grapheme (letter) to phoneme (speech sound) correspondences, and better readers tend to have more attuned language-specific speech perception allowing them to direct attention towards phonologically relevant distinctions. As a consequence of greater attention to native phonology, perception of non-native speech sounds becomes even worse at the early-reading stage. However, once reading is fluent it demands less attention, and non-native speech perception skills improve. Literacy even has implications for adult speech processing. Tyler and Burnham (2006) showed that reaction time in a phoneme deletion task is shorter (i.e. the speech is more quickly processed) when the original item and the item-minus-deleted phone are spelled similarly, for example pace-ace as opposed to cough-off. Adult listeners also need more time to decide if an item presented aurally is a word or non-word, when the item is a word and has more than one spelling (e.g. wine and whine) (Ziegler and Ferrand, 1998).

13.4 Fundamentals of auditory learning

Although the greatest changes to hearing and the auditory system occur during development, maturation, and ageing, hearing can be modified by experience throughout life. Auditory learning happens naturally, through exposure and experience with sound. For example, trained musicians are better able to discriminate sounds—they can hear a mistuned note that those who are not trained may not notice. Learning can also be induced through directed training, either in the laboratory or out of it. With training, our ability to detect, discriminate, and identify sounds can improve, often dramatically (by orders of magnitude) and rapidly (with as little as several minutes of training, and in some cases even a few presentations of the stimuli, or 'trials').

Auditory learning can be simply defined as performance improvement on an auditory task. It can be measured as an overall improvement resulting from training, or as a continual improvement as training progresses. This improvement is usually most noticeable on the trained task itself. However, learning can transfer between tasks, so that often training on one task or stimulus transfers to other, untrained tasks or stimuli. The pattern of transfer between conditions can often be used to infer important information about the auditory system, such as the level of processing at which neural changes are likely to have occurred. More interestingly from an applied point of view, however, auditory learning can generalize to improvement on other cognitive or language skills, such as phonological awareness, a skill underlying speech perception and crucial for reading development. The potential for using simple stimuli to train complex skills is an appealing one from an applied perspective, and will be addressed in the following section. This section will deal mainly with the theoretical aspects of auditory learning.

The overall improvement and the time-course over which performance gain is observed depend on task-specific factors such as task demands and task difficulty, as well as more general factors related to training such as the regimen and content of the training sessions. Moreover, learning is influenced by cognitive factors such as attention (both task-specific and general arousal) and memory, skills that characterize 'listening' rather than just 'hearing' (see Section 13.1.3).

13.4.1 Time course of auditory learning

Performance on an auditory task is often plotted as a function of the amount of training received. This plot is usually referred to as a 'learning curve' (see Fig. 13.5). Auditory learning can be observed both within a single training session and across multiple sessions. As a general rule, early learning is the most dramatic, with performance improvements becoming smaller over time. For some tasks (e.g. frequency discrimination) this is true both within (Fig. 13.5A) and across (Fig. 13.5B) training sessions. For other tasks, rapid early learning is followed by a performance plateau, when more training sessions do not lead to further improvement (Wright and Fitzgerald, 2001). Performance can also improve across sessions but not within a session (Wright and Sabin, 2007).

It is possible that the early, rapid learning and later, slower learning are indicative of different learning phases, rather than a single, continuous process. This idea fits nicely within the 'reverse

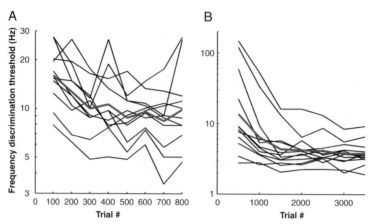

Fig. 13.5 Frequency discrimination learning curves measured (A) within a single session, using 100-trial blocks run consecutively, and (B) across multiple sessions, using 500-trial blocks (each data point is averaged over five threshold assessments run concurrently). Thin black lines denote individual listeners; thick red lines are group means. Note that the scales of both the x-axis and the y-axis are different in the two panels. (Figure 13.5(b) adapted from Amitay et al., 2005.)

hierarchy theory', originally proposed by Ahissar and Hochstein (2004) to explain visual perceptual learning. This theory posits that learning begins at higher level areas, where perceptual resolution is low, and proceeds to lower level areas when the representational resolution is insufficient to the task. The shape of the learning curve could thus be attributed to a move from higher level processing guided by top-down mechanisms to lower level processing of task- and stimulus-specific information.

Further evidence for distinct phases in auditory learning comes from physiological studies of brain activation resulting from training. For example, Atienza et al. (2002) have shown that the learning of a complex auditory pattern is accompanied by distinct changes in the auditory event-related potentials (ERPs) that develop over different time constants. In this study, mismatch negativity (MMN)[1] to the target pattern appeared immediately following training, when it became behaviourally discriminable from the standard pattern, and was enhanced further when measured 36 hours later. On the other hand, the P2 wave[2] was only enhanced 24 hours after training, coupled with an improvement in behavioural reaction time. Alain and colleagues (2007) have shown that rapid, early learning on a vowel-segregation task was accompanied by an amplitude enhancement of an early evoked response (~130 ms) localized in the right auditory cortex and a later response (~340 ms) localized in the right anterior superior temporal gyrus and/or inferior prefrontal cortex. These changes depended on active listening (as opposed to passive exposure), and were only preserved if training continued. More prolonged training (1 week) resulted in decreased N1[3] and P2 latencies as well as enhanced P2 amplitude (Reinke et al., 2003), suggesting some neural changes can only be observed once learning has started to consolidate.

[1] The MMN is an ERP response elicited by an infrequent ('deviant') sound occurring in an ongoing sequence of repetitive ('standard') sounds. It peaks 100–250 ms after sound onset.
[2] The P2 is a positive deflection of the ERP wave which occurs ~200 ms after sound onset.
[3] The N1 is a negative deflection of the ERP wave, occurring approximately 100 ms after sound onset.

Different learning patterns can be observed for the same task when using different cues. Wright and Fitzgerald (2001) have shown that sound lateralization with a binaural temporal cue (ITD) improves rapidly at first, but shows no subsequent improvement past the initial training session. On the other hand, training on the same behavioural task (lateralization) with a binaural level cue (interaural level difference, ILD) starts similarly, but continues to improve over several more training sessions. These and other results suggest that while the initial learning may generalize more readily to untrained stimuli, the slower phase of learning generalizes less well. This indicates that the initial learning occurs in brain regions where multiple cues are processed by the same neural pool, whereas subsequent learning occurs at sites where the two cues are processed separately. Thus, the shape of the learning curve can be used to infer the type of neural changes that accompany learning.

Different listeners can display markedly different learning curves for the same task and stimuli. For example, Amitay *et al.* (2005) have shown that when training on frequency discrimination where the standard (comparison) tone is widely variable and changes on a trial-by-trial basis, some listeners are unaffected by the variability and show the rapid learning observed with an unchanging comparison stimulus, while others do not. These listeners, who tend to have a poorer initial performance, display a slower improvement over a longer time (see Fig. 13.6A). Such learning also results in reduced transfer to untrained frequencies (Fig. 13.6B).

There is also evidence that the time-course of learning depends on the amount and content of each training session. Wright and Sabin (2007) have shown that too little training in each session can result in a failure of the learning to 'consolidate'. The amount of training necessary is task-dependent: 900 trials were necessary to show across-session improvement on a frequency discrimination task, whereas 360 trials failed to result in significant improvement from day to day. On the other hand, in training temporal-interval discrimination, 360 trials were sufficient, and additional training (to 900 trials) within the same session did not result in greater improvement.

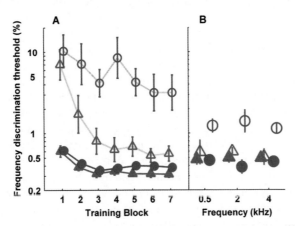

Fig. 13.6 (A) Frequency discrimination learning curves for listeners with better (filled symbols) and poorer initial performance (empty symbols), trained using a single standard frequency of 1000 Hz (red) or five different frequencies (570, 840, 1170, 1600, and 2150 Hz) varied on a trial-by-trial basis (blue). Frequency discrimination thresholds are presented as a percentage of the standard (comparison) tone frequency. For listeners trained on varying frequencies, the results are averaged across frequencies (thresholds did not differ significantly between frequencies). (B) Transfer of learning tested at various untrained frequencies. Error bars are standard errors of the means (s.e.m.). (Figure adapted from Amitay *et al.*, 2005.)

Moreover, when training on one task is followed by training on another task, 'interference' may occur—learning on the first task does not consolidate, while learning on the second task does (Wright *et al.*, 2008).

13.4.2 The 'rules' of auditory learning

The rules of auditory learning describe how the nature of the training affects the learning process and its outcome. We already know much about issues to do with the training regimen, such as variability in the training stimulus sets (see Section 13.4.1), training procedures, and higher level and cognitive issues such as attention and individual variability. This section will cover some recent findings.

Perceptual learning tasks usually take a similar form to testing psychophysical thresholds (see Amitay *et al.*, 2006a). Repeated measurements act both to test performance and to provide training. The advantage of this approach is that it allows training to be tracked continuously. However, the challenge is that performance continuously changes while it is being measured. The problem this presents can be appreciated when considering the way learning is generally assessed: performance on several conditions of interest is assessed before and after training to produce a 'learning index' for each condition. Training is given for only one of these conditions, so transfer to other conditions can be measured with a relatively small number of participants (e.g. Wright *et al.*, 1997). However, if threshold assessments in the pre-training phase involve extensive testing, they may provide significant training in and of themselves, before the actual 'training' phase of the study has started. One way to circumvent this problem is to test (briefly; Amitay *et al.*, 2006a) on a single condition and train different groups on different conditions. However, this method is labour-intensive and requires large numbers of participants (e.g. Amitay *et al.*, 2006b). Varying amounts of testing prior to the training phase may explain why different investigators observe different learning curves, even when training on the same task (e.g. frequency discrimination).

It appears that learning is largely unaffected by the exact psychophysical procedure used. In comparing two- and three-alternative forced-choice procedures, no significant differences were found in the pattern of early learning (Amitay *et al.*, 2006a; Fig. 13.7). Nor did the learning differ when two- or three-interval presentations were used. This is surprising, since additional intervals imply greater stimulus exposure and, we might predict, more learning. Moreover, we might have predicted that a procedure of gradually increasing difficulty, such as an adaptive staircase (Levitt, 1971), would be preferable to a more volatile procedure, such as a maximum-likelihood estimator (Green, 1993). In addition to the hypothesized benefit of a gradual increase in difficulty, a staircase provides an initial 'lead in' phase of trials where the target can be easily detected. However, the procedure appears to have little effect on early learning (in adults), even when using a constant set of stimuli that does not change adaptively (Amitay *et al.*, 2006b).

While training with different psychophysical procedures does not significantly affect learning, the way in which stimuli are presented within the training block does. Varying the standard stimulus slightly on a trial-by-trial basis leads to slow and protracted learning (Amitay *et al.*, 2005) compared to training with an unchanging standard. However, training on the same stimuli when they are blocked (each block uses a different standard) is no different from training with a single standard (Moore and Amitay, 2007).

Another line of evidence starts with the common assumption that a training task may be too difficult (e.g. Cansino and Williamson, 1997) or too easy to produce learning. Learning should thus be optimal when task difficulty during training is kept at a moderate level. The prediction regarding training on an easy task has been borne out (Amitay *et al.*, 2006b); when keeping the sounds to be compared so different during training that performance was at or near ceiling (100% correct), learning, though still significant, was reduced (Fig. 13.8A). However, even an impossibly

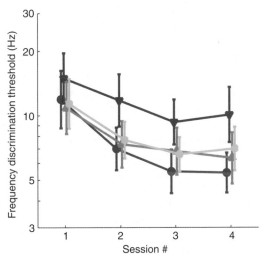

Fig. 13.7 Comparison of frequency-discrimination training with four different adaptive procedures: 3-down, 1-up staircase procedure with a 3-alternative, forced-choice 'odd-one-out' response paradigm (red); 3-down, 1-up staircase procedure with a 2-alternative, forced-choice AXB response paradigm (blue); Maximum-likelihood procedure targeting 79.4% correct with a 3-alternative, forced-choice 'odd-one-out' response paradigm (orange); Maximum-likelihood procedure targeting 79.4% correct with a 2-alternative forced-choice AXB response paradigm (cyan). Error bars are standard errors of the means (s.e.m.). (Adapted from Amitay *et al.*, 2006*a*.)

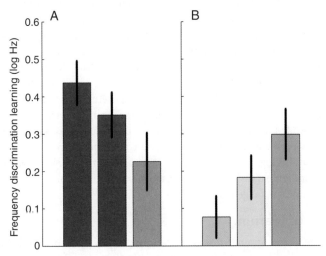

Fig. 13.8 Frequency discrimination learning of a 1-kHz tone for (A) 800 trials of frequency discrimination training using adaptive tracking of the threshold at 75% correct (blue), 800 trials of training with no frequency difference (red) and with a large difference of 400 Hz (orange); and (B) controls who did not train during the 50 minutes between threshold assessments (cyan), playing Tetris for 50 minutes without sound (yellow) and playing Tetris for 50 minutes during playback of an adaptive track from a participant doing the adaptive training, while ignoring the sounds (green). Error bars are standard errors of the means (s.e.m.). (Adapted from Amitay *et al.*, 2006*b*.)

difficult task (attempting to discriminate identical sounds) resulted in robust learning of pure-tone frequency discrimination. Thus, while a training task can be made too easy to be effective, it apparently cannot be made too difficult.

It is surprising that, despite the lack of a physical difference between the sounds, the discrimination still improved with training. However, lack of a physical difference between stimuli does not necessarily mean a lack of perceptual difference. Internal noise due to random processes in neural spike generation can mean that the representation of identical stimuli in the brain physically varies from one presentation to the next. Recent modelling studies (Micheyl *et al.*, 2009) suggest that differences in internal representations of consecutive sounds are sufficient for perceptually 'discriminating' them. Alternatively, a recent model proposed by Ahissar (2007) to explain the perceptual difficulties of dyslexics suggests that most listeners perform a perceptual discrimination task by creating and refining a representation of the standard stimulus, and then compare each presented sound to this internal representation, coined a 'perceptual anchor'. Repeated exposure to the stimulus may work to create a perceptual anchor even when there is no actual difference between the 'standard' and 'target' tones, thus improving discrimination. Moreover, if listeners do not or cannot employ such perceptual anchors (e.g. when the standard stimulus is changing with every trial), learning is disrupted. Some (poorer) listeners may be unable to handle the increased cognitive demands when more than one 'anchor' is necessary to perform the task, resulting in the different learning pattern shown in Fig. 13.6.

The findings described above suggest that attention plays a fundamental role in learning. When the training task is challenging and requires a commitment of attentional resources it results in robust learning. Further evidence for the role of attention in learning comes from a passive exposure experiment (Amitay *et al.*, 2006*b*), in which two groups of participants were instructed to play the (silent) visuospatial computer game Tetris. One group was passively exposed to a playback of the sound experienced by a participant from another group, who trained on an actual adaptive sound discrimination. The Tetris-playing group were told to ignore these sounds and concentrate on the computer game. The other group played Tetris but did not hear sounds. Both groups showed some learning, but did not differ significantly from one another (Fig. 13.8B). Interestingly, improvement in playing Tetris was correlated with the improvement in frequency discrimination (the primary task) when both groups were pooled. The most surprising aspect of these results was that training on the silent computer game produced auditory learning.

When considering the rules of auditory learning, it is useful to keep in mind that extracting these rules relies on comparing average performance for groups of listeners. Individuals whose performance lies outside the 'norm' are often excluded from study. However, individual variability in naïve auditory performance plays a significant role in the learning pattern, as seen in the previous section (see also Fig. 13.6), as well as in the pattern of transfer between tasks (see Section 13.4.3). Moreover, individual variability is often the most critical factor in applications, for example in developing clinical management strategies.

13.4.3 Transfer of learning

Transfer of learning to an untrained task is of prime importance from an applied perspective (see Section 13.5), but it also allows us to infer where neural changes might be occurring as a result of the training. The transfer of learning from playing Tetris to frequency discrimination (Fig. 13.8B) suggests that this form of learning is a high-level, cognitive effect, related perhaps to general arousal or a reward feedback mechanism (e.g. Bakin and Weinberger, 1996). Other studies have shown a transfer of learning to the untrained ear following monaural training of pitch discrimination (Demany and Semal, 2002), suggesting that neural changes occur at a level after information from the two ears is integrated. Wright *et al.* (1997) have shown that training on temporal interval discrimination did not transfer from short to long intervals, but changing the frequency of the tone bursts that demarcate the interval transferred fully. Thus, learning does not transfer to an untrained condition within the same stimulus dimension, but generalizes when another stimulus dimension is varied. This suggests that the observed learning occurs in lower level areas, where stimulus dimensions (spectral and temporal) are processed separately. Learning did not transfer from training on discrimination of complex tones to pure tones at the same frequencies as the harmonics (Demany and Semal, 2002), suggesting different processing mechanisms for complex and pure tones. Learning on backward masking (detecting a tone followed by a noise masker) did not transfer to other masked-detection tasks such as forward masking and simultaneous masking (Wright et al., 1996), suggesting that masking release in these conditions relies on different neural mechanisms. It has also been shown (Hawkey et al., 2004) that learning does not always transfer between tasks, even when the training stimulus is the same: training in intensity discrimination does not transfer to frequency discrimination when the comparison (standard) stimulus is the same in both tasks, suggesting learning depends more on attending to a specific stimulus dimension than on adaptation or sensitization to the training stimulus.

One of the main predictions of the Reverse Hierarchy Theory (see above; Ahissar and Hochstein, 2004) is that as training progresses it becomes less transferable when the training is specific to a particular task and stimulus. Thus, the frequency-discrimination learning induced by playing Tetris may be the result of changes in high-level attentional processes that are common to many types of tasks and is likely to be seen early on, but not improve considerably afterwards. On the other hand, continued improvement in frequency discrimination will result in not only stimulus specificity (e.g. reduced transfer from one frequency to another) but also stimulus-dimension specificity (e.g. training on tone level does not transfer to tone frequency for the same trained standard tone).

13.5 Applications of auditory learning

The growing interest in understanding auditory learning comes in the wake of reported success in its application. The new generation of adaptive perceptual learning-based programmes, aimed initially at improving language and 'listening' skills in children with developmental language problems, has been around for about a decade, having gained popularity following the seminal work published by Tallal, Merzenich and colleagues (Merzenich et al., 1996; Tallal et al., 1996). The main focus of this section will be on the application of auditory learning to improve language abilities, especially in children. This does not rule out other applications of auditory learning, such as ameliorating tinnitus (e.g. Flor et al., 2004), improving outcomes following hearing-aid fitting (Stecker et al., 2006) or cochlear implantation (e.g. Fu et al., 2005), or additional language learning (e.g. Bradlow et al., 1997). Perceptual training has even been used to provide cognitive enhancement for the elderly (Mahncke et al., 2006), demonstrating that it can have far-reaching effects on high-level cognition (attention and memory).

Most existing training programmes rely on intensive training regimens to produce results. Children (5–10 years of age) with language-based learning impairments (LLIs) in the Tallal et al. (1996) study trained for 3 hours a day, 5 days a week for 4 weeks in the laboratory, and additionally for 2 hours a day, 7 days a week at home. The training in this study used an early version of the 'Fast ForWord' language intervention programme, which was based on the 'temporal processing deficit' hypothesis, which suggests children with LLI have difficulty with the rapid elements of the speech signal (formant transitions; see Chapter 15). It consisted of exposure to acoustically modified speech in which the rapid elements were temporally extended and amplified, as well as tasks designed to adaptively train temporal processing of simple acoustic stimuli.

Several widely used and standardized measures of language processing improved following such training.

While benefit was demonstrated in the studies of Tallal and colleagues, it is not clear that so much training is necessary to achieve improvement in language skills, or which of the training tasks were instrumental in producing the benefit. A study in mainstream schoolchildren (8–9 years of age) trained only on phoneme discrimination, using adaptive techniques similar to the basic research described in Section 13.4.2 (Moore *et al.*, 2005) showed that a mere 6 hours of training (30 minutes, 3 times a week for 4 weeks) produced measurable improvement on four subtests of another standardized instrument, the Phonological Assessment Battery (PhAB). The improvement was retained for at least 5 weeks after the end of training. A more recent study in mainstream schoolchildren following the same design (Halliday *et al.*, 2008), but with additional training groups, found that training on auditory frequency discrimination was equivalent to training on phoneme discrimination in transferring into improvement on PhAB subtests. Interestingly, in this latter study, training on either task did not generalize to learning on the other task.

A recent study in unimpaired adults (Lakshminarayanan and Tallal, 2007) showed that training on sequencing of rising and falling frequency-sweeps for 30 minutes per day over 5 days transferred to improved consonant–vowel (CV) syllable discrimination, but only for syllables that differed on the trained parameter (frequency). The duration and presentation rate of the stimuli were also varied during training, but participants needed to attend only to frequency in order to perform the task. When tested after training, no improvement was observed on the discrimination of syllables that differed on duration and presentation. Thus, dimension-specific attention when training on non-linguistic stimuli resulted in transfer to linguistic stimuli that relied on this dimension.

Despite apparent successes of this type of training, it is still unclear how specific the training and transfer effects are to the trained programme. A recent study in over 200 children with LLI by Gillam *et al.* (2008) showed that the computerized 'Fast ForWord' language intervention programme developed by Tallal and colleagues (and discussed above) resulted in a similar improvement in standardized tests of language to that achieved using more conventional academic enrichment programmes or individualized language intervention given by a speech and language pathologist. This result questions the theoretical basis of this intervention (the 'rapid processing deficit hypothesis') but, on the other hand, suggests that such auditory training programmes can be used as a good 'value-for-money' substitute to the traditional labour-intensive, one-on-one approaches, giving at least equivalent benefit for a fraction of the price. It is possible that existing training programmes are not optimal, relying as they now do on a possibly faulty theoretical footing. The other side of the coin, however, is that should such programmes be optimized they might prove even more effective, and possibly even surpass conventional treatment.

Intervention studies in adults and children thus suggest that training using simple (including non-linguistic) stimuli that are easily controlled, can result in measurable improvement in language perception. Together with the growing body of work looking at the basic rules of learning, there is hope that training will prove to be a useful tool in the remediation arsenal for various auditory-based disorders, from specific language impairment to APD in children, improving language perception in adults and children with auditory impairments, or as a (re)habilitation tool for sensorineural hearing loss, either of itself or after the fitting of hearing-aids or cochlear implants.

13.6 Summary and conclusions

In this chapter we have emphasized that hearing initially develops *in utero* in the absence of auditory experience. For most, subsequent development occurs normally in the absence of specific reinforcement or training. However, postnatal development of native language and, presumably, other listening skills is dependent on some minimum fidelity exposure to appropriate sounds. While later deprivation may impair listening, that impairment may be reversible through auditory learning.

We have shown that the newborn infant has amazing abilities to discriminate speech sounds and recognize speech patterns that are familiar from their time *in utero*. However, auditory perception is not adult-like at birth, and while rapid and dramatic development takes place in the first year of life, especially in the first 6 months, perception of frequency and duration, perception in noise, and speech perception, is not equivalent to adult performance until approximately 10 years of age.

Infants and young children are also more easily distracted than adults by competing sound information, and are limited in how long they can or will attend in auditory tasks. Certainly, cognitive factors play a role here and methods for testing infants and children attempt to counter such limitations by presenting short sessions, reward and reinforcement, and infant and child-controlled tasks. Additionally, children have difficulty in handling multiple acoustic dimensions. Thus, discovering from separate experiments that children discriminate pitch and duration changes does not necessarily imply success at handling such cues in concert, when cues are pitted against each other.

Auditory learning tasks have great utility clinically. For example, training recipients of cochlear implants to actively discriminate acoustic cues pertinent to speech perception is one application, and any failure to learn following training has implications for the development and engineering of implant devices. A challenging problem is to develop suitable infant test methods that incorporate auditory learning techniques, although the potential is there for adaptation of training paradigms such as the head-turn (VRA-like) procedure (Section 13.2.2) to be used. Recent findings highlight that a few minutes of familiarization to a non-native speech sound continuum is sufficient to temporarily shift infants' phonetic category boundaries, emphasizing that the application of auditory learning tasks to infants is indeed possible (Maye *et al.*, 2002).

As pointed out in Section 13.5, auditory training has implications for continuous learning throughout the lifespan. Training elderly hearing-aid users to effectively perceive speech is an obvious example. A less obvious application is to train patients with Parkinson's disease who are known to present speech perception deficits in temporal processing and recognition of acoustic cues that signal affect, such as pitch inflection. Auditory training may also assist second-language speech learning (children and adults) and bilingual language acquisition (infants and children).

Exploring the properties and mechanisms of listening and learning by people at all stages of development, and their interplay with cognitive abilities will, we believe, be rich and increasingly translational avenues for future research.

References

Ahissar, M. (2007). Dyslexia and the anchoring-deficit hypothesis. *Trends in Cognitive Sciences* 11:458–65.

Ahissar, M. and Hochstein, S. (2004). The reverse hierarchy theory of visual perceptual learning. *Trends in Cognitive Sciences* 8:457–64.

Alain, C., Snyder, J. S., He, Y., and Reinke, K. S. (2007). Changes in auditory cortex parallel rapid perceptual learning. *Cerebral Cortex* 17:1074–84.

Allen, P. and Wightman, F. (1992). Spectral pattern discrimination by children. *Journal of Speech and Hearing Research* 35:222–33.

Amitay, S., Hawkey, D. J. C., and Moore, D. R. (2005). Auditory frequency discrimination learning is affected by stimulus variability. *Perception and Psychophysics* 67:691–8.

Amitay, S., Irwin, A., Hawkey, D. J. C., Cowan, J. A., and Moore, D. R. (2006a). A comparison of adaptive procedures for rapid and reliable threshold assessment and training in naive listeners. *Journal of the Acoustical Society of America* 119:1616–25.

Amitay, S., Irwin, A., and Moore, D. R. (2006b). Discrimination learning induced by training with identical stimuli. *Nature Neuroscience* **9**:1446–8.

Ashmead, D. H., Davis, A. L., Whalen, T., and Odom, R. D. (1991). Sound localization and sensitivity to interaural time differences in human infants. *Child Development* **62**:1211–26.

Aslin, R. N. (1989). Discrimination of frequency transitions by human infants. *Journal of the Acoustical Society of America* **86**:582–90.

Aslin, R. N., Pisoni, D. B., and Jusczyk, P. W. (1983). Auditory development and speech perception in infancy. In *Handbook of Child Psychology* (4th edn; ed.P. H. Mussen), Vol. II: *Infancy and the Biology of Development* (ed. M. M. Haith and J. J. Campos), pp. 573–687. New York: Wiley.

Atienza, M., Cantero, J. L., and Dominguez-Marin, E. (2002). The time course of neural changes underlying auditory perceptual learning. *Learning and Memory* **9**:138–50.

Bakin, J. S. and Weinberger, N. M. (1996). Induction of a physiological memory in the cerebral cortex by stimulation of the nucleus basalis. *Proceedings of the National Academy of Sciences USA* **93**:11219–24.

Bishop, D. V. M. (1997). *Uncommon Understanding: Development and Disorders of Language Comprehension in Children*. Hove: Psychology Press.

Bradlow, A. R., Pisoni, D. B., Akahane-Yamada, R., and Tohkura, Y. (1997). Training Japanese listeners to identify English /r/ and /l/: IV. Some effects of perceptual learning on speech production. *Journal of the Acoustical Society of America* **101**:2299–310.

Burkard, R. F., Don, M., and Eggermont, J. J. (2006). *Auditory Evoked Potentials: Basic Principles and Clinical Application*. Baltimore, MD: Lippincott, Williams and Wilkins.

Burnham, D. K. (1986). Developmental loss of speech perception: Exposure to and experience with a first language. *Applied Psycholinguistics* **7**:207–39.

Burnham, D. (2003). Language specific speech perception and the onset of reading. *Reading and Writing* **16**:573–609.

Buss, E., Hall, J. W. III, and Grose, J. H. (2006). Development and the role of internal noise in detection and discrimination threshold with narrow band stimuli. *Journal of the Acoustical Society of America* **120**:2777–88.

Cansino, S. and Williamson, S. J. (1997). Neuromagnetic fields reveal cortical plasticity when learning an auditory discrimination task. *Brain Research* **764**:53–66.

Chang, H.-W. and Trehub, S. E. (1977). Infants' perception of temporal grouping in auditory patterns. *Child Development* **48**:1666–70.

Clarkson, M. G. and Clifton, R. K. (1985). Infant pitch perception: Evidence for responding to pitch categories and the missing fundamental. *Journal of Acoustical Society of America* **77**:1521–8.

Davis, S. M. and McCroskey, R. L. (1980). Auditory fusion in children. *Child Development* **51**:75–80.

DeCasper, A. J. and Fifer, W. P. (1980). Of human bonding: Newborns prefer their mothers' voices. *Science* **280**:1174–6.

DeCasper, A. and Spence, M. (1986). Prenatal maternal speech influences newborns' perception of speech sounds. *Infant Behavior and Development* **9**:133–50.

DeCasper, A., Lecanuet, J. P., Busnel, M.-C., Granier-Deferre, C., and Maugeais, R. (1994). Fetal reactions to recurrent maternal speech. *Infant Behavior and Development* **17**:159–64.

Demany, L. and Semal, C. (2002). Learning to perceive pitch differences. *Journal of the Acoustical Society of America* **111**:1377–88.

Echols, C. H., Crowhurst, M. J., and Childers, J. (1997). The perception of rhythmic units in speech by infants and adults. *Journal of Memory and Language* **36**:202–5.

Eimas, P. D., Siqueland, E. R., Jusczyk, P., and Vigorito, J. (1971). Speech perception in infants. *Science* **171**:303–6.

Elfenbein, J., Small, A., and Davis, J. M. (1993). Developmental patterns of duration discrimination. *Journal of Speech and Hearing Research* **36**:842–9.

Elliott, L. L., Hammer, M. A., and Evan, K. E. (1987). Perception of gated, highly familiar spoken monosyllabic nouns by children, teenagers, and older adults. *Perception and Psychophysics* **42**:150–7.

Fahle, M. and Poggio, T. (2002). *Perceptual Learning.* Cambridge, MA: MIT Press.

Flor, H., Hoffmann, D., Struve, M., and Diesch, E. (2004). Auditory discrimination training for the treatment of tinnitus. *Applied Psychophysiology and Biofeedback* 29:113–20.

Folsom, R. C. and Wynne, M. K. (1987). Auditory brain stem responses from human adults and infants: Wave V tuning curves. *Journal of the Acoustical Society of America* 81:412–17.

Fu, Q. J., Galvin, J., Wang, X., and Nogaki, G. (2005). Moderate auditory training can improve speech performance of adult cochlear implant patients. *Acoustics Research Letters Online* 6:106–11. http://dx. doi.org/10.1121/1.1898345

Gerhardt, K. J. and Abrams, R. M. (1996). Fetal hearing: characterization of the stimulus and response. *Seminars in Perinatology* 20:11–20.

Gillam, R. B., Loeb, D. F., Hoffman, L. M., et al. (2008). The efficacy of Fast ForWord Language intervention in school-age children with language impairment: A randomized controlled trial. *Journal of Speech, Language, and Hearing Research* 51:97–119.

Green, D. M. (1993). A maximum-likelihood method for estimating thresholds in a yes-no task. *Journal of the Acoustical Society of America* 93:2096–105.

Halliday, L. F., Taylor, A., Edmondson-Jones, M., and Moore, D. R. (2008a). Frequency discrimination learning in children. *Journal of the Acoustical Society of America* 123:4393–402.

Halliday, L., Taylor, J., Millward, K., and Moore, D. (2008b). Speech and nonspeech auditory training enhances phonological processing in children. *Association for Research in Otolaryngology Abstracts, #456.* http:www.aro.org/abstracts/abstracts.html

Hartley, D. E. H., Wright, B. A., Hogan, S. C., and Moore, D. R. (2000). Age-related improvements in auditory backward and simultaneous masking in 6- to 10-year-old children. *Journal of Speech, Language, and Hearing Research* 43:1402–25.

Hawkey, D. J., Amitay, S., and Moore, D. R. (2004). Early and rapid perceptual learning. *Nature Neuroscience* 7:1055–6.

Hill, P. R., Hartley, D. E., Glasberg, B. R., Moore, B. C., and Moore, D. R. (2004). Auditory processing efficiency and temporal resolution in children and adults. *Journal of Speech, Language, and Hearing Research* 47:1022–9.

Hogan, S. C. M. and Moore, D. R. (2003). Impaired binaural hearing in children produced by a threshold level of middle ear disease. *Journal of Association for Research in Otolaryngology* 4:123–9.

Irwin, R. J., Ball, A. K. R., Kay, N., Stillman, J. A., and Rosner, J. (1985). The development of auditory temporal acuity in children. *Child Development* 56:614–20.

Jensen, J. K. and Neff, D. L. (1993). Development of basic auditory discrimination in preschool children. *Psychological Science* 4:104–7.

Jusczyk, P. W. (1997). *The Discovery of Spoken Language.* Cambridge, MA: MIT Press.

Jusczyk, P. W., Pisoni, D. B., and Mullenix, K. (1992). Some consequences of stimulus variability in speech processing by 2-month-old infants. *Cognition* 43:253–91.

Kisilevsky, B. S., Pang, L., and Hains, S. M. J. (2000). Maturation of human fetal responses to airborne sound in low- and high-risk fetuses. *Early Human Development* 58:179–95.

Kisilevsky, B. S., Hains, S. M. J., Lee, K., et al. (2003). Effects of experience on fetal voice recognition. *Psychological Science* 14:220–4.

Kopyar, B. A. (1997). Intensity discrimination abilities of infants and adults: Implications for underlying processes. Unpublished doctoral dissertation, University of Washington, Seattle.

Kuhl, P. K., Williams, K. A., Lacerda, F., Stevens, K. N., and Lindblom, B. (1992). Linguistic experience alters phonetic perception in infants by 6 months of age. *Science* 255:606–8.

Lakshminarayanan, K. and Tallal, P. (2007). Generalization of non-linguistic auditory perceptual training to syllable discrimination. *Restorative Neurology and Neuroscience* 25:263–72.

Lecanuet, J.-P., Granier-Deferre, C., DeCasper, A. J., Mugeais, R., Andrieu, A.-J., and Busnel, M.-C. (1987). Perception et discrimination foetales de stimuli langagien mise en évidence á partir de la réactivité cardiaque; resultants préliminaries. *Compte-Rendus de l'Academie des Sciences, Paris (III)* **305**:161–4.

Lecanuet, J.-P., Granier-Deferre, C., and Busnel, M.-C. (1995). Human fetal auditory perception. In *Fetal Development: A Psychobiological Perspective* (ed. J.-P. Lecanuet, W. P. Fifer, N. A. Krasnegor, and W. P. Smotherman), pp. 239–62. Hillsdale, NJ: Lawrence Erlbaum Associates.

Lecanuet, J. P, Granier-Deferre, C., Jacquet, A. Y., and DeCaster, A. J. (2000). Fetal discrimination of low-pitched musical notes. *Developmental Psychobiology* **36**:29–39.

Leibold, L. J. and Werner, L. A. (2006). Effect of masker-frequency variability on the detection performance of infants and adults. *Journal of the Acoustical Society of America* **119**:3960–70.

Levitt, H. (1971). Transformed up-down methods in psychoacoustics. *Journal of the Acoustical Society of America* **49**:467–77.

Liberman, A. M., Harris, K. S., Hoffman, H. S., and Griffith, B. C. (1957). The discrimination of speech sounds within and across phoneme boundaries. *Journal of Experimental Psychology* **54**:358–68.

Litovsky, T. Y. (1997). Developmental changes in the precedence effect: Estimates of minimum audible angle. *Journal of the Acoustical Society of America* **102**:1739–45.

Mahncke, H. W., Connor, B. B., Appelman, J., et al. (2006). Memory enhancement in healthy older adults using a brain plasticity-based training program: A randomized, controlled study. *Proceedings of the National Academy of Sciences USA* **103**:12523–8.

Manly, T., Robertson, I. H., Anderson, V., Nimmo-Smith, I., et al. (2001). The differential assessment of children's attention: the test of everyday attention for childen (TEA–Ch), normal sample and ADHD performance. *Journal of Applied Child Psychology and Psychiatry and Allied Disciplines* **42**:1065–81.

Mattock, K. and Burnham, D. (2006). Chinese and English infants' tone perception: Evidence for perceptual reorganization. *Infancy* **10**:241–65.

Maye, J., Werker, J. F., and Gerken, L. (2002). Infant sensitivity to distributional information can affect phonetic discrimination. *Cognition* **82**:B101–B111.

Merzenich, M. M., Jenkins, W. M., Johnston, P., Schreiner, C., Miller, S. L., and Tallal, P. (1996). Temporal processing deficits of language-learning impaired children ameliorated by training. *Science* **271**:77–81.

Metsala, J. L. (1997). An examination of word frequency and neighbourhood density in the development of spoken word recognition. *Memory and Cognition* **25**:47–56.

Metsala, J. L. and Walley, A. C. (1998). Spoken vocabulary growth and the segmental restructuring of lexical representations: Precursors to phonemic awareness and early reading ability. In *Word Recognition in Beginning Literacy* (ed. J. L. Metsala and L. C. Ehri), pp. 89–120. Mahwah, NJ: Erlbaum.

Micheyl, C., McDermott, J. H., and Oxenham, A. J. (2009). Sensory noise explains auditory frequency discrimination learning induced by training with identical stimuli. *Attention, Perception and Psychophysics* **71**:5–7.

Moon, C., Cooper, R. P., and Fifer, W. P. (1993). Two-day-olds prefer their native language. *Infant Behavior and Development* **16**:495–500.

Moore, D. R. and Amitay, S. (2007). Auditory training: Rules and applications. *Seminars in Hearing* **28**:99–109.

Moore, D. R., Rosenberg, J. F., and Coleman, J. S. (2005). Discrimination training of phonemic contrasts enhances phonological processing in mainstream school children. *Brain and Language* **94**:72–85.

Moore, D. R., Ferguson, M. A., Halliday, L. F., and Riley, A. (2008). Frequency discrimination in children: Perception, learning and attention. *Hearing Research* **238**:147–54.

Morrongiello, B. A. and Trehub, S. E. (1987). Age-related changes in auditory temporal perception. *Journal of Experimental Child Psychology* **44**:413–26.

Morrongiello, B. A., Fenwick, K. D., Hillier, L., and Chance, G. (1994). Sound localization in human infants. *Developmental Psychobiology* **27**:519–38.

Muir, D. W. and Field, J. (1979). Newborn infants orient to sounds. *Child Development* **50**:431–6.

Nittrouer, S. and Studdert-Kennedy, M. (1987). The role of coarticulatory effects in the perception of fricatives by children and adults. *Journal of Speech and Hearing Research* 30:319–29.

Nozza, R. J. (1995). Estimating the contribution of non-sensory factors to infant-adult differences in behavioral thresholds. *Hearing Research* 91:72–8.

Nozza, R. J., Miller, S. L., Rossman, R. N. F., and Bond, L. C. (1991). Reliability and validity of infants speech-sound discrimination-in-noise thresholds. *Journal of Speech and Hearing Research* 34:643–50.

Olsho, L. W., Koch, E. G., and Carter, E. A. (1988). Nonsensory factors in infant frequency discrimination. *Infant Behavior and Development* 11:205–22.

Plack, C. J. (2005). *The Sense of Hearing*. Hillsdale, NJ: Lawrence Erlbaum Associates.

Polka, L. and Rvachew, S. (2005). The impact of otitis media with effusion on infant phonetic perception. *Infancy* 8:101–17.

Polka, L., Colantonio, C., and Sundara, M. (2001). Cross-language perception of /d–ð/: Evidence for a new developmental pattern. *Journal of the Acoustical Society of America* 109:2190–200.

Poulsen, C., Picton, T. W., and Paus, T. (2007). Age-related changes in transient and oscillatory brain responses to auditory stimulation in healthy adults, 19–45 years old. *Cerebral Cortex* 17:1454–67.

Querleu, D., Renard, X., Versyp, F., Paris-Delrue, L., and Crèpin, G. (1988). Fetal hearing. *European Journal of Obstetrics, Gynecology, and Reproductive Biology* 28:191–212.

Reinke, K. S., He, Y., Wang, C., and Alain, C. (2003). Perceptual learning modulates sensory evoked response during vowel segregation. *Cognitive Brain Research* 17:781–91.

Richards, A. D., Frentzen, B., Gerhardt, K. J., McCann, M. E., and Abrams, R. M. (1992). Sound levels in the human uterus. *Obstetrics and Gynecology* 80:186–90.

Rubel, E. W., Popper, A. N., and Fay, R. R. (eds) (1998). Springer Handbook of Auditory Research; Vol. 9: *Development of the Auditory System*. New York: Springer.

Schneider, B. A., Morrongiello, B. A., and Trehub, S. E. (1990). Size of critical band in infants, children, and adults. *Journal of Experimental Psychology: Human Perception and Performance* 16:642–52.

Schneider, B. A., Li, L., and Daneman, M. (2007). How competing speech interferes with speech comprehension in everyday listening situations. *Journal of the American Academy of Audiology* 18: 559–72.

Sinnott, J. M. and Aslin, R. N. (1985). Frequency and intensity discrimination in human infants and adults. *Journal of the Acoustical Society of America* 78:1986–92.

Soderquist, D. R. and Moore, M. (1970) Effect of training on frequency discrimination in primary school children. *Journal of Auditory Research* 10:185–92.

Spetner, N. B. and Olsho, L. W. (1990). Auditory frequency resolution in human infancy. *Child Development* 61:632–52.

Stager, C. L. and Werker, J. F. (1997). Infants listen for more phonetic detail in speech perception than in word learning tasks. *Nature* 388:381–2.

Stecker, G. C., Bowman, G. A., Yund, E. W., Herron, T. J., Roup, C. M., and Woods, D. L. (2006). Perceptual training improves syllable identification in new and experienced hearing aid users. *Journal of Rehabilitation Research and Development* 43:537–51.

Stellmack, M. A., Willihnganz, M. S., Wightman, F. L., and Lufti, R. (1997). Spectral weights in level discrimination by preschool children: Analytic listening conditions. *Journal of the Acoustical Society of America* 101:2811–21.

Sweetow, R. W. (ed.) (2007). Auditory training. *Seminars in Hearing* 28:87–161.

Tallal, P., Miller, S. L., Bedi, G., Byma, G., et al. (1996). Language comprehension in language-learning impaired children improved with acoustically modified speech. *Science* 271:81–4.

Tarquinio, N., Zelazo, P. R., and Weiss, M. J. (1990). Recovery of neonatal headturning to decreased sound pressure level. *Developmental Psychology* 26:752–8.

Thompson, N. C., Cranford, J. L., and Hoyer, E. (1999). Brief-tone frequency discrimination by children. *Journal of Speech, Language, and Hearing Research* 42:1061–8.

Thorpe, L. A. (1986). Infants categorise rising and falling pitch. Presented at the *Fifth International Conference on Infant Studies*, 10–13th April, 1986, Los Angeles, CA.

Thorpe, L. A., Trehub, S. E., Morrongiello, B. A., and Bull, D. (1988). Perceptual grouping by infants and preschool children. *Developmental Psychology* 24:484–91.

Trainor, L. J. and Trehub, S. E. (1992). A comparison of infants' and adults' sensitivity to western musical structure. *Journal of Experimental Psychology: Human Perception and Performance* 18:394–402.

Tyler, M. D. and Burnham, D. K. (2006). Orthographic influences on phonemic deletion response times. *Quarterly Journal of Experimental Psychology* 59:2010–31.

Vouloumanos, A. and Werker, J. F. (2007). Listening to language at birth: Evidence for a speech bias in neonates. *Developmental Science* 10:159–64.

Walley, A. C. and Metsala, J. L. (1990). The growth of lexical constraints on spoken word recognition. *Perception and Psychophysics* 47:267–80.

Werker, J. F. and Curtin, S. (2005). PRIMIR: A developmental model of speech processing, *Language Learning and Development* 1:197–234.

Werker, J. F. and Tees, R. C. (1984). Cross-language speech perception: Evidence for perceptual reorganization during the first year of life. *Infant Behavior and Development* 71:49–63.

Werker, J., Gilbert, J. H. V., Humphrey, K., and Tees, R. C. (1981). Developmental aspects of cross-language speech perception. *Child Development* 52:349–55.

Werner, L. A. and Boike, K. (2001). Infants' sensitivity to broadband noise. *Journal of the Acoustical Society of America* 109:2103–11.

Werner, L. A. and Gray, L. (1998). Behavioral studies of hearing development. In *Springer Handbook of Auditory Research* (ed. E.W. Rubel, A. N. Popper, and R. R. Fay); Vol. 9: *Development of the Auditory System*, pp. 12–79. New York: Springer.

Werner, L. A. and Rubel, E. W. (eds) (1992). *Developmental Psychoacoustics*. Washington, DC: American Psychological Association.

Wightman, F., Allen, P., Dolan, T. R., Kistler, D. J., and Jamieson, D. (1989). Temporal resolution in children. *Child Development* 60:611–24.

Wright, B. A. and Fitzgerald, M. B. (2001). Different patterns of human discrimination learning for two interaural cues to sound-source location. *Proceedings of the National Academy of Sciences USA* 98:12307–12.

Wright, B. A. and Sabin, A. T. (2007). Perceptual learning: How much daily training is enough? *Experimental Brain Research* 180:727–36.

Wright, B. A., Johnston, P. A., and Reid, M. D. (1996). Learning and generalization in auditory backward masking. *Journal of the Acoustical Society of America* 100:2818.

Wright, B. A., Buonomano, D. V., Mahncke, H. W., and Merzenich, M. M. (1997). Learning and generalization of auditory temporal-interval discrimination in humans. *Journal of Neuroscience* 17:3956–63.

Wright, B. A., Sabin, A. T., and Wilson, R. M. (2008). Disruption of consolidation of learning on an auditory temporal-interval discrimination task. *Association for Research in Otolaryngology Abstracts*, #941. p. 120

Ziegler, J. C. and Ferrand, L. (1998). Orthography shapes the perception of speech: the consistency effect in auditory word recognition. *Psychonomic Bulletin and Review* 5:683–9.

Zimmer, E. Z., Fifer, W. P., Kim, Y.-I., Rey, H. R., Chao, C. R., and Myers, M. M. (1993). Response of the premature fetus to stimulation by speech sounds. *Early Human Development* 33:207–45.

Zlatin, M. A. and Koenigsknecht, R. A. (1976). Development of the voicing contrast: A comparison of voice onset time in stop perception and production. *Journal of Speech and Hearing Research* 19:93–111.

Chapter 14

Hearing impairment

Fan-Gang Zeng and Hamid Djalilian

14.1 Introduction

A typical normal-hearing person can process sound information over at least a 120-dB dynamic range, from detecting nanometre vibrations to understanding speech in the noisy background of a loud concert. Under controlled conditions, a listener can discriminate a one-thousandth difference in pitch while processing timing information from tens of microseconds to hundreds of milliseconds. These sharp sensitivities are accomplished by delicate and exquisite mechanical, electrical, and neural mechanisms in the normal auditory system. Unfortunately, the sharp sensitivities are also susceptible to genetic and environmental impacts, from abnormal genes and the normal aging process to exposure to ototoxic drugs and noise, resulting in hearing impairment that affects one out of every ten people on earth. This hearing impairment not only lowers personal life quality but also increases the global health burden.

Here we deal with the perceptual and functional consequences of hearing impairment at the system level. Figure 14.1 illustrates this system approach to hearing impairment. Sound, the input to the auditory system, goes through a series of processing and transformations from the outer ear to the cortex, with its output being the perceived quality, meaning, and context of that sound. Specifically, the sound vibration is shaped by the outer and middle ears to produce maximal responses at 1–2 kHz, frequencies that are important to speech recognition. The cochlea, or the inner ear, adaptively amplifies the sound via outer hair cell motility and converts mechanical vibration into electric impulses via chemical transmission from the inner hair cell to the auditory nerve fibers. The electric impulses are further processed, coded, and interpreted by the auditory brainstem and cortex to form an auditory object of the sound vibration. In addition to this forward-feeding pathway, there are backward-feeding pathways from the auditory brainstem to the auditory nerve, the cochlea, and the middle ear that modulate the forward-feeding activities.

Damage to any part or parts of the auditory system will affect normal processing and produce hearing impairment. Depending upon the degree and the site of damage, different physiological processes may be disrupted, producing not only different degrees of hearing impairment but also different perceptual and functional deficits. The remainder of this chapter will discuss the types of hearing impairment, linking structural damages to physiological changes and functional consequences. While the focus will be the perceptual and functional consequences of hearing impairment, this chapter will also briefly discuss the diagnosis and treatment of hearing impairment.

14.2 Causes

Clinically, hearing impairment is classified into two major categories: conductive loss and sensorineural loss. Both types of hearing impairment can be congenital or acquired. Congenital hearing loss is typically identified at birth via hearing screening or from the family history. It may have a genetic or non-genetic origin. Most forms of congenital hearing loss are not syndromic and are

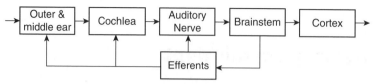

Fig. 14.1 A system approach to hearing impairment.

associated with autosomal recessive transmission: for example Alport's syndrome or Potter's syndrome may present with a family history of kidney disease. Additional causes of congenital hearing loss that are not hereditary include maternal infection, kernicterus, trauma during birth, and medication toxicity (e.g. Gurtler and Lalwani, 2002).

Although there is a genetic component, acquired hearing loss is usually related to environmental factors. Noise exposure, ototoxic medications, and presbyacusis (a general term used to describe hearing loss due to aging), are the leading causes for acquired sensorineural loss. Other forms of acquired sensorineural loss include autoimmune disorders, sudden sensorineural hearing loss, head trauma, or an acoustic neuroma. The main causes for acquired conductive hearing loss include otosclerosis, otitis media, obstruction of the ear canal, tympanic membrane perforation, cholesteatoma, or tympanosclerosis (e.g. Zadeh and Selesnick, 2001).

Here we describe the symptoms and diagnosis of several major types of hearing impairment. First, in noise-induced hearing loss, a temporary loss of hearing may occur which usually resolves after 24 hours, but a permanent hearing loss will occur with repeated exposure to loud noises. High-pitched tinnitus frequently accompanies noise-induced hearing loss. A history of noise exposure and an audiogram that demonstrates a worsened threshold at frequencies near 4 kHz typically confirms the diagnosis (Conference, 1990).

Ototoxic drugs include the following common medications: aminoglycoside antibiotics, platin-based chemotherapeutic agents (i.e. cisplatin, carboplatin), and loop diuretics. Non-steroidal anti-inflammatory drugs (NSAIDs) cause a sensorineural hearing loss as well as tinnitus, which sometimes reverse after stopping the medication. Close monitoring of a patient's hearing and dosing can reduce the risk of ototoxicity during the use of known deleterious drugs (e.g. Rybak and Ramkumar, 2007).

Autoimmune disorders, specifically polyarteritis nodosa, systemic lupus erythematosis, and Wegener's granulomatosis may cause hearing loss. Metabolic disorders such as diabetes, hypothyroidism, renal failure, and hyperlipidemia may also cause hearing loss in extreme situations. Autoimmune inner ear disorders are characterized by a progressive bilateral sensorineural hearing loss that is responsive to steroid treatment. The rate of hearing loss can be rapid (over weeks) or slower (over years). Speech understanding is generally significantly poorer than would be expected based on the degree of hearing loss (e.g. Ryan *et al.*, 2001).

Ménière's disease is characterized by episodic vertigo, tinnitus, fluctuating hearing loss, and aural pressure. There is no universally accepted cause, but histopathologic evidence shows increased hydraulic pressure in the affected inner ear's endolymphatic system. The etiology is multifactorial, as both genetic and environmental factors play a role. Treatment includes lifestyle changes such as reduced sodium intake, elimination of caffeine and alcohol from the diet, and stress reduction. Intratympanic steroids and aminoglycoside antibiotics have been used for treatment. Surgical therapy is used as a last resort (e.g. Paparella and Djalilian, 2002).

Sudden sensorineural hearing loss is a medical emergency, defined as the loss of greater than 30 dB at three or more adjacent audiometric frequencies. This loss may occur over a period of three days or less and is typically unilateral. While spontaneous recovery rates are cited to be between 32% and 70%, only 10–15% of cases are discovered to have a specific etiology. Reversible causes include perilymphatic fistula, trauma to the inner ear or ossicular chain, or the presence of an acoustic neuroma. Most sudden hearing loss cases are irreversible and may be due to an autoimmune process, or a viral or vascular etiology (e.g. Conlin and Parnes, 2007).

Acoustic tumors, or more accurately, vestibular schwannomas, often produce a unilateral, asymmetric, or sudden hearing loss. Other common symptoms include unilateral tinnitus, vertigo, or imbalance. In rare cases, acoustic tumors can occur as a familial form in neurofibromatosis type-2 with bilateral vestibular schwannomas (e.g. Daniels *et al.*, 2000). A loss resulting from an acoustic tumor is also referred to as a 'retrocochlear loss' in the literature.

14.3 Diagnosis

A diagnostic method can be subjective or objective. Subjective methods include pure-tone audiometry and speech audiometry. A pure-tone audiogram illustrates a relative measure of hearing against the averaged young and healthy subjects' hearing level (HL) by depicting the softest level that a person can hear as a function of pure-tone frequency from 250 Hz to 8000 Hz. Hearing levels are grouped in ranges of 20 dB HL to differentiate those with normal hearing from those who have a mild, moderate, severe, or profound hearing loss.

Figure 14.2 shows three audiograms from a person with normal hearing (top-left panel), a person with conductive hearing loss (top-right panel), and a person with sensorineural hearing

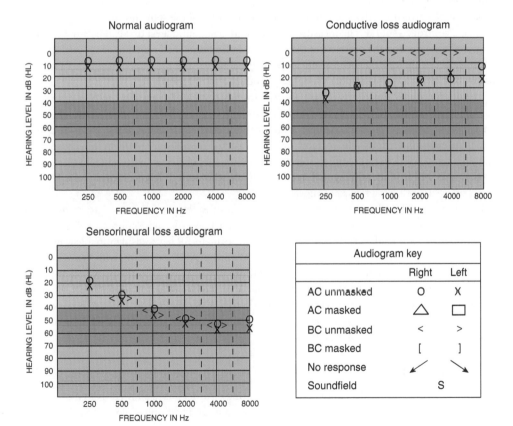

Fig. 14.2 Audiograms of normal and impaired hearing.

loss (bottom-left panel). A person with pure-tone thresholds less than 20 dB HL is considered to have normal hearing. A person with conductive loss can be identified by a >15-dB air–bone gap between air and bone conduction thresholds. In this typical case, the air–bone gap decreases from 30 dB at low frequencies to 20 dB at high frequencies. On the other hand, a person with typical sensorineural loss will have similar air and bone conduction thresholds at low and high frequencies. All three audiograms show symmetrical hearing. In the cases of unilateral hearing loss, masking is required in the better ear to prevent cross-hearing (i.e. hearing the sound in the good ear when testing the bad ear).

Because pure-tone audiograms may not always predict true hearing impairment, speech audiometry is also used. For example, the speech reception threshold (SRT) measures the lowest level at which a patient can identify 50% of spondees (a set of double-syllabic words). This threshold should be within ± 5 dB of the pure-tone average thresholds. Speech recognition scores over 90% are considered to be within normal ranges when single-syllable words are presented at 30–40 dB above the speech reception threshold. In patients with neural and central losses, there are often inconsistent results between the pure-tone audiogram and speech audiometry.

Various objective methods can also be used to differentially diagnose the integration and function of the external ear, the middle ear, the inner ear, and the auditory nervous system. First, tympanometry measures the reflection of sounds from the eardrum and can be used to measure the eardrum and middle ear function. For example, a flat tympanogram indicates that acoustic compliance does not change as a function of the ear pressure, usually signaling middle ear effusion or eardrum perforation.

Second, the acoustic reflex method measures contraction of the stapedius muscle in response to a loud controlled sound. The measure is the least intense sound level that can be administered to give a response, and the presence of the response indicates normal function of the cochlea, the auditory nerve, the ventral cochlear nucleus, the facial nerve, and the stapedius muscle. Damage to any part or parts of this feedback loop may produce absent acoustic reflexes.

Third, otoacoustic emissions (OAE) are tiny sounds generated from the cochlear outer hair cells that can be measured by placing a sensitive, low-noise microphone in the ear canal. The presence of OAE indicates normal cochlear amplification function, whereas absence can be due to either damaged outer hair cells (origin) or an obstructed middle ear (pathway). Because OAE testing is rapid and does not require subject cooperation, it has been widely used in infant hearing screening as well as in identifying malingering patients who want to feign a hearing loss. The top panel of Fig. 14.3 shows a typical OAE waveform.

Fourth, the auditory brainstem response (ABR) measures the evoked potentials, recorded by surface electrodes placed at the vertex of the head and the mastoids, in response to a click or tone pip through an air transducer or bone oscillator. The normal ABR has well-identifiable waveform peaks. The bottom panel of Fig. 14.3 shows a typical normal ABR waveform, with Wave I corresponding to activities generated at the distal auditory nerve, Wave II to the proximal auditory nerve, Wave III to the cochlear nucleus, and Wave V to the lateral lemniscus/inferior colliculus (Wave IV, not shown, corresponds to the superior olive). Abnormalities in ABR can occur due to conditions such as auditory neuropathy or tumors involving the internal auditory canal (e.g. vestibular schwannoma and Meningioma).

14.4 Classification

Recent advances in our understanding of these hearing disorders have allowed us to more accurately classify hearing impairment according to its anatomy and pathophysiology. To reflect these

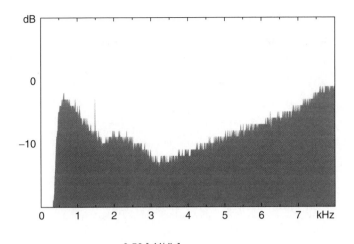

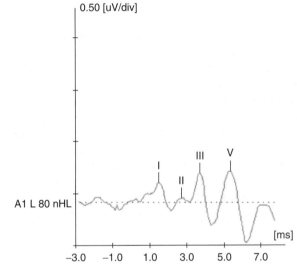

A1 L 80 nHL

Fig. 14.3 Sample otoacoustic emission (top panel) and auditory brainstem response (bottom panel) recordings. Otoacoustic emission is spontaneously recorded from a young, normal-hearing ear, showing a peak of –3 dB SPL at 1.5 kHz. Auditory brainstem response is generated by a click sound and recorded from the same young, normal-hearing ear, showing wave I, II, III, and V.

advances in both diagnosis and knowledge, here we classify hearing impairment according to the following five categories:

1 Conductive loss (damage to the outer and/or middle ears)
2 Cochlear loss (damage to the inner ear)
3 Neural loss (damage to the auditory nerve)
4 Feedback loss (damage to the backward-feed pathway)
5 Central loss (damage to the brainstem and the cortex)

Table 14.1 lists diagnosis and symptoms on each of these different types of hearing impairments. Patients with conductive loss typically have elevated thresholds with air conduction compared to bone conduction, particularly at low frequencies. The middle ear function can be affected and measured by positive results in tympanograms. Acoustic reflex and OAE should not be affected, but may not be measured because of the disrupted mechanic pathway rather than

Table 14.1 Diagnosis and symptoms of different hearing impairments

Type	Origin	Audiog	Tymp	AR	OAE	ER	Imag	Sp
1	Conductive	+	+	−*	−*	−	−	−
2a	Cochl.—OHC	+	−	−*	+	−	−	−*
2b	Cochl.—IHC	−*	−	+	−	+*	−	+
3	Neural	−*	−	+	−	+	−	+
4	Feedback	−	−	+	−	−	−	−*
5	Central	−	−	−	−	+*	+*	+

Notes and abbreviations: Cochl., cochlear; OHC, outer hair cell (damage); IHC, inner hair cell (damage); Audiog, audiogram; Tymp, tympanogram; AR, acoustic reflex; OAE, otoacoustic emission; ER, evoked responses; Imag, brain imaging, including PET, MRI and fMRI techniques; Sp, speech recognition in quiet and in noise. +, positive or abnormal result; −, negative or normal result; *, see notes in the text.

damaged neural processing. Patients with outer hair cell damage typically have elevated thresholds with both air and bone conduction, particularly at high frequencies. The OAE may disappear but the middle ear and the nerve function should be normal. Speech recognition can be compensated for with properly fitted hearing aids. Patients with inner hair cell damage could have normal thresholds, normal middle ear, and normal OAE function, but demonstrate abnormal acoustic reflex, ABR and speech recognition that are disproportionate to the hearing loss suggested by the audiogram. Patients with neural loss (e.g. auditory neuropathy) have essentially the same symptoms as those with inner hair cell damage, which needs fine diagnostic measures to differentiate them. Patients with feedback loss may have normal function in quiet but impaired function in noise. Patients with central loss have normal peripheral function but abnormal central function, as reflected by evoked potentials, brain imaging, and speech recognition.

The next five sections focus on the perceptual consequences of these hearing impairments.

14.5 Conductive loss

Conductive hearing loss can be caused by any process that impedes the conduction of sound from the auricle to the cochlea. For example, cerumen impaction or a foreign body in the ear canal is a common cause of ear canal obstruction. In addition, congenital malformations of the ear canal, as well as collapse of the ear canal can cause a conductive hearing loss of up to 30 dB.

However, the most common cause of conductive hearing loss is typically fluid accumulation in the middle ear. This fluid is generally caused by a dysfunctional Eustachian tube, a ventilation path between the middle ear and throat. If this fluid is secondarily infected, as frequently occurs in children, then it becomes a common condition called 'otitis media'. The fluid in the middle ear impedes vibration of the tympanic membrane, reducing the efficiency of sound conduction. Other similar conductive losses may involve perforation, tympanosclerosis (thickening of the fibrous layer), or atelectasis (loss of the fibrous layer) of the tympanic membrane.

Conductive loss can occur as a result of disruption of sound transmission in other parts of the middle ear or even the inner ear. For example, chronic infections of the middle ear may permanently disrupt the ossicular chain function. Overgrowth of bones in the stapes region, namely 'otosclerosis', reduces mobility of the stapes. Finally, if there is an opening into the inner ear that is uncovered, then some of the sound-induced volume velocity will be shunted away from the cochlea, creating a conductive hearing loss.

Generally, conductive loss can be corrected medically, producing nearly normal perceptual performance after correction (e.g. Snik *et al.*, 1991). The exception to this rule is auditory deprivation in early life secondary to conductive loss, which can cause abnormal development and significant hearing impairment including temporal and speech processing. However, there is evidence that prompt and proper training can correct these problems (Gravel *et al.*, 1996; Moore *et al.*, 2003).

14.6 Cochlear loss

Cochlear loss usually refers to structural damage in the inner ear, ranging from disarrayed stereorocilia to the loss of outer and inner hair cells (Liberman, 1990). While the physiological responses to these structural damages have been systematically documented, their perceptual consequences are yet to be totally delineated. Here, we consider mainly the different effects between selective loss of outer hair cells and selective loss of inner hair cells on hearing.

The main cause of cochlear loss is damage to the outer hair cells. Outer hair cells provide non-linear amplification to an incoming sound. Non-linear amplification involves amplifying a soft sound up to 1000 times (60-dB gain) while gradually decreasing gain as the sound gets louder, causing the cochlea eventually to become a linear system that provides no gain to a loud sound (Ruggero, 1992). At high frequencies the gain is also frequency-specific, such that the gain is applied only to frequencies close to the best frequency of each place on the basilar membrane. This non-linear amplification is critical to solving the dynamic range problem (Chapter 3) and sharp frequency selectivity (Chapter 2). Damage to outer hair cells, therefore, has a fundamental impact on the perception of sound.

The most apparent consequence of outer hair cell damage is loss of sensitivity (an inability to hear soft sounds). Most cochlear-impaired subjects in this category have elevated thresholds at high frequencies because there is some evidence that high-frequency hearing behaves more non-linearly than low-frequency hearing.

Outer hair cell damage also produces significant changes in suprathreshold measures, particularly in the intensity and frequency domains. Loudness recruitment is a well-known manifestation of the perceptual changes in intensity as a result of the outer hair cell damage. The top-left panel of Fig. 14.4 demonstrates this phenomenon by contrasting loudness growth as a function of sound intensity between a normal-hearing ear and a cochlear-impaired ear. Loudness grows as a power function of sound intensity in the normal ear, over at least a 100-dB dynamic range (Stevens, 1961). In the impaired ear, the dynamic range is reduced because of the loss of sensitivity to low levels rather than insufficient loudness perception at high intensities. As a consequence, loudness appears to grow more steeply near threshold but catches up at high intensities. However, the loudness recruitment function does not necessarily require a change in the slope of the loudness function. It may also be accounted for, at least in part, by an increased loudness baseline value at the threshold in the impaired ear (Buus and Florentine, 2002; see Chapter 3).

At the physiological level, outer hair cell damage makes the basilar membrane behave more like a linear system. Behavioral measures using on- and off-frequency forward-masking techniques have confirmed the linearalization of the basilar membrane vibration in the impaired ear (Oxenham and Plack, 1997). The top-right panel re-plots the Oxenham and Plack data, showing non-linear compression (roughly a 5 dB : 1 dB slope in the off-frequency masking growth function) in the normal ears, as opposed to the linear masking growth function in the impaired ears.

Outer hair cell damage also reduces frequency selectivity in the impaired ear. Frequency selectivity can be measured as psychophysical tuning curves, in which a pure tone is presented at a fixed level while the masker level is varied as a function of masker frequency, such that the masker

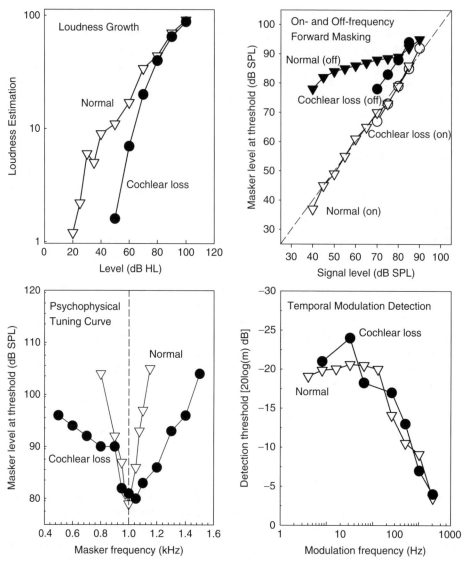

Fig. 14.4 Perceptual consequences of cochlear hearing loss (damage to outer hair cells). Top-left panel: Loudness growth from a unilaterally cochlear-impaired listener in the normal ear (open inverted triangles) and the impaired ear (solid circles). Unpublished data collected by Zeng. Top-right panel: Behavioral measurements of basilar membrane non-linearity in normal-hearing listeners (inverted triangles) and cochlear-impaired listeners (circles). The degree of compression is illustrated by the slope difference in the growth of masking function between 6-kHz on-frequency (open symbols) and 3-kHz off-frequency (solid symbols) forward maskers for a 6-kHz signal frequency. Data are re-plotted from Oxenham and Plack (1997). Bottom-left panel: Psychophysical tuning curve from a unilaterally cochlear-impaired listener in the normal ear (open inverted triangles) and the impaired ear (solid circles). Data are re-plotted from Fig. 8 in Moore and Glasberg (1986), who used a forward-masking procedure and a similar signal level in a unilaterally impaired subject PM. The signal was a 1-kHz pure tone presented at 72 and 84 dB SPL in the normal (threshold at 1 kHz = 24 dB SPL) ear and the impaired (threshold = 69 dB SPL) ear, respectively. Bottom-right panel: Temporal modulation transfer functions in normal-hearing listeners (open inverted triangles) and a cochlear-impaired listener (solid circles). Data are re-plotted from Zeng et al. (1999).

just makes the signal inaudible. Although the shape of psychophysical tuning curves is greatly influenced by the choice of signal level, masker type (pure tone vs. noise) and procedure (forward vs. simultaneous masking) (e.g. Ryan *et al.*, 1979; O'Loughlin and Moore, 1981; Nelson, 1991), there is strong evidence for broadening of the tuning curve, particularly the loss of the sharp tuning curve tip, in the cochlear-impaired ear (e.g. Moore and Glasberg, 1986). The bottom-left panel shows psychophysical tuning curves at 1-kHz frequency between the normal ear and the impaired ear in a unilaterally cochlear-impaired subject. Compared with the sharp tuning curve (10-dB bandwidth = 128 Hz) in the normal ear, the impaired ear had essentially the same characteristic frequency or tip but a three to four times wider 10-dB bandwidth. This broadened tuning curve does not necessarily worsen frequency discrimination because the cochlear-impaired listeners may utilize a temporally based cue, such as phasing locking in the auditory nerve, in frequency discrimination (e.g. Tyler *et al.*, 1983).

Indeed, outer hair cell damage may produce a relatively minor effect on temporal processing. The bottom-right panel of Fig. 14.4 shows essentially normal temporal modulation detection in a cochlear-impaired listener (adapted from Zeng et al., 1999), but similar data have been obtained in larger subject populations and different audiogram configurations (Bacon and Gleitman, 1992; Moore *et al.*, 1992). There is a known non-linear interaction between intensity and temporal processing (e.g. Penner and Shiffrin, 1980), making direct assessment of temporal processing in cochlear-impaired listeners somewhat tricky. It is generally accepted that, after taking elevated thresholds, reduced non-linear compression, and loudness recruitment into account (Oxenham and Bacon, 2003), cochlear damage usually does not impair temporal processing such as the temporal integration function (Florentine *et al.*, 1988; Plack and Skeels, 2007), temporal gap detection (Florentine and Buus, 1984; Nelson and Thomas, 1997), the temporal window (Plack and Moore, 1991), and forward and backward masking (Nelson and Freyman, 1987).

Similarly, after taking audibility and asymmetric hearing loss into account, outer hair cell damage typically has little or no effect on binaural tasks, such as sound localization using interaural level and timing differences (Hawkins and Wightman, 1980; Hausler *et al.*, 1983; Hall *et al.*, 1984; Smoski and Trahiotis, 1986). Although outer hair cell damage impairs intensity and frequency processing as well as speech recognition, particularly in noise and reverberation situations, its impairment can be remedied to a large extent by properly fitted hearing aids with dynamic range compression.

On the other hand, selective inner hair cell loss, such as that induced by the anti-cancer ototoxic drug carboplatin (Wake *et al.*, 1993), produces totally different physiological responses. As long as the outer hair cells are largely intact, significant selective loss of inner hair cells could produce relatively normal thresholds and tuning at the auditory nerve level (Wang *et al.*, 1997; Salvi *et al.*, 2000). Perceptually, selective inner hair cell loss has been studied as 'dead regions' (i.e. regions with no inner hair cell activity) in the cochlea (Moore, 2004).

The most significant difference between outer and inner hair cell damage has been the shifted tip of the psychophysical tuning curve. Figure 14.5 re-plots the Florentine and Houtsma data (1983), showing relatively unchanged tuning but an almost 2-octave shift in the tuning curve tip from 1 kHz in the normal ear to 4 kHz in the impaired ear that is indicative of inner hair cell loss. Because of the selective inner hair cell loss in the affected frequency region, signal detection relies on intact inner hair cells whose characteristic frequencies are outside the dead region (Moore and Alcantara, 2001).

Another manifestation of the presence of dead regions in the cochlea is the significantly increased threshold for detection of pure tones in suprathreshold noise. The idea is simple, because one would expect only a 3–6-dB increase in threshold, had the hearing loss been solely related to outer hair cell damage that increases the auditory filter bandwidth by a factor of 2–4. If the detection threshold is increased by 10 dB or more, then it is more likely that the inner hair

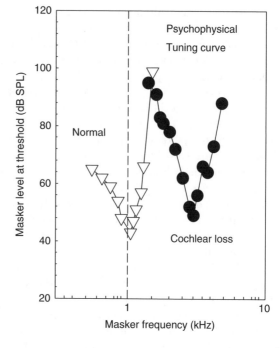

Fig. 14.5 Perceptual consequences of cochlear loss (damage to inner hair cells). Psychophysical tuning curve from a unilaterally cochlear-impaired listener in the normal ear (open inverted triangles) and the impaired ear (solid circles). Data are re-plotted from Florentine and Houtsma (1983).

cells at the signal frequency are lost, and that detection of the signal has to evoke responses by inner hair cells outside the dead region. For clinical convenience, Moore and his colleagues proposed to use 'threshold equalizing noise' (TEN) to probe the dead region, because TEN can overcome the difficulty with different audiogram configurations that may be due to either loss of sensitivity as a result of the damaged outer hair cells or the presence of dead regions associated with the selective inner hair cell loss (Moore *et al.*, 2000).

Although the presence of dead regions in the cochlea certainly affects place-based frequency perception (Huss and Moore, 2005), its associated dramatic change in psychophysical tuning curve position does not necessarily change the affected subject's pitch perception, nor does it necessarily worsen frequency discrimination (Turner *et al.*, 1983). In fact, frequency discrimination at the edge of dead regions may be enhanced compared with normal performance (Thai-Van *et al.*, 2003). This relatively unaffected, or even improved, pitch performance suggests either the usage of a temporally based pitch perception cue or cortical plasticity induced by cochlear damage.

Intensity and temporal processing have not been studied in listeners with dead regions, but they may be relatively normal as long as they can use intact inner hair cells outside the dead region to process the intensity and temporal information. The problem with this 'apparent' normal processing is that the relevant intensity and temporal information is processed in the wrong place, resulting in abnormal processing of complex temporal–spectral patterns that are typically associated with speech and music perception (see Chapters 8–10). Indeed, there is some evidence that hearing aids that amplify the sound above audibility in the dead region do not improve, and may decrease, speech intelligibility (e.g. Hogan and Turner, 1998).

14.7 Neural loss

Auditory neurons receive information from the inner hair cells via chemical synapses, and send electric information to the brainstem for further processing. Neural loss ranges from dysfunctional synapses to demyelination, axonal loss, or even cell death. Clinically, neural loss is often referred to as 'auditory neuropathy' (Starr *et al.*, 1996) or 'auditory dys-synchrony' (Berlin *et al.*, 2003). The signature of auditory neuropathy is the presence of a normal cochlear amplification function with absent or abnormal auditory brainstem responses. Functionally, neural loss differs from cochlear loss in that neural loss produces significant temporal processing deficits, which, in turn, lead to significant speech perception difficulty that cannot be accounted for by the degree of audibility (Zeng *et al.*, 1999, 2005).

Figure 14.6 shows the same sample perceptual measures in people with auditory neuropathy as shown in Fig. 14.4 for people with cochlear impairment, providing contrast between the two types of hearing impairment. The top-left panel shows nearly normal loudness-growth function in a neuropathy subject who has a normal audiogram. Intensity discrimination is also relatively normal in neuropathy subjects (Zeng *et al.*, 2005).

The top-right panel shows behavioral measures of basilar membrane non-linearity in neuropathy subjects. Similar to the Oxenham and Plack data (1997), the open inverted triangles show linear on-frequency forward-masking growth function while the solid inverted triangles show highly compressive off-frequency forward-masking growth function in normal-hearing subjects (Bai *et al.*, unpublished data). The neuropathy subjects show a similarly linear on-frequency masking function (open circles) and compressive off-frequency masking function (solid circles below 90 dB SPL). However, neuropathy subjects are 20–40 dB more susceptible to the masker, particularly for the off-frequency masker. The excessive masking has been observed in other types of masking, including simultaneous, forward, backward, onset, and steady-state masking (Zeng *et al.*, 2005). Although both neuropathy subjects and the subjects with dead regions show excessive masking, the underlying mechanisms can be totally different. The dead regions lack signal-carrying inner hair cells, while neuropathy produces temporal jitters in nerve discharge, effectively removing the phase-locking cue that is important in the detection of tones in noise.

The bottom-left panel shows psychophysical tuning curves from a normal-hearing subject (Kluk and Moore, 2004) and a neuropathy subject (Vinay and Moore, 2007). The neuropathy subject produced a slightly wider psychophysical tuning curve (a factor of 1.7 in bandwidth) than the normal-hearing subject but the same tip at 4 kHz. These tuning curve parameters are important to help differentiate between cochlear loss and neural loss. On the one hand, the neural damage and the outer hair cell damage do not change the tuning curve position, but the latter produces much wider tuning curves. On the other hand, neural damage and the inner hair cell damage produce similarly wide tuning curves, but the latter changes the tuning curve position.

The bottom-right panel shows temporal modulation transfer functions measured in a group of normal subjects and a group of neuropathy subjects (Zeng *et al.*, 1999). On average, the neuropathy subjects require an approximately 30% amplitude modulation to reach detection threshold, and their transfer functions have a bandpass characteristic. In comparison, the normal subjects require only 10% modulation for detection, and their transfer functions have a low-pass characteristic with a significantly higher low-pass cut-off frequency.

Extensive psychophysical measures (Starr *et al.*, 1996; Kraus *et al.*, 2000; Rance *et al.*, 2004; Zeng *et al.*, 2005) have shown that neural damage has minimal effects on intensity-related perception, such as loudness discrimination, frequency discrimination at high frequencies, and sound localization using interaural level differences. In contrast, neural damage significantly impairs timing-related perception, such as frequency discrimination at low frequencies, temporal integration, gap detection, temporal modulation detection, backward and forward masking, signal detection in noise, binaural beats, and sound localization using interaural time differences. These perceptual consequences are the opposite of what is typically observed in cochlear-impaired subjects, who have impaired intensity perception but relatively normal temporal processing after taking

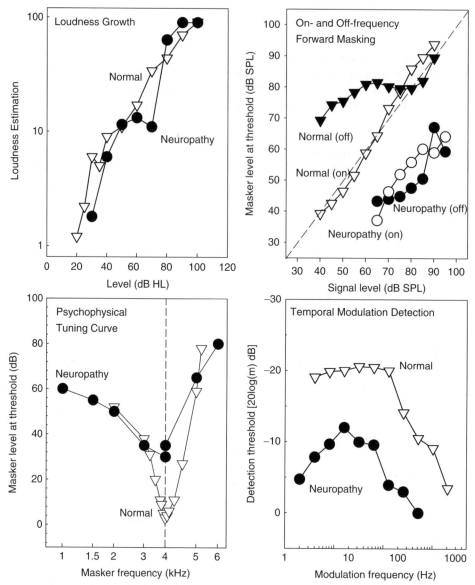

Fig. 14.6 Perceptual consequences of neural loss (auditory neuropathy, AN). Top-left panel: Loudness growth in a normal ear (open inverted triangles) and an AN ear (solid circles). Unpublished data collected by Zeng. Top-right panel: Behavioral measurements of basilar membrane non-linearity in normal-hearing listeners (inverted triangles) and AN listeners (circles). The degree of compression is illustrated by the slope difference in the growth of masking function between 6-kHz on-frequency (open symbols) and 3-kHz off-frequency (solid symbols) forward maskers. Unpublished data from Zeng, Bai, and Starr. Bottom-left panel: Psychophysical tuning curve in normal-hearing listeners (open inverted triangles) and an AN listener (solid circles). The normal data are from Kluk and Moore (2004, mean data in their Fig. 4 using a 10-dB SL, 4-kHz pure-tone signal and a 320-Hz wide masker), with permission; while the AN data are from Vinay and Moore (2007, S8 left ear data in their Fig. 8 using a 10-dB SL, 4-kHz pure-tone signal and a third-octave noise masker), with permission. Bottom-right panel: Temporal modulation transfer functions in normal-hearing listeners (open inverted triangles) and AN listeners (solid circles). Data are re-plotted from Zeng et al. (1999).

their impaired intensity perception into account. Studying perceptual differences between cochlear loss and neural loss also sheds light on the mechanisms underlying basic auditory processing.
Different neural codes are used: a suboptimal spike count code for intensity processing, a synchronized spike code for temporal processing, and a duplex code for frequency processing.

14.8 **Feedback damage**

In addition to the ascending pathway, the auditory system has a descending pathway that uses
feedback loops to control information flow and processing (see Volume 2, Chapters 3 and 11).
Damage to the feedback control can also impair auditory processing, but relatively little attention
has been paid to this impairment. Here we consider two feedback loops: the middle ear or the
stapedius muscle reflex, and the olivocochlear efferent reflex.

Physiological studies have demonstrated an anti-masking role for both the stapedius reflex and
the efferent reflex, but these two reflexes work at different intensities and frequencies (e.g.
Liberman and Guinan, 1998). The stapedius reflex is activated by loud sounds and attenuates the
sound input to the cochlea up to 20–30 dB at low-to-middle frequencies (below 1 kHz, the solid
line in Fig. 14.7). On the other hand, the efferent reflex can be activated by soft sounds and
attenuates the mechanical transmission up to 30 dB at middle-to-high frequencies (2–10 kHz, the
dashed line in Fig. 14.7). Damage to these reflexes can cause significant hearing impairment.

Borg and Zakrisson (1973) measured speech intelligibility as a function of speech level from 30
to 127 dB SPL in seven subjects with unilateral Bell's palsy and paralysed stapedius muscles. In the
normal ears, speech intelligibility maintained a high performance level at ~90% correct up to 120 dB
SPL; whereas in the affected ears with paralysed stapedius muscles, performance started to deterio-
rate at 100 dB SPL and dropped to 30% correct at 120 dB SPL. This roll-over performance-intensity
function was replicated in a large patient population with Bell's palsy and may be related to excessive
upward spread of masking from low-frequency components of speech to intelligibility-bearing

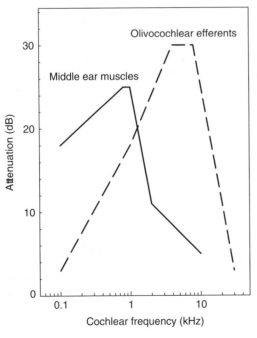

Fig. 14.7 Attenuation as a
function of cochlear frequency
caused by middle ear muscle
contraction (the solid line) or by
electrical stimulation of the
medial olivocochlear efferents
(the dashed line). The original
middle ear muscle data were
taken from Pang and Peake
(1986) with permission, and
the original olivocochlear
efferent data were taken from
Guinan and Gifford 1988) with
permission. The figure was
modified according to Liberman
and Guinan's (1998) Figure 2
with the y-axis converted into
dB values.

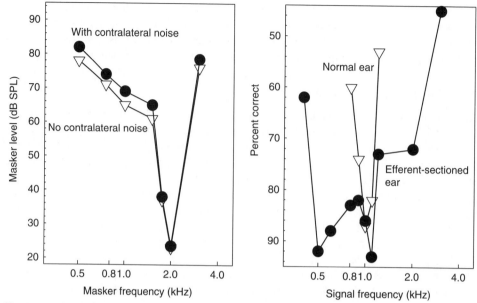

Fig. 14.8 Role of olivocochlear efferents in hearing. Psychophysical tuning curves (left panel) measured in the absence (control, open inverted triangles) and presence (solid circles) of contralateral noise. Attention filters (right panel) measured before (control, open inverted triangles) and after (solid circles) efferent section.

middle- and high-frequency components (Wormald *et al.*, 1995). The impaired stapedius muscle reflex reduces the auditory operating range by 15–20 dB at high levels.

Activation of the efferent reflex enhances frequency selectivity, whereas an impaired efferent reflex reduces frequency selectivity, impeding auditory performance in noise (Zeng *et al.*, 2000; Guinan, 2006). The left panel of Fig. 14.8 shows that activation of the efferent reflex via contralateral noise sharpens the psychophysical tuning curve, mostly by increasing the slope of the low-frequency side (Kawase *et al.*, 2000). The overall effect of the efferent reflex is relatively small, but may contribute to the changes in frequency selectivity caused by cochlear loss and neural loss. The right panel of Fig. 14.8 shows that surgical removal of the efferent reflex widens the attention filter by more than one order of magnitude (Scharf *et al.*, 1994). There are also multiple backward-feeding pathways from the cortex to the auditory brainstem, which are not discussed here because their perceptual significance has not been clearly identified (for a review, see Suga *et al.*, 2000).

14.9 **Central loss**

With few exceptions, hearing impairment related to central loss has no clearly defined physiopathology and is usually associated with, or sometimes the main culprit responsible for, symptoms such as central auditory processing disorder, language impairment, learning disability, autism, and attention deficits. Here we define central loss as hearing impairment unrelated to any apparent problems in the peripheral auditory system from the external ear to the inner ear, including the auditory nerve. This is an emergent area of research that is closely tied to aspects of neuroscience such as brain imaging and cortical plasticity. We present several hearing impairment cases related to central loss to shed light upon the common and different aspects between peripheral and central hearing impairments.

Levine *et al.* (1993) measured electrophysiological and psychophysical performance in 38 patients with multiple sclerosis (MS), a demyelinating disease in the brain. They compared these results with brain imaging data, being able to pinpoint specific abnormal performance to central lesion sites. They found that both abnormal brainstem auditory evoked potentials and abnormal interaural timing differences (see Chapter 6) using high-frequency carriers (>4000 Hz) are tightly coupled with the auditory brainstem lesion, whereas interaural level differences and interaural timing differences using low-frequency carriers (<1000 Hz) may not be tightly coupled with the auditory brainstem lesion. In contrast to neural loss in the periphery, relatively simple temporal processing such as gap detection may not be affected in patients with MS unless the degree and scope of the demyelination are extensive (Hendler *et al.*, 1990).

Auditory processing impairment has been suggested to be the main culprit causing specific language impairment in 3–6% of children who are otherwise unimpaired (e.g. Tallal and Stark, 1981). The hearing impairment is not related to audibility, as in the case of traditional sensorineural hearing loss, but related to the inability to process rapidly varying temporal information, such as detection and discrimination of brief sounds in the presence of competing sounds (e.g. Wright *et al.*, 1997). Because there are no apparent lesions in the auditory periphery in these affected children, their inability to process brief sounds is most likely to have a central origin. There have been reports that intensive and structured training in processing brief sounds can lead to improved language learning in these children, but whether temporal processing deficits are the culprit for language impairment and whether these training programs are effective are still subjects of controversy (Bishop *et al.*, 1999; Gillam *et al.*, 2008).

A final example that shows centrally related hearing impairment is autism—which typically involves the affected subjects' inability to filter out irrelevant background information. Again, children with autism typically show normal peripheral audition from pure-tone audiogram, middle ear function, acoustic reflex to otoacoustic emission (Gravel *et al.*, 2006). However, children with autism have difficulty processing suprathreshold information, including abnormal loudness perception, frequency processing, attention, and cortical processing of complex sounds such as voices (Ceponiene *et al.*, 2003; Gage *et al.*, 2003; Gervais *et al.*, 2004; Khalfa *et al.*, 2004).

14.10 Summary of perceptual consequences of hearing impairment

Table 14.2 summarizes the perceptual consequences of various hearing impairments. Conductive loss would linearly reduce loudness growth but should have negligible effects on all other perceptual functions. The three asterisks on temporal, binaural, and speech processing associated with conductive loss may indicate temporary difficulties due to deprivation of early auditory experience and unilateral loss.

Outer hair cell (OHC) damage produces loudness recruitment, linear basilar membrane response, and reduced frequency resolution and selectivity, but otherwise relatively normal perceptual functions if the elevated thresholds are properly compensated for.

Inner hair cell (IHC) damage will likely not affect loudness growth and basilar membrane nonlinearity. The two signatures of the inner hair cell damage, or the presence of dead regions, are the shifted psychophysical tuning curve position and excessive masking (>10 dB than normal or outer hair cell damage). The dead region can occur anywhere in the cochlea. As long as the adjacent inner hair cells are intact, frequency discrimination and binaural differences do not have to be compromised. However, the 'wrong place' pitch can produce a significant problem in speech and music perception.

Recall that clinical audiological diagnosis in Table 14.1 cannot differentiate between inner hair cell damage and neural damage. Here the perceptual consequences of these two impairments can

Table 14.2 Perceptual consequences of hearing impairments

Type	Origin	Loudness	BM	FDL	PTC	tMTF	Mask	Binaural	Speech
1	Conductive	+	−	−	−	−*	−	−*	−*
2a	Cochlear —OHC	+	+	+	Wide	−*	−	−	−*
2b	Cochlear —IHC	−*	−?	−*	Shift	−?	+	−?	+
3	Neural	−*	−*	+Low	−*	+	+	+ITD	+
4	Feedback	−	−	−	−*	+	+	+ITD	−*
5	Central	−	−	−	−	+	?	+	+

Notes and Abbreviations: Loudness, loudness growth; BM, basilar membrane non-linearity; FDL, frequency discrimination limen; PCT, psychophysical tuning curve; tMTF, temporal modulation transfer function; Mask, masking; Binaural, binaural hearing; ITD, interaural time difference; Speech, speech recognition. +, positive result; −, negative result; *, see notes in the text.

be differentiated because the neural damage explicitly affects spike synchrony, whereas the inner hair cell damage does not. Spike synchrony is essentially a low-frequency effect, specifically affecting frequency discrimination at low frequencies, temporal modulation transfer function, and only interaural time differences but not interaural level differences. The psychophysical tuning curve does not shift position nor does it significantly increase its breadth, especially at high frequencies. The excessive masking and speech recognition deficits are a result of impaired temporal processing.

Feedback loss produces relatively subtle changes in perception. The known effects include a 10–20-dB reduction in dynamic range as a result of the damaged middle ear muscle reflex, a reduced anti-masking function and broadened attention filters as a result of the sectioned efferent pathway.

Except for well-identified pathological conditions such as MS, where specific lesions relate to perceptual consequences, most cases of central auditory processing disorders lack correlation between structural changes and (dys)functions. Improved functional measures and brain imaging techniques are needed to provide such correlation.

The above examples are more like 'pure' cases involving only one type of hearing impairment. In reality, there are at least two difficulties challenging the diagnosis and treatment of hearing impairment. First, a patient may have mixed losses involving several types of hearing impairment. Second, different hearing impairments may produce similar perceptual consequences. For example, impaired temporal processing may be observed in patients with auditory neuropathy, multiple sclerosis, central auditory processing disorder, or specific language impairment. Systematic and strategic diagnosis is required to differentiate the origin of these hearing impairments. For example, auditory neuropathy and MS both produce abnormal auditory brainstem responses, but auditory neuropathy will have normal brain imaging whereas multiple sclerosis will not. Central auditory processing disorder may have auditory specific impairment, whereas language impairment may accompany impairment in other modalities. Proper diagnosis is important because it will lead to proper treatment.

14.11 Simulations of hearing impairment

It has always been an intriguing question: What does sound sound like to a hearing-impaired person? Simulations of hearing impairment are important not only to allow a normal-hearing person to appreciate the difficulty a hearing-impaired person faces in daily life, but also to help understand mechanisms and perceptual consequences of hearing loss. Over the years, researchers have developed audio-simulations of various hearing impairments, which are briefly summarized here.

To simulate conductive loss, the simplest way is to use fingers to plug up both ear canals. One would experience either loudness reduction (about 20 dB) for an external sound source or loudness increment for an internal sound source (e.g. chewing crunchy potato chips, the so-called 'occlusion effect').

To simulate the effect of sloping high-frequency hearing loss, low-pass filters with different cut-off frequencies can be implemented (Fig. 14.9), see: http://www.neurophys.wisc.edu/animations/ Notice the differential effects of high-frequency hearing loss on speech and music: the low-pass filtering greatly reduces speech intelligibility but has no effect on melody recognition. To further simulate suprathreshold distortions such as loudness recruitment and spectral smearing that are typically associated with cochlear loss (Moore and Glasberg, 1993), the reader is referred to the sound samples, including speech, music, and environmental sounds under quiet and more realistic listening situations, on the Phonak website: http://www.phonak.com/consumer/hearing/hearinglossdemo.htm

To simulate auditory neuropathy, different degrees of temporal smearing using actually measured modulation transfer functions are applied to speech sounds (Zeng et al., 1999), see: http://www.ucihs.uci.edu/hesp/Simulations/simulationsmain.htm

Notice in the waveforms that the natural fluctuations in amplitude are gradually flattened as the severity of auditory neuropathy is increased.

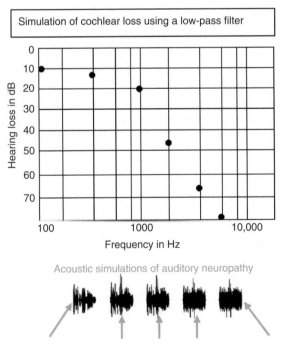

Fig. 14.9 Simulations of hearing impairment: Cochlear loss (top panel) and auditory neuropathy (bottom panel).

Finally, simulation of information overload in autism can be viewed at: http://www.youtube. com/watch?v = BPDTEuotHe0

14.12 **Treatment**

Depending upon the type and severity of hearing impairment, three treatment options are available, including hearing aids, middle ear implants, and cochlear implants. These devices all use a microphone to pick up acoustic signals, but use different signal processing techniques, and most importantly have totally different output signals (Fig. 14.10).

A hearing aid is essentially an acoustic transducer that has a sound input and a sound output. According to the degree and frequency region of hearing loss, the hearing aid selectively amplifies the sound to make otherwise inaudible frequency components of a sound audible, while at the same time ensuring that the sound is not amplified too much as to overstimulate the hearing-impaired listener. A multichannel, wide-dynamic compression circuit is typically implemented to achieve these two seemingly conflicting goals. Acoustic feedback (a loud ringing) resulting from the direct acoustic path between the microphone and the speaker can be an annoying problem for hearing-aid users who require a great deal of amplification (>40–60 dB); automatic feedback cancellation (e.g. reverse filtering at the ringing frequency) can be used to alleviate this problem. Hearing aids are most effective for hearing-impaired listeners with mild-to-severe cochlear loss.

A middle ear implant can avoid the feedback problem by bypassing air conduction altogether. The middle ear implant stimulates the cochlea via mechanic vibration delivered to either the middle ear bones or the mastoid bone. Because no speaker is needed, the implant can maintain relatively high fidelity, particularly at high output levels. Bone-conduction hearing aids are traditionally used for patients with conductive and mixed loss hearing loss, chronic infections of the ear canal or the middle ear, ear canal atresia or stenosis, and single-sided deafness. One major difference between traditional bone-conduction hearing aids and middle ear implants is that traditional bone-conduction hearing aids do not require surgery but middle ear implants do.

If the hearing-impaired listener has no functional inner hair cells, then no matter how loud a sound is amplified, the impaired listener cannot hear any sound. A cochlear implant is therefore needed to replace the function of the damaged inner ear by directly stimulating the residual auditory nerve with electric currents. The cochlear implant has two main components: an external processor, and an internal receiver and stimulator. The external sound processor takes sound, processes it digitally, breaks it down into a number of frequencies (typically 16–22) and sends the

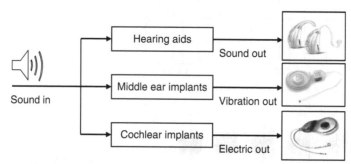

Fig. 14.10 Treatment of hearing impairment using hearing aids, middle-ear implants, and cochlear implants. The hearing aids shown are Exélia micro from Phonak (www.phonak.com). The middle-ear implant shown is Soundbridge from Med-El (www.medel.com). The cochlear implant shown is Nucleus-24 from Cochlear (www.cochlear.com).

frequencies via a radio-frequency signal to the implanted part. The internal receiver and stimulator decode the radio-frequency signal into patterned electric pulses and send them to different electrodes to stimulate the adjacent spiral ganglion cells in the cochlea.

Cochlear implants have been used by more than 130 000 hearing-impaired persons worldwide as of 2009, more than half being deaf children who have since developed normal language. Previously, a cochlear-implant candidate needed to be profoundly deaf to be eligible for implantation. At present, a person can receive a cochlear implant even if he or she has a normal audiogram but less than 50% speech intelligibility. Some success has been reported for using cochlear implants to treat patients with auditory neuropathy (e.g. Miyamoto *et al.*, 1999; Shallop *et al.*, 2001; Zeng and Liu, 2006). However, to treat patients with sectional auditory nerve and a totally deformed or ossified cochlea, a brainstem implant with electrodes placed in the cochlear nucleus or inferior colliculus would be used (e.g. Brackmann *et al.*, 1993; Lenarz *et al.*, 2006).

In addition to the device approach, there has been a strong effort towards the regeneration of hair cells for the biological treatment of hearing impairment. It is well known that hair cells can be regenerated from basal cells in birds, but recent results have demonstrated hair cell regeneration in mammals (Izumikawa *et al.*, 2005; White *et al.*, 2006). Future treatment of hearing impairment may incorporate, or combine, both engineering and biological approaches.

14.13 **Concluding remarks**

Hearing impairment may arise from genetic deficits or environmental assaults, affecting one part or many parts of the normal auditory process from the external ear to the brain. Hearing impairment has been traditionally classified into conductive loss and sensorineural loss. However, recent advances in genetics, physiology, and psychology have allowed the differentiation of at least five types of hearing impairment according to lesion site and perceptual consequences:

1 Conductive loss (elevated thresholds)

2 Cochlear loss (loudness and frequency-tuning abnormalities)

3 Neural loss (temporal processing impairment)

4 Feedback loss (anti-masking and attention deficits)

5 Central loss (temporal and complex processing deficits)

Conductive loss can be treated by either surgery or bone-conduction hearing aids. Cochlear loss, particularly that due to outer hair cell damage, can be treated with hearing aids, but cochlear loss with inner hair cell damage may require cochlear implantation. Neural loss cannot be treated effectively with hearing aids, but can be partially compensated for by cochlear implants. Feedback loss produces relatively subtle perceptual changes, which may not require aggressive intervention. Central loss can be permanent, e.g. multiple sclerosis, or temporary, such as plasticity-based changes, which may be ameliorated by training and learning. Hearing impairment may also produce other symptoms such as tinnitus and dizziness, which have no wholly effective treatment at present.

Acknowledgements

The writing of this chapter was partially supported by National Institutes of Health, United States Department of Health and Human Services. We thank Aparajita Bhattacharya for generating Fig. 14.2 and Abby Copeland for providing comments on the manuscript.

References

Bacon, S. P. and Gleitman, R. M. (1992). Modulation detection in subjects with relatively flat hearing losses. *Journal of Speech and Hearing Research* 35:642–53.

Berlin, C. I., Hood, L., Morlet, T., Rose, K., and Brashears, S. (2003). Auditory neuropathy/dys-synchrony: diagnosis and management. *Mental Retardation and Developmental Disabilities Research Reviews* 9: 225–31.

Bishop, D. V., Carlyon, R. P., Deeks, J. M., and Bishop, S. J. (1999). Auditory temporal processing impairment: neither necessary nor sufficient for causing language impairment in children. *Journal of Speech and Hearing Research* 42:1295–310.

Borg, E. and Zakrisson, J. E. (1973). Stapedius reflex and speech features. *Journal of the Acoustical Society of America* 54:525–7.

Brackmann, D. E., Hitselberger, W. E., Nelson, R. A., Moore, J., Waring, M. D., Portillo, F., *et al.* (1993). Auditory brainstem implant: I. Issues in surgical implantation. *Otolaryngology and Head and Neck Surgery* 108:624–33.

Buus, S. and Florentine, M. (2002). Growth of loudness in listeners with cochlear hearing losses: recruitment reconsidered. *Journal of the Association for Research in Otolaryngology* 3:120–39.

Ceponiene, R., Lepisto, T., Shestakova, A., Vanhala, R., Alku, P., Naatanen, R., *et al.* (2003). Speech-sound-selective auditory impairment in children with autism: they can perceive but do not attend. *Proceedings of the National Academy of Sciences USA* 100:5567–72.

Conference, N. C. (1990). Noise and hearing loss. *Journal of the American Medical Association* 263:3185–90.

Conlin, A. E. and Parnes, L. S. (2007). Treatment of sudden sensorineural hearing loss: I. A systematic review. *Archives of Otolaryngology and Head and Neck Surgery* 133:573–81.

Daniels, R. L., Swallow, C., Shelton, C., Davidson, H. C., Krejci, C. S., and Harnsberger, H. R. (2000). Causes of unilateral sensorineural hearing loss screened by high-resolution fast spin echo magnetic resonance imaging: review of 1,070 consecutive cases. *American Journal of Otology* 21:173–80.

Florentine, M. and Buus, S. (1984). Temporal gap detection in sensorineural and simulated hearing impairments. *Journal of Speech and Hearing Research* 27:449–55.

Florentine, M. and Houtsma, A. J. (1983). Tuning curves and pitch matches in a listener with a unilateral, low-frequency hearing loss. *Journal of the Acoustical Society of America* 73:961–5.

Florentine, M., Fastl, H., and Buus, S. (1988). Temporal integration in normal hearing, cochlear impairment, and impairment simulated by masking. *Journal of the Acoustical Society of America* 84: 195–203.

Gage, N. M., Siegel, B., Callen, M., and Roberts, T. P. (2003). Cortical sound processing in children with autism disorder: an MEG investigation. *Neuroreport* 14:2047–51.

Gervais, H., Belin, P., Boddaert, N., Leboyer, M., Coez, A., Sfaello, I., *et al.* (2004). Abnormal cortical voice processing in autism. *Nature Neuroscience* 7:801–2.

Gillam, R. B., Loeb, D. F., Hoffman, L. M., Bohman, T., Champlin, C. A., Thibodeau, L., *et al.* (2008). The efficacy of Fast ForWord Language intervention in school-age children with language impairment: a randomized controlled trial. *Journal of Speech, Language, and Hearing Research* 51:97–119.

Gravel, J. S., Wallace, I. F., and Ruben, R. J. (1996). Auditory consequences of early mild hearing loss associated with otitis media. *Acta Oto-laryngologica* 116:219–21.

Gravel, J. S., Dunn, M., Lee, W. W., and Ellis, M. A. (2006). Peripheral audition of children on the autistic spectrum. *Ear and Hearing* 27:299–312.

Guinan, J. J., Jr. (2006). Olivocochlear efferents: anatomy, physiology, function, and the measurement of efferent effects in humans. *Ear and Hearing* 27:589–607.

Guinan, J. J., Jr and Gifford, M. L. (1988). Effects of electrical stimulation of efferent olivocochlear neurons on cat auditory-nerve fibers. III. Tuning curves and thresholds at CF. *Hearing Research* 37:29–45.

Gurtler, N. and Lalwani, A. K. (2002). Etiology of syndromic and nonsyndromic sensorineural hearing loss. *Otolaryngologic Clinics of North America* 35:891–908.

Hall, J. W., Tyler, R. S., and Fernandes, M. A. (1984). Factors influencing the masking level difference in cochlear hearing-impaired and normal-hearing listeners. *Journal of Speech and Hearing Research* 27:145–54.

Hausler, R., Colburn, S., and Marr, E. (1983). Sound localization in subjects with impaired hearing. Spatial-discrimination and interaural-discrimination tests. *Acta Oto-Laryngologica* **400** (Suppl.):1–62.

Hawkins, D. B. and Wightman, F. L. (1980). Interaural time discrimination ability of listeners with sensorineural hearing loss. *Audiology* **19**:495–507.

Hendler, T., Squires, N. K., and Emmerich, D. S. (1990). Psychophysical measures of central auditory dysfunction in multiple sclerosis: neurophysiological and neuroanatomical correlates. *Ear and Hearing* **11**:403–16.

Hogan, C. A. and Turner, C. W. (1998). High-frequency audibility: benefits for hearing-impaired listeners. *Journal of the Acoustical Society of America* **104**:432–41.

Huss, M. and Moore, B. C. (2005). Dead regions and pitch perception. *Journal of the Acoustical Society of America* **117**:3841–52.

Izumikawa, M., Minoda, R., Kawamoto, K., Abrashkin, K. A., Swiderski, D. L., Dolan, D. F., et al. (2005). Auditory hair cell replacement and hearing improvement by Atoh1 gene therapy in deaf mammals. *Nature Medicine* **11**:271–6.

Kawase, T., Ogura, M., Hidaka, H., Sasaki, N., Suzuki, Y., and Takasaka, T. (2000). Effects of contralateral noise on measurement of the psychophysical tuning curve. *Hearing Research* **142**:63–70.

Khalfa, S., Bruneau, N., Roge, B., Georgieff, N., Veuillet, E., Adrien, J. L., et al. (2004). Increased perception of loudness in autism. *Hearing Research* **198**:87–92.

Kluk, K. and Moore, B. C. (2004). Factors affecting psychophysical tuning curves for normally hearing subjects. *Hearing Research* **194**:118–34.

Kraus, N., Bradlow, A. R., Cheatham, M. A., Cunningham, J., King, C. D., Koch, D. B., et al. (2000). Consequences of neural asynchrony: a case of auditory neuropathy. *Journal of the Association for Research in Otolaryngology* **1**:33–45.

Lenarz, T., Lim, H. H., Reuter, G., Patrick, J. F., and Lenarz, M. (2006). The auditory midbrain implant: a new auditory prosthesis for neural deafness–concept and device description. *Otology and Neurotology* **27**:838–43.

Levine, R. A., Gardner, J. C., Stufflebeam, S. M., Fullerton, B. C., Carlisle, E. W., Furst, M., et al. (1993). Binaural auditory processing in multiple sclerosis subjects. *Hearing Research* **68**:59–72.

Liberman, M. C. (1990). Quantitative assessment of inner ear pathology following ototoxic drugs or acoustic trauma. *Toxicologic Pathology,* **18**(1, Pt 2):138–48.

Liberman, M. C. and Guinan, J. J., Jr. (1998). Feedback control of the auditory periphery: anti-masking effects of middle ear muscles vs. olivocochlear efferents. *Journal of Communication Disorders* **31**:471–82; quiz 483; 553.

Miyamoto, R. T., Kirk, K. I., Renshaw, J., and Hussain, D. (1999). Cochlear implantation in auditory neuropathy. *Laryngoscope* **109**(2, Pt 1):181–5.

Moore, B. C. J. (2004). Dead regions in the cochlea: conceptual foundations, diagnosis, and clinical applications. *Ear and Hearing* **25**:98–116.

Moore, B. C. J. and Alcantara, J. I. (2001). The use of psychophysical tuning curves to explore dead regions in the cochlea. *Ear and Hearing* **22**:268–78.

Moore, B. C. J. and Glasberg, B. R. (1986). Comparisons of frequency selectivity in simultaneous and forward masking for subjects with unilateral cochlear impairments. *Journal of the Acoustical Society of America* **80**:93–107.

Moore, B. C. J. and Glasberg, B. R. (1993). Simulation of the effects of loudness recruitment and threshold elevation on the intelligibility of speech in quiet and in a background of speech. *Journal of the Acoustical Society of America* **94**:2050–62.

Moore, B. C. J., Shailer, M. J., and Schooneveldt, G. P. (1992). Temporal modulation transfer functions for band-limited noise in subjects with cochlear hearing loss. *British Journal of Audiology* **26**:229–37.

Moore, B. C. J., Huss, M., Vickers, D. A., Glasberg, B. R., and Alcantara, J. I. (2000). A test for the diagnosis of dead regions in the cochlea. *British Journal of Audiology* **34**:205–24.

Moore, D. R., Hartley, D. E., and Hogan, S. C. (2003). Effects of otitis media with effusion (OME) on central auditory function. *International Journal of Pediatric Otorhinolaryngology* 67(Suppl. 1):S63–67.

Nelson, D. A. (1991). High-level psychophysical tuning curves – forward masking in normal-hearing and hearing-impaired listeners. *Journal of Speech and Hearing Research* 34:1233–49.

Nelson, D. A. and Freyman, R. L. (1987). Temporal resolution in sensorineural hearing-impaired listeners. *Journal of the Acoustical Society of America* 81:709–20.

Nelson, P. B. and Thomas, S. D. (1997). Gap detection as a function of stimulus loudness for listeners with and without hearing loss. *Journal of Speech, Language, and Hearing Research* 40:1387–94.

O'Loughlin, B. J. and Moore, B. C. (1981). Off-frequency listening: effects on psychoacoustical tuning curves obtained in simultaneous and forward masking. *Journal of the Acoustical Society of America* 69:1119–25.

Oxenham, A. J. and Bacon, S. P. (2003). Cochlear compression: perceptual measures and implications for normal and impaired hearing. *Ear and Hearing* 24:352–66.

Oxenham, A. J. and Plack, C. J. (1997). A behavioral measure of basilar-membrane nonlinearity in listeners with normal and impaired hearing. *Journal of the Acoustical Society of America* 101:3666–75.

Pang, X. D. and Peake, W. T. (1986). How do contractions of the stapedius muscle alter the acoustic properties of the ear? In *Peripheral Auditory Mechanisms* (ed. J. L. H. J. Allen, A. Hubbard, S. I. Neely, and A. Tubis), pp. 136–43. New York, NY: Springer-Verlag.

Paparella, M. M. and Djalilian, H. R. (2002). Etiology, pathophysiology of symptoms, and pathogenesis of Meniere's disease. *Otolaryngologic Clinics of North America* 35:529–45, vi.

Penner, M. J. and Shiffrin, R. M. (1980). Nonlinearities in the coding of intensity within the context of a temporal summation model. *Journal of the Acoustical Society of America* 67:617–27.

Plack, C. J. and Moore, B. C. (1991). Decrement detection in normal and impaired ears. *Journal of the Acoustical Society of America* 90:3069–76.

Plack, C. J. and Skeels, V. (2007). Temporal integration and compression near absolute threshold in normal and impaired ears. *Journal of the Acoustical Society of America* 122:2236–44.

Rance, G., McKay, C., and Grayden, D. (2004). Perceptual characterization of children with auditory neuropathy. *Ear and Hearing* 25:34–46.

Ruggero, M. A. (1992). Responses to sound of the basilar membrane of the mammalian cochlea. *Current Opinion in Neurobiology* 2:449–56.

Ryan, A., Dallos, P., and McGee, T. (1979). Psychophysical tuning curves and auditory thresholds after hair cell damage in the chinchilla. *Journal of the Acoustical Society of America* 66:370–8.

Ryan, A. F., Keithley, E. M., and Harris, J. P. (2001). Autoimmune inner ear disorders. *Current Opinion in Neurology* 14:35–40.

Rybak, L. P. and Ramkumar, V. (2007). Ototoxicity. *Kidney International* 72:931–5.

Salvi, R. J., Ding, D., Wang, J., and Jiang, H. Y. (2000). A review of the effects of selective inner hair cell lesions on distortion product otoacoustic emissions, cochlear function and auditory evoked potentials. *Noise and Health* 2:9–26.

Scharf, B., Magnan, J., Collet, L., Ulmer, E., and Chays, A. (1994). On the role of the olivocochlear bundle in hearing: a case study. *Hearing Research* 75:11–26.

Shallop, J. K., Peterson, A., Facer, G. W., Fabry, L. B., and Driscoll, C. L. (2001). Cochlear implants in five cases of auditory neuropathy: postoperative findings and progress. *Laryngoscope* 111(4, Pt 1):555–62.

Smoski, W. J. and Trahiotis, C. (1986). Discrimination of interaural temporal disparities by normal-hearing listeners and listeners with high-frequency sensorineural hearing loss. *Journal of the Acoustical Society of America* 79:1541–7.

Snik, A. F., Teunissen, E., and Cremers, C. W. (1991). Frequency resolution after successful surgery in congenital ear anomalies. *Scandinavian Audiology* 20:265–7.

Starr, A., Picton, T. W., Sininger, Y., Hood, L. J., and Berlin, C. I. (1996). Auditory neuropathy. *Brain* 119:741–53.

Stevens, S. S. (1961). To honor Fechner and repeal his law: A power function, not a log function, describes the operating characteristic of a sensory system. *Science* 133:80–6.

Suga, N., Gao, E., Zhang, Y., Ma, X., and Olsen, J. F. (2000). The corticofugal system for hearing: recent progress. *Proceedings of the National Academy of Sciences USA* 97:11807–14.

Tallal, P. and Stark, R. E. (1981). Speech acoustic-cue discrimination abilities of normally developing and language-impaired children. *Journal of the Acoustical Society of America* 69:568–74.

Thai-Van, H., Micheyl, C., Moore, B. C., and Collet, L. (2003). Enhanced frequency discrimination near the hearing loss cut-off: a consequence of central auditory plasticity induced by cochlear damage? *Brain* 126:2235–45.

Turner, C., Burns, E. M., and Nelson, D. A. (1983). Pure tone pitch perception and low-frequency hearing loss. *Journal of the Acoustical Society of America* 73:966–75.

Tyler, R. S., Wood, E. J., and Fernandes, M. (1983). Frequency resolution and discrimination of constant and dynamic tones in normal and hearing-impaired listeners. *Journal of the Acoustical Society of America* 74:1190–9.

Vinay, [S. N.] and Moore, B. C. (2007). Ten(HL)-test results and psychophysical tuning curves for subjects with auditory neuropathy. *International Journal of Audiology* 46:39–46.

Wake, M., Takeno, S., Ibrahim, D., Harrison, R., and Mount, R. (1993). Carboplatin ototoxicity: an animal model. *Journal of Laryngology and Otology* 107:585–9.

Wang, J., Powers, N. L., Hofstetter, P., Trautwein, P., Ding, D., and Salvi, R. (1997). Effects of selective inner hair cell loss on auditory nerve fiber threshold, tuning and spontaneous and driven discharge rate. *Hearing Research* 107:67–82.

White, P. M., Doetzlhofer, A., Lee, Y. S., Groves, A. K., and Segil, N. (2006). Mammalian cochlear supporting cells can divide and trans-differentiate into hair cells. *Nature* 441:984–7.

Wormald, P. J., Rogers, C., and Gatehouse, S. (1995). Speech discrimination in patients with Bell's palsy and a paralysed stapedius muscle. *Clinical Otolaryngology and Allied Sciences* 20:59–62.

Wright, B. A., Lombardino, L. J., King, W. M., Puranik, C. S., Leonard, C. M., and Merzenich, M. M. (1997). Deficits in auditory temporal and spectral resolution in language-impaired children. *Nature* 387:176–8.

Zadeh, M. H. and Selesnick, S. H. (2001). Evaluation of hearing impairment. *Comprehensive Therapy* 27:302–10.

Zeng, F. G. and Liu, S. (2006). Speech perception in individuals with auditory neuropathy. *Journal of Speech, Language, and Hearing Research* 49:367–80.

Zeng, F. G., Oba, S., Garde, S., Sininger, Y., and Starr, A. (1999). Temporal and speech processing deficits in auditory neuropathy. *Neuroreport* 10:3429–35.

Zeng, F. G., Martino, K. M., Linthicum, F. H., and Soli, S. D. (2000). Auditory perception in vestibular neurectomy subjects. *Hearing Research* 142:102–12.

Zeng, F. G., Kong, Y. Y., Michalewski, H. J., and Starr, A. (2005). Perceptual consequences of disrupted auditory nerve activity. *Journal of Neurophysiology* 93:3050–63.

Chapter 15

Auditory basis of language and learning disorders

Lorna F. Halliday and David R. Moore

15.1 Introduction

Language and learning disorders can be defined as any delay or deviance in an individual's normal language and/or cognitive development, which cannot be explained by a lack of opportunity to learn, and which has the potential to have a negative impact upon the educational and/or psychosocial outcomes of that individual. Although there are a number of different (known and hypothesized) causes for language and learning disorders, it is well established that many have an auditory basis. We have known for some time that children with permanent hearing losses arising from cochlear damage often go on to develop poorer language skills and achieve poorer educational outcomes than their normally hearing peers. Indeed, it was an awareness of this fact that saw the introduction of specialist educational programmes for the deaf, and which spurred the development of hearing-aid and cochlear-implant technologies. So pervasive is the link between hearing and learning that many conventional definitions of known language and learning disorders (e.g. specific language impairment, dyslexia) specifically require that a hearing sensitivity impairment is ruled out. However, rather less clear is the extent to which a range of more subtle auditory deficits might contribute to difficulties in language and learning. In this chapter we take a predominantly developmental perspective, exploring the contribution of auditory function to cognitive and linguistic maturation, and focusing on how impaired hearing and listening can lead to disorders of language and learning.

15.2 Auditory basis of normal language development

Language is a complex, multifaceted skill, which comprises a number of interconnected systems (see Fig. 15.1). Although an oversimplification, in this chapter we divide language into three main domains: 'speech', the basic input and output signals of language devoid of any linguistic meaning; 'oral language', the 'higher-level' conversion of the speech stream into meaning (comprehension) and meaning into speech (expression); and 'written language', a system of shared meaning based on text. In considering speech, we can make the further distinction between 'speech perception' (see Chapter 9)—the identification and interpretation of speech sounds (from phones, the smallest units of sound, up to sentences)—and 'speech production'—the process by which linguistic information is transformed into phonological output patterns and articulation. Oral language can be similarly divided into semantics, grammar, and pragmatics. Semantics is concerned with the meaning of words and word combinations. Grammar can be divided into two domains: syntax, which is concerned with the rules underlying word orders; and morphology, which encompasses the underlying structure of words and inflections as elements of minimal meaning. Pragmatics involves the appropriate use of language in different contexts, and requires

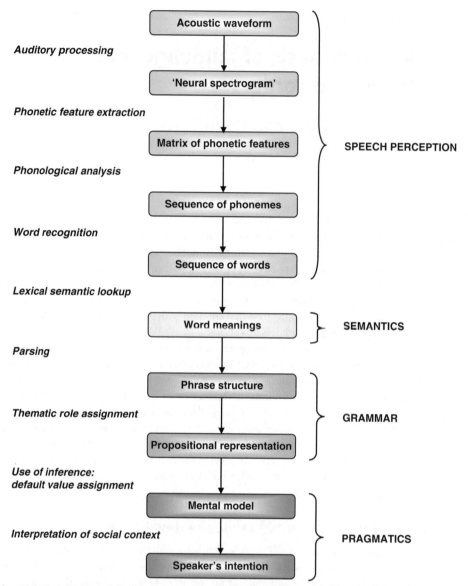

Fig. 15.1 Simplified model of the stages of processing involved in transforming an incoming sound wave into meaning. The hypothesized stages involved in language processing are described in the left-hand column, and the incremental outcomes of these processes are shown in the middle column. In the right-hand column these processes and their outcomes are divided according to the distinctions we make in this chapter between speech—here the process of speech perception—and (oral) language—'higher-level' abilities including semantics (vocabulary), grammar (syntax and morphology), and pragmatics (the understanding of social meaning). Adapted with permission from 'Uncommon Understanding' by Bishop (1997), p. 3. ©1997, Psychology Press Ltd.

the listener not only to take on the literal meaning of a particular speech act, but also its communicative function. Finally, written language comprises writing—the transfer of thoughts to orthography—and reading—the extraction of meaning from orthography.

The auditory channel forms the primary modality for language learning in the vast majority of individuals with both normal and abnormal auditory function. In spoken languages, meaning is communicated via a system of shared sounds, with speech comprising acoustic signals, expressed via the vocal tract, and received via the auditory system. That is not to say, however, that the visual modality plays no part in both typical and atypical language development. In spoken languages, visual cues provide important information about the identity of particular speech sounds, and establish a context in which semantic, grammatical, and pragmatic information can be shared. Signed languages use entirely visual cues (manual communication, body language, and lip patterns) to convey meaning. Moreover, users of both spoken and signed languages share written language as a common, and visually based, system of communication. However, a comprehensive discussion of the development of signed language in deaf children is beyond the scope of the current chapter, and readers are encouraged to see Schick *et al.* (2006) for a recent review of this topic. In the following section, we examine some of the major milestones that link audition with spoken and written language development in children with normal hearing and listening, before going on to consider what happens when hearing and/or listening go wrong.

15.2.1 Speech

As outlined in the previous section, the acquisition of a mature speech system sees the development of both speech perception and speech production processes. These processes rely on the analysis of the acoustic-phonetic properties of the speech stream. Consequently, despite following separate developmental paths, the childhood acquisition of speech perception and production processes is integrally related.

The development of speech perception is thought to progress along three levels of complexity: detection, discrimination, and identification. In acquiring a spoken language, it is first important for the language learner to have sufficient hearing sensitivity to be able to detect incoming speech sounds. These speech sounds vary according to both their temporal and spectral structure (see Fig. 15.2) and the level and type of background noise against which they are presented. The consequence of this is that a variety of auditory processing abilities are required for accurate speech–sound detection. For instance, hearing sensitivity at high frequencies is important for the detection of fricatives, which contain substantial high-frequency energy, but not nasals, which do not. Efficient temporal processing mechanisms are central to the detection of stop consonants, which are distinguished by rapid changes in formant-frequency transitions, but not vowels, for which spectral changes occur more slowly. As we saw in Chapter 13, the auditory systems of humans born with normal hearing show near adult-like sensitivity across the frequency range significant for speech by 6 months of age (Werner and Gray, 1998).

Speech discrimination refers to the process by which listeners distinguish different speech sounds. The predominant view for many years was that infants are born pre-programmed to perceive the phonetic boundaries of all the world's languages. According to this view, these sensitivities gradually sharpen and refine over the first year of life, such that only those contrasts that are meaningful in the ambient language are retained. Consistent with this idea are reports that some infants seemed to have, in one sense, *better* speech discrimination skills than adults, with infants aged 6–8 months or younger being able to discriminate a large number of phonetic contrasts, regardless of whether or not those contrasts are present in their own language (see Werker and Tees, 1999, for review). More recent research has, however, suggested that previous studies may have overestimated the speech discrimination skills of infants (e.g. Nittrouer, 2001).

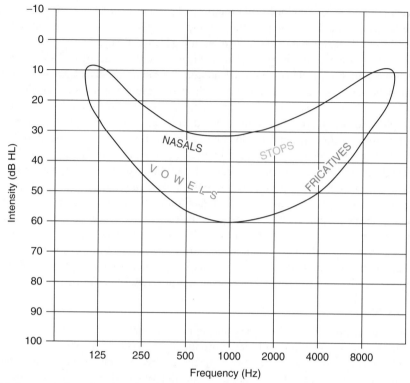

Fig. 15.2 Frequency/intensity plot, showing the region occupied by speech sounds in the English language. Reprinted with permission from 'Uncommon Understanding' by Bishop (1997), p. 53. © 1997, Psychology Press Ltd.

The theme emerging from these studies is that exposure to a child's native language affects the perceptual weight assigned to particular acoustic properties of speech (Nittrouer and Miller, 1997). Initially, children show a preferential weighting towards dynamic, spectrally changing cues that provide information about the syllabic structure of speech. With linguistic exposure, however, children gradually increase their attention towards the static properties of speech which provide information about the phonetic structure of their native language.

Speech identification denotes the process by which we categorize spoken words into their constituent parts. As skilled readers, we have no difficulty in appreciating that the word 'pat' can be broken down into three sounds—/p/, /a/, and /t/ —and that two of these sounds—/p/ and /t/-correspond to the initial and end sounds of the words 'pet', 'pit', 'pot', and 'put'. However, as we saw in Chapter 9, the acoustic structure of a consonant will vary depending on the adjacent vowel. Therefore, whilst in acoustic terms the /p/'s in 'pat' and 'pet' are not equivalent (i.e. /pʰ/ vs. /p/), in linguistic terms, they are. The perceptual challenge for young children is to learn to identify these smallest units of speech—phones—so that they know which sounds can be treated as variants of the same phone (allophones), and which signal distinct phones capable of altering word meaning (phonemes). This skill, known as 'phonological awareness', has a strong reciprocal relationship with reading. Although at least an implicit level of phonological awareness is a prerequisite for learning to read, children's explicit awareness develops further through exposure to written language (Morais et al., 1979).

Like our ability to receive speech, the process of speech production is dependent upon the speaker's knowledge about the sound structure of words (e.g. Levelt, 2001; see Fig. 15.3). In typical development, infants make the progression from primitive vocalizations such as crying and cooing, which occur within the first 6 months, to complex vocal utterances (babbling) at 6–14 months (see Eisenberg, 2007, for a review). Legal phonemic or syllabic speech patterns occur later, with spoken words emerging between 12 and 15 months of age. Importantly, the phonemic and articulatory codes involved in all stages of speech production development are refined by the language learner, both through auditory feedback and through exposure to their native language (e.g. Rvachew *et al.*, 2006).

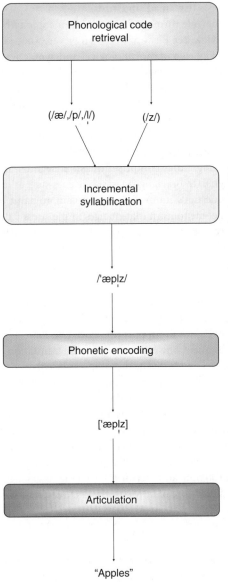

Fig. 15.3 Model of the stages of speech production. In order to produce the word 'apples', the skilled speaker must retrieve a set of phonological codes corresponding to the morphemes that make up that word (e.g. <apple> and <z>), spell these phonological codes out as an ordered sequence of phonological segments (e.g. (/æ/,/p/,/l/) (/z/), order these segments into syllables that obey rules of prosody (e.g. /'æplz/), retrieve a set of articulatory routines ['æplz], and execute these via their laryngeal and supralaryngeal apparatus to result in overt speech. Adapted with permission from 'Spoken word production: a theory of lexical access' by Levelt (2001), *Proceedings of the National Academy of Sciences*, 98, p. 13465. ©2001 National Academy of Sciences, USA.

15.2.2 Oral language

In contrast to the development of speech perception and production, which is generally thought to be complete by the end of childhood, vocabulary continues to develop throughout a person's life. In older (literate) children and adults, this growth occurs through exposure to new words that are encountered in either the spoken or the written form. For infants and young children, who do not have access to the written code, this word learning is confined to the spoken form. Thus, to acquire a new entry to their lexicon, a child must be able to identify both recurring phonological sequences in the speech stream, and the concepts that those sequences represent, and map the first domain (phonology) onto the second (word meaning). Consequently, it is important for the child to have sufficient auditory information to extract a stable phonological representation of the sequence of sounds contained within that word in order to avoid the potential confusion of similar sounding words (e.g. 'mad' and 'mat').

Both the processes and the timescale through which children come to have a knowledge of grammar are still debated (for review, see Bishop, 1997). However, some researchers have suggested that audition may play a key role in morphological and syntactical development. For instance, it has been suggested that syntax can be bootstrapped by prosodic cues in speech—stress, timing, and intonation—which provide additional information about the structure and grouping of an utterance (Morgan *et al.*, 1987). It has also been proposed that the acquisition of grammar may be dependent on the perception of morphological inflections, such as plural '-s', and past tense '-ed' in the English language, which tend to be unstressed and brief, and therefore of low perceptual salience in the speech stream (Leonard, 1989).

Finally, the auditory basis of pragmatics comprises the suprasegmental phonology (stress, rhythm, tempo) of the speech signal. In oral languages, subtle cues such as intonation can signal a speaker's intent to apologize, question, command, or complain, to name but a few examples. In typical development, children come to learn that changes in the stress patterns of a statement can be used to modify meaning (compare 'Does HE want that?' to 'Does he want THAT?').

15.2.3 Written language

In addition to oral language acquisition, the majority of language learners in the developed world also acquire a system of written language, in which they learn to read and write. Although it may seem counterintuitive to suggest that reading, a seemingly visual skill, is dependent on an auditory code, there is considerable evidence to support this assertion. First, as outlined above, it is generally accepted that the development of word decoding—the translation of the orthographic code into its phonological properties and hence its meaning—is heavily dependent upon phonological processing skills. This is evident in Fig. 15.4, which shows an influential model of reading development. In theory, a child learning to read could have difficulty with any of the representations shown in Fig. 15.4 or the connections between them. However, research has shown that poor reading ability is, in practice, most commonly associated with deficits in phonology. Second, in order to extract meaning from a passage of text (reading comprehension), the reader must draw upon his or her knowledge of the 'higher-level' aspects of language (semantics, grammar, pragmatics) that are involved in listening and speaking. Given that oral language development is so dependent upon audition, it is therefore of little surprise that reading comprehension appears to follow suit.

15.2.4 Summary

We need to be able to receive language in order to learn to speak, and to otherwise communicate and act on our knowledge. To acquire a spoken language, a child must build up a mental representation

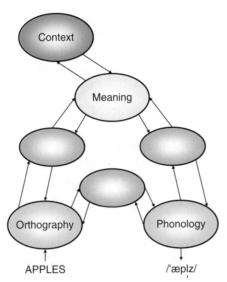

Context

Meaning

Orthography

Phonology

APPLES

/ˈæplz/

Fig. 15.4 The triangle model of reading. Phonological, semantic, and orthographic units are connected via a series of (green) mappings which are modified by learning. In the untrained model, the network first establishes connections between orthography and phonology (corresponding to the development of letter–sound correspondence skills in children and the reading of regular and nonsense words (e.g. 'skriflunaflistrop')). As training proceeds the model strengthens the mappings between orthography and semantics, enabling the processing of words with irregular grapheme–phoneme correspondences (e.g. 'pint') and a more economic reading pathway. Adapted with permission from 'A distributed, developmental model of word recognition' by Seidenberg and McClelland (1989), *Psychological Review*, 96, p. 526. © 1989 by the American Psychological Association, Inc.

of the speech sounds—phonemes—that are specific to their language. To build a vocabulary, they must be able to conceptualize the specific and arbitrary sequences of the phonemes that correspond to particular referents, and store those sequences first in short-term auditory memory and later in long-term lexical memory. In developing a system of grammar, a child must be exposed to examples of word orders—syntax—that are legal in their language, and develop an understanding of how morphological inflections, many of which are of low perceptual salience in the English language, can change the meaning of an inflected word. Finally, in order to develop an understanding of speaker intention in language—pragmatics—a child must learn to listen for subtle auditory cues such as intonation and stress which can modify the meaning of a sentence. It is no wonder then that impairments to the input of auditory information to the system are likely to have an impact on the oral language learner. In the following sections, we consider what happens to cognitive and/or language development when the auditory system is compromised.

15.3 Effects of hearing impairment on language development

15.3.1 Conductive hearing loss

Hearing impairment is traditionally divided into two types, 'conductive' and 'sensorineural' (see below), as detailed in Chapter 14. Conductive hearing loss is, briefly, a reduction in sound energy at the site of sensory transduction, usually produced by an occlusion of the sound conduction pathway in the outer or middle ear. The most common causes, in children, are a build up of ear wax or other material (cerumen) in the ear canal, and middle ear disease, leading to pressure changes and/or fluid in the middle ear. Excess ear wax usually occurs infrequently and is easily and quickly diagnosed and treated. Middle ear disease, on the other hand, is common, pervasive, and still quite poorly understood, despite much research activity over the last 30 years (Rosenfeld and Bluestone, 2003).

Otitis media with effusion

Middle ear disease may be divided into two main types, acute otitis media (AOM) and otitis media with effusion (OME). AOM involves a bacterial infection and an inflammatory response of the middle ear, and is often associated with pain and/or fever. It typically results in a visit to the family physician and the prescription of antibiotics. Although repeated AOM episodes may lead, in some cases, to a substantial amount of time away from school and, hence, to interruptions in learning, there are to the authors' knowledge no data on the effects on academic performance of missing school through this route. A much more common problem, and one that has been the subject of considerably more research, is OME in which the middle ear fluid, if visible, is serous; there is no clear infection or inflammatory response. The child is otherwise symptom-free, aside from the presence of negative middle ear pressure and, in most but not all cases, a relatively flat conductive hearing loss of 5–50 dB (median 10 dB). Several large-scale epidemiological studies (e.g. Engel *et al.*, 1999) have shown a high prevalence of OME, especially during the first few years of life. Those findings are corroborated by smaller, but more sensitive studies that have shown OME to be present in nearly all children at some stage during development, with one study showing that around 15% of otherwise healthy children have OME in at least one ear for more than 50% of their first 5 years of life (Hogan and Moore, 2003; Fig. 15.5).

Because OME produces an intermittent, persistent, slight to mild, and typically asymmetric hearing loss in a large number of children, concerns have been expressed that it may contribute to language and learning disorders. These could take the form of both shorter term, actual hearing loss, when the fluid is in place during the critical years for language acquisition, and longer term, especially binaural effects produced by maladaptive brain plasticity. There is, in fact, evidence for both of these consequences but, to summarize the following presentation, OME appears to have a long-term negative impact only when there are other exacerbating circumstances, such as an impoverished home communication environment.

Methodological challenges

There has been considerable debate about whether OME has any impact on language development, primarily because it is usually a very mild and at least a somewhat intermittent form of hearing loss. Consequently, the ear and brain continue to receive adequate levels of acoustic and neural stimulation, respectively. Providing speech is presented at a typical level (e.g. >50 dB SPL at the ear) and adequate signal-to-noise level, it should be audible by a child who has active bilateral OME. In general, the brain will form its connections normally based on a genetic programme, and sensory experience is an issue only if the impairment is dramatic (e.g. eye cataracts). However, a well-recognized exception is if the two eyes are misaligned at birth (congenital strabismus). This results in lifelong impaired vision (amblyopia) in the turned eye unless treated early. In hearing, there is good evidence of impaired binaural function that outlasts the ear fluid by at least two years following early, severe OME (Hall *et al.*, 1995; Hogan and Moore, 2003). This is thought to result from an imbalance of binaural input and timing (see Chapter 6) caused by an interaural asymmetry of the hearing loss. But the later recovery, even in extreme cases of unilateral, congenital conductive loss (see Wilmington *et al.*, 1994), and the finding of similar effects in adults

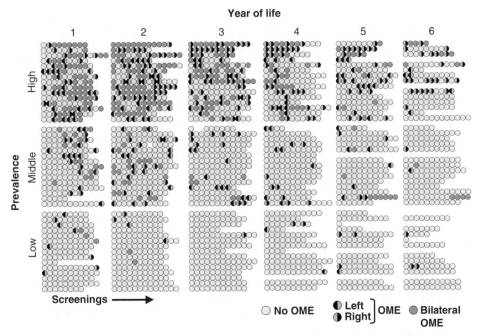

Fig. 15.5 Prevalence of otitis media with effusion (OME) in early life of typically developing children. Each row represents repeated screening of one child for OME. Screening (tympanometry and otoscopy) was performed bilaterally during home visits at approximately monthly intervals (circles) for up to 6 years. Pale (yellow) circles represent OME-free in both ears, and fillings show instances of OME in one (blue/black) or both (pink) ears. The rows are arranged in order of overall prevalence in about half the studied sample ($n = 112$; for further details of the sample and their hearing, see Hogan et al., 1997; Hogan and Moore, 2003). The 15 individuals closest to the median prevalence are shown in the 'Middle' set of rows, and the 15 individuals with the highest and lowest prevalence are shown, respectively, in the 'High' and 'Low' set of rows. Only three children in this sample were OME-free for all screenings, whilst those at the high-prevalence end of the continuum had OME in one or both ears for around one half of their first six years. (S. C. M. Hogan and D. R. Moore, unpublished data.)

with asymmetric conductive loss (Hall and Grose, 1993) suggests that severe OME may lead to a reversible re-learning of the auditory cues associated with certain aspects of perception, including spatial release from masking and aspects of spectral processing relevant to language (Roberts et al., 2004; Eapen et al., 2008). Despite increased understanding of the acoustic and neurological consequences of OME, its effect on language and learning in children remains controversial. As discussed elsewhere in this chapter, comorbidity is a general problem in ascribing language problems to hearing deficits. This is partly a problem of recruitment. Most studies are retrospective—they rely on clinical or parental reports of OME that are often inaccurate. They often include, or fail to exclude, selection criteria that bias the sample towards children with language or other learning problems. Because the OME is 'silent'—asymptomatic—it is usually those learning problems (or AOM) that lead to referral. A child experiencing or suspected of language difficulties may well, on otological examination, turn out to have active OME. However, a random sampling of children aged 2–4 years may reveal an equal or higher prevalence of OME (Fig. 15.5), making a positive association difficult to interpret. In addition, while a child who has active OME may have transient language difficulties, the OME will, in most cases, not last long enough to produce a permanent problem. Finally, if a clear association is made, it may not be causal. Both the OME and the language problem could, for example, be the result of a common genetic predisposition. Below, we consider some of the evidence relating OME to speech, language, and other developmental difficulties.

Speech

As introduced above, speech development normally requires access to high-fidelity and reproducible acoustic signals. In OME, the acoustic signal fluctuates, both within and between the ears. While the immediate impact this has on speech perception and production does not appear to have been examined, a few studies have reported poorer or otherwise transformed speech perception following a history of OME. While these have generally been difficult to interpret because of poor design, including low sensitivity, one recent study (Eapen *et al.*, 2008) showed a clear relation between speech spectrum weighting and OME history. Speech production, however, has not been found to be markedly affected by OME (Roberts *et al.*, 2004). Because speech is heavily redundant, and the auditory system can rapidly adapt to quite marked variations in its spectrotemporal characteristics, it may not be too surprising that a fluctuating, mild hearing loss has little long-term effect. On the other hand, the methodological difficulties discussed above may have prevented the detection of mild impairment. It may be that more sensitive methods, such as those used by Eapen *et al.* (2008), will produce further convincing evidence of mild impairment in the future.

Oral and written language

Despite the scant and equivocal literature relating OME to speech, many studies have suggested that OME disrupts language processing. Generally, these studies have examined performance on a battery of language tests in children with a clinical history of OME. Performance is compared with a control group of children with no known OME, but matched for age and other factors.

In reviewing this literature, Roberts *et al.* (2004) concluded that the relation between children's language skills and OME is 'negligible to mild in degree, accounting for none to a small part of the variance [on tests of language]' (p. 115). In other words, there is no clear link between a history of OME and language, either in small-scale studies that have relied on retrospective diagnosis of OME, or in much larger, often prospective studies. However, a small number of well-conducted and recent prospective studies have used correlation analysis to suggest an interaction between OME and home and childcare environments to produce problems with language development. Children who came from low-income, communicatively unresponsive homes or who experienced low-quality child-care facilities, had expressive language problems that were exacerbated by OME. Apparently, the combined effect of a mild hearing loss and a poor communication environment was sufficient to produce a language deficit. These community-based studies are consistent with prospective laboratory studies (e.g. Hogan and Moore, 2003) in suggesting that a high level and persistence of conductive hearing loss and/or auditory deprivation is needed to produce long-term problems of auditory processing and language. These findings are, in turn, consistent with many observations of brain plasticity in animals showing that, while continuous sensory deprivation (e.g. congenital eye cataracts), especially during a sensitive period in early life, can lead to profound and permanent impairment, a surprisingly low level of normal sensory experience is sufficient for the sensory brain to develop normally (Sanes *et al.*, 2006).

Learning difficulties and behaviour

Building on the previous evidence suggesting an interaction between OME and the listening environment on language skills, several well-conducted studies have reported that a similar interaction may adversely affect academic achievement, attention, and behaviour. Although the evidence in support of this idea is, typically, mixed, it is noteworthy that one large, prospective study that failed to find almost any lasting consequences of persistent OME earlier in childhood concluded that adolescents with a history of persistent OME were more prone to poor reading, verbal IQ, and behaviour than their low-OME peers (Bennett *et al.*, 2001).

Summary

The effects of conductive hearing loss on listening, language, and learning have been extensively studied in children with a history of OME. The literature is fraught with methodological difficulties that render the majority of studies inconclusive. Of the remainder, the evidence appears to support some modest negative effects of OME, both during and following the presence of middle ear fluid. The strongest evidence shows persistent effects of OME on aspects of binaural and spectrotemporal hearing and, in combination with more generally impoverished listening environments, on language and learning. Surprisingly, longer term effects of OME on aspects of intelligence and behaviour have also been found. A model that summarizes these findings from an auditory learning perspective suggests that the poor hearing produced by OME leads to inappropriate associations between auditory cues and the child's environment. Following resolution of the OME, typically around 5–7 years, the older child can gradually relearn appropriate associations between sound and environment. However, the early impact of the OME may result in a modest, long-term disadvantage for the child relative to his or her peers.

15.3.2 Sensorineural hearing loss

Sensorineural hearing loss (SNHL) is defined as a permanent hearing loss caused by damage to the hair cells of the inner ear (cochlea) or to the neural pathways from the inner ear to the brain (retrocochlear) (American Speech-Language-Hearing Association, 2007). Although there is no universally accepted classification system for the degree of loss, here we adopt a fairly representative system that has been advocated by the British Society of Audiology (BSA, 2004; see Table 15.1) in which SNHL is seen as falling into one of four categories—mild, moderate, severe, or profound—depending on the 'severity' of the loss. These descriptors are based on the average decibel loss for an individual's better ear, derived from pure-tone audiometry across the speech frequencies (250, 500, 1000, 2000, and 4000 Hz). As such, they constitute a relatively crude reflection of an individual's level of disability for (at least) two reasons. First, the configuration of SNHL, in terms of the loss of sensitivity at different frequencies, can and does vary widely between individuals. Second, although SNHL is typically defined in terms of loss of sensitivity, this definition neglects the existence of additional physiological changes—including broadening of auditory filters, a reduction in auditory filter non-linearity, changes in the propagation time of auditory stimuli

Table 15.1 Audiometric descriptors for degrees of sensorineural hearing loss

Audiometric descriptor	Pure-tone average threshold[a] (dB HL)
Mild hearing loss	20–40
Moderate hearing loss	41–70
Severe hearing loss	71–95
Profound hearing loss	> 95

[a] Average hearing threshold obtained by a pure-tone audiogram over the frequencies 250, 500, 1000, 2000, and 4000 Hz, obtained in the better ear.
Reprinted with permission from 'Pure tone air and bone conduction threshold audiometry with and without masking and determination of uncomfortable loudness levels' by British Society of Audiology (2004).

along the basilar membrane, and broadening of the 'temporal envelope'—that are likely to accompany SNHL (for reviews see Moore, 1995; and Chapter 14). The result of these changes is that, in addition to reductions in hearing sensitivity, individuals with SNHL are also likely to experience a wide range of perceptual consequences associated with their loss, including reductions in frequency selectivity and discrimination, temporal resolution and integration and—for individuals with asymmetrical losses—poorer sound localization and lateralization.

The proportion of children born with a moderate or worse bilateral SNHL is approximately 0.91/1000 (Fortnum *et al.*, 2001). However, many (16–38%) cases of childhood SNHL are acquired (Davis *et al.*, 1997). The consequence of this is that the prevalence of childhood SNHL is closer to 1.65/1000 for children aged 9–16 years (Fortnum *et al.*, 2001). There is currently no cure for SNHL. Once identified, children enter a system of provision aimed to manage, and therefore minimize, the impact of their loss. Depending on the aetiology, degree, and age of onset/identification of the loss, this management generally consists of the fitting of (uni- or bilateral) hearing aids and/or cochlear implants and, in some cases, behavioural interventions. However, although both approaches are designed to increase the hearing-impaired child's sensitivity to sound, they do not overcome many of the perceptual consequences associated with cochlear and retrocochlear damage.

Because of its marked impact on hearing sensation and perception, childhood sensorineural damage has, historically, had a marked and negative impact on the learning of speech-based languages. In the past, many children (particularly those with severe to profound SNHL) required specialist education and, despite this, often went on to develop poorer language skills and achieve poorer educational outcomes than those with normal hearing. However, the past two decades have seen the emergence of two important developments in the field. First, recent advances in hearing-aid technology and, in the 1980s, the advent of the cochlear implant, have led to improvements in the auditory sensitivity of a whole generation of hearing-impaired children. In the case of children with profound losses, the cochlear implant has given access to auditory information that would otherwise not have been possible. Second, a major breakthrough has been the earlier identification of childhood SNHL. Until recently, around 50% of children born with a SNHL were not identified until they were 18 months old, with 25% remaining undiagnosed at 3 years. The last decade has seen the introduction of universal newborn hearing-screen programmes designed to increase the rates of early detection of childhood SNHL. The consequence of these two developments has been the provision of earlier and, arguably, better management strategies for childhood SNHL. Because language acquisition takes time, the impacts of these developments on language outcome are just coming to light. Nevertheless, the optimistic picture emerging from these studies (reviewed in the subsections on 'Speech', 'Oral language', and 'Written language') is that, provided children with SNHL are identified at an early age and given appropriate support, they may have the potential to go on to develop language at the same rate as their normal-hearing peers.

Methodological challenges

Teasing apart the link between SNHL and language difficulties presents a serious challenge to clinicians, educators, and researchers alike. As outlined above, the reductions in hearing sensitivity associated with sensorineural damage range from mild (20–40 dB HL) to profound (>95 dB HL), show different within- and between- ear configurations, and may be congenital or acquired. For those children who were born before the introduction of universal newborn screening, or whose loses are aquired, some may have gone undetected for some time. When hearing losses are detected, they can be managed in different ways, although there is marked variability in the extent to which individuals benefit from or comply with their particular management strategies. Some children with more severe hearing losses will be bilingual in both signed and oral language, while others will not. Moreover, children will vary with respect to the communication method through which they are taught and which is used at home. Finally, in some cases the factors that caused the hearing loss in the first place may have other consequences for the child's learning and development. Given then that there is no such thing as the 'typical' child with hearing impairment it is perhaps not surprising that the outcomes for language learning in children with hearing impairment are so heterogeneous.

In general, research has identified two main factors that appear to have a marked impact upon language learning in children with SNHL—severity of loss, and age of identification. In contrast to the large body of research on children with severe to profound SNHL, very few studies have investigated language development in children with milder losses. Nevertheless, of those that have, the majority have indicated that children with mild to moderate losses tend to have better outcomes than those with severe or profound losses. Accordingly, in this chapter we make the distinction between children who have some residual hearing (mild to moderate) versus those who have little or none (severe to profound). It is also generally accepted that early identification is better than later identification, in children with SNHL. However, because many of the published studies available focus on children whose hearing loss was diagnosed before the introduction of newborn hearing screening, we have yet to see the full benefits of this scheme. Consequently, although the review below focuses primarily on research published in the last decade, it is possible that future investigations will paint an even more optimistic picture of the communication outcomes of children with SNHL.

Speech

It is a truism to say that children with SNHL have poorer speech *detection* abilities than those with normal hearing. More informative have been those studies looking at the speech *discrimination* skills of children with SNHL. Although limited in number, these studies have been summarized in two recent reviews (Eisenberg, 2007; Jerger, 2007), which have identified a number of trends in the literature. In reviewing the phonetic contrast discrimination abilities of this group, Eisenberg (2007) reported that (1) performance tends to decrease with increasing hearing loss, (2) discrimination abilities are generally better when additional visual (speechreading) input is available, and (3) children with, at most, moderate levels of SNHL have the potential to show normal phonetic contrast discrimination skills. This latter conclusion is further supported by studies reviewed in Jerger (2007), which reported that children with up to a moderate degree of hearing loss show perceptual weighting strategies and phonetic boundaries for voice onset time that are, in general, comparable to those of normally hearing children.

In addition to detection and discrimination, we can also ask how well children with SNHL can identify and manipulate aspects of the speech stream. Here, research suggests that even children with mild SNHL show poorer phonological processing skills relative to hearing controls (Briscoe *et al.*, 2001; Wake *et al.*, 2006). For severe to profound SNHL, however, the picture is even bleaker, and it remains an open question as to whether these children are capable of using a phonological code at all. Nevertheless, a study by Sterne and Goswami (2000) found that, although worse than their hearing peers, children with profound SNHL were capable of making judgements at the level of both rhyme and phoneme. However, the hearing-impaired group were more likely than their hearing peers to use the orthographic forms of words to influence their judgements of phonological similarity. Based on these findings, Sterne and Goswami (2000) concluded that '(children with profound SNHL) can develop phonological awareness, but … their phonological skills lag (behind) those of hearing children and may develop in different ways' (p. 609).

Given the poorer speech perception skills of children with SNHL, we might expect their speech production to follow suit. As a general rule, this prediction can be confirmed. As reviewed by Eisenberg (2007), children with SNHL (1) have a more prolonged stage of primitive vocalizations, (2) show both deviant and delayed babbling behaviour, and (3) experience delays in their development of phonemic and/or syllabic speech patterns, particularly those required for conso-nantal contrasts, relative to their normal-hearing peers. Speech production abilities tend to dete-riorate with increasing levels of hearing loss, although deficits have been reported in children with even mild levels of SNHL (Eisenberg, 2007). Nevertheless, despite these developmental delays, the eventual outcome of speech production in children with SNHL is not all bad. The majority of children with mild to moderate losses, as they mature, go on to produce intelligible speech. Cochlear implants provide at least the potential for normal speech production in children with severe to profound SNHL, through providing a channel for speech perception (e.g. Geers, 2004).

Oral language

As with speech perception and production, the outcome of children with SNHL on measures of oral language is strongly linked to the degree of loss. Of the few studies that have examined the oral language abilities of children with mild to moderate SNHL, outcomes have been mixed (for a review, see Moeller *et al.*, 2007). Whereas some studies have found evidence for relatively spared performance on measures of vocabulary, syntax, and morphological development, others have not. The picture that is emerging from these studies is one of marked individual differences in the oral language skills of this group. For instance, three studies have reported impairments in vocabulary and/or the production of morphological inflections in a *subset* of children with mild to moderate SNHL (Briscoe *et al.*, 2001; Hansson *et al.*, 2007; Norbury *et al.*, 2001). These subsets were charac-terized by children who, in general, had poorer hearing thresholds, poorer phonological process-ing, and/or were younger than their non-language-impaired peers. Our tentative conclusion from these studies is that although the majority of children with mild to moderate SNHL will go on to develop age-appropriate oral language skills, as a group these children may show a marginally higher incidence of language difficulties than would be expected for the general population.

As outlined above, although historically children with severe to profound SNHL have been at significant risk for delays in oral language development, recent developments in technology and healthcare provision have led to improved prospects for these children. Research detailing the impact of these developments on oral language outcomes is just emerging. Nevertheless, a number of key trends can be identified. In general, children with severe to profound SNHL who have received a cochlear implant have better outcomes compared to those who have not, or to those who have been fitted with conventional hearing aids (e.g. Tomblin *et al.*, 1999). Moreover, many of these children show oral language skills that are commensurate with, or develop at the same rate as, those of their hearing peers (e.g. Geers, 2004). However, there are large individual differences in performance outcomes, and upwards of 50% of these children do not achieve such positive outcomes (Geers, 2004). Research aimed at identifying the factors predicting oral lan-guage success in these children is ongoing, although the age at implantation has been strongly implicated, as has the language environment of the child. For instance, studies have shown that children implanted below the age of 2.5 years tend to show the greatest benefit (e.g. Connor *et al.*, 2006). Future studies are needed to help us understand the additional factors contributing to these individual differences, and to guide management strategies aimed at improving the oral language outcomes of this group.

Written language

Despite a long history of studies reporting poor reading achievement (see Moeller *et al.*, 2007, for a review), recent findings suggest that children with mild to moderate SNHL show age-appropriate reading skills (e.g. Briscoe *et al.*, 2001). In contrast to those with milder losses, however, the major-ity of children with severe to profound SNHL experience considerable difficulty in learning to read. This finding has largely been put down to the poorer phonological skills of this group which, for hearing children, are the precursors of learning to read. Recent research has aimed to identify the factors contributing to reading success in children with severe-profound SNHL (Harris & Moreno, 2006; Kyle & Harris, 2006). Together these studies suggest that (at least) two factors in particular might be important. In their cross-sectional study, Kyle and Harris (2006) showed that both expressive vocabulary and speechreading ability were significant predictors of reading in a sample of severe-profound hearing-impaired children, once degree of hearing loss and nonverbal intelligence had been accounted for. Consistent with this finding, Harris and Moreno (2006) found speechreading to be the only factor that discriminated between 'good' and 'poor' readers with severe-profound SNHL. These findings have led to the suggestion that, as for hearing children, a phonological code may underpin the reading of children with severe-profound SNHL, but that this code may be acquired via the visual modality in the absence of auditory input.

Summary

Children with SNHL show variable outcomes on measures of speech perception and production, and oral and written language. A distinction can be made between children with mild to moderate losses, and those whose losses are more severe. In general, children with mild to moderate SNHL show impaired phonological skills, in the absence of any wider difficulties in oral or written language ability. However, a subset of children with mild to moderate SNHL have poorer vocabulary and grammar than would be expected for their age, suggesting that the perceptual difficulties experienced by these children may contribute to their greater risk of language impairments. Deficits in almost all aspects of language development have been reported in children with severe to profound SNHL. However, cochlear implant technologies have meant that their prospects for language development are significantly improved in this group. Nevertheless, many of these children still experience delays in language development that are sufficiently marked to impact upon their communicative, social, and academic development. More research is needed to understand the factors that contribute to the language success or otherwise of children with severe to profound SNHL but it may be that early intervention, combined with a period of appropriate rehabilitation, is sufficient to confer significant advantage.

15.4 Specific language impairment and dyslexia

15.4.1 Definition

Specific language impairment (SLI) and dyslexia are developmental language disorders that are characterized by respective failures in spoken and written language acquisition. Both are relatively common, with prevalence rates for both ranging between 3 and 10% (Tomblin *et al.*, 1997; Snowling, 2000). However, despite their common occurrence, there is still no general consensus on what might cause these disorders and, consequently, both are still typically defined negatively, and at the behavioural level. SLI can be defined as late-developing and impaired language abilities, and dyslexia as impaired reading abilities, in those children who otherwise have adequate hearing and vision, at least average non-verbal IQ, and no known neurological, physical, emotional, or socio-economic problems which might account for their symptoms (McArthur and Bishop, 2001). Note that our preference to include normal non-verbal IQ as a diagnostic criterion is purely academic and, in common parlance, these rather stringent definitions are commonly ignored or distorted. The consequence of this is that, in practice, the terms 'SLI' and 'dyslexia' are often applied to children who do not have a substantial mismatch between language and non-verbal abilities.

15.4.2 Comorbidity

Although SLI and dyslexia are conventionally defined as separate disorders, there is strong evidence for high comorbidity between written and oral language problems. Many children with a preschool diagnosis of SLI later go on to experience problems in learning to read (e.g. Catts, 1991), and many children with dyslexia show difficulties with spoken language (Anderson *et al.*, 1993). Moreover, recent estimates suggest that approximately 50% of children with a diagnosis of either SLI or dyslexia would meet criteria for both disorders (e.g. McArthur *et al.*, 2000). At the behavioural level, this overlap appears to be due to the fact that both groups tend to experience difficulty with tasks that involve phonological processing. This has led some researchers to argue that rather than constituting distinct disorders, SLI and dyslexia may instead fall on a continuum, and has resulted in the introduction of the umbrella term 'language-learning impairments' (LLI) to include children with both oral and/or written language impairments. Furthermore, given the extent of this overlap, a number of researchers have conceptualized these phenotypically distinct disorders as different manifestations of the same underlying deficit. Specifically, it has been argued that the phonological impairment observed in SLI and dyslexia derives from a domain-general deficit in auditory processing.

15.4.3 Auditory processing theories of SLI and dyslexia

By far the most influential theory advocating a link between auditory processing and LLI has been put forward by Tallal and colleagues in what is now known as the 'rate-processing constraint hypothesis' (e.g. Tallal, 2004). Although initially put forward as an account of SLI, this theory now encompasses written as well as oral language disorders and therefore constitutes a general model of LLI. According to Tallal, deficient auditory processing mechanisms, particularly those involved in processing dynamic spectral and/or temporal change, lead to difficulty in analysing the incoming speech stream. In turn, this interferes with the acquisition of segmental phonological representations and, consequently, hinders grammatical and vocabulary development (SLI). Subsequently, it is argued, this impairment leads to difficulty analysing the letter–sound correspondences thought to be important in learning to read (dyslexia) (see Fig. 15.6).

Behavioural basis

Substantial behavioural evidence points to the existence of auditory processing difficulties in many children and adults with LLI. Early evidence of this sort was obtained using a modified version of a temporal order judgment task that has become known as the 'Auditory Repetition Test' (ART). In this task, listeners are initially presented with two, clearly distinguishable sounds, and are trained either to associate each sound with a different button press, or to associate two identical sounds with one button press, and two different sounds with another button press. Once this association has been learned, listeners are presented with a series of two-sound sequences at variable inter-stimulus intervals. The task is for listeners either to press the buttons corresponding to the sequence of sounds they heard (i.e. A-A, A-B, B-B, or B-A) (sequencing task) or to decide whether the two sounds were the same or different (same vs. different task). Using this paradigm, Tallal and colleagues showed that children with SLI had difficulty in identifying and discriminating both speech and non-speech stimuli, but only when they were brief or rapidly presented (reviewed in Tallal, 2004). These findings were later replicated in a subset of children with dyslexia (Tallal, 1980).

The last decade has seen an explosion of studies investigating the link between behaviour-based deficits in auditory processing and LLI. Although findings have been mixed, these studies have given rise to at least two key developments in the field. First, evidence for poor performance on tasks incorporating a temporal processing component in some children and adults with SLI and/or dyslexia has been largely confirmed using standard psychophysical tasks, including backward masking as well as 'beat', frequency-, and amplitude-modulation detection (for review see Rosen, 2003). However, the notion that LLI is linked to a *selective* deficit in processing brief, rapid,

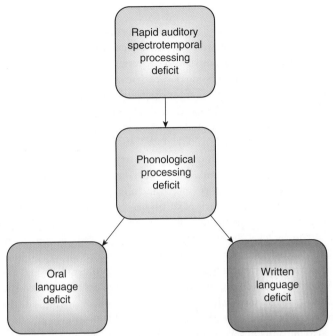

Fig. 15.6 The rate-processing constraint hypothesis of language-learning impairments (e.g. Tallal, 2004). Deficits in the processing of rapid spectrotemporal auditory stimuli lead to the development of imprecise phonological representations. In turn, phonological processing deficits lead to difficulties in learning grammar and vocabulary in the case of SLI, and to difficulties in learning to read in the case of dyslexia. Note that the high comorbidity of SLI and dyslexia means that, in practice, there is likely to be significant overlap of these two outcome categories.

and/or dynamic auditory signals has been called into question by some. Specifically, recent findings have identified deficits in both children and adults with SLI and/or dyslexia on tasks that involve (predominantly static) *spectral* processing and that may be more robust to methodological and sample change (e.g. McArthur and Bishop, 2004; Halliday and Bishop, 2006). On the basis of these and other findings, new incarnations of auditory processing theories of LLI may need to be extended to include deficits in the processing of spectral, as well as temporal, information.

Second, in addition to questions regarding the nature of the auditory processing deficit(s) are those concerning the profile of these deficits in LLI. A recurrent challenge to any theory advocating a link between auditory processing deficits and LLI has come from those studies which have failed to find evidence of such impairments, or which have found evidence of a deficit but only in a subset of individuals (Ramus, 2003). Key to addressing this issue have been a recent spate of longitudinal studies that have tracked over time the development of auditory processing abilities of both typically developing children and those with LLI (e.g. Bishop and McArthur, 2005; Hill, Hogben, and Bishop, 2005). The picture that is emerging from these studies is one of a changing profile of auditory processing deficits in LLI with age. Indeed, according to Bishop and McArthur (2005), whether or not we find evidence for a particular deficit in auditory processing is likely to depend on both the age of the child, and the developmental trajectory of the task being assessed. This raises the possibility that a child may have had an underlying deficit in auditory processing that had nonetheless resolved by the time of testing, or that behavioural measures were no longer sufficiently sensitive to detect.

Neural basis

Given the evidence for a behavioural deficit in auditory processing in children and adults with SLI and/or dyslexia, a major question is whether this deficit can be traced at the neural level. Although still in its early days, research to date has yielded converging evidence for a significant overlap in the brain regions involved in the processing of speech and non-speech auditory signals designed to mimic the transient spectrotemporal changes of speech. Various electrophysiological and neuroimaging studies have reported similar patterns of activation to such stimuli in the left superior temporal and inferior frontal cortex—regions which, traditionally, have been associated with language processing (e.g. Zatorre and Belin, 2001). Other studies have found that these regions may show lower levels of activation to rapidly changing non-speech acoustic stimuli in individuals with LLI relative to controls (e.g. Temple et al., 2000). Together, these studies provide evidence for a shared network of rapid temporal auditory (speech and non-speech) processing within the superior temporal and inferior frontal cortex, parts of which may be disrupted in individuals with LLI.

In parallel to the literature on abnormal cortical processing is a growing body of research that points to the role of lower level, auditory pathway encoding defects in contributing to the auditory perceptual deficits associated with LLI. This research has focused on a population of children who are afflicted with some type of language-based learning problem (LP) and therefore includes children with attention deficit hyperactivity disorder and/or auditory processing disorder (see Section 15.5 below) as well as those with dyslexia and/or SLI. Findings indicate that, regardless of clinical diagnosis, many children with language-based LP show evoked auditory brainstem responses (ABRs) to the onset of speech sounds that are shallower and/or delayed relative to those of typically developing children, and which correspond to 'weaker' patterns of activation at the level of the cortex (Wible et al., 2005). Although these findings have been interpreted as reflecting abnormal coding in the region of the lateral lemniscus and/or inferior colliculus, the possibility remains that these might be traced to more peripheral (cochlear and low-brainstem; Muchnik et al., 2004) or central sources.

Intervention

The proposal that LLI may be caused by deficient auditory processing mechanisms has led to a spate of commercially available programmes offering remediation for a variety of language-based disorders. Evidence from neurophysiology suggests that the auditory system remains plastic into adulthood, with animal studies showing evidence for cortical remapping at the cellular level following intensive behavioural training (Dahmen and King, 2007). These findings therefore give rise to the possibility that training designed to improve auditory processing skills could also improve language and literacy in children with LLI. One such training programme that has received considerable attention in this regard is Fast ForWord® (Scientific Learning Corporation). In this programme children are trained, among other things, to discriminate acoustically modified speech in which rapid spectrotemporal changes are enhanced in intensity and duration. Initial findings were promising, with studies reporting marked improvements in the (rapid) auditory processing (Merzenich et al., 1996), oral (Tallal et al., 1996), and written (Temple et al., 2003) language abilities of children with SLI and/or dyslexia following training with Fast ForWord®.

Despite some positive results, however, the efficacy of Fast ForWord® has been called into question. There are now two large, randomized controlled trials, neither of which has shown a significant advantage for Fast ForWord® over a 'waiting list' control condition, or over computer-assisted-language interventions similar to Fast ForWord® but without modified speech (Cohen et al., 2005; Gillam et al., 2008). Added to this are claims that the programme fails to provide a valid test of the rate-processing constraint hypothesis. Fast ForWord® trains multiple functions including those designed to explicitly redress the grammatical and written language difficulties characteristic of LLI. This makes it difficult to isolate the specific aspect(s) of training responsible for particular outcomes.

Nevertheless, despite the shortcomings of some commercially available training programmes, studies have reported evidence for robust improvements in auditory processing abilities, particularly in adult listeners, following auditory training (e.g. Amitay *et al.*, 2006; see Chapter 13). Moreover, recent findings suggest that even quite specific auditory training may lead to more general improvements in phonological processing in typically developing children (Moore *et al.*, 2005). Together, these findings indicate that auditory learning remains an important potential tool in the quest for the remediation of auditory processing deficits in children, and is likely to yield more targeted intervention packages for language-learning impairments such as SLI and dyslexia in the not too distant future.

Controversies

In the years since it was first put forward, the rate-processing constraint hypothesis has generated considerable, and sometimes heated, debate. At least three major criticisms have been levelled. First, as outlined above, there has been a lack of replication in the field, with many studies failing to find evidence of—particularly 'rapid'—auditory processing deficits in children and adults with LLI. Moreover, where deficits have been reported they are typically only seen in about one-third of the LLI population. Second, despite early claims that deficits in auditory processing were particular to the temporal domain, it is now clear that these deficits extend to spectral processing. Although these findings do not call into question the validity of the rate-processing constraint model *per se*, they do pose a challenge to those trying to reconcile the multiple symptoms of LLI into a unifying deficit. To this extent it is becoming increasingly difficult to predict what auditory processing tasks a child with LLI might be expected to struggle with if the theory was correct. Finally, and most crucially, a number of researchers have questioned the *causal* nature of the relationship between deficits in auditory processing, language, and literacy. Critical to this argument have been those studies that have shown evidence for a dissociation between auditory processing and language development. A case in point is children with clinically significant levels of hearing loss caused by SNHL and/or OME (Sections 15.3.2 and 15.3.1, respectively), many of whom show unimpaired oral and written language acquisition despite difficulties with auditory perception. These and other findings led Rosen (2003), in a recent review, to conclude that 'auditory deficits appear not to be causally related to language disorders, but only occur in association with them' (p. 509).

Nevertheless, that both behavioural and neurological abnormalities of auditory perception appear to be over-represented in children and adults with LLI relative to the normal population does need explaining. One possibility, suggested by Bishop (2006), is that childhood deficits in auditory processing do not act in isolation, but rather increase the risk that an underlying (genetic, environmental) predisposition to LLI will be expressed in the phenotype (see 'Methodological challenges' in Section 15.3.1 for a similar account of the language difficulties seen in some children with OME). According to this model, auditory processing deficits are neither necessary nor sufficient to cause LLI. Rather, they increase the likelihood that a particular individual will go on to develop the disorder. This could account for why many children with LLI do not show evidence of auditory impairments, as well as accommodating the reported higher risk of language difficulties in children with SNHL relative to the general population (see Fig. 15.7).

Summary

An influential theory holds that LLIs such as SLI and dyslexia are caused by deficits in auditory processing, particularly of dynamic spectral and/or temporal change. A large body of behavioural and neurophysiological data supports the claims of aberrant auditory processing mechanisms in

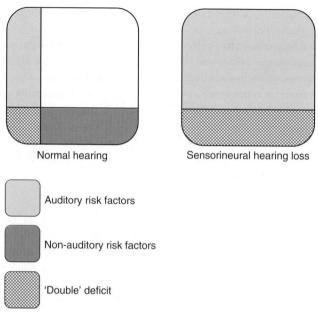

Fig. 15.7 Model of the frequency of underlying language-learning impairments in children with unimpaired hearing versus those with mild to severe sensorineural hearing loss (SNHL). Each square represents the whole population of individuals in that category. Auditory risk factors, including auditory processing deficits, only manifest as a language-learning impairment in the presence of additional (non-auditory) risk factor(s). All the SNHL group has an auditory deficit, contributing to the higher incidence of language-learning impairments in this group than in the normally hearing population. Adapted with permission from 'Developmental cognitive genetics: How psychology can inform genetics and vice versa' by Bishop (2006), *The Quarterly Journal of Experimental Psychology*, 59, p. 1162. © 2006 Taylor & Francis Ltd, http://www.informaworld.com.

LLI, at least in a subset of individuals, and at particular points during development. These findings have led to the emergence of intervention programmes which, through training individuals to discriminate the auditory contrasts relevant to speech, aim to remediate 'higher level' functions such as language and literacy. However, considerable controversy still surrounds the hypothesized link between auditory processing and language impairments. Failures to replicate and, recently, the trend for LLI to be linked with increasingly more and more deficient processes have meant that the field is running the risk of spiralling out of control, with a wealth of findings but no clear unifying concepts. Nevertheless, one model may be able to account for the body of seemingly contradictory findings, and thereby offer a way forward. This model suggests that auditory processing deficits may go on to cause LLI, but only in the presence of additional risk factors. Further research is needed to identify these additional risk factors and to understand how they, in conjunction with an auditory processing deficit, might contribute to the development of childhood LLI.

15.5 Auditory processing disorder

15.5.1 Definition

A significant proportion (estimated at 5%; Saunders and Haggard, 1989) of patients of all ages referred to audiology clinics with self-reported hearing or listening problems are found to perform within the 'normal' range, at least in one ear, on standard tests. In addition, an increasingly large number of primary school-age children (5–11 years) who, likewise, are subsequently found to be audiometrically normal are also suspected of having listening problems. Both these groups have audiometric sensitivity of better than 20 dB HL across a range of speech frequencies (250–4000 Hz). The clinical presentation is, typically, a difficulty in understanding speech in noisy and otherwise challenging environments (Keith, 2000). However, the audiological underpinnings of these problems, now known almost universally as 'auditory processing disorder' (APD) are poorly understood. There are several possibilities. The first and widely accepted hypothesis is that, while the sound detection machinery in the ear is working well, the brain processing of sound is not, either at the coding or at some higher level. One possibility is that auditory perception makes a primary contribution to higher level cognitive processing and that APD could thus impair that cognition. This theory has parallels to auditory processing theories of LLIs, although the cognitive impairments following on from APD would not necessarily be confined to the language domain. However, a second possibility is that the perceptual problems may be secondary to a higher level speech or other cognitive deficiency (Moore *et al.*, 2008b). If this is the case, the use of an additional label of APD may be misleading; the real problem may be LLI, as discussed in the previous section. Here, we might expect auditory processing deficits to be confined to those processes specifically involving speech and/or language. Finally, it is possible that the APD is a secondary consequence of a mild but subclinical peripheral dysfunction. APD has been referred to in the literature as 'central' auditory processing disorder (CAPD) but the involvement of peripheral pathology is difficult to rule out.

Because of this complexity and lack of knowledge, APD is sometimes defined negatively as impaired auditory function that is not explained by a known problem with the ear or the central auditory system. However, most researchers believe that APD has its origin in the brain, and that the question is whether it is separable from designated language (SLI, dyslexia) or other cognitive (attention deficit, autistic spectrum) problems in which auditory dysfunction has been implicated.

The American Speech, Language and Hearing Association (ASHA, 2005) and the British Society of Audiology (BSA, 2007) have defined APD primarily in terms of basic properties of auditory function, but with certain exclusions. These differ somewhat between the two organizations, but the succinct BSA definition that follows encapsulates three principles. First, that APD is due to impaired neural function; second, that it needs to be observed in impaired perception of non-speech sounds; and, third, that it is not solely due to a problem in supra- or multimodal cognition.

> APD results from impaired neural function and is characterized by poor recognition, discrimination, separation, grouping, localization, or ordering of *non-speech* sounds. It does not result *solely* from a deficit in general attention, language or other cognitive processes.
>
> (BSA, 2007)

15.5.2 Diagnosis

There is no generally agreed test profile for the clinical diagnosis of APD, other than the negative criterion outlined above. The concept of APD has, in fact, developed from clinical demand rather than from scientific principles or constructs. There are many clinical tests that purport to provide a diagnosis, of which the best known is probably the 'SCAN' (e.g. Keith, 2009). This and most other presently available APD tests are based on clinical observation and have not received full scientific validation. Many use linguistic stimuli, resulting in measures that rely on both listening and language skills. Attempts are currently underway to develop scientifically validated diagnostic tests for APD that do not use linguistic stimuli and are based on the ASHA and BSA definitions. The challenge will be to simplify test interpretation, including the integration of perceptual and cognitive data, while maintaining scientific rigour and capturing the clinical presentation.

15.5.3 **Intervention**

Because there is no generally agreed measure of APD it is currently impossible to gauge quantitatively the effectiveness of intervention programmes. However, there are two promising approaches for which indirect evidence is compelling. One type of intervention focuses on improving the listening environment for these children. Children with suspected APD are encouraged to sit near target speakers and focus their attention on the speaker in order to benefit from both auditory and visual cues. The listening environment should ideally be low noise and have low reverberation. Personal amplification systems resembling hearing aids are available for children with APD and these may help by improving signal-to-noise levels.

Auditory training has been suggested as another form of intervention for APD. A working hypothesis (Moore, 2006) is that the main underlying problem of APD is with unimodal (auditory) attention rather than with more 'bottom-up' aspects of auditory 'processing' as the name implies. In support of this proposal, recent evidence (Moore *et al.*, 2008*b*) has shown that the poor tone frequency discrimination seen in some children is usually due to poor sustained attention, with performance oscillating between age-appropriate and age-retarded over relatively short periods of time. This proposal is further corroborated by the lack of correlation, of both performance and variability, between procedurally matched visual and auditory frequency discrimination tasks by children who have a clinical diagnosis of APD (Moore *et al.*, 2008*a*). This suggests that the auditory frequency discrimination difficulties of such children are not due to impaired multimodal attention, since a generalized attention problem would be expected to produce poor performance in both modalities. Auditory training has been shown in adults to draw on both general arousal and specific auditory attention resources (Amitay *et al.*, 2006), and may thus be an effective intervention for APD. However, further research is required to draw these various observations together and to seek training-induced gains in tasks reported clinically to be indicative of poor listening, such as the perception of target sentences against a background of irrelevant speech.

15.5.4 **Summary**

A large and growing number of people are thought to have listening difficulties suggestive of APD, defined as a problem in the perception of non-speech sounds in people with normal audibility. The clinical presentation and diagnosis of APD is highly variable, but recent research suggests that it may be due more to problems of auditory attention than to problems with the sensory aspects of auditory perception. Good management of APD includes improvement of listening strategy and environment. Auditory training shows promise as another effective intervention.

15.6 **General summary**

In this chapter we have reviewed the auditory basis of language and learning impairments in childhood. Although well accepted, links between audition, language development, and academic achievement are still poorly understood. We have seen that normal auditory function plays an important role for the language learner, whose exposure to their native language comes primarily via the auditory modality. It is also clear that if unmanaged, a severe and permanent hearing loss, such as that caused by SNHL, is likely to lead to poorer language and academic outcome. However, the impact of more subtle impairments in auditory function on language and/or learning remains less certain. On the one hand, recurrent/permanent reductions in auditory sensitivity as seen in childhood OME and mild to moderate SNHL have been linked to relatively marginal (and not inevitable) impairments in language and learning. On the other hand, poorly defined deficits in 'auditory processing' have been blamed for a whole range of symptoms as diverse as deficits in reading (dyslexia), oral language (SLI), and general academic achievement (APD). It is currently unclear why some types of auditory dysfunction lead to, or, indeed, why some individuals go on to develop, particular profiles of language and/or learning disorder, although a model which sees abnormal auditory function as one of a number of risk factors is perhaps most likely to account for this heterogeneity. The challenge for researchers is to find out what these (auditory and non-auditory) risk factors are, and how to identify them in young children, so that effective interventions can be put in place.

Acknowledgements

Thanks to Dorothy Bishop for helpful comments on an earlier draft of this chapter. Thanks to Jenny Taylor for formatting the Figures in Chapter 15. Thanks also to Bronwen Evans for advising on the phonetic transcription.

References

American Speech-Language-Hearing Association (2005). *(Central) Auditory Processing Disorders—The Role of the Audiologist*. http://www.asha.org/docs/html/PS2005-00114.html [Viewed 1 June, 2007.]

American Speech-Language-Hearing Association (2007). *Type, Degree, and Configuration of Hearing Loss*. http://www.asha.org/public/hearing/disorders/types.htm [Viewed 1 June, 2007.]

Amitay, S., Irwin, A., and Moore, D. R. (2006). Discrimination learning induced by training with identical stimuli. *Nature Neuroscience* 9:1446–8.

Anderson, K. C., Brown, C. P., and Tallal, P. (1993). Developmental language disorders – evidence for a basic processing deficit. *Current Opinion in Neurology and Neurosurgery* 6:98–106.

Bennett, K. E., Haggard, M. P., Silva, P. A., and Stewart, I. A. (2001). Behaviour and developmental effects of otitis media with effusion into the teens. *Archives of Disease in Childhood* 85:91–5.

Bishop, D. V. M. (1997). *Uncommon Understanding*. Hove, E. Sussex: Psychology Press.

Bishop, D. V. M. (2006). Developmental cognitive genetics: how psychology can inform genetics and vice versa. *The Quarterly Journal of Experimental Psychology* 59:1153–68.

Bishop, D. V. M. and McArthur, G. M. (2005). Individual differences in auditory processing in specific language impairment: a follow-up study using event-related potentials and behavioural thresholds. *Cortex* 41:327–41.

Briscoe, J., Bishop, D. V. M., and Norbury, C. F. (2001). Phonological processing, language, and literacy: a comparison of children with mild-to-moderate sensorineural hearing loss and those with specific language impairment. *Journal of Child Psychology and Psychiatry* 42:329–40.

British Society of Audiology (2004). *Pure Tone Air and Bone Conduction Threshold Audiometry with and without Masking and Determination of Uncomfortable Loudness Levels*. http://www.thebsa.org.uk/docs/bsapta.doc/ [Viewed 1 June, 2007.]

British Society of Audiology (2007). *Working Definition of APD*. http://www.thebsa.org.uk/apd/Home.htm [Viewed 1 June, 2007.]

Catts, H. W. (1991). Early identification of dyslexia: evidence from a follow-up study of speech–language impaired children. *Annals of Dyslexia* 41:163–77.

Cohen, W., Hodson, A., O'Hare A., et al. (2005). Effects of computer-based intervention through acoustically modified speech (Fast ForWord) in severe mixed receptive–expressive language impairment: Outcomes from a randomized controlled trial. *Journal of Speech, Language, and Hearing Research* 48:715–29.

Connor, C. M., Craig, H. K., Raudenbush, S. W., Heaver, K., and Zwolan, T. A. (2006). The age at which young deaf children receive cochlear implants and their vocabulary and speech-production growth: is there an added value for early implantation? *Ear and Hearing* 27:628–44.

Dahmen, J. C. and King, A. J. (2007). Learning to hear: plasticity of auditory cortical processing. *Current Opinion in Neurobiology* 17:456–64.

Davis, A., Bamford, J., Ramkalawan, T., Forshaw, M., and Wright, S. (1997). *A Critical Review of the Role of Neonatal Screening in the Detection of Hearing Impairment*. Nottingham: Institute of Hearing Research.

Eapen, R. J., Buss, E. G., Grose, J. H., Drake, A. F., Dev, M., and Hall, J. W. (2008). The development of frequency weighting for speech in children with a history of otitis media with effusion. *Ear and Hearing* 29:718–24.

Eisenberg, S. (2007). Current state of knowledge: Speech recognition and production in children with hearing impairment. *Ear and Hearing* 28:766–72.

Engel, J., Anteunis, L., Volovics, A., et al. (1999). Prevalence rates of otitis media with effusion from 0 to 2 years of age: healthy-born versus high-risk infants. *International Journal of Pediatric Otorhinolaryngology* 47:243–51.

Fortnum, H. M., Summerfield, A. Q., Marshall, D. H., Davis, A. C., and Bamford, J. M. (2001). Prevalence of permanent childhood hearing impairment in the United Kingdom and implications for universal neonatal hearing screening: questionnaire based ascertainment study. *British Medical Journal* 323:536–8.

Geers, A. E. (2004). Speech, language, and reading skills after early cochlear implantation. *Archives of Otolaryngology, Head and Neck Surgery,* 130:634–8.

Gillam, R. B., Loeb, D. F., Hoffman, L. M., et al. (2008). The efficacy of Fast ForWord language intervention in school-age children with language impairment: A randomized control trial. *Journal of Speech, Language, and Hearing Research* 51:97–119.

Hall, J. W. and Grose, J. H. (1993). Short-term and long-term effects on the masking level difference following middle ear surgery. *Journal of the American Academy of Audiology* 4:307–12.

Hall, J. W., Grose, J. H., and Pillsbury, H. C. (1995). Long-term effects of chronic otitis media on binaural hearing in children. *Archives of Otolaryngology—Head and Neck Surgery* 121:847–52.

Halliday, L. F. and Bishop, D. V. M. (2006). Auditory frequency discrimination in children with dyslexia. *Journal of Research in Reading* 29:213–28.

Hansson, K., Sahlén, B., and Mäki-Torkko, E. (2007). Can a 'single hit' cause limitations in language development? A comparative study of Swedish children with hearing impairment and children with specific language impairment. *International Journal of Language and Communication Disorders* 42: 307–23.

Harris, M. and Moreno, C. (2006). Speech reading and learning to read: a comparison of 8-year-old profoundly deaf children with good and poor reading ability. *Journal of Deaf Studies and Deaf Education* 11:189–201.

Hill, P. R., Hogben, J., and Bishop, D. V. M. (2005). Auditory frequency discrimination in children with Specific Language Impairment: A longitudinal study. *Journal of Speech, Language, and Hearing Research* 48:1136–46.

Hogan, S. C. M. and Moore, D. R. (2003). Impaired binaural hearing in children produced by a threshold level of middle ear disease. *Journal of the Association for Research in Otolaryngology* 4:123–9.

Hogan, S. C. M., Stratford, K. J., and Moore, D. R. (1997). Duration and recurrence of otitis media with effusion in children from birth to 3 years: Prospective study using monthly otoscopy and tympanometry. *British Medical Journal* 314:350–3.

Jerger, S. (2007). Current state of knowledge: perceptual processing by children with hearing impairment. *Ear and Hearing* 28:754–65.

Keith, R. W. (2000). Audiology: Diagnosis, treatment strategies, and practice management. In *Diagnosing Central Auditory Processing Disorders in Children* (ed. R. Roeser, H. Hosford-Dunn, and M. Valente), pp. 337–55. New York: Thieme Medical and Scientific Publishers.

Keith, R. W. (2009). *SCAN-3C: Tests for Auditory Processing Disorders for Children*. San Antonio, TX: The Psychological Corporation.

Kyle, F. E. and Harris, M. (2006). Concurrent Correlates and Predictors of Reading and Spelling Achievement in Deaf and Hearing School Children. *Journal of Deaf Studies and Deaf Education* 11:273–88.

Leonard, L. (1989). Language learnability and specific language impairment in children. *Applied Psycholinguistics* 10:179–202.

Levelt, W. J. M. (2001). Spoken word production: a theory of lexical access. *Proceedings of the National Academy of Sciences USA* **98**:13464–71.

McArthur, G. M. and Bishop, D. V. M. (2001). Auditory perceptual processing in people with reading and oral language impairments: current issues and recommendations. *Dyslexia* **7**:150–70.

McArthur, G. M. and Bishop, D. V. M. (2004). Which people with specific language impairment have auditory processing deficits? *Cognitive Neuropsychology* **21**:79–94.

McArthur, G. M., Hogben, J. H., Edwards, V. T., Heath, S. M., and Mengler, E. D. (2000). On the 'specifics' of specific reading disability and specific language impairment. *Journal of Child Psychology and Psychiatry and Allied Disciplines* **41**:869–74.

Merzenich, M. M., Jenkins, W. M., Johnston, P., Schreiner, C., Miller, S. L., and Tallal, P. (1996). Temporal processing deficits of language-learning impaired children ameliorated by training. *Science* **271**:77–81.

Moeller, M. P., Tomblin, J. B., Yoshinaga-Itano, C., McDonald Connor, C., and Jerger, S. (2007). Current state of knowledge: Language and literacy of children with hearing impairment. *Ear and Hearing* **28**:740–53.

Moore, B. C. J. (1995). *Perceptual Consequences of Cochlear Damage*. Oxford: Oxford University Press.

Moore, D. R. (2006). Auditory processing disorder (APD): definition, diagnosis, neural basis, and intervention. *Audiological Medicine* **4**:4–11.

Moore, D. R., Rosenberg, J. F., and Coleman, J. S. (2005). Discrimination training of phonemic contrasts enhances phonological processing in mainstream school children. *Brain and Language* **94**:72–85.

Moore, D. R., Ferguson, M. A., Riley, A., and Halliday, L. F. (2008a). Auditory processing disorder (APD) in children. *Proceedings of the International Symposium on Auditory and Audiological Research*, 2007, Denmark.

Moore, D. R., Ferguson, M. A., Halliday, L. F., and Riley, A. (2008b). Frequency discrimination in children: perception, learning, and attention. *Hearing Research* **238**:147–54.

Morais, J., Cary, L., Alegria, J., and Bertelson, P. (1979). Does awareness of speech as a sequence of phones arise spontaneously? *Cognition* **7**:323–31.

Morgan, J., Meier, R. P., and Newport, E. L. (1987). Structural packaging in the input to language learning: contributions of prosodic and morphological marking of phrases to the acquisition of language. *Cognitive Psychology* **19**:498–550.

Muchnik, C., Roth, D. A. E., Othman-Jebara, R., Putter-Katz, H., Shabtai, E. L., and Hildesheimer, M. (2004). Reduced medial olivocochlear bundle system function in children with auditory processing disorders. *Audiology and Neuro-Otology* **9**:107–14.

Nittrouer, S. (2001). Challenging the notion of innate phonetic boundaries. *Journal of the Acoustical Society of America* **110**:1598–605.

Nittrouer, S. and Miller, M. E. (1997). Predicting developmental shifts in perceptual weighting schemes. *Journal of the Acoustical Society of America* **101**:2253–66.

Norbury, C. F., Bishop, D. V. M., and Briscoe, J. (2001). Production of verb morphology: a comparison of SLI and moderate hearing impairment. *Journal of Speech, Language and Hearing Research* **44**:165–78.

Ramus, F. (2003). Developmental dyslexia: Specific phonological deficit or general sensorimotor dysfunction? *Current Opinion in Neurobiology* **13**:212–8.

Roberts, J. E., Hunter, L., Gravel, J., et al. (2004). Otitis media, hearing loss, and language learning: controversies and current research. *Journal of Developmental and Behavioral Pediatrics* **25**:1–13.

Rosen, S. (2003). Auditory processing in dyslexia and specific language impairment: is there a deficit? What is its nature? Does it explain anything? *Journal of Phonetics* **31**:509–27.

Rosenfeld, R. M. and Bluestone, C. D. (2003). *Evidence Based Otitis Media*. Hamilton, Ontario: B.C. Decker.

Rvachew, S., Mattock, K., Polka, L., and Menard, L. (2006). Developmental and cross-linguistic variation in the infant vowel space: The case of Canadian English and Canadian French. *Journal of the Acoustic Society of America* **120**:2250–9.

Sanes, D. H., Reh, T. A., and Harris, W. A. (2006). *Development of the Nervous System* (2nd edn). Amsterdam: Academic Press.

Saunders, G. H. and Haggard, M. P. (1989) The clinical assessment of obscure auditory dysfunction—1. Auditory and psychological factors. *Ear and Hearing* 10:200–8.

Schick, B., Marschark, M., and Spencer, P. E. (eds) (2006). *Advances in the Sign Language Development of Deaf Children*. New York: Oxford University Press.

Seidenberg, M. S. and McClelland, J. (1989). A distributed, developmental model of word recognition. *Psychological Review* 96:523–68.

Snowling, M. J. (2000). *Dyslexia*. Oxford: Blackwell Publ.

Sterne, A. and Goswami, U. (2000). Phonological awareness of syllables, rhymes, and phonemes in deaf children. *Journal of Child Psychology and Psychiatry* 41:609–25.

Tallal, P. (1980). Auditory temporal perception, phonics, and reading disabilities in children. *Brain and Language* 9:182–98.

Tallal, P. (2004). Improving language and literacy is a matter of time. *Nature Reviews Neuroscience* 5:721–8.

Tallal, P., Miller, S. L., Bedi, G., et al. (1996). Language comprehension in language-learning impaired children improved with acoustically modified speech. *Science* 271:81–4.

Temple, E., Poldrack, R. A., Protopapas, A., et al. (2000). Disruption of the neural response to rapid acoustic stimuli in dyslexia: evidence from functional MRI. *Proceedings of the National Academy of Sciences USA* 97:13907–12.

Temple, E., Deutsch, G. K., Poldrack, R. A., et al. (2003). Neural deficits in children with dyslexia ameliorated by behavioral remediation: evidence from fMRI. *Proceedings of the National Academy of Sciences USA* 100:2860–5.

Tomblin, J. B., Smith, E., and Zhang, X. (1997). Epidemiology of specific language impairment: prenatal and perinatal risk factors. *Journal of Communication Disorders* 30:325–44.

Tomblin, J. B., Spencer, L., Flock, S., Tyler, R., and Gantz, B. (1999). A comparison of language achievement in children with cochlear implants and children using hearing aids. *Journal of Speech, Language, and Hearing Research* 42:497–511.

Wake, M., Tobin, S., Cone-Wesson, B., et al. (2006). Slight/mild sensorineural hearing loss in children. *Pediatrics* 118:1842–51.

Werker, J. and Tees, R. C. (1999). Influences on infant speech processing: Toward a new synthesis. *Annual Review of Psychology* 50:509–35.

Werner, L. A. and Gray, L. (1998). Behavioural studies of hearing development. In *Development of the Auditory System. Volume 5, Springer Handbook of Auditory Research* (ed. E. W. Rubel, A. N. Popper, and R. R. Fay), pp. 12–79. New York: Springer-Verlag.

Wible, B., Nicol, T., and Kraus, N. (2005). Correlation between brainstem and cortical auditory processes in normal and language-impaired children. *Brain* 128:417–23.

Wilmington, D., Gray, L., and Jahrsdoerfer, R. (1994). Binaural processing after corrected congenital unilateral conductive hearing-loss. *Hearing Research* 74:99–114.

Zatorre, R. J. and Belin, P. (2001). Spectral and temporal processing in human auditory cortex. *Cerebral Cortex* 11:946–53.

Chapter 16

The acoustic environment

William J. Davies

16.1 Introduction

This chapter gives an overview of what shapes the acoustic signals that arrive at the ear. It is structured as an account of the journey of a sound wave, from first generation, then propagation outdoors, followed by transmission into a building and indoor reverberation to its final reception, perception, and assessment. In doing so, I seek to shed some light on such questions as, How are the signals that arrive at the ear generated? How does the environment around us influence the characteristics of these signals? How is sound in the environment perceived, controlled, and assessed? Information is given on basic principles, common measurements and current modelling techniques.

16.2 Sound sources

There are three physical processes which are capable of generating audible sound: a vibrating surface, a turbulent fluid, and a rapid pressure change. A loudspeaker diaphragm, the body of a guitar, and the casing of a machine are examples of vibrating surfaces. As the surface moves back and forth, the medium in contact with it is 'pushed' and 'pulled' and regions of increased and decreased pressure are created which propagate through the medium as a sound wave. A jet engine and a hairdryer are examples of turbulent sound sources. These create sound by bringing high-velocity air into contact with stationary air. At the interface, mixing takes place and turbulence is created. The turbulence is characterized by pressure changes which are propagated through the air and can be heard as sound. The final generation mechanism is a rapid pressure change, sometimes caused by rapid local heating of the air, such as thunder or an explosion. This creates a sudden local increase in pressure followed by a decrease, and the resulting impulse propagates through the air.

16.2.1 Spectra

Real sound sources of interest are often composed of several instances of the basic types mentioned above and are usually extremely complex. For example, vehicle noise is an important source in the outdoor environment. The noise of a car or lorry is composed of engine noise, road/tyre interaction, and air turbulence as the vehicle passes. At low speeds, engine noise predominates, while at high speeds, the tyre/road interaction is often the most significant. The engine noise can itself be broken down into several sources: inlet, exhaust, engine wall vibration, gearbox vibration, and transmission vibration. For railways, there is a similar mix of engine noise, rail noise, and turbulence. A typical measured spectrum of motorway traffic is shown in Fig. 16.1. Peaks around 80 Hz, due to engine noise, and 1 kHz, due to tyre/road noise, can be seen.

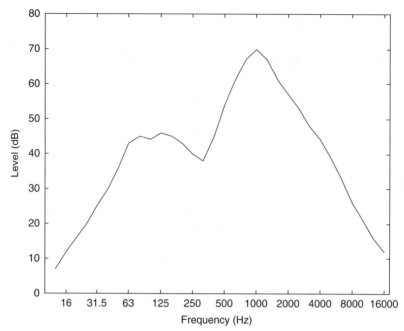

Fig. 16.1 Motorway traffic noise $L_{eq,5\,min}$ measured 100 m from the carriageway.

The constituent source parts of complex machines like cars have, in general, been researched quite thoroughly and in some cases numerical models are available to predict their acoustic characteristics. From the point of view of the designer, however, while it is usually possible to visualize what a complete machine will look like before it is made, listening to it is another matter. In order to hear, or 'auralize' a design, computational models of all the constituent mechanical parts must be developed and then combined. This goal is sometimes called 'virtual acoustic prototyping' (VAP; Moorhouse, 2005). Considerable effort is required to characterize all the many excitation and transmission mechanisms of even quite simple machines, and investigate the transfer functions that connect them. Most numerical models produce a magnitude–frequency spectrum, so producing temporal signals to listen to involves generating a phase spectrum. The current generation of VAPs assume that phase is of second-order importance and simply randomize phase, perhaps followed by time-domain shaping. Research continues to develop phase models, particularly for transient sounds. In most machines there are also active components and some nonlinear transfers, for which models do not usually exist. Current virtual acoustic prototypes therefore usually incorporate a mixture of simulated and measured data. While the ultimate goal is complete simulation, this mixture does enable the effect of several possible design decisions to be quickly heard, and so the technique is becoming more common. An example of the output of a mixed VAP of a washing machine is shown in Fig. 16.2.

Of course, the contemporary acoustic environment may not just be dominated by noisy mechanical devices. The music of others may be a problem as well. As the availability of powerful amplifiers grows, music is becoming a more prevalent source type in many environments. There are important differences between sounds, often described as noise and music. Individual musical notes are usually harmonic or pseudoharmonic; that is, they are composed of a fundamental and several harmonic frequencies at integer multiples of the fundamental.

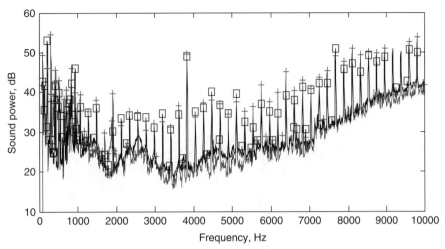

Fig. 16.2 Comparison of measured (black) and predicted (blue) sound power level for a washing machine with an unloaded motor. (After Moorhouse, 2005.)

Harmonicity in the frequency domain implies periodicity in the time domain and vice versa. Hence, a Fourier series can be used as a simple model of a musical note, according to eqn 16.1.

$$x(t) = A_0 + \sum_{n=1}^{\infty} A_n e^{j2n\pi f_1 t} \tag{16.1}$$

where A_n is the complex amplitude of the nth harmonic with a frequency n times the fundamental frequency, f_1, and j is the square root of -1.

By altering the relative amplitudes of the harmonics we can create different musical timbres. Real musical notes usually deviate from this simple additive synthesis in several ways. For example, Fig. 16.3 shows the spectrum of a piano note. In fact, the frequency components are not exact harmonics—these pseudoharmonics are usually referred to as 'partials'. The higher order partials are progressively higher (sharper) than a true harmonic. This is one of the characteristics that make a piano recognizable as a piano.

There is a large literature concerned with modelling musical instruments and the sounds they produce (Roads, 1996). Simple methods such as additive and subtractive synthesis are often motivated by a desire to synthesize sounds for musical performance or recordings. The several variants of additive synthesis are all based on eqn 16.1, while subtractive synthesis is essentially a filtering process. On the other hand, musical instruments have been studied as physical systems for longer than acoustics has existed as a separate discipline, and there are now several numerical and analytical models available for most common classes of pseudoharmonic instruments (Smith, 2004). The rapid growth in computer processing power has led to the two subfields of musical synthesis and the physics of musical instruments converging somewhat. This is represented by recent physical instrument models which are used to produce realistic sound. Interestingly, one still has to learn to control (play) a successful physical model of an instrument!

In the everyday environment, it is not usually single notes from a single musical instrument that we are exposed to. The spectrum of amplified music is shaped by the frequency response characteristics of the equipment that it is played through, but it is possible to identify characteristic

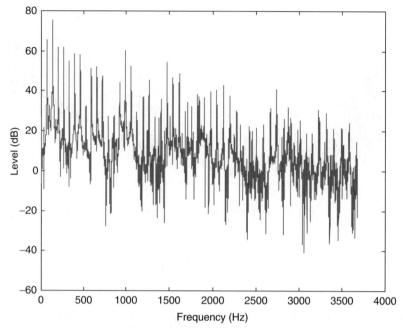

Fig. 16.3 Spectrum of a low-C piano note.

spectra of different types of music. Indeed, spectral variation during a piece is one of the features that can be used to classify music by genre. If we look at the average spectrum over a whole song or movement, though, a striking similarity appears. Figure 16.4 shows some time-averaged spectra of common genres. This shape appears to be very widespread. Several authors have found *1/f* spectra in music (Voss and Clarke, 1975), other sounds (De Coensel *et al.*, 2003), and even paintings (Alvarez-Ramirez *et al.*, 2008).

16.2.2 Temporal characteristics

Looking at the frequency spectrum of a source seems a natural way of studying a sound source (perhaps because of the ear's role as a frequency analyser). However, sources and signals have other important characteristics in other domains. The properties of a signal in the time domain contain many important cues. For example, the simple additive synthesis of eqn 16.1 fails to produce subjectively realistic musical notes partly because the output is steady-state. Real musical sounds have complex time histories. In musical synthesis, these are often usefully simplified using an amplitude envelope which can be used as a gain function for a Fourier series. For example, Fig. 16.5 shows the time history of the piano note from Fig. 16.3.

The time history *x(t)* of a source is related to its frequency spectrum *X(ω)* by the Fourier Transform pair:

$$X(\omega) = \int_{-\infty}^{\infty} x(t)e^{-j\omega t} dt$$

$$x(t) = \frac{1}{2\pi} \int_{-\infty}^{\infty} X(\omega)e^{j\omega t} d\omega \qquad (16.2)$$

where *ω* is the radial frequency and equals the natural frequency *f* multiplied by 2π.

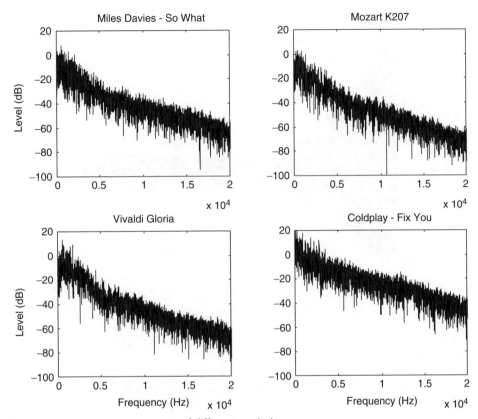

Fig. 16.4 Long-term average spectra of different musical genres.

16.2.3 Directivity

Another important characteristic of a sound source is its directivity—that is, the spatial directions in which it radiates sound. The simplest and widely used models of source directivity are those of the point and line sources. A point source can be thought of as a small pulsating sphere. We assume that it radiates sound equally in all directions, so it will generate spherical wavefronts centred on itself. This allows us to say something about the strength of the sound field generated. If the source has an acoustic power of W watts then it generates W joules of energy per second. This acoustic energy will be evenly distributed over the surface of the expanding spherical wavefront. The intensity of the sound field is defined by the power of the source divided by the area over which it radiates, so at a distance r from the source, the intensity is given by:

$$I = \frac{W}{4\pi r^2} \tag{16.3}$$

This inverse square relationship for a point source is often expressed in decibel form, where it becomes:

$$L_I = L_W - 20\log_{10}(r) - 11 \tag{16.4}$$

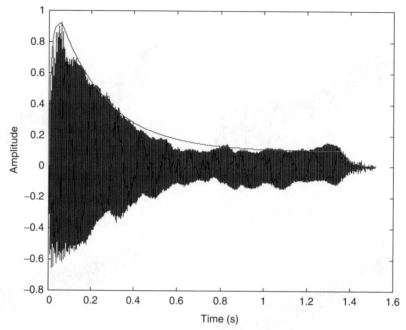

Fig. 16.5 Time history of the piano note in Fig. 16.3. A simple exponential attack–decay–release envelope is superimposed.

where L_I is the sound intensity level, and where L_W is the sound power level, defined thus:

$$L_I = 10\log_{10}\left(\frac{I}{10^{-12}}\right)$$

$$L_W = 10\log_{10}\left(\frac{W}{10^{-12}}\right) \tag{16.5}$$

Equation 16.4 indicates that a point source should produce a sound level which drops by 6 dB for each doubling of distance r away from the source. The point source model is often used as the default approximation in environmental noise problems where it works surprisingly well, as long as r and the wavelength are large compared with the real dimensions of the source.

The other common simple directivity model is a line source. This can be thought of as an infinitely long vibrating wire, radiating sound radially. If the radiation is radially even, then cylindrical wavefronts are generated. Proceeding in the same way as for the point source, we see that the intensity per unit length of the source is:

$$I = \frac{W}{2\pi r} \tag{16.6}$$

and the intensity level is given by:

$$L_I = L_W - 10\log_{10}(r) - 8 \tag{16.7}$$

Note that eqn 16.7 indicates that we expect a drop of 3 dB per doubling of r, in contrast with a point source. Line source models are often used for free-flowing traffic on a road.

Of course, real sources do not usually radiate sound perfectly evenly in all directions. (Although we might still expect to find a 6-dB per distance doubling in a particular direction.) In particular, source directivity is usually a function of frequency. Most sources become more directional at high frequencies. For example, a single loudspeaker set into a plane is often modelled as a vibrating circular piston. The piston radiates acoustic pressure in front of it, and the way in which the pressure varies with angle is expressed by a directivity function. It can be shown that the directivity function D for a rigid circular piston of radius a in an infinite baffle is given by:

$$D = \frac{2J_1(ka\sin\theta)}{ka\sin\theta} \qquad (16.8)$$

where a is the radius of the piston, k is the wave number of the radiated sound and is equal to ω/c, and J_1 means a Bessel function of the first kind. Figure 16.6 plots the directivity in decibels for increasing ka. At low frequencies, the sound source is omnidirectional, radiating evenly over all angles. As ka increases, the sound energy is confined into a narrower beam or lobe. As the frequency is increased still further, the main lobe becomes narrower but increasing numbers of side lobes develop.

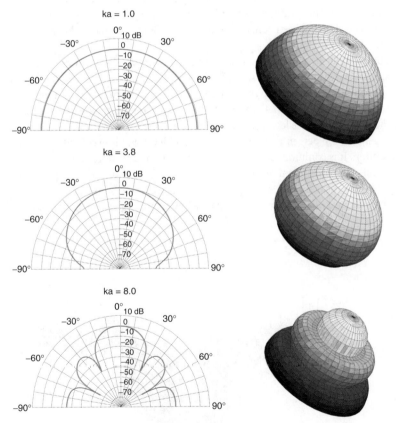

Fig. 16.6 Directivity plots of a piston set into a large plane (baffle). These model the variation of intensity level with angle in front of a single loudspeaker. The left column shows a polar plot of intensity level in dB against angle, while the right column shows a three-dimensional directivity 'balloon'. For a given size a of loudspeaker, ka increases with frequency. The sound field becomes increasingly directional as ka increases. (For a loudspeaker of radius 10 cm, the frequencies corresponding to the three values of ka shown here are 546, 2074, and 4367 Hz.)

Analytical models of directivity exist for most types of loudspeaker and some other simple sound sources. Many real environmental noise sources, such as vehicles, contain many radiating components, each with their own directivity. The resulting radiation pattern is sufficiently complicated that measurements are usually preferred to models.

16.2.4 Amplitude domain

The fourth and last basic characteristic of sources and signals is their amplitude distribution. We have already noted that, in contrast to many synthesized sounds, real sounds tend to vary over time. One way of distinguishing different signals and their impact on us is to ask questions about the range and probability of different amplitude values. Figure 16.7 shows the time history of the sound level ($5\,\mathrm{s}\,L_{Aeq}$) from a location close to a busy road over 24 hours. We can see clear variations in level at different times of day. Levels are lower but with more variation during the night. There are a small number of isolated peaks, but rush-hour traffic gives a small range of about 70–80 dB.

Figure 16.7 shows us the range of sound level values. But this is just the most basic statistic of the amplitude distribution. If we divide up this amplitude range into equal bins, and then sample the amplitude of Fig. 16.7 at regular short intervals, we can obtain a view of this signal in the amplitude domain. This has been done in Fig. 16.8 and scaled to give the probability and cumulative density functions of the signal.

The probability density function shows us the distribution of amplitude values. The data in Fig. 16.8 are not a symmetrical Gaussian distribution. Instead, the dominant traffic noise gives a lop-sided distribution, with a sharp modal peak at 76.1 dB. The much wider range of night-time levels gives the long low tail from 45 to 65 dB. (Rather different shapes would appear if we examined just the night-time noise levels.). The cumulative density function allows us to calculate percentiles. In general, the percentile level L_n is the sound level that is exceeded for n per cent of the analysis duration. It is common to pay particular attention to the more extreme ends of the distribution: L_{10} and L_{90} (and sometimes L_1 and L_{99}). Procedures for evaluating environmental noise often require some measure of the background sound level and also of the disturbing noise level. To avoid the influence of a single unrepresentative low or high value, we do not usually simply use

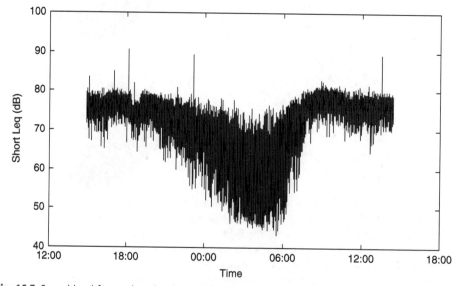

Fig. 16.7 Sound level from a location in Manchester.

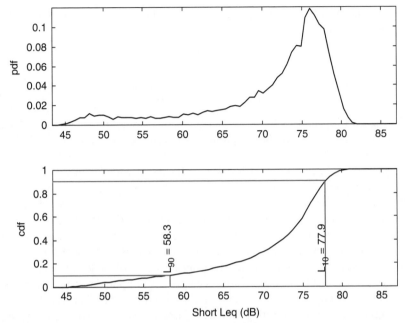

Fig. 16.8 Probability density function and cumulative density function of the sound level from a location in Manchester.

the maximum and minimum levels recorded. (Only three of the 16 944 sound levels in Fig. 16.7 are above 89 dB.) Instead, L_{90} is often used as a proxy for background level and L_{10} is often used to rate traffic (Department of Transport and Welsh Office, 1988) because it has been found to correlate well with community response (variously measured as annoyance, disturbance, or perceived noisiness).

16.3 **Transmission outdoors**

The simple models of a point and line source discussed above assume that the source radiates into free space. While there are some environments that approach this, in most cases there will be surfaces or obstacles which alter the acoustic signal on its way to the receiver.

16.3.1 **Ground effects**

The simplest situation is a single source and receiver above an empty hard plane. In this case, we can modify the point source model introduced above. The sound will reflect at the ground with no loss of amplitude. From the point of view of the receiver, it is as if there are now two sources: the real one above the ground, and a virtual source which is the acoustic mirror image of the real one reflected in the ground. Figure 16.9 illustrates this.

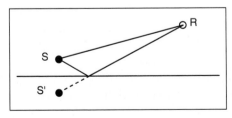

Fig. 16.9 A point source, S, is mirrored by a hard-ground plane.

The real source now radiates into a hemisphere, a solid angle of 2π steradians. This alters eqns 16.3 and 16.4 thus:

$$I = \frac{W}{2\pi r^2} \qquad (16.9)$$

$$L_I = L_W - 20\log_{10}(r) - 8 \qquad (16.10)$$

Comparing eqns 16.4 and 16.10 we see that changing from a completely absorbent-ground plane (no reflection) to a completely hard ground (perfect reflection) has increased the level at the receiver by 3 dB.

While some environments are modelled well by the hard-ground plane, in many others the ground is neither a perfect reflector nor a perfect absorber. In these cases it may be sufficient to adopt eqn 16.4 with a ground correction interpolated between 0 and 3 dB according to the percentage of ground between source and receiver that is assumed to be soft (BS5228-1, 1997). Where more accuracy is needed, we must take into account the fact that the impedance of the ground is likely to vary with frequency. In fact, real ground is often composed of more than one layer, each with different acoustic properties. Because a direct measurement of the acoustic impedance of real ground outdoors is difficult, calculations are often based on computational models of impedance adjusted to fit measured sound pressure levels (Attenborough, 1992). In particular, long-range propagation is often predicted by fitting a model to measurements made over a short range.

The effect of the ground on the sound level at the receiver is often presented as excess attenuation. This is the difference between the measured level at the receiver and that which would be obtained in a free field. It is usually normalized to remove the effect of spherical spreading (the $20\log_{10}(r)$ term). Figure 16.10 shows the measured excess attenuation for a single point source propagating over grassland to a receiver. The main feature is the strong attenuation just above

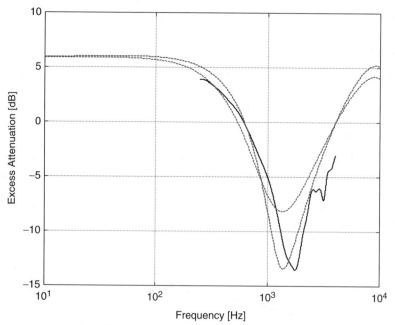

Fig. 16.10 Measured excess attenuation over long grass (black), compared to prediction models from Delany and Bazley (1970; red) and Attenborough (1992; blue).

1 kHz due to destructive interference of the incident and reflected waves. Further dips will occur at multiples of the first frequency. Predictions from two simple models are also shown. Delany and Bazley (1970) assume that the ground is a single homogeneous layer of infinite thickness where the porosity (and hence impedance) is constant with depth. Attenborough's hard-backed layer impedance two-parameter model, named '2PA' (Attenborough, 1992), allows the porosity to vary with depth and fits the measured data slightly better in this case.

16.3.2 Air absorption

As well as ground attenuation, sound waves also lose energy from propagating through air. This process is additional to the effective attenuation due to spherical spreading accounted for in eqns 16.3 and 16.9. Air attenuation is due to heat losses as the sound wave passes from molecule to molecule. It depends on atmospheric pressure, humidity, temperature, and frequency. Figure 16.11 plots an empirical expression for the attenuation due to Bass *et al.* (1995). Note that the attenuation rises logarithmically with frequency, so that, for 40% relative humidity and 20 °C, it is only 0.04 dB/100 m at 100 Hz, but rises to 19.3 dB/100 m at 10 kHz. We can therefore expect environmental sounds to experience a low-pass filter effect as they travel increasing distance through the air. This of course explains why the hiss of tyres on a wet motorway becomes a dull hum at a distance of a couple of kilometres.

16.3.3 Multiple reflections

In urban locations, there are often many reflections arriving at the receiver from each sound source. In particular, where a street is lined by tall buildings, multiple reflections between building

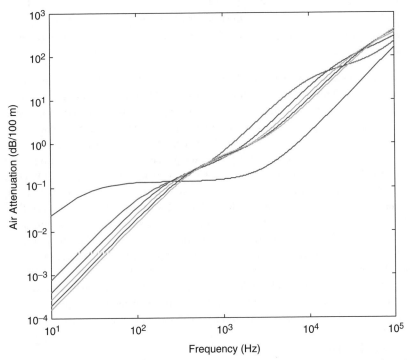

Fig. 16.11 Attenuation due to atmospheric absorption, for every 100 m travelled, as a function of relative humidity: blue, 0%; dark green, 20%; red, 40%; cyan, 60%; magenta, 80%; light green, 100%. Atmospheric pressure is standard (10^5 Pa) and temperature is 20 °C.

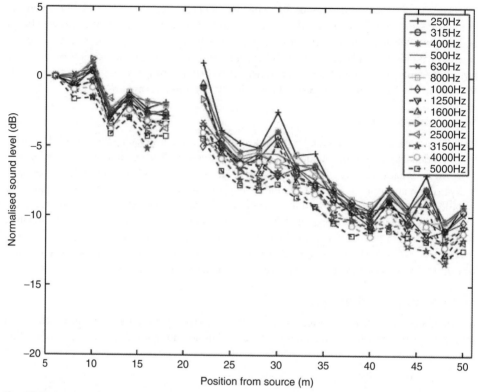

Fig. 16.12 Measured sound propagation curves along a narrow street as a function of frequency. (After Picaut *et al.*, 2005.)

facades produce a kind of reverberation. This urban canyon effect is like a room or corridor with an absorbent ceiling. The parameter of interest is usually the change in sound pressure level with distance, sometimes called the 'sound propagation curve'. In a free field, eqn 16.4, we expect a drop of 6 dB per doubling of distance. In a truly diffuse indoor reverberant field, eqn 16.22, we expect the sound level to be constant with distance away from the source. Street canyons are examples of disproportionate reflective spaces which produce a sound propagation curve somewhere between these two extremes. Figure 16.12 shows some measured examples. Other examples of disproportionate spaces which exhibit similar characteristics are corridors and underground railway platforms (one-dimensional) and large, flat factories (two-dimensional). In these cases, successful numerical models are adapted from room acoustics and consider the corpus of energy contained in the build-up of multiple reflections, the reverberation. The simplest model is an extension of the image source diagram in Fig. 16.9. This predicts all the reflections between two street facades, but assumes geometric reflection. Many real street surfaces scatter significant amounts of sound energy, so a model which takes this into account is often more successful. Kang (2000) has developed a radiosity model for street canyons which allows for a proportion of sound energy to be scattered on every reflection and has been shown to match measured data well.

16.3.4 Noise barriers

Sound radiating outdoors often encounters an obstacle or barrier on its way to the receiver. Unless the object is much smaller than the wavelength, diffraction will occur at the edges. The simplest

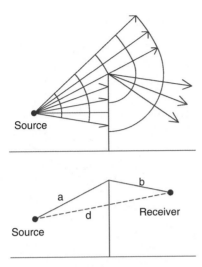

Fig. 16.13 Geometry for Maekawa's barrier attenuation model.

and most widely used treatment of this is due to Maekawa (1968) who contributed a model of the sound field around a single thin barrier, based on Fresnel diffraction. This model is two-dimensional as shown in Fig. 16.13.

The effect of a barrier is usually given in terms of insertion loss—the drop in sound pressure level at the receiver when the barrier is introduced. Maekawa's model for insertion loss is:

$$IL = 10\log_{10}\left(3 + 20N\right) \tag{16.11}$$

where the Fresnel number N is given by:

$$N = \frac{2\left(a + b - d\right)}{\lambda} \tag{16.12}$$

where the letters refer to Fig. 16.13.

Figure 16.14 plots the insertion loss against frequency for various values of path-length difference $(a + b - d)$, and we see that the barrier acts as a low-pass filter. Maekawa's model is widely used in environmental noise standards for prediction and assessment. Sometimes it is simplified further by assuming a source spectrum and giving the barrier attenuation in terms of an A-weighted loss (BS5228-1, 1997; Department of Transport, 1995).

Some real barriers do not conform very well to the assumptions in Maekawa's model of a thin, single, infinitely wide simple barrier. It is possible to apply the method to a finite thin barrier by predicting diffracted sound around the three free edges—top, left, and right—and then summing the signals as incoherent sources at the receiver. However, this has been shown to overpredict insertion loss by up to 10 dB (Takagi, 1990). Similarly, many different profiles have been suggested for barriers, and some examples are shown in Fig. 16.15. These can be approximated by a Maekawa barrier but, again, the error can be 10 dB. An exact analytical model exists for some particular barrier profiles but these are not easy to generalize and so have limited application.

A better way to predict insertion loss for complicated barrier profiles is offered by the boundary element method (BEM). This is a numerical solution of the Helmholtz–Kirchhoff integral equation which describes exactly the interaction of a sound field with a solid body. In general, the method can be used either for interior problems (a room, for example) or exterior problems such

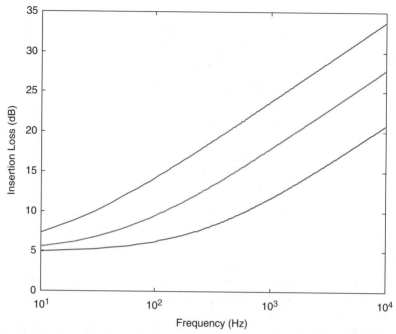

Fig. 16.14 Insertion loss of a single simple barrier as a function of path length difference ($a+b-d$): blue line, 0.1 m; green line, 0.5 m; red line, 2 m. (After Maekawa, 1968.)

as a sound wave scattering from a barrier. The general geometry for the BEM is shown in Fig. 16.16. The pressure $P(r)$ for one point source is given by:

$$\int_S P(\underline{r}_s)\nabla G(\underline{r},\underline{r}_s).\underline{n}_s(\underline{r}_s)\,dS + P_i(\underline{r},\underline{r}_0) = \begin{array}{ll} P(\underline{r}) & \underline{r}\in\Omega \\ \frac{1}{2}P(\underline{r}) & \underline{r}\in S \\ 0 & \underline{r}\in\Omega_0 \end{array} \tag{16.13}$$

where $P_i(\underline{r},\underline{r}_0)$ is the sound pressure direct from the source; $\underline{n}_s(\underline{r}_s)$ the outward pointing unit vector normal to the surface at $\underline{r}_s$, and $G(\underline{r},\underline{r}_s)$ the Green's function. The Green's function is the standard two-dimensional form:

$$G(\underline{r},\underline{r}_s) = -\frac{i}{4}[\,H_0^{(1)}(k\,|\underline{r}-\underline{r}_s|) + H_0^{(1)}(k\,|\underline{r}-\underline{r}_s'|)\,] \tag{16.14}$$

where $H_0^{(1)}(x)$ is the Hankel function of the first kind of order zero.

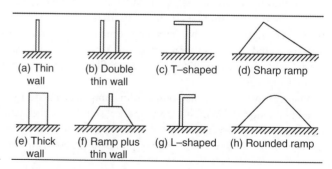

Fig. 16.15 Some barrier profiles.

(a) Thin wall
(b) Double thin wall
(c) T-shaped
(d) Sharp ramp
(e) Thick wall
(f) Ramp plus thin wall
(g) L-shaped
(h) Rounded ramp

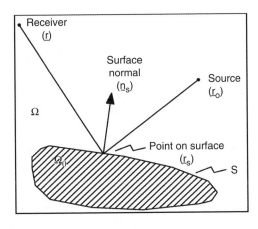

Fig. 16.16 BEM geometry and vectors.

The BEM solution technique involves first subdividing the surface into a set of elements across which the pressure is assumed constant. Once the surface is subdivided the calculation proceeds in two steps: first an evaluation of the surface pressures is made via simultaneous equations; then the pressures at the external receiver positions are calculated by a simple surface integral. Extension of the BEM to a three-dimensional barrier is straightforward, but the significant increase in the number of elements may make the calculation time impractical.

The BEM can be used as a tool to make empirical explorations of the attenuation spectra of many different barrier profiles. An example of a novel barrier profile prediction is shown in Fig. 16.17. This shape is an attempt to design a barrier with better low-frequency attenuation than the standard shapes. It was inspired by the low-frequency attenuation observed in many concert halls when sound grazes over the multiple edges of rows of seats (Davies, 2002).

16.4 **Transmission indoors**

We now move indoors. As sound generated outdoors passes through the envelope of a building it passes through a wall, door, or window. How does this affect its characteristics? The sound insulation of a wall is first described in terms of its intensity transmission coefficient, τ, which is the ratio of acoustic intensity transmitted through the wall to the incident intensity. It is usually more convenient to use the logarithmic form of this, the sound reduction index:

$$R = 10\log_{10}\left(\frac{1}{\tau}\right)$$ (16.15)

For a single-skin partition (wall or window) there is a useful model which results in an equation for R commonly called the 'Mass Law':

$$R = 20\log_{10}(Mf) - 48$$ (16.16)

where M is the surface density of the partition, in kg m^{-2}, and f is frequency.

Equation 16.16 predicts that sound insulation will improve by 6 dB per octave as frequency rises. Straightaway, this explains our common experience of walls reducing high-frequency levels while transmitting most of the low-frequency energy. (This may be why the bass drum of our neighbour's rock music is so annoying.) It also explains why massive walls give better sound insulation than lightweight partitions.

In practice, we find that the Mass Law is only an approximation to some quite complicated wave mechanics. The performance of a single-leaf partition approaches that predicted by the

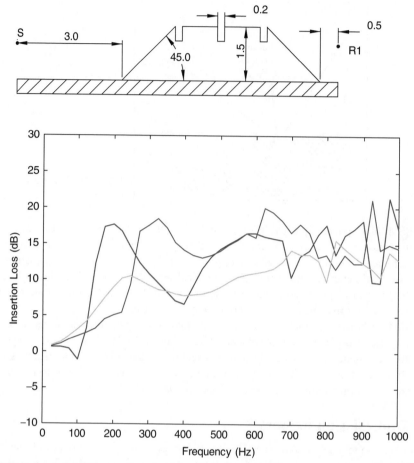

Fig. 16.17 A 'broadband' barrier insertion loss predicted with the BEM. The parameter is the depth of trench cut into the top of the bund: cyan, no trench; red, 0.2 m deep; blue, 0.5 m.

Mass Law over a finite frequency range. The main deviations from ideal Mass Law behaviour come from (1) coincidence, and (2) panel resonances.

Both effects result from the fact that the incident sound wave in air sets up travelling waves inside the wall. Coincidence occurs when the wavelength of the incident sound in air matches the wavelength of the bending wave in the partition. When this happens, the impedance of the wall is lowered, transmission will be efficient and R will be reduced. The critical frequency at which this occurs is given by:

$$f_c = \frac{c^2}{2\pi}\sqrt{\frac{12M\left(1-v^2\right)}{Eh^3}} \tag{16.17}$$

where M is the mass per unit area of the panel (or surface density) (kg m^{-2}), v is Poisson's ratio, E is Young's modulus and h the wall thickness.

Above f_c R increases again, but typically does not reach Mass Law values. One design response to this might be to build a lightweight partition, so that the coincidence dip is at a high frequency. Mass Law reduction is then achieved below the dip.

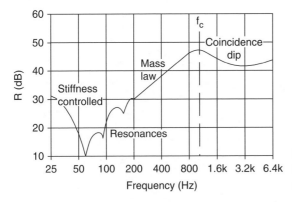

Fig. 16.18 Sound reduction index of a typical finite single-leaf partition.

There is also a low-frequency limit on Mass Law performance: the resonant modes of a finite stiff panel. We have already seen that sound impinging on the partition gives rise to bending waves travelling within it. In a finite partition, these waves will be reflected from the edges. Interference between incident and reflected bending waves produces standing waves, giving rise to increased motion of the panel at these frequencies, and hence a reduced sound reduction index. It can be shown (by analysing the vibration of a rectangular plate model) that the resonant frequencies at which this happens are given by:

$$f_{mn} = \frac{\pi}{2}\sqrt{\left(\frac{B}{M}\right)\left(\left(\frac{m}{L_x}\right)^2 + \left(\frac{n}{L_y}\right)^2\right)}$$

(16.18)

where B is the bending stiffness of the panel (N m^{-2}), m and n are integers (1,2,3, ...), and L_x and L_y are the panel dimensions (metres).

The bending stiffness is given by:

$$B = \frac{Yh^3}{12(1-v^2)}$$

(16.19)

Most energy is radiated in the (1, 1) mode. These resonances typically have an effect on the SRI at low frequencies.

The finite panel resonances and coincidence frequencies act to limit the Mass Law range in the manner of Fig. 16.18. Like the noise barrier, we see that a wall, window, or door is roughly another low-pass filter, attenuating high-frequency sound while letting lower frequencies through.

16.4.1 Multiple-leaf partitions

Equation 16.16 indicates that better sound insulation should result from increasing the density or thickness of a single partition. In practice, this is not a very efficient strategy, for two reasons: firstly, the increase is only 6 dB for each doubling of surface density and secondly, increasing M increases the fundamental panel resonance f_{11} and lowers the coincidence frequency f_c thus reducing the frequency range of good Mass Law insulation. More efficient acoustic (and thermal) insulation can be achieved by lightweight double- or triple-leaf partitions and so these are common building elements. In a double-leaf construction, the partition is constructed from two panels in parallel with each other, separated by an air gap. Here we exploit the impedance mismatch of the air–panel–air–panel–air system to achieve a good sound reduction index. With this more complicated system, performance is harder to predict than for a single panel (Fahy, 1985),

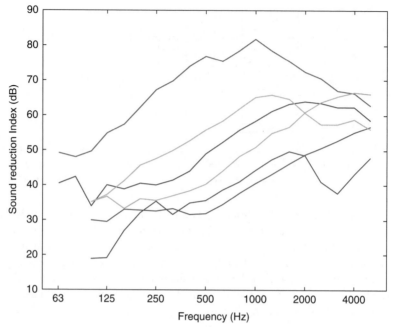

Fig. 16.19 Measured sound reduction index of some common wall constructions. Red line: lightweight blockwork wall pointed both sides; cyan line: lightweight blockwork wall pointed and plastered both sides; blue line: 100-mm brick + 127-mm cavity with 50-mm fibreglass (100 kg m^{-3}) + 100-mm brick; dark green line: 330-mm blockwork + 70-mm cavity with 50-mm fibreglass + 330-mm blockwork; magenta line: 12.5-mm plasterboard (11 kg m^{-2}) either side of 70-mm stud (wood), 30-mm 16 kg m^{-2} acoustic blanket in cavity; light green line: two layers of 15-mm plasterboard (12.5 kg m^{-2}) with 540-mm cavity.

and insulation is usually measured. An example of the measured SRI for some double partitions is shown in Fig. 16.19.

The frequency range can be divided as follows:

- At very low frequencies, the two leaves move together, and the transmission loss is equivalent to that of a single wall with the same mass and stiffness. This region is below the usual frequency range of interest for airborne sound.

- At slightly higher frequencies, the two leaves move independently against a restoring force supplied by the air 'spring' between them. This system has a simple resonance given by:

$$f_d = \frac{1}{2\pi} \sqrt{\frac{\gamma P_0 (M_1 + M_2)}{M_1 M_2 d}} \qquad (16.20)$$

where γ is the ratio of specific heats for air (= 1.4), P_0 is the atmospheric pressure, M_1 and M_2 are the surface densities of the two leaves and d is the width of the cavity; f_d should be well below 100 Hz (not difficult to achieve).

- At mid-frequencies, air resonances are established and the cavity behaves like a two-dimensional reverberant space; some of this sound is transmitted through to the other side. The solution here is to fill the cavity with absorbent material. In this region, the insulation approaches that of a 'double' Mass Law, with a slope of 12 dB/octave.

◆ At high frequencies we still have a coincidence dip—one for each leaf. If the leaves are of the same material, we can make the dips occur at different frequencies by using different thicknesses. This will usually result in a better single-figure rating for SRI. This is why good double-glazed windows usually use different thicknesses of glass.

16.5 **Room acoustics**

Thus far we have established some characteristics of common outdoor sound sources and have examined how their acoustic signals might be altered by features in the outdoor environment and the envelope of buildings. We now turn to the effect of a room on the signals arriving at our ears, both for sound travelling into the room through a wall, and for sounds originating in the room.

16.5.1 **Reverberation**

The subject of room acoustics is dominated by reverberation. It is probably the most important percept of a particular room's acoustic and it was the first to be successfully modelled. General models of reverberation are high-frequency models: they characterize sound waves as rays. We imagine a sound source in a room to emit a large number of rays omnidirectionally. Each ray will travel in a straight line. When it meets a surface it will be reflected and some energy will be lost due to absorption at the surface. Very soon after the sound source is switched on, the room will be full of very many rays travelling in all directions. The set of all the rays can be described as a sound field with a certain acoustic energy density (the energy per unit volume) which can change over time as the field builds up or dies away. This is a dynamic process first modelled by Sabine (1993). The source continually supplies acoustic energy into the room and energy is continually lost by absorption at the boundary. It can be shown that the amount of energy falling on a unit area of the room walls per second is given by: $\frac{ScD}{4}$ where S is the total surface area of the room, c is the speed of sound, and D is the acoustic energy density in the room. Thus, Sabine's energy balance equation is

$$\frac{d(DV)}{dt} = W - \frac{\alpha ScD}{4}$$
(16.21)

where V is the volume of the room, W is the acoustic power of the source (energy per second), and α is the absorption coefficient of the room surfaces; that is, the fraction of energy striking unit area of a wall which is absorbed.

Equation 16.21 states that the rate of change of energy in the room is equal to the rate at which the source supplies it minus the rate at which it is removed. Solving it leads to an expression for the way the energy density in the room changes as a function of time. The solution we get depends on the initial conditions. We can choose to look at what happens when the sound source is first switched on, when the sound field reaches a steady state, or when the source is switched off again and the field decays. Perhaps surprisingly, our perception of room acoustics is dominated by the third case—what happens when the sound source suddenly stops. Solving for this case gives:

$$D(t) = D_0 e^{\frac{-\alpha Sct}{4V}}$$
$$where \quad D_0 = \frac{4W}{\alpha Sc}$$
(16.22)

This is the classic exponential decay of a reverberant room, illustrated in Fig. 16.20.

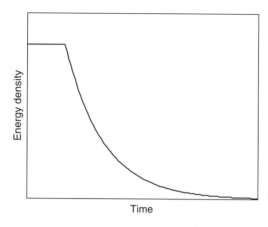

Fig. 16.20 Exponential decay of diffuse reverberation.

Note that it can be shown that, for a steady-state reverberant sound field, the mean square acoustic pressure is simply related to the energy density thus:

$$D_0 = \frac{\overline{p^2}}{\rho_0 c^2} \tag{16.23}$$

Hence, the exponential decay shown in Fig. 16.20 is expected for the square of pressure, or the acoustic intensity in the room. If this is expressed in decibels, by converting the decay to sound pressure level, then the exponential decay becomes a straight line. It is the rate of this slope which we hear as reverberance. (Current research discriminates between the physical process of reverberation and its perceptual correlate of reverberance.) The gradient of the decay is usually expressed as the reverberation time. This is defined as the time taken for the energy density to decay by a factor of a million (that is, by 60 dB). Applying this condition to eqn 16.22 shows that reverberation time is given by:

$$T = 0.161 \frac{V}{\alpha S} \tag{16.24}$$

where a value of $343\,\mathrm{m\,s^{-1}}$ has been assumed for c.

Equation 16.24 is known as Sabine's equation. It is a strikingly simple model of a complex process. It tells us that reverberation is governed only by the volume of a room and its absorption. This is, of course, not completely accurate in real rooms. Sabine's model requires that the sound field in the room is diffuse; specifically that the energy density is the same throughout the room (homogeneous) and that equal intensity travels in all directions at any instant in time (isotropic). These conditions are never completely fulfilled in a real room. One of the consequences of this is that measured reverberation time does usually vary a little from one place to another within a room; another is that sound decays are not always perfectly exponential, particularly at low frequencies. Nevertheless, Sabine's equation is accurate enough to form the basis of many room designs.

A slightly different reverberation equation, developed by Eyring (1930) is more accurate for rooms with high absorption coefficients. The theoretical development and underlying assumptions are similar, except that, where Sabine imagines a bundle of sound rays meeting all the room surfaces simultaneously, Eyring imagines a sound ray meeting one room surface after another sequentially.

$$T = 0.161 \frac{V}{-S \log_e (1 - \alpha)} \tag{16.25}$$

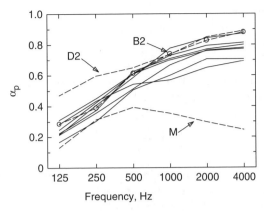

Fig. 16.21 Random incidence absorption coefficient for ten different kinds of auditorium seating (after Davies *et al.*, 1994). Type B2 was a typical well-upholstered, cloth-covered seat; M was unusually unabsorbent due to its impervious vinyl covering; while D2 had a hollow seat base producing a low-frequency resonance.

In real rooms, the surfaces do not all have the same absorption coefficient and α should be interpreted as the (area-weighted) mean absorption coefficient of the room. Furthermore, the absorption coefficient of a surface generally varies with frequency, and so the reverberation time of a room will vary with frequency (unless designed not to). This is important because it affects our perception of the reverberation that the room applies to sounds heard in it. Many common room surfaces are essentially porous absorbers, converting sound energy to heat through friction within many small pores. Examples are carpet, clothes, seat cushions, curtains, and ceiling tiles. Porous absorbers typically absorb efficiently at high frequencies and much less so at low frequencies. Figure 16.21 shows the measured absorption coefficient for ten different types of concert hall seating.

Low-frequency absorption often appears in the form of resonant absorbers, whether specially designed cavities or decorative wood panels laid over an air gap. Simple mass-spring models can be used to predict the resonant frequencies (where absorption will be at a maximum) and the sharpness of the resonant peak controlled by damping.

In performance spaces, the profile of reverberation time (RT) with frequency is an important part of the perception of the room and it is usually desirable to design the RT to keep to a constant value across frequency, appropriate to the type of performance.

16.5.2 Room modes

The reverberation models discussed so far point to room acoustics being a time-domain process, and this certainly agrees with a large area of our perception of the sound of a room. However, it is not the whole story. If we are dissatisfied with the high-frequency approximation of a sound wave as a ray, then we might seek a more accurate model of the room by setting up a three-dimensional wave equation for the room and solving it. In three dimensions, the linear acoustic wave equation can be expressed as:

$$\frac{\partial^2 p}{\partial x^2} + \frac{\partial^2 p}{\partial y^2} + \frac{\partial^2 p}{\partial z^2} = \frac{1}{c^2}\frac{\partial^2 p}{\partial t^2} \tag{16.26}$$

In a rectangular room of dimensions L_x, L_y, and L_z and with boundary conditions imposed by rigid walls, the steady-state solution of eqn 16.26 is:

$$p(x,y,z,t) = A\cos(k_x x)\cos(k_y y)\cos(k_z z)e^{j2\pi ft} \tag{16.27}$$

where:

$$k_x = \frac{m\pi}{L_x}; \quad k_y = \frac{n\pi}{L_y}; \quad k_z = \frac{p\pi}{L_z} \tag{16.28}$$

where m, n, and p are positive integers.

The k's can be thought of as vector components of the wave number k, so that

$$k = \sqrt{k_x^2 + k_y^2 + k_z^2} \tag{16.29}$$

Where this gets really interesting is that for eqn 16.27 to work as a solution of the wave eqn 16.26, then the frequency and wave number have to be related thus:

$$f = \frac{kc}{2\pi} = \frac{c}{2}\sqrt{\left(\frac{m}{L_x}\right)^2 + \left(\frac{n}{L_y}\right)^2 + \left(\frac{p}{L_z}\right)^2} \tag{16.30}$$

This means that the solution to the wave equation in a room requires quantized frequencies. The pressure shapes in eqn 16.27 now occur at specific resonant frequencies given by eqn 16.30. These resonances are often called 'room modes'. Some lower-order modes are plotted in Fig. 16.22.

The response of a room thus seems to vary strongly as we move around it, and this seems to strongly contradict the diffuse field assumptions necessary for a simple reverberant field. However, this contradiction can be resolved. The modal frequencies predicted by eqn 16.30 are indeed all separate resonances. However, as we move up in frequency, the number of modal frequencies increases quite rapidly, and the individual modes start to overlap. It can be shown that the modal density—the number of modes per hertz at a frequency f—is given by:

$$\frac{dN_f}{df} = \frac{4\pi V f^2}{c^3} \tag{16.31}$$

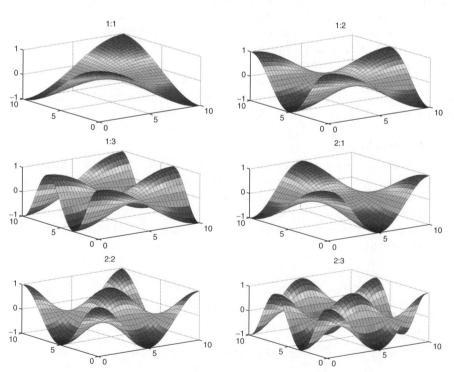

Fig. 16.22 Room modes of a 10 × 10-m room. Each surface is a snaphot of how pressure varies across the room for a fixed value of height ($z = 0$) and time ($t = 0$). The label of each plot is the m:n mode number and the vertical axis is pressure. In general, the response of the room to a broadband sound source will be a superposition of many mode shapes.

Once we have many modes overlapping in a small frequency band, it is not sensible to predict or measure the response of individual modes. So the wave equation is a low-frequency model of room acoustics and diffuse reverberation is a high-frequency model. The frequency f_s where one should change models was suggested by Schroeder as being that where, on average, three modal frequencies occur within the half-bandwidth of one modal resonance. This is given (Kuttruff, 2000) by:

$$f_s \approx 2000\sqrt{\frac{T}{V}} \tag{16.32}$$

where the units of f_s are hertz, T is the reverberation time of the room (seconds), and V its volume (m^3).

At low frequencies, the resonant response of room modes is subjectively significant in time, frequency, and spatial domains. Several authors have shown that listeners can detect spatial variations in pressure due to room modes, within a broadband, complex signal like music. In the time domain, the effect of isolated modes can be heard as a ringing reverberation rather like the twang of a spring. With a constant broadband signal, the frequency-domain effects of modes can be heard as tonal coloration. Fazenda *et al.* (2005) have explored the perceptual trade-offs of room modes and have found that the characteristics of the signal exciting the modes are just as important as the modes themselves.

16.5.3 Room impulse response

We have already seen that the time-domain response of a room is very significant in our perception of its acoustics. If we borrow from signal processing theory, we can treat the room as a linear acoustic filter and study its time response further. The output of a linear filter to any input signal can be predicted if one knows the impulse response of the filter. The impulse response is defined as the response of the filter (or room) to a perfect impulse. (This impulse, a Dirac delta function, has zero duration, infinite magnitude, and has an integral area equal to one. In measurements of real systems it must be approximated, or the impulse response must be measured indirectly.) Formally, the output signal $y(t)$ results from the convolution of the input signal $x(t)$ with the impulse response $g(t)$:

$$y(t) = \int_{-\infty}^{\infty} g(\tau)x(t-\tau)d\tau \tag{16.33}$$

This means that the impulse response contains all information about the acoustics of the room, at least between the particular source and receiver positions chosen. For example, the envelope of the tail of the impulse response will yield the reverberation time of the room. Measuring and predicting the impulse response of rooms is therefore of much interest. People sometimes do this in an informal way when they enter a new room and clap once to listen to the subsequent sound decay. Figure 16.23 shows the measured impulse response of a small concert hall. We can see the arrival of the direct sound, the first wave travelling straight from the source to the receiver. Soon after, early reflections arrive, resulting from a single reflection at the walls. Then the reflections quickly increase in number while their magnitude decreases approximately exponentially (as Sabine predicted).

16.5.4 Perception

The questions of how sound, especially music, is perceived in a room and why one room sounds different from another, have been pursued for a long time, indeed for longer than room acoustics became a science with the quantification of RT by Sabine. At first, these discussions were dominated by reverberation (time), but soon it was recognized that two concert halls might have the same measured RT and yet sound very different when we listen to music in them. Investigation of

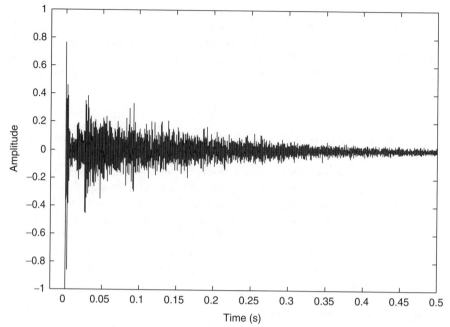

Fig. 16.23 Impulse response of a small concert hall.

the factors underlying the perceived differences has mainly been done by experiment. These experiments typically take the form of subjecting a listener to a sound field and asking her to make a judgement about what she hears. The sound field might be 'real' (e.g. an orchestra playing in a real hall), or it might be simulated (e.g. an anechoic recording of music played over loudspeakers in an anechoic chamber). The judgement required might be very specific (e.g. 'which of these two snatches of music sounds more reverberant?') or they might be more general (e.g. 'which of these two concert halls do you prefer?'). An example of the simulated sound field technique appears in the paper by Cox *et al.* (1993). Each experimental method has advantages and disadvantages. Many of these come from trading accuracy and experimental control against realism. For example, the simulated sound field can be easily controlled, but it can be difficult to make a simulated impulse response as rich in reflections as that from a real room.

Many classical experiments have been conducted with simple simulated sound fields to discover the perceptual effects of reflected sound. These generally take place in an anechoic chamber with one loudspeaker simulating the direct sound from the stage and another fed by a delayed signal simulating the reflection. Experimenters have varied reflection delay, level, and angle of incidence to uncover perceptual effects for both music and noise signals. The simplest experiments use only one reflection, but others have used several (with different delays, etc.). The main effects can be summarized thus (Kuttruff, 2000):

◆ In most 'normal' rooms, a reflection will not be perceived as a distinct echo: this depends mainly on the delay time and level of the reflection.

◆ For delay times of less than 20 ms, the reflection will almost never be perceived as an echo (the Haas, 'precedence', effect; see Chapter 6).

◆ If the reflection is not perceived as an echo, then it will either not be perceived at all, or it will be perceived as altering the character of the direct sound.

- The threshold of perception of a single reflection depends on its delay and level.
- The alteration of the character of the direct sound will usually be reported as tonal (the reflection 'colours' the direct sound) or spatial (lateral reflections make the sound source seem wider than a point source).
- Strong coloration is usually seen as undesirable in a hall for music or speech, but spatial broadening is usually seen as desirable (especially for music).

The Haas effect is very useful in sound reinforcement system design. Imagine a hall with a person speaking on the stage. We wish to make the speaker sound louder to the audience, but without making them feel that a loudspeaker at the edge of the stage is the sound source. This can be done by exploiting the Haas effect. We simply introduce a small delay into the amplification chain, so that the audience hears the direct, unamplified sound from the person speaking first, and then a louder 'reflection' from the loudspeaker 10 ms later. As long as the relative delay at the listener is less than about 20 ms, he or she will integrate the two sound sources into one, and will perceive this single sound to come from the direction of the first arrival, namely the person speaking on the stage. (Note that this becomes harder to achieve if multiple loudspeakers are installed around the hall.)

The impulse response of a typical room is very rich, with many thousands of reflections. It seems reasonable that the ear should be sensitive to changes in this which do not alter the overall decay rate as measured by the reverberation time.

It has been found that our perceptions are influenced strongly by the *early reflections* in a room (Cox *et al.*, 1993). Near the beginning of an impulse response, the reflection density is low. After the direct sound, we typically receive first a reflection from one side wall, then from the other, then one from the ceiling, perhaps followed by one from the rear wall, and so on. The timing, level, and frequency content of these reflections can alter the perceived character of the sound in the room considerably. Because there are so many reflections in an impulse response, we need a way of boiling down these reflection distributions into values of a few parameters which will (we hope) correlate with our subjective impressions. But what are the most important perceptions? Schroeder and his students attempted to answer this question by exposing test subjects to the same music signal performed in different halls (Schroeder *et al.*, 1974). Paired comparisons of the halls allowed subjects to judge the effect of the hall acoustics. The musical performance itself was removed as a variable by using the same anechoic music recording convolved with the binaural impulse response of each hall. Factor analysis of the results was used to identify the number of significant orthogonal percepts. This work has been continued and extended by Ando and collaborators (Ando, 1985) and there is now good agreement that there are four main perceptual dimensions of the acoustics of a room: *reverberance*, *level*, *clarity*, and *spaciousness*:

Reverberance correlates with RT (measured over 60-dB decay) but even better (Farina, 2001) with Early Decay Time, measured over the first 10 dB of decay. Preferred RT varies for the type of performance (romantic classical music, symphonic classical music, speech, etc.), size of hall, from one country to another, and from one listener to another (Barron, 1988).

Level varies over a hall (they are not perfectly diffuse), it is important that it sounds loud enough, and level affects the other percepts (louder halls sound more reverberant).

Clarity (important for both music and speech) is controlled by the energy in the early reflections, and has several correlates based on the measured impulse response $g(t)$: for speech D_{50} is used, for music C_{80} is favoured:

$$D_{50} = \frac{\int_0^{50\,ms} [g(t)]^2 dt}{\int_0^\infty [g(t)]^2 dt} \times 100\% \qquad (16.34)$$

$$C_{80} = 10\log_{10}\left[\frac{\int_0^{80\,ms}\left[g(t)\right]^2 dt}{\int_{80\,ms}^{\infty}\left[g(t)\right]^2 dt}\right] dB \qquad (16.35)$$

Spaciousness, in contrast to the above monaural attributes, is caused by dissimilar signals arriving at the two ears (see Chapter 6). There are currently thought to be at least two different subpercepts: apparent source width and envelopment. Dissimilarity in the signals at the left and right ears is mainly caused by early lateral reflections. The two main objective parameters which attempt to measure this are the early lateral energy fraction, LEF, and interaural cross-correlation.

$$LEF = \frac{\int_5^{80\,ms}\left[g(t)\cos\theta\right]^2 dt}{\int_0^{80\,ms}\left[g(t)\right]^2 dt} \qquad (16.36)$$

where θ is the angle between the axis through the listener's ears and the angle of sound incidence. Interaural cross-correlation (IACC) is defined in terms of the impulse response arriving at the left and right ear (eqn 16.37). It is usually measured using a dummy head which has microphones in place of eardrums. IACC is defined as the maximum value of $|\Phi_{rl}|$ within the range $|\tau| < 1$ ms.

$$\Phi_{rl} = \frac{\int_0^{100\,ms} g_r(t)g_l(t+\tau)dt}{\sqrt{\int_0^{100\,ms}\left[g_r(t)\right]^2 dt \times \int_0^{100\,ms}\left[g_l(t)\right]^2 dt}} \qquad (16.37)$$

All these parameters and their associated percepts vary over the seats of a typical hall and from one hall to another; these variations are generally audible, according to Cox *et al.* (1993) who measured the smallest perceptible changes in the objective parameters.

Note that we only require additional monaural parameters to RT because real rooms (especially concert halls) do not have perfectly exponential decays (i.e. they are not perfectly diffuse). If they did, then EDT would be identical to RT, and we could predict values for C_{80} and D_{50} (and so on) from the RT.

16.5.5 Modelling

Modelling in room acoustics centres on prediction of the room impulse response, either as a single channel from the source to the receiver within the room, or as a binaural prediction from the source to each of the listener's ears. Current models are mainly based on the assumption that sound can be modelled as rays instead of waves and so diffraction and phase can be neglected. This suggests possible errors in low-frequency predictions. The two classical algorithms are the image-source model and the ray-tracing model. The image source model was first described thoroughly by Allen and Berkley (1979) and it imagines that each sound reflection comes from a virtual or image source sited outside the real room. The position of the image source is such that the sound it generates arrives at the receiver at the same time as would the real reflection. The position of each image source is simply found by reflecting the real source in the walls of the room. Higher-order reflections are generated by multiply-reflected image sources. For a two-dimensional rectangular room, this process results in a plane tiled perfectly with image rooms and sources, as shown in Fig. 16.24. The correct amplitude of each reflection is simply calculated by inverse square law and multiplying by the wall reflection coefficient each time the pulse from the image source crosses a virtual wall. This process can be easily generalized to three dimensions, giving the expression in eqn 16.38 for the energy impulse response of a rectangular room with uniform absorption coefficient α.

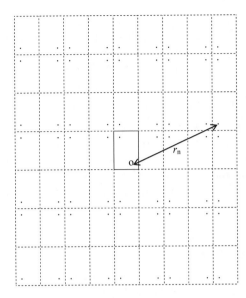

Fig. 16.24 The construction of image sources (·) to predict the impulse response of a two-dimensional room at a receiver (o). The image rooms continue outwards infinitely to cover the plane.

$$g(t) = \sum_n \frac{P}{4\pi c r_n^2} (1 - \alpha)^i \, \delta\left(t - \frac{r_n}{c}\right)$$

(16.38)

where r_n is the distance of the nth image with order i, and P is the power of the source.

The main disadvantage of the image source model is that, for a room which is not a simple rectangle, ensuring that the image sources would actually be visible to the receiver is a time-consuming calculation (Borish, 1984). This problem gets significantly worse as the reflection order gets higher, so the image source algorithm is usually only used to predict the earliest reflections in a room impulse response. The ray-tracing algorithm does not suffer from the image visibility problem. In ray tracing (Krokstad et al., 1968), we imagine that the sound source emits a large number (at least 100 000) rays in all directions at time $t = 0$. Each ray is tracked as it travels in straight lines around the room, reflecting off surfaces and losing energy as it goes. If the ray crosses a receiver sphere of finite size, we log its energy and arrival time and add it to the predicted room impulse response. Most rays, of course, do not encounter the receiver, and we track them until their energy falls below some predetermined cut-off level. Ray-tracing is quicker than the image source model for higher-order reflections, but it is not as accurate. One problem is that a very large number of rays are needed to sufficiently illuminate (or insonify) the room surfaces. There are several variants of ray-tracing which address this problem, such as beam-tracing (Drumm and Lam, 2000). Most commercially available room acoustic-modelling programs combine at least two different types of algorithm for different stages of the impulse response, for example the Odeon model (Naylor, 1993).

Ray-tracing, image source, and other similar models share several other inaccuracies. Being high-frequency models, they generally ignore the wave properties of sound and thus do not accurately handle phase changes, diffraction, and scattering at rough surfaces. Phase has been shown to be less significant (Kuttruff, 1993), but the other two problems mean that results at low frequencies should be interpreted with caution. Nevertheless, modern programs are accurate enough to give a clear impression of what an unbuilt room will sound like. This extension to the room impulse prediction is achieved by modelling the receiver as a human head with a binaural transfer function (usually measured separately). Each incoming reflection is then filtered to give the correct signal at the entrance to the ear. The resulting two-channel impulse response (left and right ears) can then be used as a filter through which anechoically recorded music is played. This process of auralization (Kleiner *et al.*, 1993) is becoming increasingly common in building design since it enables the results of design decisions to be easily conveyed to non-experts.

16.6 Sound reproduction

We now have a reasonable picture of what shapes sounds in the outdoor and indoor environments. One type of sound perhaps deserves special mention because of its increasing availability— reproduced sound, radiated from loudspeakers. Loudspeakers are becoming almost ubiquitous, certainly in urban environments. Mobile phones, personal music players, car stereos, televisions, personal computers, and public address systems all radiate sound from loudspeakers. Since these sound signals are such a common feature of modern life, it is worth examining the characteristics of loudspeakers.

16.6.1 How loudspeakers work

There are several transduction methods that can be used to make a loudspeaker, but the most common is one of the oldest—the moving coil. Figure 16.25 illustrates how it works. The moving-coil loudspeaker consists of a light rigid cone attached to a coil placed in a ring magnet. Current flowing in the coil causes the cone to move and radiate pressure waves. The suspension of the cone is carefully tuned to minimize its resonances so that it acts as a uniform piston. The goal of the designer is to make the pressure wave a precise analogue of the electrical signal. Designs usually seek to maximize either a wide flat-frequency response and linearity, or high power. In high-fidelity systems more than one loudspeaker with different radii are generally used to cover the audible frequency range. The directivity of a moving-coil loudspeaker approaches omnidirectionality for a small radius cone at low frequencies. At higher frequencies, lobes are found in the directivity, as shown in Fig. 16.6. If a more directional device is needed, several loud-speakers can be combined into a column, where mutual interference between them creates much sharper lobes along the axis of the column.

Moving-coil loudspeakers are used in a wide range of sizes, from the earbuds used with an MP3 player to the subwoofer in a hi-fi system. However, they are not ideal for some applications because it is difficult to make them very thin. The trend in visual displays towards flat screens calls for similarly flat loudspeakers. A recent development has attempted to answer this with the distributed mode loudspeaker (DML) (also called the 'flat panel' loudspeaker). Here, a rigid flat panel is excited to produce bending waves. The exciter is often a moving-coil motor. Unlike the moving-coil loudspeaker, as many panel resonances as possible are excited. Above a lower cut-off frequency, the modal density is sufficient that the panel vibration is distributed approximately randomly across its surface. This gives a transducer which is more efficient than the moving-coil loudspeaker (and hence potentially suitable for low-power electronics). The directivity also varies less with frequency and it can be built into the display (the DML can be used as a projection

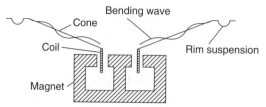

Fig. 16.25 Simplified section through a moving-coil loudspeaker.

screen, for example). To date, high-fidelity applications still use moving-coil loudspeakers in preference to DMLs, partly because the DML does not work well at low frequencies.

16.6.2 Loudspeakers in rooms

When a loudspeaker system is used in a room, what the listener hears can be modelled as a convolution of the loudspeaker response and the room impulse response. At high frequencies, this is straightforward and the listener hears the high-frequency roll-off of the loudspeaker superimposed onto the room. At low frequencies, things are more complicated. Individual room modes start to become dominant and there can also be a feedback path, where a room mode loads the loudspeaker, changing the impedance it sees as it radiates into the room. The effects of this are heard in all three domains: ringing in the time domain, coloration in the frequency domain, and variance in loudness across the room (Fazenda et al., 2002). Equation 16.30 indicates that, for a given bass frequency, a smaller room will have a sparser distribution of modes in the frequency domain. The effect of individual modes is thus likely to become more noticeable in a smaller room. This finding is of particular significance to those wanting to reproduce low frequencies in a small room, as in many modern recording-studio control rooms.

16.6.3 Speech intelligibility

One aspect of the loudspeaker-room system that is often important is speech intelligibility. In transport stations, shopping malls, theatres, and other public spaces, it is important that intelligible speech can be heard by large numbers of people. To understand the factors at work we need to consider the characteristics of rooms, loudspeakers, and speech signals. For our purposes, a useful simple model of speech is of a high-frequency carrier signal modulated by a low-frequency signal. Examples of the high-frequency signal are the periodic glottal pulse (as in a singing vowel sound like 'aaah') and the more broadband signal made by a rush of breath (as in 'ssss'). In speech, these are shaped into individual syllables (more properly, we should say individual phonemes) at a rate of a few hertz. Most of the information in the speech signal is contained in the envelope, the outer shape, rather than in the carrier signal. Thus, for good speech intelligibility, we want to preserve the modulation. Transmitting speech through a room tends to reduce intelligibility through two main mechanisms. Firstly, due to reverberation, the listener receives multiple copies of the speech signal, all slightly delayed. The reflections tend to fill in the troughs of the modulated speech envelope, so the difference between peak and trough in the modulation is reduced. Figure 16.23 illustrates this effect. (In fact, our ears improve on the performance suggested by this model. Room reflections arriving within about 50 ms of the direct sound are integrated to form a single sound and actually improve the loudness and hence intelligibility of the signal. This is acknowledged in the theatre metric D_{50} given in eqn 16.34 above.) The second mechanism that tends to degrade speech modulation is background noise. Uncorrelated noise will tend to fill in the troughs of the signal in a similar way to reverberation. Houtgast and Steeneken (1973) proposed a way of characterizing the effect of the room on speech-like signals, by using the modulation transfer function (MTF). The MTF describes, as a function of frequency, the fraction of the original modulation that is preserved when the signal is transmitted from one point to another in the room. It can be shown that, for a room with reverberation and background noise, the MTF is given by eqn 16.39:

$$m(F) = \frac{1}{\sqrt{1 + \left(\frac{2\pi FT}{13.8}\right)^2}} \cdot \frac{1}{1 + 10^{\frac{-S}{10}}} \tag{16.39}$$

where $m(F)$ is the MTF at modulation frequency F, T is the reverberation time, and S the signal-to-noise ratio in dB.

Houtgast and Steeneken used MTF as the basis of their metric speech transmission index (STI), which correlates well with subjectively perceived intelligibility (Houtgast and Steeneken, 1985). For STI, one measures or predicts MTF for a range of octave band noise signals modulated by a range of low-frequency sine waves. The resulting values of m are weighted to reflect the relative importance of certain combinations of carrier and modulator in real speech, and combined to give a single number between 0 and 1, the speech transmission index. Subsequent variants of STI reduced the number of measurements needed and attempted to cater for non-linear systems, such as public address speakers with compressors. The success of STI shows us that the main determinants of intelligibility are the room and the speech signal. Any loudspeakers in the system (STI can be used to rate a room for unamplified speech, such as a classroom) are important mainly for their directivity. Having observed that we would like to maximize direct sound at the expense of reverberation, an obvious step is to make our loudspeakers directional. Thus, a well-designed system will attempt to beam sound only onto the listeners and try to avoid exciting the reverberant field as far as possible. A large market of loudspeakers is available with defined directivities to help designers.

16.6.4 Spatial reproduction

In a critical listening application, as well requiring a good frequency response and appropriate directivity, we may also need to consider the spatial performance of a loudspeaker reproduction system. Often it is not sufficient to use a single loudspeaker and radiate as if from a point source. Instead we might want to synthesize a complex sound field around the listener, perhaps so that they can hear the acoustics of the space in which the recording was made, or perceive a set of sound sources at defined locations in space. Thus one goal here is to accurately recreate the signals arriving at the ears of the listener when he or she is sitting in a particular seat at a performance. There are several different approaches to achieving this effect. The most common, stereo, aims to give an illusion of a distributed sound source stretching between the two loudspeakers. In this, it is quite successful, though it should be noted that much commercially available material is closer to two-channel mono than stereo. (The reason for this may be that most of it will be listened to not by a listener in an equilateral triangle with his loudspeakers, but in a car or on headphones.) An improvement over stereo might be offered by domestic 5.1 systems, which augment the stereo pair with a central loudspeaker, two rear ones, and a separate low-frequency subwoofer speaker. The subwoofer takes advantage of the poor localization of low-frequency sources and means that the rest of the speakers can be much smaller. The main problem with 5.1 is that there is no defined encoding method with which an engineer can sample a real spatial sound field and capture the correct signals for each of the five loudspeakers. Therefore 5.1 seems to be generally used as a sort of 'stereo plus effects' system.

Better spatial reproduction results from the aim of capturing the exact signals arriving at a listener from all directions: two notable techniques are binaural and ambisonic. To make a binaural recording, one simply needs a dummy head with small microphones placed at the entrance to the ear canals (see Chapter 6). Reproducing the signals through headphones results in good spatial accuracy. A variant is to measure a pair of impulse responses from a point source to the left and right ears, in an anechoic chamber. This is repeated over a full range of elevation and azimuth angles of the source. The resulting set of head-related impulse responses can then be used to synthesize (by convolution) a virtual sound source at any point in space around the listener. Residual errors in binaural systems mainly stem from differences between the head-related transfer function of the listener's head and that used to make the recordings.

The ambisonic system was invented by Gerzon (1973) and uses four microphone capsules arranged on orthogonal axes within a single shell, to sample a spatial sound field at a single point. The recordings are later reproduced from an array of loudspeakers around the listener in an acoustically dead room. One of the advantages of the ambisonic system is that encoding and decoding functions are defined for several different arrangements of loudspeakers. One might use five loudspeakers equally spaced around the horizontal plane containing the listener's head. Another might place the listener at the centre of a cube with a loudspeaker at each corner. There is now plenty of experimental evidence to suggest that reproduction of a spatial sound field (outdoors or indoors) is much more realistic with an ambisonic or binaural system or one of their variants (e.g. Kleiner *et al.*, 1993; Bauck and Cooper, 1996; Guastavino *et al.*, 2005).

16.7 Assessment of noise

We have now completed our overview of how sound signals are generated and modified by the environment around us before they arrive at our ears. We are now in a position to consider how to assess and measure these sounds. Why should we do this? Well, all of us have been affected by unwanted sound, by noise, to some extent. Most of the sound around us is generated or modified by human activity, after all, so we should expect to be able to devise sensible rating systems. In fact, this simply stated exercise turns out to be one of the most intractable in acoustics, mainly because of the massively complex interaction between the stimulus and the listener. A detailed account of the mechanisms that drive auditory perception are, of course, given in the rest of this volume, so here we shall restrict ourselves to the relatively 'high-level' percepts and effects of environmental acoustics, such as annoyance and disturbance.

16.7.1 Single-figure metrics

In everyday noise problems, we often need a single-figure measurement of the noise. A complainant may ask how loud his neighbour's stereo system is, a politician may want to set a limit for night-time noise level in a residential zone, and a law court may need to know if this limit was breached. But different noise signals may show significant variation in the time, frequency, and amplitude domains, and the response of the auditory system is far from linear, so fairly reducing this to a single figure involves many compromises. The classical approach is to seek a dose–response relationship, as Bradley (1993) did for air-conditioner noise, for example. One begins by defining a subjective response variable of interest, such as annoyance. The human population or community affected by the noise is then defined, and surveyed in some way to establish the magnitude of their response. The most common method is for a field survey to be undertaken with interviewers asking subjects to rate their own annoyance on some scale. Physical measurements of the noise are made at the same time, using a wide range of acoustic metrics. The experimenters then look for correlations between the objective-dose metrics and the subjective response values. Several different single-figure acoustic metrics have been proposed for different kinds of noise over the last 50 years, the most common of which are summarized in Table 16.1.

By far the most common single-figure noise metric is the A-weighted equivalent continuous-sound pressure level, or L_{Aeq}. With A-weighting, our nuanced loudness perception is simplified to a single frequency response which can be implemented in a linear filter. (The A-weighting curve was derived by simplifying the 40-phon equal loudness contour—see Chapter 3—to a shape which could be easily implemented in the portable electronics of the time.) The output of the A-weighting filter is summed energetically as a single, broadband decibel. That takes care of

Table 16.1 Examples of single-figure metrics used in environmental noise assessment

Metric	Description	Example use
$L_{pA,max}$	Maximum recorded A-weighted sound pressure level	Construction site noise (BS5228-1, 1997)
L_{peak}	Peak acoustic pressure, converted to sound pressure level	Impulse noise in industry (European Commission, 2003)
$L_{Aeq,T}$	Averages $L_{p,A}$ over time (see text)	Most environmental noise (BS7445-1, 2003), including for planning (Department of the Environment, 1994), rail noise (Department of Transport, 1995) and individual cars (BSISO362, 1998)
L_{AE}	Sound exposure level, a $L_{Aeq,1\ second}$ for a noise event	Vehicle pass-by (Department of Transport, 1995), gunshot
$L_{A10,T}$	$L_{p,A}$ exceeded for only 10% of the measuring time T—near maximum	Road traffic noise (Department of Transport and Welsh Office, 1988)
$L_{A90,T}$	$L_{p,A}$ exceeded for 90% of the measuring time T	Approximate background level of environmental noise (BS4142, 1997)
L_{den}	$L_{Aeq,T}$ modified to weight evening(1900–2300) levels 5 dB higher and night (2300–0700) 10 dB higher, than day (0700–1900)	General environmental noise (European Commission, 2002)

the frequency domain. Measured A-weighted sound pressure levels can, of course, be seen to vary from one moment to the next, so some sort of time-averaging is needed for a single figure. This is provided by averaging the square of the acoustic pressure over time, in approximately the same way in which the ear averages sound energy. Thus L_{Aeq} is defined by eqn 16.40.

$$L_{Aeq,T} = 10 \log_{10} \left(\frac{1}{T} \int_0^T \frac{p_A^2(t)}{p_0^2} \, dt \right) \, dB \qquad (16.40)$$

where p_A is the A-weighted acoustic pressure, p_0 is the reference pressure, 2×10^{-5} Pa, and T is the averaging time. Note that T must be stated for the measurement to be useful.

That L_{Aeq} is a good predictor of hearing loss for higher-level sound has been known since the 1960s, and L_{Aeq} is now the basis for legislation controlling noise at work in most developed countries (e.g. the EU Physical Agents directive; European Commission, 2003). At lower levels, more subjective factors come into play and dose–response correlations are not so good. For some noise types, there is evidence that annoyance is predicted by $L_{A,10}$ and this makes intuitive sense: people complain about the loudest sounds in their environment. Assessment of road traffic noise is based on $L_{A,10}$ in the UK (Department of Transport and Welsh Office, 1988). Other noise types have a history of quite complex assessment schemes. For example, aircraft noise has been evaluated with many different assessment schemes, such as effective perceived noise level, based on a modified measured noise spectrum, and the UK noise-and-number-index. A general trend is discernable, however, towards using $L_{Aeq,T}$ wherever possible. Miedema and Vos (1998) conducted a meta-analysis of data on annoyance due to transport noise. They found clear quadratic dose–response curves between the percentage highly annoyed and day–night level (DNL). DNL is a version of L_{Aeq}, with a 10-dB night-time penalty, defined in eqn 16.41. It is very clear from Miedema's work that annoyance rises much less quickly for rail than for road or aircraft noise.

In the UK, aircraft noise is now assessed using separate daytime and night-time L_{Aeq}, with the time limits as set in DNL.

$$DNL = 10\log_{10}\left(\frac{15 \times 10^{\frac{L_{Aeq,0700-2200}}{10}} + 9 \times 10^{\frac{L_{Aeq,2200-0700}+10}{10}}}{24}\right)$$

(16.41)

16.7.2 Exposure and targets

If we accept that $L_{Aeq,T}$ is a reasonable way to indicate overall noise level, we can ask what the appropriate target levels might be for different activities or settings in the environment. This question was addressed by the widely cited WHO report by Berglund *et al.* (1999). Berglund's team reviewed the available data on annoyance and health effects to synthesize the targets reproduced in Table 16.2. The targets are quite stringent when compared with actual values of noise levels, as the authors note:

> In the European Union about 40% of the population is exposed to road traffic noise with an equivalent sound pressure level exceeding 55 dB(A) daytime, and 20% are exposed to levels exceeding 65 dB(A). When all transportation noise is considered, more than half of all European Union citizens is estimated to live in zones that do not ensure acoustical comfort to residents. At night, more than 30% are exposed to equivalent sound pressure levels exceeding 55 dB(A), which are disturbing to sleep.

It is notable that the report defines annoyance as a critical health effect.

In England and Wales, environmental noise levels have been usefully documented by a large-scale survey of levels outside dwellings, undertaken in 1990 and repeated in 2000 (BRE, 2002). Table 16.3 shows the distribution of noise levels at the 1020 measurement sites from the 2000 survey, expressed as the percentage of the population exposed to a certain level or greater. Compared to the WHO targets, the levels are quite high: 93% of the population are exposed to an L_{Aeq} of more than 50 dB, while 75% of people are exposed to a background daytime level of 40 dB (L_{A90}). In fact, the precise figure at the WHO external daytime limit of 55 dB is 54 ± 3% of population, while the WHO night-time limit of 45 dB is exceeded for 67 ± 3% of people.

The existence of data from 1990 and 2000 allows an interesting comparison of noise levels, and some salient comparisons from BRE (2002) are repeated in Table 16.4. Perhaps counter-intuitively, decreases are found in daytime and evening levels, both in average (L_{Aeq}) levels and near-maximum (L_{A10}) levels. However, a statistically significant increase is found between 1990 and 2000 for the night-time background (L_{A90}) level. These changes, though significant at the 5% level, are small—on the order of 1 dB. Nevertheless, they suggest that the environment is becoming less noisy, but also less quiet. As the authors of the survey note, this change is consistent with a model in which noise events are more numerous but each on average quieter.

Reporting of environmental noise in Europe has now moved on since the BRE survey. European directive 2002/49/EC, commonly called the European Noise Directive (European Commission, 2002), mandates the use of a metric called day–evening–night level L_{den}. L_{den}, defined in eqn 16.42 is a weighted combination of the day, evening, and night L_{Aeq} as used in the tables above. It is supposed to be used to produce public noise maps of all significant urban areas and to identify quiet areas to be protected.

$$L_{den} = 10\log_{10}\left(\frac{12 \times 10^{\frac{L_{Aeq,0700-1900}}{10}} + 4 \times 10^{\frac{L_{Aeq,1900-2300}+5}{10}} + 8 \times 10^{\frac{L_{Aeq,2300-0700}+10}{10}}}{24}\right)$$

(16.42)

Table 16.2 Guideline values for community noise in specific environments (after Berglund *et al.*, 1999)

Specific environment	Critical health effect(s)	$L_{Aeq,T}$ (dB)	T (h)	$L_{Amax:fast}$ (dB)
Outdoor living area	Serious annoyance, d + e	55	16	–
	Moderate annoyance, d + e	50	16	–
Dwelling, indoors	Speech intelligibility and moderate annoyance, d and e	35	16	
Inside bedrooms	Sleep disturbance, night-time	30	8	45
Outside bedrooms	Sleep disturbance, window open (outdoor values)	45	8	60
School classrooms and pre- schools, indoors	Speech intelligibility, disturbance of information extraction, message commun.	35	during class	–
Pre-school bedrooms, indoors	Sleep disturbance	30	sleep-time	45
School, playground outdoor	Annoyance (external source)	55	during play	–
Hospital, ward rooms, indoors	Sleep disturbance, night-time	30	8	40
	Sleep disturbance, d + e	30	16	–
Hospitals, treatment rooms, indoors	Interference with rest and recovery	as low as possible		
Industrial, commercial shopping, and traffic areas— indoors and outdoors	HI	70	24	110
Ceremonies, festivals, and entertainment events	HI (patrons:< 5 times/year)	100	4	110
Public addresses, in- + outdoors	HI	85	1	110
Music through headphones/earphones	HI (free-field value)	85	1	110
Impulse sounds from toys, fireworks, and firearms	HI (adults)	–	–	L_{peak} = 140
	HI (children)	–	–	L_{peak} = 120
Outdoors in parkland and conservation areas	Disruption of tranquility	Quiet areas preserved and intruding noise kept low		

Abbreviations: d, daytime; e, evening; commun., communication; HI, hearing impairment.

16.7.3 Low-frequency noise

Though L_{Aeq} is becoming more universal, there are specialist criteria for some types of noise. Low-frequency environmental noise is a good example. There is evidence that low-frequency noise is a growing problem, partly due to the increased deployment of powerful bass loudspeakers (e.g. in pubs and clubs) and the increased use of double- and triple-glazing (Davies *et al.*, 2005). Sound insulation which performs well on reducing A-weighted sound level will still typically offer low insulation at low frequencies, as predicted by eqn 16.16. Amplified music will typically pass through

Table 16.3 Percentage of the population of England and Wales exposed to noise levels exceeding the indicated level (after BRE, 2002)

Index	30 dB	40 dB	50 dB	60 dB	70 dB
$L_{Aeq,0700-1900}$	100	100	93	27	3
$L_{A10,0700-1900}$	100	100	90	28	6
$L_{A90,0700-1900}$	100	75	17	2	1
$L_{Aeq,1900-2300}$	100	99	66	17	1
$L_{A10,1900-2300}$	100	99	60	18	3
$L_{A90,1900-2300}$	97	51	6	1	–
$L_{Aeq,2300-0700}$	100	95	30	5	–
$L_{A10,2300-0700}$	100	82	22	3	–
$L_{A90,2300-0700}$	76	20	1	–	–

two building envelopes giving a steep low-pass filter. In the complainant's house, much of the high-frequency masking noise is removed by the walls. The resulting low-level background hum can be very annoying for some people. The annoyance is increased by two properties of the ear. low-frequency noise is more difficult to localize, and the loudness gradient is steepest at Low frequencies. In laboratory experiments of low-frequency noise, Moorhouse *et al.* (2005) found that self-identified sufferers from low-frequency noise set their 'acceptability' threshold only 2–3 dB above their audibility threshold. Several countries have developed specific methods for rating low-frequency noise, and most of these use a rating curve. The procedure is essentially to record the L_{eq} of the noise in third-octave bands and compare this spectrum to the rating curve. If the noise breaches the reference curve at any frequency, then this indicates that it may be disturbing. Figure 16.26 compares some rating curves used in different national standards with the ISO threshold for audibility of pure tones. It is striking that the curves are close to or even below the threshold.

16.8 Soundscapes

The discussion above indicates that we have a partially satisfactory situation regarding environmental noise. On the stimulus side, engineers have made progress in understanding and controlling

Table 16.4 Noise levels outside dwellings in 1990 and 2000 (after BRE, 2002)

Index	1990	2000	Significant change (5% level)
$L_{Aeq,0700-1900}$	57.6	57.1	Decrease
$L_{A10,0700\ 1900}$	58.1	57.5	Decrease
$L_{A90,0700-1900}$	44.9	44.9	–
$L_{Aeq,1900-2300}$	54.1	53.1	Decrease
$L_{A10,1900-2300}$	54.0	53.3	Decrease
$L_{A90,1900-2300}$	40.5	40.8	–
$L_{Aeq,2300-0700}$	48.3	48.2	–
$L_{A10,2300-0700}$	45.3	45.6	–
$L_{A90,2300-0700}$	34.4	35.3	Increase

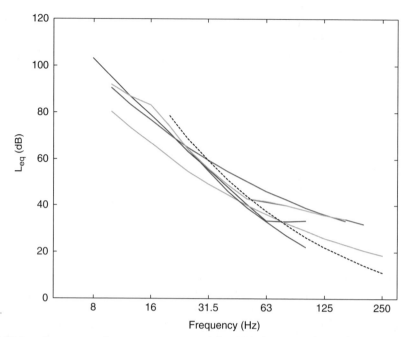

Fig. 16.26 Low-frequency noise assessment curves (after Moorhouse *et al.*, 2005). Blue line, Germany; green line, Denmark; red line, Sweden; cyan line, Poland; magenta line, The Netherlands; yellow line, proposed UK; black dashed, ISO pure-tone threshold.

noise sources. In some areas, such as the internal combustion engine, the technology is mature and future gains likely to be small. The number of vehicles is increasing in most developed and developing nations. On the other hand, new engine technology may allow much quieter power sources. On the response side, looking for correlations with single-figure metrics gives only fair agreement and a suspicion that L_{Aeq} is becoming universal, partly because the correlation scatter is so large in most experiments. Furthermore, treating all environmental sound as noise seems crude and may give rise to undue pessimism.

A very different approach to characterizing environmental sound exists which seeks to address these problems. The concept of the soundscape is generally credited to Schafer (1977) as part of an ecological ideology. Schafer defined a soundscape as 'the total acoustic environment'. The concept is somewhat fluid, perhaps reflecting the multidisciplinary interest in it. Thompson (2002) defines a soundscape as an auditory landscape, while Truax (1999) defines it as an environment of sound where the emphasis is on the way the sound is perceived and understood by an individual, or by a society. Despite their differences, these authors and others share a desire to account for both positive and negative aspects of the sound environment. One key idea is that the binary division of all environmental sound into noise or not-noise is too simple. Mainstream acoustics has, over the last 15 years or so, attempted to integrate some of the concepts of soundscapes. It may offer a way out of the L_{Aeq} impasse because it allows us to treat sounds in a more nuanced way and so incorporate more features of listener response. From the perspective of acoustic science, we might think of the soundscape of a location as consisting of all the sounds arriving at your ear, analogous to the landscape perceived by your eyes. Each sound may have several attributes, some physical (spatial location and frequency content, for example), some perceptual (e.g. loudness and roughness), and some cognitive (association or meaning, for example). Some attributes may also be properties of the whole soundscape rather than individual sounds—the 'meaning' of the soundscape in a train station, for example. Davies *et al.* (2007) have pointed out that we might expect the experience of hearing sound in the environment to be multidimensional because we know that listening in a concert hall has four or five orthogonal subjective dimensions (Schroeder *et al.*, 1974). Scientific characterization of all the factors involved in perceiving a soundscape is a very large task and we are a long way from a complete account. The research summarized here must therefore be taken as fragmentary and incomplete.

The largest body of experimental work to date is probably that of Kang and his co-workers (Kang, 2007). Concentrating mainly on fieldwork, they have surveyed over 9000 users of 14 urban open public spaces across Europe. The work used brief questionnaires to capture individual user's evaluation of a quiet/noisy scale and their three favourite sounds (from a defined list of 15). In two sites, further questions were asked on acoustic comfort and source identification. Correlations were found between measured L_{Aeq} and both noisiness and acoustic comfort scores. Evidence was also found that the introduction of a sound rated pleasant can considerably improve acoustic comfort, even when its sound level is high. Subsequent similar work in China (Kang, 2007) found that preferred sounds could be divided into sounds from human activity and sounds from landscape elements, and that the former were more important in overall preference.

Several research teams have attempted to characterize the perceptual space involved in listening to a soundscape. Kang (2007) used 18 semantic differential scales with 223 subjects in two urban squares. He extracted four principal factors. All the factors have significant relationships with many of the 18 scales, so attempting to summarize the factors in one word leads to some generalization. Nevertheless, Kang's perceptual factors can be described as: relaxation, communication, spatiality, and dynamics. Guillén and López-Barrio (2007*a*) conducted a similar investigation using the same method and found three dimensions which explained 66% of the variance in sound quality judgements. They named the dimensions, emotional evaluation and strength (42%), activity (14%), and clarity (10%). Separately, Guillén and López-Barrio (2007*b*) also investigated the effect that physical context and attitudinal variables had on rating soundscape pleasantness. They found that pleasantness was related to source identification and meaning to listener noise sensitivity and attitudes to environmental and noise pollution, and to visual stimuli. A related group of studies focuses on the perceptual dimensions of single sounds from a soundscape. A good example is due to Gygi *et al.* (2007) who researched the similarity and categorization of 50 sounds such as rain, typewriters, and birds. They found that the sounds grouped into harmonic sounds, continuous sounds, and discrete impact sounds. The similarity space was characterized by three dimensions with fairly good acoustic correlates: pitch strength, low-frequency level, and duration. Dubois *et al.* (2006) showed that people categorized sounds based on semantic meaning, and that these semantic concepts were important for sound quality evaluation. That is, people judged sounds based on what the sounds meant to them. Specifically, soundscapes involving human activity were more pleasant than those where mechanical sounds dominated.

Several authors have focused on cognitive listening states as being a key determinant of an individual's response to a soundscape. The listening state can be associated with activity state: what we are doing determines how we are listening to the sounds around us. Truax (2000) defines three listening states: *listening in search*—or *analytical listening*—is an active, conscious activity where the listener is 'tuned in' to whatever they are listening to, for example concentrating on what a train station announcer is saying. *Listening in readiness* is an intermediate type of listening where the listener's attention is ready to receive significant information but where the focus of attention is directed elsewhere. An example might be hearing and recognizing your phone ring, when others' phones are ringing around you. Truax's third state is *background listening*—or

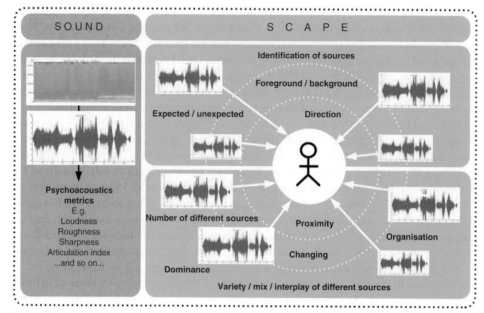

Fig. 16.27 Conceptual model of soundscape perception (after Cain *et al.*, 2008).

distracted listening—where the listener is engaged in another activity, 'tuning out' the sound, e.g. concentrating on reading a book. Raimbault (2006) has found evidence from fieldwork of the existence of two listening states, which he calls 'descriptive listening' and 'holistic hearing'. These seem very close to Truax's first and third states listed above. For Raimbault, the key difference between his two modes seems to be whether semantic processing of the sounds is involved.

Few attempts have been made thus far to draw all the strands of research in soundscape perception into a single framework; but two exceptions are due to Zhang and Kang (reported in Kang, 2007) and Cain *et al.* (2008). Cain *et al.*'s framework is reproduced in Fig. 16.27. Both models incorporate physical features of each sound source, characteristics of the physical space, and the relationship between the listener and soundscape. They differ mainly in the emphasis: Cain *et al.*'s framework is intended to be used with an emphasis on the activity or purpose (and hence listening mode) of the listener, while Zhang and Kang's model focuses more on the physical characteristics of the soundscape and location. At the time of writing, both models are just outlines, since the authors have not yet quantified or characterized the large number of factors they have identified.

If the soundscape research bears fruit, in terms of a better understanding of how people perceive environmental sound, then new tools for measuring soundscapes and designing them will undoubtedly be needed. Subjective evaluation of real or simulated soundscapes is a slow, expensive business and often results in data that need expert interpretation. The dream of an objective meter for measuring a soundscape is therefore attractive. To measure L_{Aeq} or L_{den}, an ordinary sound level meter is needed. To measure a soundscape, one would at least need a meter which can distinguish between different sound sources or different soundscapes. The bottom-up approach of identifying individual sources first is pursued by Karatsovis and Dyne (2008), with some promising initial results, based on blind source-separation techniques. A top-down approach is taken by Aucouturier and Defreville (2007) who use the 'bag-of-frames' method to represent signals as the long-term statistical distribution of their local spectral features. This results in an algorithm that can distinguish between a park and a street without having to identify individual sources. The authors point out that the success of these techniques apparently contradicts the idea that high-level cognitive processing of concepts, such as meaning, is important in soundscape perception.

16.9 **Conclusion**

Our external environment is complex and the acoustic signals arriving at our ear bear witness to this complexity by carrying information about their production, their interaction with the environment, and their transmission through it. In some cases—like room reverberation—we have a good understanding of the systems involved and can model them sufficiently well to explain most of the significant perceptual features. In others—complex sound sources or soundscapes—we can model individual elements well enough and correlate the perception of one element to its physical features. There is, however, much work still to be done to understand the interaction of these elements in systems like a rich outdoor soundscape and particularly in how they map to perception and cognition. In reviewing what we know about how the acoustic environment is shaped, it is striking that we have a good understanding of almost all the physical principles involved. However, there are much larger gaps where the physical models connect to the human listener, and it is here that there seems to be scope for significant progress in the future.

References

Allen, J. B. and Berkley, D. A. (1979). Image method for efficiently simulating small-room acoustics. *Journal of the Acoustical Society of America* **65**:943–50.

Alvarez-Ramirez, J., Lbarra-Valdez, C., Rodriguez, E., and Dagdug, L. (2008). 1/f-noise structures in Pollocks's drip paintings. *Physica a—Statistical Mechanics and Its Applications* **387**:281–95.

Ando, Y. (1985). *Concert Hall Acoustics*. Berlin: Springer.

Attenborough, K. (1992). Ground parameter information for propagation modeling. *Journal of the Acoustical Society of America* **92**:418–27.

Aucouturier, J.-J. and Defreville, B. (2007). Sounds like a park: A computational technique to recognise soundscapes holistically, without source identification. *19th International Congress on Acoustics*, 2–7 September, Sociedad Espanola de Acustica, Madrid.

Barron, M. (1988). Subjective study of British symphony concert halls. *Acustica* **66**:1–14.

Bass, H. E., Sutherland, L. C., Zuckerwar, A. J., Blackstock, D. T., and Hester, D. M. (1995). Atmospheric absorption of sound – further developments. *Journal of the Acoustical Society of America* **97**:680–3.

Bauck, J. and Cooper, D. H. (1996). Generalized transaural stereo and applications. *Journal of the Audio Engineering Society* **44**:683–705.

Berglund, B., Lindwell, T., and Schwela, D. (1999). *Guidelines for Community Noise*. Geneva: World Health Organization.

Borish, J. (1984). Extension of the image model to arbitrary polyhedra. *Journal of the Acoustical Society of America* **75**:1827–36.

Bradley, J. S. (1993). Disturbance caused by residential air-conditioner noise. *Journal of the Acoustical Society of America* **93**:1978–86.

BRE (2002). *The National Noise Incidence Study 2000 (England and Wales)*. London.

BS4142 (1997). *Rating Industrial Noise Affecting Mixed Residential and Industrial Areas*. London.

BS5228-1 (1997). *Noise and Vibration Control on Construction and Open Sites. Code of Practice for Basic Information and Procedures for Noise and Vibration Control*. London.

BS7445-1 (2003). *Description and Measurement of Environmental Noise. Guide to Quantities and Procedures*. London.

BSISO362 (1998). *Acoustics. Measurement of Noise Emitted by Accelerating Road Vehicles. Engineering Method*. London.

Cain, R., Jennings, P., Adams, M., *et al.* (2008). A framework for characterising positive urban soundscapes. *Acoustics 08*, 29 June–4 July, Paris, France.

Cox, T. J., Davies, W. J., and Lam, Y. W. (1993). The sensitivity of listeners to early sound field changes in auditoriums. *Acustica* **79**:27–41.

Davies, W. J. (2002). From concert halls to noise barriers: Attenuation from interference gratings. *Proceedings of the Institute of Acoustics*, 25–27 March, Salford, **24**.

Davies, W. J., Orlowski, R. J., and Lam, Y. W. (1994). Measuring Auditorium Seat Absorption. *Journal of the Acoustical Society of America* **96**:879–88.

Davies, W. J., Hepworth, P., Moorhouse, A., and Oldfield, R. (2005). *Noise from Pubs and Clubs – Final Report*. London: Department for Environment Food and Rural Affairs.

Davies, W. J., Adams, M. D., Bruce, N. S., *et al.* (2007).The Positive Soundscape Project. *19th International Congress on Acoustics*, 2–7 September, Sociedad Espanola de Acustica, Madrid.

De Coensel, B., Botteldooren, D., and De Muer, T. (2003). 1/f noise in rural and urban soundscapes. *Acta Acustica United with Acustica* **89**:287–95.

Delany, M. E. and Bazley, E. N. (1970). Acoustical properties of fibrous absorbent materials. *Applied Acoustics* **3**:105–16.

Department of the Environment (1994). *Planning Policy Guidance 24 (PPG24) – Planning and Noise*. London: HMSO.

Department of Transport (1995). *Calculation of Railway Noise*. London: HMSO.

Department of Transport and Welsh Office (1988). *Calculation of Road Traffic Noise*. London: HMSO.

Drumm, I. A. and Lam, Y. W. (2000). The adaptive beam-tracing algorithm. *Journal of the Acoustical Society of America* **107**:1405–12.

Dubois, D., Guastavino, C., and Raimbault, M. (2006). A cognitive approach to urban soundscapes: Using verbal data to access everyday life auditory categories. *Acta Acustica United with Acustica* **92**:865–74.

European Commission (2002). Directive 2002/49/EC of the European Parliament and of the Council of 25 June 2002 relating to the assessment and management of environmental noise. *Official Journal of the European Communities* **L189**, 12–25.

European Commission (2003). Directive 2003/10/EC of the European Parliament and the Council of 6 February 2003 on the Minimum Health and Safety Requirements Regarding the Exposure of Workers to the Risks Arising from Physical Agents (Noise). *Official Journal of the European Communities* **L42**, 38–44.

Eyring, C. F. (1930). Reverberation time in 'dead' rooms. *Journal of the Acoustical Society of America* **1**:217–41.

Fahy, F. (1985). *Sound and Structural Vibration*. London: Academic Press.

Farina, A. (2001). Acoustic quality of theatres: correlations between experimental measures and subjective evaluations. *Applied Acoustics* **62**:889–916.

Fazenda, B. M., Avis, M. R., and Davies, W. J. (2002). Low frequency room excitation using Distributed Mode Loudspeakers. *21st International Conference of the Audio-Engineering-Society*, 1–3 June, St Petersburg, Russia.

Fazenda, B. M., Avis, M. R., and Davies, W. J. (2005). Perception of modal distribution metrics in critical listening spaces – Dependence on room aspect ratios. *Journal of the Audio Engineering Society* **53**:1128–41.

Gerzon, M. A. (1973). Periphony – with-height sound reproduction. *Journal of the Audio Engineering Society* **21**:2–10.

Guastavino, C., Katz, B. F. G., Polack, J. D., Levitin, D. J., and Dubois, D. (2005). Ecological validity of soundscape reproduction. *Acta Acustica United with Acustica* **91**:333–41.

Guillén, J. D. and Lopez-Barrio, I. (2007a). The soundscape experience. *19th International Congress on Acoustics*, 2–7 September, Sociedad Espanola de Acustica, Madrid.

Guillén, J. D. and Lopez-Barrio, I. (2007b). Soundscape perception: Importance of non-acoustical variables. *Spanish Journal of Psychology* **10**:493. [Abstracts from CIP 2007.]

Gygi, B., Kidd, G. P. K., and Watson, C. S. (2007). Similarity and categorization of environmental sounds. *Perception and Psychophysics* **69**:839–55.

Houtgast, T. and Steeneken, H. J. M. (1973). Modulation transfer-function in room acoustics as a predictor of speech intelligibility. *Acustica* **28**:66–73.

Houtgast, T. and Steeneken, H. J. M. (1985). A review of the MTF concept in room acoustics and its use for estimating speech-intelligibility in auditoria. *Journal of the Acoustical Society of America* **77**:1069–77.

Kang, J. (2000). Sound propagation in street canyons: Comparison between diffusely and geometrically reflecting boundaries. *Journal of the Acoustical Society of America* **107**:1394–404.

Kang, J. (2007). *Urban Sound Environment*. London: Taylor and Francis.

Karatsovis, C. and Dyne, S. J. C. (2008). Instrument for soundscape recognition, identification and evaluation: An overview and potential use in legislative applications. *Proceedings of the Institute of Acoustics*, 10–11 April, Reading, UK.

Kleiner, M., Svensson, P., and Dalenback, B.-I. (1993). Auralization – an overview. *Journal of the Audio Engineering Society* **41**:861–75.

Krokstad, A., Strom, S., and Sorsdal, S. (1968). Calculating acoustical room response by use of a ray tracing technique. *Journal of Sound and Vibration* **8**:118–125.

Kuttruff, H. (1993). Auralization of impulse responses modeled on the basis of ray-tracing results. *Journal of the Audio Engineering Society* **41**:876–80.

Kuttruff, H. (2000). *Room Acoustics*. London: Spon Press.

Maekawa, Z. (1968). Noise reduction by screens. *Applied Acoustics* **1**:157–73.

Miedema, H. M. E. and Vos, H. (1998). Exposure–response relationships for transportation noise. *Journal of the Acoustical Society of America* **104**:3432–45.

Moorhouse, A. (2005).Virtual acoustic prototypes: listening to machines that don't exist. *ACOUSTICS 2005*, 9–11 November, Busselton, Western Australia.

Moorhouse, A., Waddington, D., and Adams, M. (2005). *Proposed Criteria for the Assessment of Low Frequency Noise Disturbance*. London: Department for Environment Food and Rural Affairs.

Naylor, G. M. (1993). Odeon – another hybrid room acoustical model. *Applied Acoustics* **38**:131–43.

Picaut, J., Le Polles, T., L'Hermite, P., and Gary, V. (2005). Experimental study of sound propagation in a street. *Applied Acoustics* **66**:149–73.

Raimbault, M. (2006). Qualitative judgements of urban soundscapes: Questionning questionnaires and semantic scales. *Acta Acustica United with Acustica* **92**:929–37.

Roads, C. (1996). *The Computer Music Tutorial*. Cambridge, MA: MIT Press.

Sabine, W. C. (1993). *Collected Papers on Acoustics*. Los Altos, CA: Peninsula Publishing.

Schafer, R. M. (1977). *The Tuning of the World*. New York: Knopf.

Schroeder, M. R., Gottlob, D., and Siebrasse, K. F. (1974). Comparative study of European concert halls: correlation of subjective preference with geometric and acoustic parameters. *Journal of the Acoustical Society of America* **56**:1195–201.

Smith, J. O. (2004). Virtual acoustic musical instruments: Review and update. *Journal of New Music Research* **33**:283–304.

Takagi, K. (1990). Some remarks on practical methods for calculating acoustical diffraction. *Applied Acoustics* **31**:119–32.

Thompson, E. (2002). *The Soundscape of Modernity: Architectural Acoustics and the Culture of Listening in America 1900–1933*. Cambridge, MA: The MIT Press.

Truax, B. (1999). *Handbook for Acoustic Ecology*. Cambridge, MA: Cambridge Street Publishing.

Truax, B. (2000). *Acoustic Communication*. Santa Barbara, CA: Greenwood Publishing Group.

Voss, R. F. and Clarke, J. (1975). 1-F-Noise in Music and Speech. *Nature* **258**:317–18.

Index